MW01199654

ADVANCES IN PHARMACEUTICAL

CELL THERAPY

Principles of Cell-Based Biopharmaceuticals

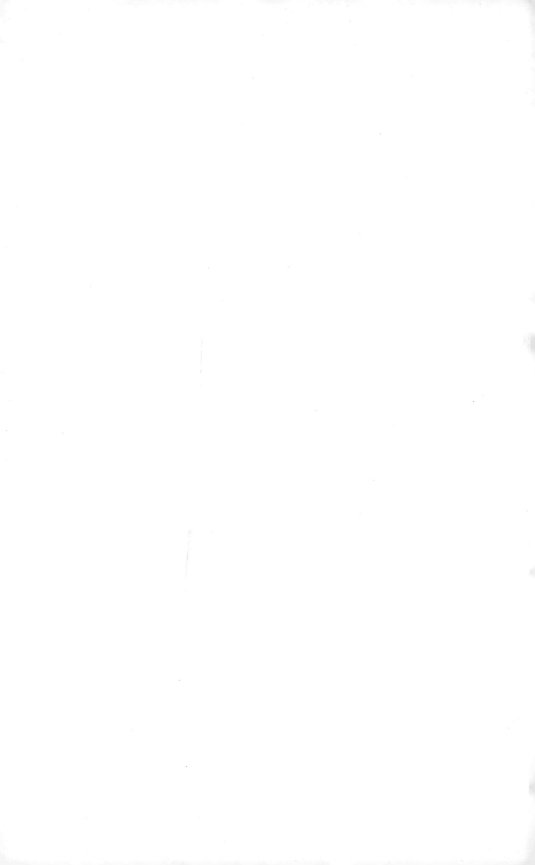

ADVANCES IN PHARMACEUTICAL

CELL THERAPY

Principles of Cell-Based Biopharmaceuticals

Christine Günther
Apceth GmbH & Co KG, Germany

Andrea Hauser
University Hospital Regensburg, Germany

Ralf Huss
Apceth GmbH & Co KG, Germany
and
University College Dublin, Ireland

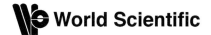

World Scientific

NEW JERSEY · LONDON · SINGAPORE · BEIJING · SHANGHAI · HONG KONG · TAIPEI · CHENNAI · TOKYO

Published by

World Scientific Publishing Co. Pte. Ltd.

5 Toh Tuck Link, Singapore 596224

USA office: 27 Warren Street, Suite 401-402, Hackensack, NJ 07601

UK office: 57 Shelton Street, Covent Garden, London WC2H 9HE

Library of Congress Cataloging-in-Publication Data
Günther, Christine, author.
    Advances in pharmaceutical cell therapy : principles of cell-based biopharmaceuticals /
Christine Günther, Andrea Hauser, Ralf Huss.
        p. ; cm.
    Includes bibliographical references and index.
    ISBN 978-9814616782 (hardcover : alk. paper)
    I. Hauser, Andrea, 1976–   , author. II. Huss, Ralf, author. III. Title.
    [DNLM: 1. Biopharmaceutics--methods. 2. Cell- and Tissue-Based Therapy--methods.
3. Drug Delivery Systems--methods. 4. Genetic Therapy--methods. QV 35]
    RM301.4
    615.7--dc23
                                2015024081

British Library Cataloguing-in-Publication Data
A catalogue record for this book is available from the British Library.

Typeset by Stallion Press
Email: enquiries@stallionpress.com

Printed in Singapore

Contents

Foreword   xxi

Contributing Authors   xxiii

Abbreviations   xxvii

Glossary   xxxiii

1. About this Book: Why Cell Therapy?   1

2. Regulatory Landscape and Risk-Based Approach   9
    2.1   Introduction: Regulatory Landscape   9
    2.2   Regional Definitions and Requirements   10
          2.2.1   Europe   10
          2.2.2   USA/Food and Drug Administration (FDA)   11
          2.2.3   Japan   12
    2.3   Quality, Safety, and Efficacy Regulatory Requirements in the
          European Commission (EC)   13
    2.4   Risk-Based Approach   13
          2.4.1   Introduction: Risk-based approach   13
          2.4.2   General discussion   14
          2.4.3   Risk-based approach in quality/development
                  and manufacturing   15
          2.4.4   Risk-based approach in safety/preclinical
                  toxicological investigations   16
          2.4.5   Risk-based approach in efficacy/clinical setting   17
          2.4.6   Risk-based approach in regulatory affairs   19

2.5   Environmental Risk Assessment (ERA)   20
       2.5.1   ERA in the EC   20
2.6   Pharmacovigilance in the EC   21
References   23

3. Non-Clinical Development of Cell-Based Products   25
3.1   Introduction   25
3.2   Legal Background and Regulatory Guidance for Cell and Gene
       Therapies   26
       3.2.1   The European Union (EU)   27
       3.2.2   The US regulatory frame work   28
       3.2.3   International harmonization   28
3.3   The Process is the Product: The Link between Manufacturing
       and Non-Clinical Development   29
3.4   Development Stages for GTPs and CTPs   30
       3.4.1   Discovery stage/prototype definition   31
       3.4.2   Non-clinical development for first-in-human
                application   32
       3.4.3   Non-clinical development accompanying clinical
                phases   33
3.5   Animal Models to Study Cell-Based Products   33
       3.5.1   Rodent-models   34
       3.5.2   Non-rodent mammals (NRM) models   35
                3.5.2.1   Pigs emerging as superior models
                           in regenerative medicine   35
                3.5.2.2   Cardiac and cardiovascular diseases, e.g.,
                           myocardial infarction   36
                3.5.2.3   Infectious diseases, e.g., human
                           immunodeficiency virus (HIV)   37
                3.5.2.4   Neurological diseases, e.g., Parkinson's
                           disease   37
                3.5.2.5   Musculoskeletal diseases, e.g.,
                           osteoarthritis   38
3.6   Primary Pharmacodynamics: Proof-of-concept and Efficacy
       Studies   39
3.7   Pharmacokinetics (PK)   39
       3.7.1   Monitoring distribution and engraftment   39
3.8   Toxicity Studies   40
       3.8.1   Tumorigenicity and genotoxicity studies for CTP
                and GTP   42

3.9   Dose Finding   42
3.10   Conclusion   42
References   43

4.   Quality Management   49
4.1   Introduction   49
4.2   Principles of GMP   51
4.3   Pharmaceutical Quality System (PQS)   54
        4.3.1   Quality manual   54
        4.3.2   Site master file (SMF)   61
        4.3.3   Quality Risk Management (QRM)   62
        4.3.4   Deviation management   64
        4.3.5   Change control management   64
        4.3.6   Corrective action/preventive action (CAPA)   65
        4.3.7   Product Quality Review (PQR)   66
4.4   Personnel   67
        4.4.1   Human resources, organization,
                 and responsibilities   67
        4.4.2   Training   68
4.5   Documentation   69
        4.5.1   Required GMP documentation   69
        4.5.2   Generation and control of documentation   73
        4.5.3   Good documentation practice   76
4.6   Outsourced Activities . . . . ,   77
4.7   Complaints and Product Recall   79
4.8   Self Inspections (SIs)   80
4.9   Qualification and Validation   81
        4.9.1   Qualification   81
        4.9.2   Validation   83
4.10   Supplement on Required Documentation   85
References   88

5.   Process Development and Manufacturing   91
5.1   Introduction   91
5.2   Process Development   94
        5.2.1   Scale-up   95
        5.2.2   Scale-out   96
5.3   Premises and Equipments   96
        5.3.1   Production area and clean rooms   97
                 5.3.1.1   Clean room design   99

5.3.1.2 Clean room grades 100

5.3.1.3 Personnel and material flow 103

5.3.1.4 Clothing 104

5.3.1.5 Gowning procedures and qualification
of gowning 105

5.3.1.6 Cleaning and disinfection 105

5.3.1.7 Personnel hygiene and health control
of personnel 109

5.3.2 Equipments and premises 110

5.3.3 Storage rooms and warehouses 111

5.3.4 Qualification of clean rooms 113

5.3.5 Qualification of equipments 115

5.3.6 Isolator technique for ATMP manufacturing 116

5.4 Manufacturing/Production 117

5.4.1 Primary human cells as starting material
for ATMP production 120

5.4.2 Isolation and selection of target cells
for ATMP manufacturing 123

5.4.2.1 Procurement of starting material 123

5.4.2.2 Processing of starting material 124

5.4.2.2.1 Density gradient
centrifugation 124

5.4.2.2.2 Mechanical break-up 125

5.4.2.2.3 Magnetic-activated cell sorting
(MACS) 125

5.4.2.2.4 FACS 127

5.4.3 Cell culture 128

5.4.3.1 Adherent (anchorage dependent) cell culture
and its scale-up potential 129

5.4.3.1.1 Classical two-dimensional cell
culture 130

5.4.3.1.2 Carrier-based systems 131

5.4.3.2 Suspension cell culture and its scale-up
potential 133

5.4.3.3 Cell culture media and media
components 133

5.4.4 Activation and stimulation 136

5.4.5   Genetic modification using viral vector systems 138
        5.4.5.1   Introduction 138
        5.4.5.2   General consideration with regard to producer
                  cell lines 139
                  5.4.5.2.1   Qualification of producer cell
                              lines 139
                  5.4.5.2.2   Serum-free vs. serum containing
                              cell culture systems 141
                  5.4.5.2.3   Inadvertent generation
                              of replication competent
                              viruses 141
        5.4.5.3   Integrating vector systems: The retroviral
                  family 141
                  5.4.5.3.1   Retroviral biology and vector
                              design 141
                  5.4.5.3.2   Production of gamma-retroviral
                              vectors 143
                  5.4.5.3.3   Production of lentiviral
                              vectors 144
        5.4.5.4   Non-integrating systems 144
                  5.4.5.4.1   Adenovirus biology and vector
                              design 144
                  5.4.5.4.2   Production of first generation
                              vectors 146
                  5.4.5.4.3   Production of second generation
                              vectors 146
                  5.4.5.4.4   Production of helper dependent
                              vectors 146
                  5.4.5.4.5   Adeno-associated viral vector
                              biology 147
                  5.4.5.4.6   Production of AAV 147
                  5.4.5.4.7   Down-stream processing of AAV 148
5.4.6   Examples for GMP manufacture of ATMPs 149
        5.4.6.1   Tissue-engineered ATMP 149
        5.4.6.2   Somatic cell therapy/tumor vaccine
                  products 150
        5.4.6.3   Gene therapy products 151

	5.4.7	Formulation of finished product	152
	5.4.8	Cryopreservation	153
	5.4.9	Labeling	156
	5.4.10	Transport and shipping	160
	5.4.11	On-site preparation and administration	162
5.5	Validation		162
	5.5.1	Process validation	162
	5.5.2	Validation of aseptic handling via media fills	163
	5.5.3	Cleaning validation after employment of viral particles for ATMP production	165
References			167

6. **Quality Control** — 173

6.1	Introduction		173
6.2	QC of Materials		174
	6.2.1	Terms and definitions	174
	6.2.2	Starting material	175
		6.2.2.1 Primary cells and tissues as starting material	175
		6.2.2.2 Primary cell lines from banking systems as starting material	180
		6.2.2.3 Vectors and plasmids as starting material for CBMPs	182
	6.2.3	Donor testing and traceability	185
		6.2.3.1 Rules and regulations for procurement and testing of blood, tissues and cells	185
		6.2.3.2 Donor selection and testing	189
		6.2.3.3 Traceability	190
	6.2.4	Ancillary Materials (AMs)/Raw materials	192
		6.2.4.1 Regulatory situation for raw materials in Europe	194
		6.2.4.2 Regulatory situation for AMs in the USA	196
		6.2.4.3 Raw materials of animal origin	200
	6.2.5	Excipients	202
	6.2.6	Reagents and materials for QC	202
	6.2.7	Quality agreement	203
6.3	Assay Development		205
6.4	Analytical Methods for QC of CBMPs		207

6.5   In-Process Controls 207
6.6   Specifications and Release Criteria 219
       6.6.1   Terms and definitions 219
                6.6.1.1   Acceptance criteria 219
                6.6.1.2   Specification 219
                6.6.1.3   Release specification 220
                6.6.1.4   Shelf life specification 220
       6.6.2   Choice and justification of specifications and acceptance
                criteria 220
       6.6.3   Identity 229
       6.6.4   Purity 230
       6.6.5   Impurities 231
                6.6.5.1   Product-related impurities 231
                6.6.5.2   Process-related impurities 232
                6.6.5.3   Adventitious (microbial) agents 237
       6.6.6   Quantity 237
       6.6.7   Viability 239
       6.6.8   Potency 240
       6.6.9   Microbiology 242
                6.6.9.1   Sterility testing and microbiological
                           control 242
                6.6.9.2   Pyrogens 253
                6.6.9.3   Bacterial endotoxins 255
                6.6.9.4   Mycoplasma 257
       6.6.10   Certificate of Analysis (CoA) 259
6.7   Genetic Stability and Tumorigenicity 259
       6.7.1   Overview and methodologies 261
                6.7.1.1   Karyotyping/FISH 261
                6.7.1.2   Molecular-based techniques 262
                6.7.1.3   Telomere length and telomerase activity . . . 263
                6.7.1.4   Soft agar colony formation assay 264
       6.7.2   Status quo of the scientific and regulatory opinion . . . 264
6.8   Environmental Control of Microbial Contamination 266
       6.8.1   Routine microbial monitoring 266
       6.8.2   Alert and action levels 267
       6.8.3   Media growth promotion 268
6.9   Reference and Retention Samples 269
       6.9.1   Principles 269

6.9.2	Duration of storage	269
6.9.3	Location of storage	270
6.9.4	Sample size	271
6.9.5	Written agreements	271
6.9.6	Reference and retention samples for CBMPs	272
6.10	Stability	272
6.10.1	General requirements for stability testing and relevant guidelines	272
6.10.2	Specifics of cell-based products	277
	6.10.2.1 Fresh versus cryopreserved cell products	279
	6.10.2.2 Potency assays	280
	6.10.2.3 Small batch size-reduced design	280
6.11	Validation of Analytical Procedures	282
6.11.1	Validation principles	282
6.11.2	Validation characteristics	283
	6.11.2.1 Accuracy and precision	284
	6.11.2.2 Accuracy	286
	6.11.2.3 Precision	287
	6.11.2.4 Specificity	288
	6.11.2.5 Detection limit	290
	6.11.2.6 Quantitation limit	292
	6.11.2.7 Linearity	293
	6.11.2.8 Range	293
	6.11.2.9 Robustness	294
6.11.3	System suitability test (SST)	295
6.11.4	Method transfer	295
	6.11.4.1 Transfer of documentation/knowledge transfer	296
	6.11.4.2 Criteria for the successful transfer	296
	6.11.4.3 Gap analysis	297
	6.11.4.4 Staff training	297
	6.11.4.5 Written transfer plan	297
	6.11.4.6 Execution	297
	6.11.4.7 Method transfer for CBMPs	298
6.11.5	Reference material and reference standards	299
6.11.6	Standards and controls	301
	6.11.6.1 Principles	301

6.11.6.2   Standards and controls in flow
cytometry 302
6.12   Deviation Management and OOS Results 304
6.13   Round Robin and Proficiency Tests 307
References 309

7. Cell Banking   317
7.1   Introduction and Overview 317
7.2   Definitions and Guidelines 319
7.3   MCB and WCB 320
7.4   Alternative Banking Strategies: Banking of Blood and Tissue as a
Source of Therapeutic Cells 321
7.5   Summary 323
References 324

8. Product Release   325
8.1   Introduction 325
8.2   General Principles 326
8.3   Required Qualification to Act as QP 328
8.4   Batch Record Review (BRR) 331
8.5   Batch Certification and Product Release 335
8.6   Specifics of CBMPs 335
8.7   Specific Guidance for IMPs 341
8.8   Batch Release of Short Shelf-Life Products 344
8.9   Deviations, OOS Results and other Non-Conformances 346
References 348

9. Clinical Development of Cell-Based Products   351
9.1   Clinical Application of Mesenchymal Stem Cells (MSCs) 351
9.2   Legislation and Guidance 352
9.3   Legal Basis of ATMP Classification 352
9.4   Regulatory Definitions for ATMPs 353
9.4.1   SCTMP 353
9.4.2   TEP 353
9.4.3   Combined ATMP 353
9.5   Regulatory Framework in the EU 354
9.6   Application and Evaluation Procedure for ATMPs 356
9.7   EU Marketing Procedure 357
9.8   CAT 358
9.9   CHMP 358

9.10   Gene Therapy Working Party (GTWP)   358

9.11   Specific Rules for Post-Authorization Surveillance
of ATMPs   359

    9.11.1   Safety concerns   359

    9.11.2   Risks to living donors   359

9.12   Dynamics of the Disease and Effects of the Product   361

9.13   Considerations on Safety Follow-Up of Living Donors   361

9.14   Regulatory Framework in the US   362

9.15   The Orphan Drug Act and the Development of SCBPs for Rare
Diseases   363

    9.15.1   Rare diseases at a glance   364

9.16   Application Procedure   364

    9.16.1   Pre-submission meeting   364

    9.16.2   Submission   365

    9.16.3   Validation   365

    9.16.4   Evaluation   365

    9.16.5   Opinion   366

    9.16.6   Decision   366

9.17   The Hospital Exemption for Specific ATMPs   366

    9.17.1   Scope of the hospital exemption   366

    9.17.2   The hospital exemption for specific ATMPs
in Germany   368

9.18   From Preclinics to Clinics   368

    9.18.1   Bridging the gaps from discovery to medicine   368

9.19   Clinical Development of ATMPs   369

    9.19.1   Communication with authorities/agencies   369

       9.19.1.1   National or international scientific
advice   369

       9.19.1.2   Scientific advice meeting and follow up . . .   370

    9.19.2   CRO selection   371

       9.19.2.1   Choose wisely the right CRO   371

       9.19.2.2   Selection/qualification criteria   371

       9.19.2.3   Review and ongoing evaluations   372

    9.19.3   Selecting the right investigator   372

    9.19.4   Hosting an investigator meeting   373

9.20   Request for Authorization for a Clinical Trial in the EU   373

    9.20.1   Request for CTA   374

    9.20.2   Application to the ethics committee (EC)   375

9.20.3   Substantial and non-substantial amendments 377
9.21   Author's Outlook on Clinical Trial Regulation 378
9.22   Development of Key Study Documents 379
   9.22.1   Objectives of a clinical trial 379
      9.22.1.1   Design of a clinical trial 379
   9.22.2   Preparation of the Investigator's Brochure (IB) 380
   9.22.3   Preparation of an Investigational Medicinal Product
           Dossier (IMPD) 381
9.23   During the Conduct of a Clinical Trial 381
   9.23.1   Trial management & monitoring 381
   9.23.2   Data monitoring committee (DMC) 382
   9.23.3   Day to day monitoring 382
      9.23.3.1   Day to day management should be carried out
               to check 382
      9.23.3.2   On site monitoring/co-monitoring 383
      9.23.3.3   Protection of personal data of the patient . . 383
9.24   Clinical Study Report and Publication 384
   9.24.1   The role of peer-review and traditional journals 385
References 385

10. Pharmacovigilance and Look-Back Procedures   389
10.1   Basic Principles of Pharmacovigilance for Advanced Therapy
      Medicinal Products (ATMPs) 389
   10.1.1   Traceability 389
   10.1.2   Active surveillance 389
   10.1.3   Pharmacovigilance and risk assessment in cell and gene
           therapy 390
10.2   Qualified Person for Pharmacovigilance (QPPV) 390
10.3   Pharmacovigilance during Development Phase 390
   10.3.1   Reporting procedure from clinical trials in Europe . . . 390
   10.3.2   Development safety update report (DSUR) 392
   10.3.3   Responsibilities and tasks of a DSMB 393
10.4   Post Approval Pharmacovigilance 394
   10.4.1   Surveillance plan 394
   10.4.2   RMP for ATMPs 395
   10.4.3   Periodic Benefit-Risk Evaluation Report (PBRER) . . . 397
10.5   Pharmacovigilance Inspections 398
10.6   Reported Side-Effects of Cell-Therapy Products 398
References 399

11. Personalized Cell Therapy — Biomarker & Companion Diagnostics 401
    11.1 Introduction 401
    11.2 Biomarker 402
    11.3 Disease- and Drug-Related Biomarkers 403
    11.4 Companion Diagnostics 404
    11.5 Biomarker Requirements 405
    11.6 Biomarker Classification and Application 406
    11.7 Discovery of Biomarkers 406
        11.7.1 Genomics 406
        11.7.2 Proteomics 407
        11.7.3 Metabolomics 407
        11.7.4 Lipidomics 407
        11.7.5 Tissue-based biomarkers 408
        11.7.6 Imaging biomarkers 408
    11.8 Biomarker in Cell Therapy 409
    11.9 Quality Management 411
    11.10 Personalized Medicine 411
    References 412

12. Mesenchymal Stem Cells 415
    12.1 Stem Cells/Mesenchymal Stem or Stromal Cells (MSCs)
        for Therapy 415
    12.2 The Development of MSCs 416
    12.3 The Biology of MSCs 417
    12.4 Properties of MSCs 418
        12.4.1 Nomenclature & definition 418
        12.4.2 Cultivation of MSCs 420
    12.5 MoA of MSCs 420
        12.5.1 MicroRNAs (miRNAs) and exosomes 422
        12.5.2 In inflammation and immunity 423
        12.5.3 In kidney disease 424
        12.5.4 In organ fibrosis 426
        12.5.5 In cardio-vascular diseases 429
        12.5.6 In cancer therapy 429
    12.6 Clinical Applications 430
    References 433

13. Next Generation Cell Therapies 439
    13.1 Introduction 439
    13.2 Early Products 439

13.3 First Improvements 440

13.4 Changes to the Characteristics of the Cells by Culture
Conditions 440

13.5 Genetic Modification 441

    13.5.1 Introduction 441

    13.5.2 Hematopoietic stem cell (HSC) engineering 441

    13.5.3 T-Cell engineering 442

    13.5.4 Engineered MSCs 443

13.6 Genetic Modification Technologies and Methodologies 444

13.7 Summary 445

References 445

14. Cell-Based Gene Therapy 449

14.1 Definition: What is Gene Therapy? 449

    14.1.1 Somatic and germline gene therapy 450

    14.1.2 *In vivo* versus *Ex vivo* gene therapy 450

    14.1.3 Indications of gene therapy 452

14.2 Approaches 452

    14.2.1 Gene addition — Restoring cellular functions 452

    14.2.2 Targeted integration — Gene editing 453

    14.2.3 Instructing novel cellular functions — Suicide
        gene therapy 454

    14.2.4 Gene therapy vectors 455

14.3 Viral Vectors 456

    14.3.1 Integrating viral vectors 456

        14.3.1.1 Gamma-retrovirus 456

        14.3.1.2 Lentivirus 458

    14.3.2 Non-integrating viral vectors 459

        14.3.2.1 Adenoviruses 459

        14.3.2.2 AAV 460

14.4 Safety Issues 461

    14.4.1 Insertional transformation 461

    14.4.2 Strategies to increase safety 461

14.5 Historical Milestones: The Rocky Road to Success 463

    14.5.1 The early ages 463

    14.5.2 1980s 464

    14.5.3 1990s 464

    14.5.4 2000s 466

14.6   Synopsis and Outlook 467
References 469

15. Exosomes and their Therapeutic Applications   477
15.1   Introduction 477
15.2   Exosomes are Well-Positioned as Therapeutic Agents 478
15.3   Exosomes with Intrinsic Therapeutic Activity 479
       15.3.1   Characteristics of MSC exosomes 481
       15.3.2   Biological activity of MSC exosomes correlates with their
                therapeutic activity 484
                15.3.2.1   Enhancing bioenergetics and redox
                           homeostasis 484
                15.3.2.2   Immune regulation 485
                15.3.2.3   Activating pro-survival signaling
                           pathways 486
       15.3.3   Advantages of exosome-based over cell-based
                therapies 487
15.4   Exosome Modification for Drug Delivery 488
       15.4.1   Cell source 488
       15.4.2   Safety profile of exosomes 489
       15.4.3   Exosome purification 489
15.5   Conclusion 490
References 491

16. Commercial and Business Aspects of Cell Therapy —
     Start-Up to Market   503
16.1   Introduction 503
16.2   Financing and Funding Operations 504
       16.2.1   Investment 504
                16.2.1.1   Private investors 504
                16.2.1.2   Public investors 504
                16.2.1.3   Investment approaches 505
       16.2.2   Non-dilutive public grants 505
       16.2.3   Partnering 506
16.3   Cell Therapy Commercial Landscape 508
       16.3.1   Overview 508
       16.3.2   Company landscape 509
       16.3.3   Commercial CTPs 512
16.4   Commercial Considerations 514
       16.4.1   Target product profile (TPP) 514

16.4.2   Autologous vs. allogeneic cell therapy   515

16.4.2.1   Autologous cell products   515

16.4.2.2   Allogeneic cell products   516

16.4.2.3   Discussion   517

16.4.3   Cost of goods sold (COGS)   517

16.4.4   Pricing and reimbursement   517

16.5   Summary   518

References   519

Index   521

Foreword

To transplant living cells from one individual to another was met with great skepticism when it was first carried out in the 1950s. Only with the understanding of the HLA system and the identification of HLA identical siblings could it be proved that hemopoietic stem cell transplantation is feasible: the first cell therapy to benefit patients was born and has since been refined to become standard in the treatment of hemopoietic disorders and malignant diseases.

Since then, scientists and clinicians have dreamed of following up with other cell types able to treat patients. In rodent models adoptive transfer of *ex vivo* generated immune cells cured spontaneous and transplanted tumors, reconstituted failed immunity and eradicated viral infections in immunocompromised hosts. Somatic stem cell products isolated from different sources and organs started the field of regenerative medicine and tissue engineering.

Yet, from the first clinical studies in humans it took more than two decades and the event of T-cell receptor engineering technology helped by T-cell transfer, to get progress made in tumor immunology awarded the prestigious "Breakthrough of the Year 2013" by Science the world leading scientific journal.

Nowadays transfer of autologous and allogeneic cells with or without additional modifications is performed in hundreds of clinical study protocols, e.g. to fight leukemia, lymphomas and other malignancies, to restore pathogen-specific immunity and treat fatal infections in stem cell transplant patients, to down-modulate graft-versus-host reaction and autoimmune diseases, to regenerate or repair damaged tissues in heart, pancreatic islet cells, cartilage and central nervous system as well as to correct inherited metabolic disorders.

Thus, the field of cell therapy has come of age, with biotech and pharma industries entering the field and a rapidly growing interest in all aspects of cell therapy is evident: manufacture, quality measures, compliance with regulatory requirements, study design, economic aspects and marketing authorization.

A comprehensive compilation on the subject for the cell therapy community has thus been long overdue. This book satisfies the community's needs admirably.

Christine Günther, Andrea Hauser and Ralf Huss should be congratulated for having taken up this important task: they have covered all items of pharmaceutical cell therapy from bench to bedside to marketing in a perfect performance, with in-depth focus on the quality of a cell-based product and detailed descriptions when appropriate and pointing out to the essentials when necessary.

This book is a must-read, not only for scientists studying one or more aspects of cell technology but also for clinicians and pharmaceutical professionals alike.

Reinhard Andreesen
Professor Emeritus of Hematology/Oncology
University of Regensburg,
Germany

Contributing Authors

Reinhard Andreesen, MD, PhD
Professor emeritus
Center for Interventional Immunology
University of Regensburg
Regensburg, Germany.

Sabine Geiger
Senior Scientist: Preclinical Development
apceth GmbH & Co. KG
Munich, Germany.

Christine Guenther, MD
Chief Executive & Medical Officer
apceth GmbH & Co. KG
Munich, Germany

Andrea Hauser, PhD
Head of Operations
José-Carreras-Center for Somatic Cell Therapy
Department of Internal Medicine III- Hematology & Oncology
University Hospital Regensburg
Regensburg, Germany.

Carolin Hermann, PhD
Senior Scientist: Manufacturing
apceth GmbH & Co. KG
Munich, Germany.

Felix Hermann, MD, PhD
Head of Preclinical Development

apceth GmbH & Co. KG
Munich, Germany.

Daniela Hirsch, PhD
Senior Scientist: Preclinical Development
apceth GmbH & Co. KG
Munich, Germany.

Josef M. Hofer, PhD
Managing Director
Exdra GmbH
Grafing near Munich, Germany.

Ralf Huss, MD, PhD [a,b]
[a] Professor of Pathology & Regenerative Medicine Consultant
apceth mbH & Co. KG
Munich, Germany;
[b] Adjunct Professor
University College Dublin
School of Medicine and Medical Science
Belfield, Dublin 4, Ireland.

Stephanie Knoerzer
Pharmacist: Quality Management
apceth GmbH & Co. KG
Munich, Germany.

Sai Kiang Lim, PhD [a,b]
Professor
[a] Institute of Medical Biology, A*STAR, 8A Biomedical Grove, 138648 Singapore;
[b] Department of Surgery, YLL School of Medicine, NUS, 5 Lower Kent Ridge Road, 119074 Singapore.

Elena Meurer, PhD
Head of Translational Sciences
apceth GmbH & Co. KG
Munich, Germany.

Nadja Noske, PhD
Senior Scientist & Project Leader
apceth GmbH & Co. KG
Munich, Germany.

Christoph Peter, PhD
Head of Quality Management
apceth GmbH & Co. KG
Munich, Germany.

Sylvia Peter, PhD
Senior Scientist: Clinical Development
apceth GmbH & Co. KG
Munich, Germany.

Christoph Prinz
Pharmacist: Preclinical Development
apceth GmbH & Co. KG
Munich, Germany.

Volker Scherhammer, PhD
Head of Clinical Development
apceth GmbH & Co. KG
Munich, Germany.

Stefanos Theoharis, PhD
Chief Business Officer
apceth GmbH & Co. KG
Munich, Germany.

Ronne Wee Yeh Yeo
Scientist
Institute of Medical Biology
A*STAR, 8A Biomedical Grove
138648, Singapore.

Abbreviations

7-AAD	7-Aminoactinomycin D
AAV	Adeno-Associated Virus
ADME	absorption, distribution, metabolism and excretion
AIDS	Acquired Immunodeficiency Syndrome
AM	Ancillary Material
AP	Authorised Person
APC	Antigen Presenting Cell
API	Active Pharmaceutical Ingredient
ATMP	Advanced Therapy Medicinal Product
BM-MNC	bone-marrow mononuclear cells
BRR	Batch Record Review
BSE	Bovine Spongiform Encephalopathy
CA	Competent Authority
CAPA	Corrective Action/Preventive Action
CAR	Chimeric Antigen Receptor
CAT	Committee for Advanced Therapies
CBER	Center for Biologics Evaluation and Research
CBMP	Cell-based medicinal product
CD	Cluster of Differentiation
CE	Conformité Européenne (engl. European Conformity)
CFR	Code of Federal Regulations
CFSE	Carboxyfluorescein succinimidyl ester
CFU	Colony Forming Unit
CGH	Comparative Genomic Hybridization
cGMP	current Good Manufacturing Practice
cGTP	current Good Tissue Practice
CHMP	Committee for Medicinal Products for Human Use

CMC	Chemistry, Manufacturing, and Control
CMO	Contract Manufacturing Organization
CMV	Cytomegalovirus
CoA	Certificate of Analysis
CoC	Certificate of Compliance
COMP	Committee for Orphan Medicinal Products
CPMP	Committee for Proprietary Medicinal Products
CRF	Case Report Form
CRO	Contract Research Organization
CSR	Clinical Study Report
CTA	Clinical Trial Authorization
CTL	Cytotoxic T Lymphocytes
CTM	Clinical Trial Manager
CTP	Cell Therapy Product
CV	Coefficient of variation
DAPI	4′,6-Diamidino-2-Phenylindole
DC	Dendritic Cells
DLI	Donor Lymphocyte Infusion
DMC	Data Monitoring Committee
DMF	Drug Master File
DMSO	Dimethyl Sulfoxide
DNA	Deoxyribonucleic Acid
DQ	Design Qualification
DSMB	Data and Safety Monitoring Board
EBV	Epstein−Barr Virus
EC	Ethics Committee or European Commission
EDQM	European Directorate for the Quality of Medicines and Health Care
EDTA	Ethylenediaminetetraacetic acid
EEA	European Economic Area
ELISA	Enzyme-Linked Immunosorbent Assay
EMA	European Medicines Agency
ESC	Embryonic Stem Cell
EU	European Union
FACS	Fluorescence Activated Cell Sorter
FAT	Factory Acceptance Test
FBS	Fetal Bovine Serum
FDA	Food and Drug Administration
FIH	First-in-Human

FISH	Fluorescence *in situ* Hybridization
FMEA	Failure Mode and Effects Analysis
FSC	Forward Scatter
G−(M)-CSF	Granulocyte−(Macrophage)-Colony Stimulating Factor
GCP	Good Clinical Practice
GDP	Good Distribution Practice
GLP	Good Laboratory Practice
GMO	Genetically Modified Organism
GMP	Good Manufacturing Practice
GOI	Gene of Interest
GSP	Good Storage Practice
GT	Gene Therapy
GTMP	Gene Therapy Medicinal Product
GTP	Good Tissue Practice or Gene Therapy Product
GTWP	Gene Therapy Working Party
GvHD	Graft-*versus*-Host Disease
HBV	Hepatitis B Virus
HCV	Hepatitis C Virus
HEPA	High Efficiency Particulate Air
HES	Hydroxy-Ethyl-Starch
hESC	Human Embryonic Stem Cell
HIV	Human Immunodeficiency Virus
HLA	Human Leukocyte Antigen
HPLC	High Performance Liquid Chromatography
HSA	Human Serum Albumin
HSC	Hematopoietic Stem Cell
HTLV	Human T-Lymphotropic Virus
HVAC	Heating, Ventilation, and Air Conditioning
IB	Investigator's Brochure
IC	Informed Consent
ICH	International Conference on Harmonisation
IDM	Infectious Disease Marker
IFN-γ	Interferon gamma
IIT	Investigator Initiated Trial
IL	Interleukin
IMP	Investigational Medicinal Product
IMPD	Investigational Medicinal Product Dossier
IND	Investigational New Drug

IPC	In-process Control
iPSC	induced Pluripotent Stem Cell
IQ	Installation Qualification
ISCT	International Society for Cellular Therapy
ISO	International Organization for Standardization
JP	Japanese Pharmacopoeia
LAF	Laminar Air Flow
Kb	Kilobase
LAL	Limulus Amebocyte Lysate
LOD	Limit of Detection
LOQ	Limit of Quantitation
LPS	Lipopolysaccharide
MA	Marketing Authorization
MACS	Magnetic Activated Cell Sorting
MAH	Marketing Authorization Holder
MAT	Monocyte Activation Test
MCB	Master Cell Bank
Mb	Megabase
MLR	Mixed Lymphocyte Reaction
MLV	Murine Leukemia Virus
MNC	Mononuclear Cells
MP	Medicinal Product
MRA	Mutual Recognition Agreement
MRI	Magnetic Resonance Imaging
MSC	Mesenchymal Stem/Stromal Cell
NAT	Nucleic-Acid Amplification Technique
NCA	National Competent Authority
NOAEL	No Observed Adverse Effect Level
NOD	Non-obese diabetic
NRM	Non-Rodent Mammal
OOS	Out-of-Specification
OQ	Operational Qualification
PBMC	Peripheral Blood Mononuclear Cell
PBSC	Peripheral Blood Stem Cell
PEI	Paul-Ehrlich-Institut (Federal Institute for Vaccines and Biomedicines in Germany)
PET	Positron Emission Tomography
Ph. Eur.	Pharmacopoea Europaea (engl. European Pharmacopoeia)

PHS	Public Health Service
PK	Pharmacokinetics
PMT	Photomultiplier tube
POC	proof-of-concept
PQ	Performance Qualification
PQR	Product Quality Review
PSF	Product Specification File
PSUR	Periodic Safety Update Report
PV	Pharmacovigilance
QA	Quality Assurance
QC	Quality Control
QM	Quality Management
QP	Qualified Person
QPPV	Qualified Person for Pharmacovigilance
QRM	Quality Risk Management
R&D	Research and Development
RA	Regulatory Affairs or Risk Analysis
RBC	Red Blood Cell
RCR	Replication Competent Retrovirus
RCV	Replication Competent Virus
RMCE	Recombinase-Mediated Cassette Exchange
RMM	Rapid Microbiological Method
SAE	Serious Adverse Event
SAR	Serious Adverse Reaction
SCBP	Stem Cell Based Product
SCID	Severe Combined Immunodeficiency
SCT	Somatic Cell Therapy
sCTMP	somatic Cell Therapy Medicinal Product
SIN	Self-Inactivating (Vector)
SIV	Simian Immunodeficiency Virus
SME	Small and Medium-sized Enterprise
SMF	Site Master File
SOP	Standard Operating Procedure
SSC	Side Scatter
SUSAR	Suspected Unexpected Serious Adverse Reaction
TE	transendocardial (muscle injection)
TEP	Tissue Engineered Product
TMF	Trial Master File

TNF	Tumor Necrosis Factor
TSE	Transmissible Spongiform Encephalopathy
UAE	Unexpected Adverse Event
URS	User Requirement Specification
USP (−NF)	United States Pharmacopeia (−National Formulary)
VMP	Validation Master Plan
WBC	White Blood Cell
WCB	Working Cell Bank
WHO	World Health Organization

Glossary

Term	Definition
Acceptance Criteria	Numerical limits, ranges, or other suitable measures for acceptance of the results of analytical procedures, which the drug substance or drug product or materials at other stages of their manufacture should meet. *ICH Q6B*
Active Pharmaceutical Ingredient (API) or Drug Substance	Any substance or mixture of substances intended to be used in the manufacture of a drug (medicinal) product and that, when used in the production of a drug, becomes an active ingredient of the drug product. Such substances are intended to furnish pharmacological activity or other direct effect in the diagnosis, cure, mitigation, treatment, or prevention of disease or to affect the structure and function of the body. *ICH Q7*
Advanced Therapy Medicinal Product (ATMP)	'Advanced therapy medicinal product' means any of the following medicinal products for human use: — A gene therapy medicinal product as defined in Part IV of Annex I to Directive 2001/83/EC [see definition somatic cell therapy medicinal product], — A somatic cell therapy medicinal product as defined in Part IV of Annex I to Directive 2001/83/EC [see definition somatic cell therapy medicinal product],

Term	Definition
	— A tissue engineered product as defined in point (b) [*Note*: Regulation 1394/2007, Chapter 1, Article 2, 1b; see definition tissue engineered product]. *Regulation 1394/2007, Chapter 1, Article 2*
Analytical Procedure	The analytical procedure refers to the way of performing the analysis. It should describe in detail the steps necessary to perform each analytical test. This may include but is not limited to: The sample, the reference standard and the reagents preparations, use of the apparatus, generation of the calibration curve, and use of the formulae for the calculation, etc. *ICH Q2 (R1)*
Batch (or Lot)	A specific quantity of material produced in a process or series of processes so that it is expected to be homogeneous within specified limits. In the case of continuous production, a batch may correspond to a defined fraction of the production. The batch size can be defined either by a fixed quantity or by the amount produced in a fixed time interval. *ICH Q7*
Clinical Trial/Study	Any investigation in human subjects intended to discover or verify the clinical, pharmacological and/or other pharmacodynamic effects of an investigational product(s), and/or to identify any adverse reactions to an investigational product(s), and/or to study absorption, distribution, metabolism, and excretion of an investigational product(s) with the object of ascertaining its safety and/or efficacy. The terms clinical trial and clinical study are synonymous. *ICH E6 (R1)*

Term	Definition
Drug Product (Dosage Form; Finished Product)	A pharmaceutical product type that contains a drug substance, generally, in association with excipients. *ICH Q6B*
Drug Substance (Bulk Material)	The material which is subsequently formulated with excipients to produce the drug product. It can be composed of the desired product, product-related substances, and product- and process-related impurities. It may also contain excipients including other components such as buffers. *ICH Q6B*
Excipient	An ingredient added intentionally to the drug substance which should not have pharmacological properties in the quantity used. *ICH Q6B*
Gene Therapy Medicinal Product (GTMP)	Gene therapy medicinal product means a biological medicinal product which has the following characteristics: a. It contains an active substance which contains or consists of a recombinant nucleic acid used in or administered to human beings with a view to regulating, repairing, replacing, adding, or deleting a genetic sequence; b. Its therapeutic, prophylactic or diagnostic effect relates directly to the recombinant nucleic acid sequence it contains, or to the product of genetic expression of this sequence. Gene therapy medicinal products shall not include vaccines against infectious diseases. *Directive 2009/120/EC*
Good Manufacturing Practice (GMP)	The part of quality assurance which ensures that products are consistently produced and controlled in accordance with the quality standards appropriate to their intended use. *Directive 2003/94/EC*

Term	Definition
Good Clinical Practice (GCP)	A standard for the design, conduct, performance, monitoring, auditing, recording, analyses, and reporting of clinical trials that provides assurance that the data and reported results are credible and accurate, and that the rights, integrity, and confidentiality of trial subjects are protected. *ICH E6 (R1)*
Pharmacovigilance	Pharmacovigilance is defined as the science and activities relating to the detection, assessment, understanding, and prevention of adverse effects or any other medicine-related problem. *WHO*
Pharmacovigilance System	A system used by the marketing authorization holder and by Member States to fulfill the tasks and responsibilities listed in Title IX [*Note*: Of Directive 2001/83/EC] and designed to monitor the safety of authorized medicinal products and detect any change to their risk–benefit balance. *Directive 2001/83/EC*
Investigational Medicinal Product (IMP)	A pharmaceutical form of an active ingredient or placebo being tested or used as a reference in a clinical trial, including a product with a marketing authorization when used or assembled (formulated or packaged) in a way different from the approved form, or when used for an unapproved indication, or when used to gain further information about an approved use. *ICH E6 (R1)*
Investigator	A person responsible for the conduct of the clinical trial at a trial site. If a trial is conducted by a team of individuals at a trial site, the investigator is the responsible leader of the team and may be called the principal investigator. *ICH E6 (R1)*

Term	Definition
Manufacture	All operations of receipt of materials, production, packaging, repackaging, labeling, relabeling, quality control, release, storage, and distribution of APIs and related controls. *ICH Q7*
Medicinal Product	Any substance or combination of substances presented for treating or preventing disease in human beings or animals. Any substance or combination of substances which may be administered to human beings or animals with a view to making a medical diagnosis or to restoring, correcting or modifying physiological functions in human beings or in animals is likewise considered a medicinal product. *Glossary EU GMP Guidelines*
Mesenchymal Stem/Stromal Cell (MSC)	MSC are widely used for clinical cell therapy administration. MSC can be isolated and expanded from bone marrow, adipose tissue, umbilical cord, and other tissues. MSCs are characterized by their adherence to plastic, specific surface antigen expression, and differentiation potential into different lineages. Minimal Consensus criteria have been defined In 2006 by the International Society for Cellular Therapy (ISCT, Position paper: Minimal criteria for defining multipotent mesenchymal stromal cells. M. Dominici, K LeBlanc, I Mueller, I Slaper-Cortenbach, FC Marini, A Keating, DJ Prockop, EM Horwitz. *Cytotherapy* 2006, Vol 8, 315–317)
Pharmaceutical Quality System (PQS)	Management system to direct and control a pharmaceutical company with regard to quality. *ICH Q10 based upon ISO 9000: 2005*

Term	Definition
Product Specification File (PSF)	A reference file containing, or referring to files containing, all the information necessary to draft the detailed written instructions on processing, packaging, quality control testing, batch release, and shipping of an investigational medicinal product. *EU GMP Guidelines, Part I, Annex 13*
Production	All operations involved in the preparation of an API from receipt of materials through processing and packaging of the API. *ICH Q7*
Qualification	Action of proving and documenting that equipment or ancillary systems are properly installed, work correctly, and actually lead to the expected results. Qualification is part of validation, but the individual qualification steps alone do not constitute process validation. *ICH Q7*
Qualified Person (QP)	The person defined in Article 48 of Directive 2001/83/EC and Article 52 of Directive 2001/82/EC. *EU GMP Guidelines, Part I, Annex 16*
Quality Assurance (QA)	The sum total of the organized arrangements made with the objective of ensuring that all APIs are of the quality required for their intended use and that quality systems are maintained. *ICH Q7*
Quality Control (QC)	Checking or testing that specifications are met. *ICH Q7*
Quality Management (QM)	Accountability for the successful implementation of the quality system. *Guidance for Industry: Quality Systems Approach to Pharmaceutical cGMP Regulations, FDA*
Quality Risk Management (QRM)	A systematic process for the assessment, control, communication, and review of risks to the quality of the drug (medicinal) product across the product lifecycle. *ICH Q9*

Term	Definition
Somatic Cell Therapy Medicinal Product (SCTMP)	Somatic cell therapy medicinal product means a biological medicinal product which has the following characteristics: a. Contains or consists of cells or tissues that have been subjected to substantial manipulation so that biological characteristics, physiological functions or structural properties relevant for the intended clinical use have been altered, or of cells or tissues that are not intended to be used for the same essential function(s) in the recipient and the donor; b. Is presented as having properties for, or is used in or administered to human beings with a view to treating, preventing or diagnosing a disease through the pharmacological, immunological or metabolic action of its cells or tissues. For the purposes of point (a), the manipulations listed in Annex I to Regulation (EC) No 1394/2007, in particular, shall not be considered as substantial manipulations. *Directive 2009/120/EC*
Specification	A specification is defined as a list of tests, references to analytical procedures, and appropriate acceptance criteria which are numerical limits, ranges, or other criteria for the tests described. It establishes the set of criteria to which a drug substance, drug product or materials at other stages of its manufacture should conform to be considered acceptable for its intended use. "Conformance to specification" means that the drug substance and drug product, when tested according to the listed analytical procedures, will meet the acceptance criteria. Specifications are critical quality standards that are proposed and justified by the manufacturer and approved by regulatory authorities as conditions of approval. *ICH Q6B*

Term	Definition
Sponsor	An individual, company, institution, or organization which takes responsibility for the initiation, management, and/or financing of a clinical trial. *ICH E6 (R1)*
Tissue Engineered Product (TEP)	'Tissue engineered product' means a product that: — Contains or consists of engineered cells or tissues, and — Is presented as having properties for, or is used in or administered to human beings with a view to regenerating, repairing or replacing a human tissue. A tissue engineered product may contain cells or tissues of human or animal origin, or both. The cells or tissues may be viable or non-viable. It may also contain additional substances, such as cellular products, bio-molecules, biomaterials, chemical substances, and scaffolds or matrices. Products containing or consisting exclusively of non-viable human or animal cells and/or tissues, which do not contain any viable cells or tissues, and which do not act principally by pharmacological, immunological or metabolic action, shall be excluded from this definition. *Regulation 1394/2007, Chapter 1, Article 2*
Validation	A documented program that provides a high degree of assurance that a specific process, method, or system will consistently produce a result meeting pre-determined acceptance criteria. *ICH Q7*

About this Book: Why Cell Therapy?

1

Christine Guenther, Andrea Hauser, and Ralf Huss

Pharmaceutical industry quests for innovation to maintain their leadership in a competitive business and provide new therapies to those patients to whom they have currently nothing or nothing appropriate to offer. As stated by the Boston Consulting Group: "*There are no old roads to new directions*" or citing Albert Einstein: "*if they always do what they always did, they will always get what they always got*", innovations are difficult to obtain. Many present "innovations" in the existing market place are not truly considered break-through and do not deliver adequately, neither medically nor commercially.

Despite everybody's aspiration to improve the medicines for tomorrow, cell and gene therapy is still unknown territory to almost all stakeholders with a lot of uncertainties. In principle, however cell therapy is not new but presently experiences a scientific and clinical renaissance by utilizing the entire and broad potential of a biological genius that can rebuild tissue, modulate disease conditions and shuttle drugs to the desired destination in the body with insofar negligible or acceptable complications. The origin of such a therapeutic approach was initially the first attempt to treat leukemia with hematopoietic stem cells (HSCs) more than half a century ago. What initially was considered to be a mere replacement of cells after high-dose chemotherapy turned out to be also the first effective immunotherapy.

While this prime example of cell therapy was developed mainly by clinicians, the *non-GMP* manufacturing of such therapeutic cells was mainly restricted to academic centers and university hospitals. Maybe this is one reason why the pharmaceutical industry is still shy from a broad investment in such complex and yet unstandardized pharmaceutical development process, where also an off-the-shelf concept was not yet readily available.

On the other hand, the possibility to find a way into such a disruptive technology requires a new assessment of the situation, which reminds us of an old business tale: *The first shoe salesman wires back to London office: "Situation hopeless. No one is wearing shoes". The second shoe salesman says instead: "Glorious times ahead of us. No one is wearing shoes YET!"*

Biotech and pharmaceutical industry only slowly adopt the emerging field of cell therapy because of its complex biology with yet sometimes unknown mode-of-action, no current well-defined target profile, strict process dependency, existing donor restriction, lack of standardization, not yet established business model, etc.

But with an increasing demand for new therapies for diseases like cancer, diabetes, dementia, and other age-related health conditions and with an inevitable demand for a competitive portfolio including cell-based therapeutics, there is now a need for standardized procedures, harmonization, and regulation in this field. This also applies in particular for combination therapies including gene delivery.

Consequently "cell and gene therapies" start to become regulated as **"advanced therapies"** in EU and US with an increasing body of documents, regulations, guidelines, rules, procedures, acts, directives, manuscripts, etc., which are sometimes premature or just not aligned among various competent authorities. Here the authors show a way to develop, implement and commercialize advanced therapeutics like cell-based medicinal products, based on the current knowledge and understanding (please see Figure 1.1).

It is the purpose of this book to provide direction and guidance in this new field of **"advanced therapeutics"**, where yet no well-established and widely accepted state-of-the-art exists. Here we provide a critical path how to develop and implement a standardized and approved process for cell-based therapies, exemplified by mesenchymal stem cells (MSCs) as source for a "second generation" and commercial viable cell-based therapeutics.

This book is based on many discussions and interactions with stakeholders, review of the literature and own experiences. It is presented and structured in different chapters including many illustrations, tables, and references. However it cannot be complete at this point given the natural complexity of the existing topics still under discussion in different parts of the world and among various stakeholders which are still in a state of flux, but this book is intended to guide the reader to the necessary next steps during the entire development process.

Figure 1.2 shows the guided flow of activities to start a development of a cell-based product including the GMP-grade manufacturing and its implementation into a clinical development program all the way to possibly commercialization.

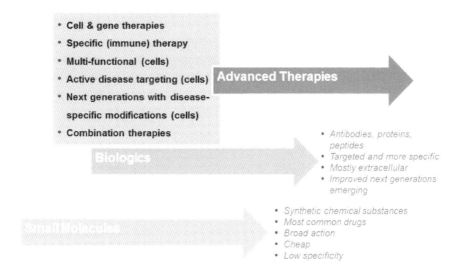

Figure 1.1: Advanced Therapies Including Cell and Gene Therapies are the next Level of "Standard of Care" for Patients Suffering from Diseases, with yet Unmet Medical Need, despite of Its Unprecedented Complexity.

After the assessment of a potential unmet medical need and an identified commercial interest in cell-based therapeutics in selected disease areas to maintain a competitive portfolio, it is necessary to explore the regulatory landscape for such a cell therapy product (please see *Chapter* 2). The landscape is not only globally highly diverse, but also within individual European member states. The introduction of the term "*advanced therapy medicinal products* (*ATMP*)" in EU legislation significantly changed the regulatory situation and affected mainly academic centers that were used to produce "their" cell products without complying with full GMP standards. There are of course different perspectives coming from academia and/or industry. While the latter is rather interested in the realization of profits based on the exclusive rights to develop and market, academia mainly wants to test scientific hypothesis and provide clinical benefits to the patients. *Chapter* 2 also deals with the different regulatory perspectives of academia *versus* industry which also includes the "hospital exemption clause" that should not lead to lower product quality, but could offer perspectives for products and treatments in which industry is not (yet) interested. One crucial aspect in an emerging and innovative field, such as cell-based therapeutics is the assessment of a "risk-based approach" defining the limits of acceptable uncertainties for patients with different diseases.

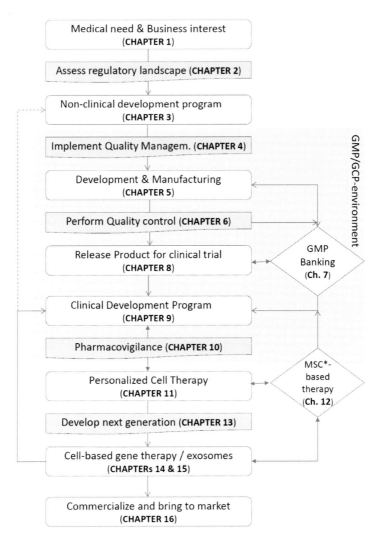

Figure 1.2: Flow Chart Depicting the Rationale of this Book, Starting from the Idea to Enter Cell Therapy until a Personalized Cell Product on the Market, with Consideration on a Next-Generation Cell-Based Product.

Any development requires a thorough non–clinical development program with *in vitro* and adequate *in vivo* models (please see *Chapter* 3). Such required activities are based on the legal background for cell and gene therapies in many places, which are currently not yet harmonized between the EU and the US regulatory framework or other parts of the world. But any pre-clinical program needs to be closely aligned with the intended clinical trial including pharmacokinetics and dose finding studies.

If the decision has been made to develop and manufacture a cell-based therapeutic for clinical use in patients, the implementation of an adequate quality management system is crucial to guarantee patient safety as well as a sustainable efficacy in the clinical setting (please see *Chapter* 4). Such Quality Management with its different pillars (documentation, training, change and deviation management, etc.), also provides the foundation to effectively deal with the still constantly changing regulatory environment, including all the gathered experiences along the way.

The process and GMP manufacturing of an IMP (EU) or IND (US) is at the core of every new development, particular for such a disruptive modality like an advanced therapy (please see *Chapter* 5). Such a cell-based product not only consists of a biological substance as starting material (cells), but can also be modified by the addition of genetic or other material. It might even change its biological behavior during the manufacturing process. It is one of the major challenges to scale-up a lab-scale protocol to a GMP-compliant and industrial process that provides enough material for larger trials and a common market.

The management of the GMP process development and manufacturing is therefore diligently accompanied by a thorough quality control (please see *Chapter* 6), which includes the survey of all materials as well as the analytical methods, specifications and release criteria. This chapter is certainly at the center of this book, describing the importance of quality measures in general and the quality control in particular for the success of advanced therapies in the clinic and in the market.

The storage of manufactured IMP/IND products (please see *Chapter* 7) and its release for clinical testing or market distribution (please see *Chapter* 8) also follows strict guidelines which are based on the general principles of quality management and several regulations.

The clinical implementation of any new therapeutic modality is the final proof of the diligently executed scientific work during non-clinical development and the equally robust manufacturing of the active substance (please see *Chapter* 9). Here it is of pivotal importance to align with the competent national or central (e.g., EMA) authorities as early as possible to reach a common understanding on the scope of the intended clinical trial in accordance with the valid regulatory landscape. While industry follows a designated critical path to comply with active regulations to eventually obtain (exclusive) market authorization, academia might pursue other opportunities to bring such therapies to the patients.

Pharmacovigilance is a crucial function during every clinical development, particularly in such innovative therapies where a lot of experience is still lacking (please see *Chapter* 10). Active surveillance substance by a Qualified Person of any event related to the new therapy is of pivotal importance to anticipate any threat to the patient's well-being as early as possible and to adopt the protocol or even stop the treatment.

After many years of trial-and-error to identify the right patient population for a treatment, personalized medicine or health care has been implemented, particularly in expensive therapies like biologics and advanced therapies (please see *Chapter* 11). This however requires the identification of biomarkers to predict the safety and clinical response of a substance in a selected cohort and stratify the patients accordingly.

Although cell therapy started decades ago with HSCs or progenitor cells, we here exemplify the non-clinical and clinical development of an advanced, cell-based medicinal product using MSCs (please see *Chapter* 12). These adult cells are already widely used in hundreds of clinical trials for many different indications by various routes of administration, providing insights into possible pitfalls or upsides of cell therapies.

Many academic centers and some companies already pursue next generation cell therapies (please see *Chapter* 13), also modifying immune cells for an altered or improved efficacy or redirected mode of action. One possible therapeutic strategy is the genetic modification of cells to imprint additional features to a cell or to delete unwanted functions (please see *Chapter* 14). Here, we focus on the engineering of MSCs for drug delivery.

Other cell-based substances of current interest are extracellular vesicles (EVs) or exosomes (please see *Chapter* 15). They can be derived also from MSCs and might perform different or additional functions than their foster cell itself.

Finally, it is of course the ultimate object for any new pharmaceutical development also to commercialize an innovative (advanced) therapy and place it on the market (please see *Chapter* 16). This requires the allocation of substantial funding (financials and resources) as well as the strategic positioning regarding pricing and reimbursement.

Although this book is a comprehensive overview on the development and implementation of advanced cell-based therapies with a strong emphasis on quality management and quality control as well as the GMP manufacturing of cellular therapeutics, it cannot substitute for consulting the respective and current guidelines, rules and regulations put into effect by the competent authorities responsible for the site of manufacturing, the clinical trial or the marketing authorization.

The authors, therefore advice the readers also to consult with the responsible agencies and experienced regulatory consultants in the field. This book can only provide guidance on the permutation of a scientific-based cell therapy into a clinically validated product on the market place.

Regulatory Landscape and Risk-Based Approach

2

Josef M. Hofer

2.1 Introduction: Regulatory Landscape

All over the International Conference on Harmonization (ICH) regions, regulations on Advanced Therapy Medicinal Products (ATMPs) are still in a process of development. Whereas the learning curve is increasing, the legislation has to provide sufficient flexibility in order to accommodate the rapid evolution of science and technology in this field.

In general, same regulatory principles apply to ATMPs as for other types of biotechnology medicinal products. However, all technical conditions and prerequisites, especially the kind and the depth of preclinical and clinical investigations necessary to demonstrate the safety and efficacy of an ATMP, are highly specific and make any strategy for regulatory authorization just unique as the product itself.

There are numerous specific issues that should be thoroughly investigated in non-clinical studies with ATMPs, such as viability, longevity, distribution, growth, differentiation, and migration of somatic cellular products, potential for germline transmission and/or re-activation of vector for gene therapy products, the duration of post administration observations etc. Other important factors to consider are determining the most useful animal model and extrapolation from animals to the human situation.

A clinical development program for an investigational ATMP should proceed through a series of exploratory and confirmatory clinical studies. The amount of clinical studies as well as the specific study design requirements for each of these trials depends on various factors, including the characteristics of the investigational product, the route of administration, the characteristics of the target patient population and the proposed indications. Due to the singular and multifactorial properties of ATMPs, their development should be subject to case–by–case risk analysis and may require product–dependent designs for clinical studies.

It is interesting that ICH is mostly concentrating on general guidance in regard to quality, safety, and efficacy but the regions themselves are providing detailed information on definitions, procedures, and requirements to get ATMPs approved.

2.2   Regional Definitions and Requirements

2.2.1   *Europe*

The framework of the Regulation 1394/2007/EC of the European Parliament and of the European Council on ATMPs ("ATMP Regulation") was reviewed in the Report from the Commission to the European Parliament and the Council [COM (2014) 188 final][1] showing that there is still potential for improvement to assure the balance between necessary requirements for clinical trials approvals/marketing authorizations and public health protection.

Classification, Certification scheme and Scientific Advice Procedures at the European Medicines Agency (EMA) are introduced, especially in order to support Small and Medium-Sized Enterprises (SMEs) and non-profit organizations in the complicated regulatory environment. The Classification enables findings in regard to the categorization, e.g., into somatic cell-based or tissue engineered ATMPs, whereas the certification procedure evaluates quality and non-clinical data independent of any marketing authorization application. The certification by the Committee of Advanced Therapies (CAT) can be used for facilitating the evaluation of any future application for clinical trial and marketing authorization based on the same data. For this reason, according to the Regulation, the evaluation of all certification applications will be conducted in accordance with the same scientific and technical requirements as are applicable to a marketing authorization application.

The discussion on 'Hospital Exemption' is still a very critical issue as there are large differences between the various European countries, e.g., in regard to the number of patients defined as non-routine. Initially, the hospital exemption was adopted to support the availability of new cell-based therapies for a defined and small patient cohort in hospitals and was mainly applied by academic institutions. Academic institutions are not expected to develop for the market but should have the access to innovative therapies and manufacture for limited application within a specialized clinical institution. As the medicinal and commercial translation of ATMPs into market authorization is far behind the expectations and the medical need, the role of hospital exemption is currently under discussion. It may be critical for any market application by companies if clinical development should be performed mainly under the hospital exemption rule. The lack of clear Good Clinical Practice (GCP)-requirements for the application within the hospital exemption rule may influence the quality of clinical data and may have direct negative effect on patient's safety. The Good Manufacturing Practice (GMP)-requirements for the product must be fulfilled. It is still not clear if data obtained by treating patients within the hospital exemption rule can form part of the dossier for market authorization.

In regard to the regulatory requirements on preclinical, pharmaceutical and clinical studies there is still a need for acceptance of flexibility and science based activities. Risk-based approach and quality by design have to be defined as the golden regulatory standards in development of ATMPs.

2.2.2 *USA/Food and Drug Administration (FDA)*

The FDA and mainly the Center for Biologics Evaluation and Research (CBER) is responsible for the regulation of Human Cells, Tissues, Cellular and Tissue-Based products (HCT/P's) and the human gene therapy products. For those products defined as medical devices, the Center for Devices and Radiological Health (CDRH) takes care.

Human somatic cell therapy and gene therapy products are regulated by CBER under Section 351 of the PHS Act and/or the FD&C Act. This grouping includes products that FDA has determined as not fulfilling all of the criteria in 21 CFR 1271.10 (a) and are regulated as drugs and/or biological products like;

- Cultured Cartilage Cells.
- Cultured Nerve Cells.
- Lymphocyte Immune Therapy.
- Gene Therapy Products.
- Human Cloning.
- Human Cells Used in Therapy Involving the Transfer of Genetic Material (cell nuclei, oocyte nuclei, mitochondrial genetic material in ooplasm, genetic material contained in a genetic vector).
- Unrelated Allogeneic Hematopoietic Stem Cells.
- Unrelated Donor Lymphocytes for Infusion.

CBER also regulates the HCT/P's solely as "361 products" when they meet all of the criteria in 21 CFR 1271.10 (a), e.g., like cartilage, ocular tissues (Corneas & Sclera), skin, amniotic membrane [when used alone (without added cells) for ocular repair], but also Hematopoietic Stem Cells derived from peripheral or umbilical cord blood, as well as semen, oocytes and embryos, whereas the CDRH regulates Devices composed of Human Tissues under the FD&C Act and device regulations like corneal lenticules, preserved umbilical cord vein grafts, human collagen, femoral veins intended as A–V Shunts.

For Combination products, a differentiation for alignment is needed, e.g., cultured cells (fibroblasts/keratinocytes/nerve/ligament/bone marrow) on synthetic membranes or combined with collagen may be regulated as Medical Devices or as Biological Products.

Earlier than all the European competent authorities, the FDA provided the first guidline on Advanced Therapies like the Guidance for Human Somatic Cell Therapy and Gene Therapy published in 1998.[2] But as today product development is globally oriented and international harmonization is ongoing, international guidance has to be taken into consideration.

2.2.3 *Japan*

In Japan at the Pharmaceutical and Medical Device Agency (PMDA), the Office of HCT/P's undertakes preliminary reviews for applications for verification of regenerative medicinal products (HCT/P's), gene therapy products, and medical devices using cells and tissues.

The general principles for handling and use of HCT/P's were notified in the Notification No. 1314 (December 26, 2000) and further guidance followed in the form of guidelines on Ensuring Quality and Safety of Products Derived from Processed Human Cell/Tissue (for autologous products, No. 0208003 (February 8, 2008), and for allogeneic products, No. 0912006 (September 12, 2008).

In regard to Clinical Trial for ATMPs, relevant guidelines exist like the Principles of Good Cell- and Tissue-Practice: MHLW Notice No. 266, the Guideline for the Quality and Safety of Human (autologous) and (allogeneic) HCT/P's, Standard for Biological Raw Material and Point-to-consider for Process Control/Quality Control of Human (autologous) HCT/P's (2010 Yakushokukanmatatsu No. 0327025), and the Guideline for Stem Cell Clinical Research (including somatic cell products).

The Japanese Government realized the big chance of College of Veterinary Medicine and Biomedical Sciences (CVMBS) and the competent authorities initiated an amendment to the pharmaceutical law to provide a separate approval channel for regenerative medicines by introducing non-phased clinical trial schemes.

2.3 Quality, Safety, and Efficacy Regulatory Requirements in the European Commission (EC)

Although the primary objectives of quality, non-clinical and clinical testing of ATMPs does not essentially differ from any other medicinal product, various and specific biological activities and functionalities have to be considered for development.

Detailed aspects and risk factors to be addressed therefore are discussed in the chapters: Non-clinical development of cell-based products, Clinical development, Quality management, Quality Control and Manufacturing, and specific guidance have to be evaluated and followed.

2.4 Risk-Based Approach

2.4.1 Introduction: Risk-based approach

Somatic Cell Therapy and its evaluation of quality, safety, and efficacy represents an extremely high level of complexity. The only adequate method of resolution can be a risk based approach This regulatory pathway is now accepted worldwide by competent authorities, pharmaceutical R&D, and academia.

The increase in knowledge especially in the biological, biotechnological, biopharmaceutical and bioanalytical science and industry created new opportunities that provide insights into the elusive space of cell therapy.

High variability of data evolves from the biological diversity during the development of cell-based therapeutic agents. The information cannot be presented in standard regulatory format. There is a need for creativity to exhibit the essential results and conclusions in a framework designed by targets and outcomes. The improvements in data management by electronic systems and statistical assessments enable the mining and manifestation of immense information.

2.4.2 *General discussion*

Risk-based Approach is intrinsically connected with the principles of risk management, as shown in the four columns:

Risk Assessment	Risk Control	Risk Communication	Risk Review
Risk Identification	Risk Reduction	Risk Communication	← ____ Risk Acceptance
Risk Analysis	Risk Acceptance ↓	↓	↑
Risk Evaluation ↓		Output/Results of Risk Management ⟹ Risk Events Process	Risk Events

The key step is the identification of risks which can be established only by experts experienced in all fields of development and research and by collecting information including historical data, theoretical analyses, opinions, concerns of stakeholders, etc.

Planning of a risk management process involves, at the minimum, the introduction of the following aspects:

- Defining the problem/risk question and the potential for risk.
- Assembling data/information on the potential hazard and human health impact.
- Defining how decision makers will use the assessment and conclusions.
- Specifying project issues (leadership, resources, timelines, and deliverables).

In regard to risk analysis, various tools can be used like Failure Mode Effects Analysis (FMEA), Failure Mode Effects and Criticality Analysis (FMECA), Fault Tree Analysis (FTA), Hazard Analysis and Critical Control Points (HACCP), Risk ranking and filtering, etc. The best way is always the one which is mostly used in the organizational unit.

As important as identification, are the implementation of risk reduction measurements — which probably may introduce new risks — and the definition of acceptable level of risks, which is always a case-by-case decision!

The Guideline on the risk-based approach came into effect on February 12, 2013[3] and concentrates on the methodology of a risk-based approach, i.e., definition of risk, risk factors and risk profiling and on the presentation of fictitious examples to illustrate the approach.

Although this is only a guideline, the risk-based approach is already introduced as an option by the legislation with the revision of Annex 1, Part IV of Directive 2001/83/EC as amended by Directive 2009/120 EC. It is important to know that the guidance is applicable to all ATMPs, as characterized in Directive 2001/83/EC, Part IV, Annex 1 (somatic cell therapy and gene therapy medicinal products) and in Regulation 1394/2007/EC (tissue engineered products and combination products).

Any detailed discussion on risk management has to be initiated in connection with the regulatory information provided in the ongoing evolution of the pharmacopeias and the current guidelines, e.g., for cell-based and gene therapy medicinal products, i.e., the Guideline on human cell-based medicinal products (EMEA/CHMP/410869/2006) and the Note for guidance on the quality, preclinical and clinical aspects of gene transfer medicinal products (CPMP/BWP/3088/99).

In detail, any risk-based approach is based on the management of various intrinsic risk factors with respect to quality, safety, and efficacy of the medicinal product or the medical device.

2.4.3   Risk-based approach in quality/development and manufacturing

Starting materials, but also media, buffers, solutions, excipients may have an early impact on the manufacturing of a homogenous drug product. Culture conditions and manufacturing steps like cell harvesting and cryoconservation may bear risk for cell transformation and even have the potential to introduce genetic instability

Process validation and/or evaluation on a multifactorial design basis are therefore as essential as intelligent analytical methods used for in-process control at critical steps or at screening of starting material as well as for control of final product.

Risk-based approach is hereby characterized by defining the right biological risk response and finding an adequate analytical parameter to ensure structural/functional integrity and batch to batch homogeneity.

Product and/or process related impurities are major risks to be mitigated, minimized, or eliminated. Morphological deviations may be easier to handle than genetic aberrations, which are mostly not adequately classified by standard atlas or catalogues.

Microbiological contamination by aerobic and anaerobic bacteria, fungi, endotoxins, and mycoplasma are most critical as they can be introduced by source material (e.g., bone marrow), all culture medium supplements, from manufacturing environment and last but not the least through application conditions at the clinical site.

As an example of specific risk minimization approaches, the microbiological testing strategy has to be adapted. The intention to develop a test procedure for the drug product according to Ph. Eur. 2.6.1 in general for cell-based products is not successful. This is due to an insufficient filter-flow-through of the biological media used. The necessary volume of 10% through a single filter could not be reached according to the particle size of medium components.

Therefore, a testing method on microbiological control according to Ph. Eur. 2.6.27 has to be developed for suitability of these specific medicinal products. Already the pharmacopeial monograph considers this test preferable for cellular products. The test method is validated for the volumes employed (amount of culture media to be tested by microbiological control procedure is $\geq 7.5\%$). The minimum inoculum volume is 1% for total product volume of ≥ 10 ml, so that the employed amount equals a factor of 750%. Another approach could be to test the intermediate and final drug product for microbial contamination. These sampling points correspond to the major handling steps in manufacturing. As the final results from sterility testing may first be available some days after application of the cell product (immediate administration necessary due to short stability); at the microbiological laboratory, a visual inspection is performed every workday followed by an immediate notification in case of any contamination.

2.4.4 Risk-based approach in safety/preclinical toxicological investigations

Toxicological investigations of cell-based products: The standard models are mostly not predictive enough for the safety and efficacy in human, especially in regard to immunogenicity and tumorigenicity. Animal models may not be predictive for treatment failure due to differences in the disease status of animal and patients. Even if the immune status of the animal model has been matched to the patient's situation (e.g., pre-treatment with a vector to induce seroconversion), a multifactorial and biological diversity can never be obtained under full control.

In addition, the risk in differences in the biodistribution of cells ("famous fade away") between animal and human organs and tissues has to be evaluated and controlled.

Translatability from preclinical to clinical trials attracted attention after the so-called TeGenero case. The serious adverse reactions (cytokine storm) that occurred in TeGenero's first-in-man trial, led almost immediately to press speculations on whether the company had appropriately tested the product in animals prior to transition to humans. Many press commentaries rather dwelled on findings like swollen lymph nodes in monkeys or on a dog that died during non-clinical testing of

TGN141227 than making efforts to explain that the clinical trial had not been an 'out of the blue' experiment, but was preceded by intensive non-clinical development, unfortunately not following adequate risk-based approach.

The follow up discussion on the "Guideline on Requirements for First-In-Man Clinical Trials for Potential High-Risk Medicinal Products"[4] defined factors of risks located in the mode-of-action, nature of the target and especially in the relevance of animal species and models.

Risk mitigation strategies discussed in regard to further clinical investigations were justified for estimation of the first dose in humans and a sufficient lag time between applied doses which had to be calculated individually and were risk-based.

The following risks have to be discussed in the preclinical section of a dossier, e.g., in case of a genetically modified cell-based medicinal product:

- Risk of generating replication competent vector.
- Risk of vector mobilization.
- Risk of insertional mutagenesis and oncogene-activation in the target cell.
- Risk of migration into non-targeted tissues.
- Risk of vector shedding.
- Risk of inadvertent immune responses as target or effector cells.
- Risk of genetic instability and tumorigenicity.
- Risk of any unintended biological response of the product.

All these risks reviewed in preclinical research have one single target which is to assure patient safety and also to identify specific patient eligibility criteria and indices to be monitored in trials in humans.

The scientific community acknowledges that, for some specific cell based medicinal products, animal models might not be representative of the clinical situation and consequently might not provide interpretable data, e.g., for immunotoxicity. In these cases, the use of homologous animal models is encouraged. In addition to non-clinical immunogenicity studies, eligibility criteria and immunogenicity studies have to be carefully planned at the clinical level.

2.4.5 *Risk-based approach in efficacy/clinical setting*

In the clinical setting, it is essential to avoid risks in regard to treatment failure and/or adverse drug reactions. The respective risk factors can be related to the

- Situation and constellation of the patient;
- Underlying disease(s);
- Overall medical procedure and treatment;

- Concomitant medication;
- Posology of the new medicinal product;
- Modes of administration of the new medicinal product, e.g., direct injection into the target organ.

These risks have to be assessed within the broad environment of the intended indication, the exclusion criteria/contraindications and minimized by stratification and preventive measures.

Potential risks in toxicity are in general dose related. The starting dose, dose escalation schemes, maximum tolerated doses, supra-therapeutic dose and/or ectopic administration may introduce excessive production of adverse drug reactions.

The risk-based approach in clinical studies is determined by the design of the clinical protocol and the performance of the clinical trials. The critical issues are

- Choice of study population;
- Form and route of administration;
- Posology: Starting dose and dose escalation increments;
- Number of subjects per dose;
- Sequence and interval between administrations within the same increment;
- Stopping rules;
- Definition of responsibilities for decisions in regard to subject dosing and dose escalation;
- Trial sites, facilities and personnel.

The cooperation between the sponsor, the contract research organization (CRO) and the investigators during protocol development is a key process in risk management within clinical studies. The expertise gained here already provides, at an early stage, appropriate level of understanding, e.g., of the mechanism-of-action and training for the later staff conducting the trial. This enables opportunities for alternative monitoring approaches (e.g., centralized monitoring) that can improve the quality and efficiency of the sponsor's oversight of clinical investigations. A risk-based monitoring approach provides not less vigilance but focuses the attention on preventing critical processes and findings. Moreover, a risk-based procedure offers the chance of continuous adaptations, amendments or other potentially risk mitigating actions like introduction of further training programs and overall clarifications in the clinical trial protocol.

2.4.6 *Risk-based approach in regulatory affairs*

Regulatory Affairs assure risk minimization by implementation of explicit requirements and specifications in the marketing authorization dossier for the upcoming information to the prescribers [Summary of Product Characteristics (SmPC)] and patients [package information leaflet (PIL)]. During R&D, the risk management strategies are discussed with the competent authorities in scientific advice, during the application process of clinical trials, in case of marketing authorization application within the obligatory Risk Management Plan (RMP) and at the time of marketing of educational material and training instructions for physicians and patients.

The RMP is today a key document of the dossier and the total Pharmacovigilance System. The Guideline on Good Pharmacovigilance Practices (GVP) Module V: Risk management systems[5] describes in detail the principles, the requirements and operational processes for pharmaceutical companies and competent authorities. The contents of RMPs are shown in Table 2.1.

For ATMPs, there are special chapters included, e.g., in SVII module "Details of important identified and potential risks (ATMP)", where explicitly risks on procurement, risks on quality characteristics of cell products, etc. are mentioned and have to be discussed. For ATMPs, more flexibility in headings and descriptions is allowed explicitly.

Table 2.1: RMP.

Part I	Product(s) overview
Part II	Safety specification
	Module SI Epidemiology of the indication(s) and target population(s)
	Module SII Non-clinical part of the safety specification
	Module SIII Clinical trial exposure
	Module SIV Populations not studied in clinical trials
	Module SV Post-authorisation experience
	Module SVI Additional EU requirements for the safety specification
	Module SVII Identified and potential risk
	Module SVIII Summary of the safety concens
Part III	Pharmacovigilance plan
Part IV	Plans for post-authorisation efficacy studies
Part V	Risk minimisation measures (including evaluation of the effectiveness of risk minimisation measures)
Part VI	Summary of the risk management plant
Part VII	Annexes

2.5 Environmental Risk Assessment (ERA)

The scope of an ERA is the environment at large, excluding the patient but including people in the patient's environment.

In general, the current ERA follows the methodology described in the EU Directive 2001/18/EC.[6] For cell therapy medicinal products, e.g., containing genetically modified organism (GMO) as defined in Directive 2001/18/EC1, the risk of dissemination is normally low as all processes run under highly controlled conditions.

No systemic spread of vector particles will occur, e.g., if the vector is designed as replication deficient. These vector particles can only be synthesized by a special packaging cell line containing essential structural and regulatory genes for vector production.

By introduction of work safety measurements for manufacturing and application at the hospital including GMP Management, training, hygiene plan, personal protective equipment and prevention of infection by suitable measurements (e.g., laminar flow), the overall risk mostly can be considered negligible.

2.5.1 *ERA in the EC*

Product innovations such as GMO, but also coming from nanotechnology entering the environment have to be carefully evaluated, especially in regard to their potential risk and sustainability.

A Risk Management Strategy has to be developed based on the characteristic of GMO potentially causing adverse effect, and its consequences, as described in the following list:

• Hazard identification.
• Likelihood of occurrence.
• Risk impact and the likelihood of detection.

For ATMPs, the evaluation is directed toward any risk of damage to the environment during the clinical trials or marketing period and includes all knowledge gained during preclinical and clinical development. For example, for Cell-Based Medicinal Products, it is of prominent importance, that no genetic information or moieties of added gene sequences, e.g., from the genetically modified somatic cells will be transferred into any other somatic or germline cell for the therapeutic purpose of correction, replacement, manipulation, addition or induction of deleted, mutated or dysfunctional genes.

For the purpose of hazard identification, the characteristics of the cells that may cause a harmful effect on human health or the environment should be identified and the potential consequences of these harmful effects should be evaluated. To identify and evaluate harmful effects that could arise from the use, a worst-case scenario can be defined. In this scenario, a number of parameters are maximized. This scenario does not necessarily correspond to the characteristics and intended use, but is useful as it yields to a maximum valuation of the potential hazards. The actual situation is taken into account subsequently in the evaluation of the likelihood to determine whether the occurrence of a harmful effect is expected.

The pathogenicity, oncogenicity and immune–reactions of the medicinal product and its formulation, viral infections, horizontal gene transfers (HGT)/lateral gene transfers (LGT) to bacteria are critical issues to be evaluated.

Uncontrolled spreading, e.g., of a vector in the patient and in the environment has to be discussed and sufficient precaution and warning should be implemented in manufacturing, distribution and application of the medicinal product. This can be realized by keeping all processes under defined conditions, sterilizing any waste at $121°C/20$ minutes and cleaning with H_2O_2 disinfection, so that no viable material from manufacturing should enter the environment. The primary packaging material should be tested in regard to mechanical stability. Double bag systems should be used for the thawing procedure at the administration site. The product should be infused directly from the primary packaging. No substantial manipulations which may bear the risk of dissemination should be performed. All staff handling the ATMP should be trained in all respective procedures.

In order to get approval, the overall risk has to be determined and Risk management strategies including a 'Monitoring Plan' must be established

General surveillance is incorporated in the monitoring plan. From the start of clinical trial or marketing, all hospitals can be advised to keep a registry of individuals who handle the medicinal product. These include pharmacy staff, operating theatre staff, personnel who care for the patients, and staff involved in cleaning. The gathered information is retained in the hospital. This plan has to be sufficient to monitor unanticipated effects on human health in general.

2.6 Pharmacovigilance in the EC

Pharmacovigilance is the top priority project in all ICH regions and worldwide exchange of safety information is one major task of authorities and companies. Nevertheless, this is also one of the most difficult issues as long as the medical philosophy and practice as well as social and patients' care systems are not harmonized.

Within the individualized medicine in ATMPs for pharmacovigilance traceability, the possibility to trace each individual unit of an ATMP from the donor and/or source material to the patient and *vice-versa* and active surveillance are the most prominent issues to be discussed, listed and elaborated as

- Traceability;
- Active Surveillance;
- Adverse Event/Adverse Reaction reporting, assessment and consequences applicable for other medicinal products during development and marketing have to be followed; special focus is directed on awareness of long-term treatment and experience. In the European Community, the Guideline on Safety and Efficacy Follow-Up — Risk Management of ATMPs EMEA/149995/08 is part of the Good Vigilance Practice system and has listed several points to be considered for efficacy of post-authorization studies. It is acknowledged that considering the nature of ATMPs, only limited efficacy and safety information may be available at the end of pre-authorization clinical trials and full benefit-risk assessment may need several years of follow-up. Rationale for conducting such studies might include following situations:

(a) ATMPs incorporating living organisms.
     Efficacy of such ATMPs may change after long periods of time. This may result in an increase (e.g., over expression of a gene of interest) or decrease of efficacy. Pre-existing immunity to the vector and its change with potential repeated administrations at later stages can also alter the clinical course of efficacy and safety.

(b) ATMPs incorporating tissue that may need years to be fully functional.
     In such cases, proof-of-concept and a positive clinical outcome in clinical trials using surrogate endpoints might be sufficient for the evidence of efficacy required for granting a marketing authorization. Nevertheless, the efficacy profile, including clinical endpoints, might need to be confirmed in the post-authorization phase.

(c) ATMPs expected to be used once a life-time.
     Efficacy of such products over time can only be answered by long-term follow-up.

(d) Efficacy of many ATMPs is highly dependent on the quality of the administration procedure. This may differ significantly between a clinical trial setting, and post-authorization normal healthcare, as well as between various healthcare establishments. These issues may be addressed *via* post-authorization efficacy follow-up system.

(e) Cell therapy products with limited life-time may require a follow-up that monitors the efficacy. This should help to determine the need of re-application of the product.

This guideline is primarily focused on post-authorization issues and describes specific aspects of pharmacovigilance, risk management planning, safety and efficacy follow-up of authorized ATMPs, as well as some aspects of clinical follow-up of patients treated with ATMPs.

But it should be clearly stated that the generation of post-approval data is not a substitute for the need for safety and efficacy data at the time of marketing authorization application.

Pre- and post-authorization pharmacovigilance of ATMPs is characterized by a continuous Benefit/Risk-Evaluation, reflecting all aspects of the advantages of treatment, for the patient at a given level of tolerability.

More detailed discussion and descriptions on GVP for ATMPs are presented in Chapter 4.

References

1. COM (2014) 188 final, 28.3.2014, Report from the Commission to the European Parliament and the Council in Accordance with Article 25 of Regulation (EC) No. 1394/2007 of the European Parliament and of the Council on Advanced Therapy Medicinal Products and Amending Directive 2001/83/EC and Regulation (EC) No. 726/2004.
2. Guidance for Industry: Guidance for Human Somatic Cell Therapy and Gene Therapy. US Department of Health and Human Services, Food and Drug Administration, Center for Biologics Evaluation and Research, March 1998.
3. EMA/CAT/CPWP/686637/2011; Guideline on the risk-based approach according to annex 1, part IV of Directive 2001/83/EC applied to Advanced therapy medicinal products.
4. EMEA/CHMP/SWP/28367/07; Guideline on Requirements for First-in-Man Clinical Trials for Potential High-Risk Medicinal Products.
5. EMA/838713/2011; Guideline on Good Pharmacovigilance Practices (GVP) Module V Risk management systems; February 20, 2012.
6. Directive 2001/18/EC of the European Parliament and of the Council on the deliberate release into the environment of genetically modified organisms and repealing Council Directive 90/220/EEC; 17.4.2001.

Non-Clinical Development of Cell-Based Products

3

Felix Hermann, Daniela Hirsch, and Christoph Prinz

3.1 Introduction

Cell-based therapeutics can be divided into cell therapy products (CTPs) and somatic cell-based *ex vivo* gene therapy products (GTPs). They are the latest addition in the tool box for drug development, which until recently contained nearly exclusively small molecules and proteins. CTPs are cells which are isolated *in vitro* from respective tissue and "are more than minimally manipulated". In general, the manipulation is an extended *in vitro* cultivation period. In principle, production of GTP follows that of CTP: Cells are isolated and cultured *in vitro*, but additionally the cells are genetically modified with the help of gene transfer vectors, which may be viral or non-viral (see Figure 3.1).

The pharmaceutical industry has established development strategies for conventional small molecule drugs to allow efficient transfer to the market. Non-clinical development is the first step on the path to routine clinical application of a new therapeutic entity. It starts with the identification of new drug candidates. Subsequently, data is collected to ensure an acceptable toxicity profile and sufficient efficacy before clinical trials in humans are initiated. The current methodological instruments have been especially tailored over the years to study the interaction of a single molecular entity within a model system, which may either be an *in vitro* system (e.g., cell culture) or *in vivo* (e.g., rodent animal model). Compared to small molecule and protein drugs, CTPs and GTPs are considerably more complex modalities as their therapeutic function does not rely on the properties of a single molecule but on the overall function of an entire cell. In the case of CTPs, the therapeutic effect in the patient is directly related to intrinsic cellular function(s), which may

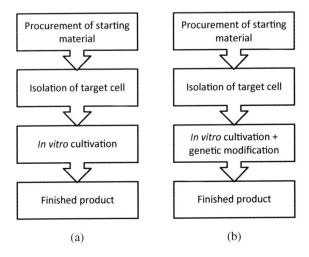

Figure 3.1: (a) CTP; (b) GTP.

have been enhanced due to specific treatment during the manufacturing process. Even more complex are GTPs as they combine the intricacy of living cells with gene transfer vector systems in order to implement therapeutic function(s) in the modified cells.

Therefore, non-clinical development of advanced therapies presents additional challenges compared to small molecules. These are especially related to the toxicity profile, the structure–function relationship and potential immunogenicity of cell-based products. In the following sections, the regulatory environment for preclinical development programs for GTP and CTP products will be outlined. Furthermore, development strategies for advanced cell-based products will be discussed with regard to the applicable regulatory guidelines. Owing to space constraints, *in vivo* gene transfer products (non-cell-based) are not reviewed in this chapter.

3.2 Legal Background and Regulatory Guidance for Cell and Gene Therapies

As advanced therapies like CTPs and GTPs are relatively new modalities, the development and implementation of generally accepted manufacturing procedures and analytical tools for these products are under way. This situation presents considerable challenge with regard to non-clinical development and requires considerable effort from the industry and the regulatory authorities to handle these products. The competent authorities in general have decided to adopt a case–by–case approach with regard to the regulation of cell-based products.[1,2] In the absence of generally accepted procedures for non–clinical assessment of advanced therapy products, this approach allows for maximum flexibility.

3.2.1 *The European Union (EU)*

The EU has recognized medicinal GTPs and somatic CTPs as new entities of medicinal products and has classified them, along with tissue engineered products as "Advanced therapy medicinal products (ATMPs)" (EC No. 1394/2007). Until the aforementioned regulation, ATMPs were regarded from a regulatory viewpoint to be non–different from standard small molecule pharmaceuticals. The new regulation was put in place to separate ATMPs from standard small molecules and biologics (antibodies), foreseeing that new and specific regulatory requirements are applicable to these products. In the Directive 2009/120/EC amending the Directive 2001/83/EC, GTPs and CTPs have been defined.

GTPs are products

- Which contain an active substance comprising a recombinant nucleic acid used in or administered to human beings with a view to regulating, repairing, replacing, adding, or deleting a genetic sequence;
- Whereas their therapeutic, prophylactic, or diagnostic effect (in a patient) relates directly to the recombinant nucleic acid sequence it contains, or to the product of genetic expression of this sequence.

According to this definition, a GTP may consist of recombinant DNA, genetically modified bacteria, genetically modified viruses (viral vectors), or genetically modified cells. Vaccines are explicitly excluded from the definition as they are specifically regulated elsewhere.

CTPs are products

- Which contain or consist of cells or tissues that have been subject to substantial manipulation so that biological charactcristics, physiological functions, or structural properties relevant for the intended clinical use have been altered, or of cells or tissues that are not intended to be used for the same essential function(s) in the recipient and the donor;
- Which have properties for, or are used in or administered to human beings with a view to treating, preventing, or diagnosing a disease through the pharmacological, immunological, or metabolic action of their cells or tissues.

The EU has implemented the European Medical Agency (EMA) as the central regulatory body, which is responsible for marketing authorization of new medicinal products in the EU. It has to be pointed out that clinical trials are regulated by the local governments of the individual counties. Within the EMA, the Committee for Medicinal Products for Human Use (CHMP) is responsible for the assessment of new products for marketing authorization. In general, ATMPs have to adhere to the same rules with regard to preclinical testing as non-ATMPS. Nevertheless, CHMP has issued various guidelines concerning the preclinical development for cell-based therapeutic products to address special issues relating to these products.

3.2.2 *The US regulatory frame work*

Within the Department of Health and Human Services, the Food and Drug Administration (FDA) is responsible for the authorization of clinical trials and marketing authorization for new medicinal products. Within the FDA, the Center for Biologics Evaluation and Research (CBER) regulates CTPs and human GTPs.

Biologics are defined in Section 351 of the Public Health Service (PHS). FDA regulations and policies have established that the biological products include cell and gene therapy products if they are more than minimally manipulated (i.e., cultured and/or genetically modified), if they are combined with an article other than a preservation or a storage agent, if they are used in a way that is not homologous to their normal function, or if they have a systemic effect and depend on the metabolic activity of living cells for their primary function. Biologic regulations (21 CFR 600) are applied to cell-based products along with the FDA's current Good Manufacturing Practice (cGMP) regulations (21 CFR Parts 210 and 211) and the Investigational New Drug (IND) regulations (21 CFR 312). Furthermore, the current Good Tissue Practice (cGTP) rules in 21 CFR part 1271 is applied to cell-based products including GTPs. The FDA has issued several documents to guide preclinical development of CTPs.

3.2.3 *International harmonization*

The International Conference on Harmonization of Technical Requirements for Registration of Pharmaceuticals for Human Use (ICH) facilitates discussion between the regulatory authorities of Europe, Japan, and the United States and experts from the pharmaceutical industry. Although the proposals of ICH are not legally binding, it is the aim of the ICH to internationally standardize requirements for the pharmaceutical development to eliminate redundancy.

Due to the rapid development in the field of cell and gene therapy, the ICH had difficulties to develop generally accepted guidelines and therefore offers little guidance on CTPs and GTPs development (see Table 3.1). Several guidelines have been

Table 3.1:   Compilation of international guidelines regarding cell-based products.

Agency	Title/Scope
ICH	Non-Clinical Safety Studies for the Conduct of Human Clinical Trials and Marketing Authorization for Pharmaceuticals (Current version).
ICH	Guideline on Virus and Gene Therapy Vector Shedding and Transmission (Concept paper).
ICH	Preclinical Safety Evaluation of Biotechnology-Derived Pharmaceuticals (Current version).
ICH	Safety Pharmacology Studies for Human Pharmaceuticals (Current version).
EMA	Guideline on the Non-Clinical Studies Required Before First Clinical Use of Gene Therapy Medicinal Products (Current version).
EMA	Guideline on the risk-based approach according to annex 1, part IV of Directive 2001/83/EC applied to Advanced therapy medicinal products (Current version).
EMA	Guideline on Strategies to Identify and Mitigate Risks for Firstin-Human Clinical Trials with Investigational Medicinal Products (Current version).
EMA	Preclinical Assessment of Investigational Cellular and Gene Therapy Products (Current version).
EMA	Guideline on Human Cell-Based Medicinal Products (Current version).
EMA	Guideline on quality, non-clinical and clinical aspects of medicinal products containing genetically modified cells (Current version).
EMA	Reflection paper on stem cell-based medicinal products (Current version).
FDA	Preclinical Assessment of Investigational Cellular and Gene Therapy Products (Current version).
FDA	Content and Review of Chemistry, Manufacturing, and Control (CMC) Information for Human Somatic Cell Therapy Investigational New Drug Applications (INDs) (Current version).
FDA	Content and Review of Chemistry, Manufacturing, and Control (CMC) Information for Human Gene Therapy Investigational New Drug Applications (INDs) (Current version).

released describing generally accepted approaches toward preclinical development, whose content is also useful for advanced medicinal products.

3.3   The Process is the Product: The Link between Manufacturing and Non-Clinical Development

Due to the complex nature of cell-based products, the implemented specifications inaccurately describe the products in their entirety. Product specifications define a few parameters, which have been identified as important but ignore the majority of the cell's properties. Changes in the manufacturing process may significantly alter the resulting product. These alterations may not be reflected in the parameters (specifications) that are measured for release, but may nevertheless significantly change the behavior of the product in the patient and may lead to unwanted side effects or reduced efficacy *in vivo*. Because of this, changes in the manufacturing process should be accompanied by comparability studies to ensure that results of previous (non-clinical) studies have not been invalidated by the change. The need for comparability studies may severely delay the entire clinical development program for a cell-based product and cause considerable costs. Keeping in mind that cell-based products are a black box to a large degree with regard to their properties, it becomes clear that the best way to ensure consistent quality is to thoroughly define and to strictly control the manufacturing process.

As the preclinical development program is dependent on manufacturing to provide test items for the non-clinical studies, it is paramount to strategically plan and define the manufacturing process as early as possible in the non-clinical development stage. Already at the earliest stage, non-clinical development is tightly interwoven with the development of a suitable manufacturing process. A special challenge arises in this respect as the manufacturing process has to be planned in advance for several years to satisfy a broad scope of requirements: A fundamental need is the potential to achieve GMP-compliance for the process. Apart from supplying test items for the non-clinical studies, the process should be capable of providing enough products for all clinical phases. Furthermore, the potential for scale up/scale out should be included into the latest strategic planning during marketing authorization and commercialization.

Although it is understood that changes will have to be implemented during the life cycles of cell-based products for various reasons (quality improvement, cost reduction, scale up, etc.), it should be the aim of a strategic long-term planning to keep comparability studies to a minimum and to ensure that none of the changes carries the risk of altering the basic nature of the cell-based product.[3]

3.4 Development Stages for GTPs and CTPs

On the way to marketing authorization for a CTP or GTP, the non-clinical development program can be divided in to three stages. The first stage is the research program based on which the prototype is generated (Discovery/prototype generation). It is followed by a development program with the aim to provide all necessary non-clinical data for the first clinical trial in human subjects (non-clinical development/first-in-man). The third stage encompasses the non-clinical program

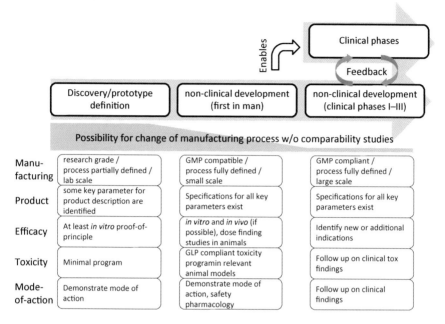

Figure 3.2: Overview of aims in the non–clinical development stages and the relationship to product characterization.

accompanying subsequent clinical development phases, until marketing authorization (see Figure 3.2).

3.4.1 *Discovery stage/prototype definition*

In the discovery stage, suitable isolation and cultivation methods are established to generate the cell type of interest as basis for the advanced therapy product. For gene therapy products, an appropriate vector system and genetic modification methods are implemented. A set of minimal parameters should be defined to describe the resulting prototype meaningfully with regard to its desired therapeutic function and identity. These parameters form the basis for the release specification for the later product stages. Furthermore, the prototype product is used to collect proof–of–principle data on the intended therapeutic application. The general aim of this stage is to determine if the product is developable. When the phase has been completed a go/no go decision for entering the next stage is taken.

A basic characterization program is initiated in this phase to describe the prototype with regard to safety/toxicity and efficacy to ensure that the prototype is suitable for further development. Safety/toxicity in this early phase, relates primarily to the viability of the cell product itself under culture conditions and on any safety issues that may arise during early *in vivo* proof-of-concept studies. Although a GMP-compliant production process is neither necessary nor required at this stage, nevertheless it should be ensured that the manufacturing process has the potential to be transferred to a GMP-environment. This precaution facilitates the later development stages.

3.4.2 *Non-clinical development for first-in-human application*

It is the aim of the non-clinical development phase for first-in-man clinical trial to provide all required data necessary to initiate a first clinical trial. Of special importance in this regard, is a comprehensive description of the safety/toxicity profile of the product, including off-target effects. The non-clinical package comprises proof-of-concept data and should support the assumed mode-of-action of the CTP. Taken together, it needs to be shown that the product can be assumed to be effective in humans. The combined results of non-clinical studies are essential to allow the selection of a safe and effective dose for clinical trials. Also, pharmacokinetic properties of the product should be assessed. These include mainly the bio-distribution pattern and (in some cases) the potential long-term engraftment of the cell-based product. Data from these studies is essential to support the mechanism of action and also helps to predict potential off-target effects. Furthermore, non-clinical studies should identify and establish parameters to be measured during the clinical trial to assess toxicity and efficacy (Biomarker program).

A prerequisite for this is that the manufacturing process of the cell-based product has been defined and specifications for the product have been set. At this stage, the process should be GMP-compatible: Although it is not necessary to have the entire GMP-qualification and -validation program completed for the preclinical testing phase, a well-controlled manufacturing process should be locked in and the respective scientifically sound quality control assays should be established including specification for the product.[4] This approach ensures that the manufactured test items are sufficiently characterized to provide reassurance that the non-clinical studies are conducted with material, which is representative of that to be administered to humans in the clinical studies.[5]

3.4.3 *Non-clinical development accompanying clinical phases*

During the clinical stage, the parallel non-clinical program is aimed to follow up on findings (e.g., new insight into mode-of-action or adverse events), to implement new treatment regimens or to evaluate new indications to be treated with the product. This stage forms a feed-back loop with ongoing clinical trials. Findings in the clinical trial will be analyzed in the subsequent preclinical studies. The results of the studies influence design of later clinical trials. In this stage, thorough understanding of all product properties has to be achieved to enable marketing authorization.[6]

3.5 Animal Models to Study Cell-Based Products

It is required to study the pharmaceutical product as part of the non–clinical development in relevant animal models to gather data on their toxicity profile, pharmacokinetics, and efficacy. The majority of cell-based products is derived from human cells and is therefore xenogeneic in relation to potential recipient animals. Application of these products to recipient animals therefore leads in general to the immune rejection of the cells and invalidates the model.

One possible solution is to use immunodeficient recipient animals to study the cell-based product. Various well-established immunocompromised rodent models exist, which are suitable recipients for xenografts and have been successfully used to study human cell-based products. The disadvantage of these models is that rodents are not closely related to humans and may therefore not mimic the human situation accordingly. Furthermore, questions concerning immunology cannot be answered in these models.

On the other hand, non-rodent models (NRMs) like dogs, pigs, and non-human primates often show more similarities to human (patho-) physiology including life span, in comparison to rodents. Furthermore, drug dosing more comparable to human patients can be performed. Despite the fact that NRMs resemble the clinical situation better, several major limitations are present in these models: Besides ethical concerns, high costs per animal and less statistical significance; it is practically not possible to test the human cell-based product in these models, as immunodeficient NRMs are scarce.

Although it is possible to suppress the immune system in large animals by pharmaceuticals to allow application of human cells, this approach is questionable as effects on the cell-based product cannot be excluded. Therefore, NRMs are more frequently used for proof-of-concept studies with homolog cell-based products. In this case, a homolog cell-based product is established using the respective animal cells. Comparability of the homolog product and the human cell-based product is of course the major concern with this approach. In the case of GTPs, this may include the exchange of the human therapeutic gene (e.g., human cytokine) for the corresponding animal variant.[2,4,7]

Regardless of the chosen animal species for studying a cell-based product, the relevance of the model should be thoroughly justified. It is important to understand that any animal model will have limitations for predicting human safety and efficacy. These may either be associated to the above mentioned reasons (immunology *vs.* homolog product) or due to product-specific considerations.

3.5.1 *Rodent-models*

Immunocompromised mouse strains are most frequently used as recipients for *in vivo* testing of human cell-based products and to prevent immunological rejection of these products. Different mouse strains with varying degrees of immunological impairment are commercially available. Immunodeficient mouse strains are a well-established model system and allow large group sizes for studies.[8]

The mouse strains originate from spontaneous mutations or have been genetically engineered with the aim to remove immunological functions. Some of the most commonly used strains are: Athymic nude mice, which lack functional T cells. Because of this, B cell function is also severely reduced. Severe Combined Immunodeficiency (SCID) mice are deficient for T and B cells. While Non–obese diabetic (NOD)/SCID-mice, besides T and B cells also lack NK cells. All described mouse strains accept application of human cell-based products to a varying degree and have been used successfully for toxicity, proof-of-concept or efficacy studies. For example, T cell and Mesenchymal stem cell (MSC) products have been successfully studied in immunodeficient mice to collect proof-of-concept data for various indications.[9–15] and to analyze their bio–distribution pattern.[13,14,16–18] and toxicity profile.[19,20] in various immunodeficient mouse strains.

A new development is the so called humanized mice. An example is the NOG (NOD/Shi- SCID IL2rγ^{null}) mouse strain, where a common gamma–chain knock out of the IL2 receptor has been bred into the NOD/SCID background. These mice allow engraftment of human hematopoietic stem cells (HSCs) and the subsequent development of a partially functional human immune system.[21–23] In these mice, cell-based products can be tested in the presence of a human immune system. Additionally, they allow studying the function of products, which are based on human HSCs in an *in vivo* model.[23,24] Due to the complexities of these models they are not generally used in the field yet and also are in many cases not good laboratory practice (GLP) compliant, which reduces their value for toxicological studies.

Although models based on immunodeficient mice have been improved in the recent years, there are still considerable drawbacks associated with them. In toxicity studies, the total absence of the immune system may potentially lead to the underestimation of immunotoxicity profile of a product. Furthermore, in proof-of-concept studies the presence of human immune cells may be needed to enable full functionality of a human cell-based product (e.g., human antigen–presenting cells for a human T cell product). Therefore, use of homolog syngenic animal models is generally encouraged by regulatory authorities.[7,25]

For example, the assessment of the genotoxic potential of integrating retroviral vectors in HSCs for gene therapy applications is often done in syngenic murine models as these studies require long follow up periods or even serial bone marrow transplantation.[26–31]

3.5.2 *Non-rodent mammals (NRM) models*

While rodent models mainly focus on mice, the field of NRMs or large animal models (LAM) faces a heterogeneous group of animals: Primates, dogs, pigs, but also sheep or rabbits can be found. Every species has its own model history for its typical field of diseases. Dogs and primates are widely associated with hematopoietic, while pigs are often related to cardiovascular or metabolic diseases. Although, the numerical use of NRMs make up the smallest group of animals for scientific use,[32] relevant contributions to special questions, e.g., infection with the human immunodeficiency virus (HIV), neuronal or cardiovascular diseases are mainly answered by NRMs. As mentioned before, the question of the immunological barrier has to be answered in every single model for the chosen cell-based therapy.

In Section 3.5.2.1, the pig and its role as biomedical model in regenerative medicine will be presented, followed by accordant NRM models for different fields of diseases. The focus lies on the cell as therapeutic unit in the model's environment.

3.5.2.1 *Pigs emerging as superior models in regenerative medicine*

Pigs (*Sus scrofa domestica*), especially mini-pigs, progressively evolve as one of the best models to mimic human physiology and diseases.[33,34] Since the whole genome was sequenced,[35] transgenic animals are available and the ability to replicate models through somatic cell cloning exists.[36,37] In contrast to dogs or monkeys, the high interest in pigs as breeding farm animals has caused a great effort in understanding

Table 3.2: Overview of the chosen models and their therapeutic approach.

Frequency of Chosen Approach	Type of Animal	Type of Cells	Donor/ Recipient Relation	Route of Delivery	Immunological Status
Prevalent	Pig	MSC	autologous	surgical[b] TE[d]	competent
Less frequent	Sheep	BM-MNC[a]	Allogeneic (MSC)	i.c.[c]	very rare: suppressed
	Dog	Skeletal myoblasts ESC[f]		i.v.[e]	

Notes: Data based on.[24]
BM-MNC[a]: Bone-marrow mononuclear cells. Surgical[b]: Surgery and local administration by injection. i.c.[c]: Intra-coronary arteries. TE[d]: Trans-endocardial muscle injection. i.v.[e]: Intra-venous. ESC[f]: Embryonic stem cell.

the swine's physiology, diseases, and genetics in order to yield a higher commercial profit. In addition, ethical considerations regarding pigs are noticed less critically in public compared to primates or dogs. Actually, porcine model and porcine stem cell research are ongoing: SCID pigs,[38] skin inflammatory diseases,[39] cystic fibrosis,[40] and also induced pluripotent cells from the pigs are available.[41] The genetic modification of pigs has developed very fast over the last decade.[42] Completing these disease model evaluations, the mini-pig resembles a representative model in toxicity testing for regulatory demands.[43]

3.5.2.2 Cardiac and cardiovascular diseases, e.g., myocardial infarction

As humans and NRMs have a similar systolic pressure and tick rate of their hearts, NRMs are favorable over rodents.[44,45] Especially the pig's heart and its coronary arteries are highly analogous in structure and distribution.[46] and in the size-to-body weight ratio.[47] Also, the cardiac cells metabolism is directly comparable to humans.[48]

Following these physiological evaluations, a systematic review of several pre-clinical studies involving an improvement of ischemic heart diseases by cell-based therapies confirmed the pig as a well-functional model.[49] Table 3.2 should give a simplified summary of the chosen approaches.

For ischemic diseases of the heart, MSCs are mainly used due to their well-known tissue-regenerative properties. Based on the review, the most commonly used

NRM model is the autologous, surgical transplantation of MSC into immunocompetent pigs. But also the intravenous or intra-arterial injection of cells is a functional option. The immune-evasive properties of MSC additionally obviate the need for immunosuppression in allogeneic NRM.[50] Although, the success of cell-based therapies in the field of cardiac diseases is limited, the toxicological and efficacy predictive relevance of NRM models could be confirmed by these studies.[49]

3.5.2.3   *Infectious diseases, e.g., human immunodeficiency virus (HIV)*

In spite of all efforts in the high active antiretroviral therapy (HAART) of HIV and potential HSC gene therapy approaches, the disease remains incompletely curable. NRM are still necessary to research the infection and its consequences. Since HIV originated as SIV (simian immunodeficiency virus) in primates, immunologic suitable models are easily found: E.g., pig-tailed macaques (*Macaca nemestrina*) are used for preclinical research. The advantages of NRM are obvious: Control over the time point of infection, close monitoring, search for latent virus reservoirs, and the understanding of HAART interruptions give more insight into the disease.

Novel HSC-based approaches include the introduction of HIV-resistant genes into the genome resulting in HIV resistant lymphocytes. C–C chemokine receptor type 5 (CCR5), an important co-receptor for the entry of HIV into the cell, is a potential target since a bone marrow transplant recipient of a CCR5-negative donor seemed to be cured of HIV.[51] To utilize this advancement in HIV-resistance, primates are needed to research and develop potential clinical protocols. Latest publications underline the feasibility of non-human primates for HSC-based approaches and highlighted the translational quality into clinical trials: Pre-stimulating for bone marrow aspiration, CD34+ cell enrichment, lentiviral transduction, and re-transplantation conditions are highly comparable. This same preclinical and clinical strategy and the high similarity in infection and disease progression of humans and primates allow a valuable testing with HSC containing the therapeutic unit.[52]

3.5.2.4   *Neurological diseases, e.g., Parkinson's disease*

The very complex neuronal system of humans limits the selection of an accordant model for the research of neuronal diseases. As an animal of choice, primates contribute to neuroscience since many similarities between monkeys and humans can be identified.[53] Neurological diseases, e.g., Parkinson's disease are often longstanding, degenerative disorders. To observe a cell-based therapeutic benefit, a longer life-span of the chosen model is necessary. In contrast to rodents, primates facilitate longer monitoring for positive influence on the disease development but also for side effects and hence increase the significance of potential therapies.

A common way to mimic Parkinson's disease in NRM is to administer the neuron-toxin, 1-methyl-4-phenyl-1, 2, 3, 6-tetrahydropyridine (MPTP), which causes a non-reversible destruction of dopaminergic neurons in the *substantia nigra*. This loss of dopaminergic functional structures leads to malfunctioned motor skills and are comparable to Parkinson's symptoms. Cell-based approaches aim to regenerate the lost functions by replacing the non-functional areas with stem-cell derived dopaminergic neurons by intracranial transplantation into the affected region.

In MPTP-treated macaques (*Macaca fascicularis*), a behavioral improvement with intracranial transplanted dopaminergic neurons could be shown. These cells were embryonic stem cells removed from other intraspecies monkeys and differentiated into dopaminergic neurons before introduced into the brain.[54] This advance of allogeneic transplantation led to preclinical studies trying to transplant xenogeneic, human cells in primates. Therefore, immunosuppressed macaques received intracranial human embryonic stem-cell derived dopaminergic neurons. The survival and function of these cells in this primate model could be approved and an attenuating of the symptoms of Parkinson's disease could be shown.[55] This proof-of-concept could have paved the way for future cell-based clinical trials due to the benefits gained by non-human primate model testing.

3.5.2.5 *Musculoskeletal diseases, e.g., osteoarthritis*

Widespread diseases, e.g., osteoarthritis are a major challenge in orthopedics. The rodent's anatomy is at a disadvantage, since the size and volume of defects are inadequate and not representative for humans. Particularly, long-term effects are necessary to evaluate the potential benefits of stem cell therapy. Treatment approaches in canines were successful, as could be seen in the experiments with dog models with chronic osteoarthritis in their humero-radial joints that were treated with autologous adipose-tissue derived MSCs.[56] Even though no breakthrough of cartilage repair could be achieved in these dog models, significant effects of autologous MSCs transplanted in goats[57] and rabbits[58] could be achieved. The immunoresponse avoiding properties of MSCs was shown by Vieira *et al.* in 2012, transplanting human adipose-derived MSCs into immunocompetent muscular dystrophy dogs, demonstrating muscle homing, and detection of human dystrophin expression.[59] MSCs with their regenerative potential are useful in NRMs and therefore favorable for long-term renewable approaches in osteoarthritic defects.

3.6 Primary Pharmacodynamics: Proof-of-concept and Efficacy Studies

Data of proof-of-concept studies provides support for the intended clinical effect of the CTP. The studies should be carried out in a relevant disease model, to assess efficacy, optimize the treatment regimen, and also to determine an effective dose (range) as a basis for clinical testing. Mode-of-action should be determined. For this, *in vitro* accompanying the *in vivo* studies or stand-alone *in vitro* approaches are recommended.

Various different immunocompromised mouse models exist to test efficacy of human cell-derived products: Engraftment and differentiation of human HSC products can be analyzed in the above mentioned humanized mice.[21–23] The efficacy of several MSC-based products (GTPs and CTPs) has been assessed in immunocompromised mouse models.[9, 60–63] It has to be pointed out that immunodeficient mouse models do not only allow use of human cell-based products, but also accept human tumor xenografts. This characteristic has been used to demonstrate anti-tumor activity of human T cells, which express a chimeric antigen receptor (CAR).[64, 65]

In the cases where relevant disease models are not available, regulators suggest collecting efficacy data *in vitro*. It is also encouraged to generate animal-derived substitute product for testing in homologous animal models.[1, 2] Whenever homolog models are used, the comparability to the human product should be justified.

3.7 Pharmacokinetics (PK)

Classical PK studies analyze the adsorption, distribution, metabolism, and excretion (ADME) of a drug. In the case of cell-based products, PK refers primarily to the distribution and persistence (if applicable) of the product over time. It is the aim of PK studies to confirm the intended target tissue/organ of the treatment and to identify potential distribution to unwanted sites. Therefore, also non-target organs should be analyzed for presence of the cell-based product. Results of these studies are helpful to predict off-target effects for the clinical application. It may therefore be useful to combine bio-distribution studies within the general toxicity studies.

3.7.1 *Monitoring distribution and engraftment*

As human cell-based products are xenogeneic in relation to the recipient animal, PCR-based methods, which specifically recognize human DNA-sequences, may be employed to detect the applied cells.[19] Furthermore, immunohistological methods can be applied to detect human cellular proteins within the animal tissue. In the case of GTP, the transgene can be used in many cases as specific marker for detection (PCR and/or immunohistology).[66] Both methods are highly sensitive and allow, in principle, the detection of single human cells. Nevertheless, it is not possible to perform in-life measurements (apart from blood), as organs and tissues have to be harvested to apply the methods. To analyze the distribution over time, groups of animals have to be sacrificed at different time points, which increase work load and costs of the entire study. Both methods are relatively cumbersome and thereby limit the number of samples which can be processed.

Several non-invasive techniques are available to monitor bio-distribution of cell-based products: Positron emission tomography (PET), Bioluminescence imaging, and magnetic resonance imaging (MRI). In contrast to the above described end-point methods, all non-invasive techniques require modification of the cells in order to apply the methods (reviewed in Ref. 67). This poses the risk that characteristics of the cell-based product will be altered leading to a different distribution or persistence pattern compared to the unaltered product.

Non-invasive monitoring approaches may be most relevant for gene therapy applications, as in some cases the therapeutic gene also can be used as marker genes for PET or MRI. Several therapeutic genes encode enzymatically active proteins for which compatible *in vivo* tracer molecules exist,[68,69] thereby allowing the detection of the cell-based product without further modifications.

Cell-based products can also be loaded with iron oxide non-particles to allow *in vivo* tracking by MRI. However, this method does not discriminate between living and dead cells. Also, iron tracer that has dissociated from cells is detected.[70]

3.8 Toxicity Studies

The goal of the general safety/toxicology program within the preclinical development is to define a safe starting dose for clinical trials and to analyze tolerance, especially to identify organs which may be affected by toxicity. The extent of the non-clinical safety studies should be determined with a risk-based approach taking into account the indication to be treated (severity, availability of alternative treatment options), patient population (children, adults), persistence of the cell-based product (transient, long-term, life-long) and product specific characteristics (genetic modification, degree of modification, similarity to known products). In the following discussion, a non-exhaustive compilation of potential product related risks is described. Toxicity of a cell-based product may be associated with the formulation of the cell-based product (excipients or contaminants), the route of application, distribution to and/or long-term engraftment at unwanted sites, level of transgene expression (in the case of GTP), unwanted differentiation of the cell-based product *in vivo*, (overshooting) immune reactions and tumor formation.

Toxicity studies have to comply with Good Laboratory Practice (GLP)-standards: The testing facility needs to be certified and the test item should be representative for the product to be used in clinical application and sufficiently characterized. Regulatory requirements dictate that the cell-based products should be tested in a relevant animal model. The choice of the relevant model and read-out parameters for toxicology studies will largely depend on product-specific considerations. The design of the studies should in principle reflect the clinical intended treatment protocol (Route of application, dosing schedule, and duration). Any deviation should be thoroughly justified. Animals should be closely monitored of toxicity during the in-life phase (food intake, weight, clinical blood chemistry, behavior) and a comprehensive macroscopic and histopathological analysis of the major organs, tissues, and lesions is expected at the end of the study or in case of unscheduled deaths. The European Medicines Agency (EMA) guideline on toxicity studies may facilitate study design especially with regard to the parameters that should be measured.[71]

For the development of small molecule pharmaceuticals, safety testing is generally required in a rodent and a NRM[72] to increase the probability to detect relevant toxicities. Regulatory authorities are aware that testing of human cell-based products in NRMs is in many cases not feasible due to immune rejections. Immunocompromised mouse strains are therefore in many cases the first choice for toxicity testing.[19] The need to assess immunotoxicity of the product may warrant the establishing of homolog animal cell-based product to be used in immunocompetent recipients. The comparability of the human cell-based product and homolog animal version should be justified.

Although humanized mouse models have been improved in the recent years and in principle allow assessment of human HSC-based products, it is still problematic to engraft human cells in humanized mice for long follow-up studies.[21–23] Therefore, homolog models may also be advisable for cell products where long-term engraftment is expected in the patient.

It is desirable to combine the toxicological analysis and efficacy study in a relevant disease model, if possible, as indication specific toxicities can be identified. Although adherence to the GLP principles may not be possible, if complex animal models are used, this does not automatically preclude the toxicity data from being used for clinical trial application or market authorization.

3.8.1 *Tumorigenicity and genotoxicity studies for CTP and GTP*

The tumorigenic potential of all cell-based products is a major safety concern. Potentially the *in vitro* cultivation process may transform the cell-based product, leading to tumor formation in the patient after application. In several non–clinical studies the tumorigenic risk associated with cell-based products has been demonstrated.[73–77] In the case of gene therapy products, it has been shown that integrating vectors (e.g., retroviral vectors and transposons) have a genotoxic potential and may cause transformation of cells. In several gene therapy trials in which HSCs had been transduced with retroviral vectors, clonal imbalances in the leukocytes compartment and leukemia were observed.[78–80]

Currently, EMA refers to Eur. Ph. 5.2.3 "Cell substrates for the production of vaccines for human use" to help in study design for tumorigenicity assessment.[1] In the described *in vivo* tumorigenicity test, 1×10^7 cells are injected s.c. into immunodeficient mice. The mice are followed for a period over three months for tumor development. Recently, Kanemura *et al.* have described an improved version of the assay which allows a more quantitative assessment of tumorigenicity.[81] The challenges to develop meaningful tumorigenicity assays *in vivo* and *in vitro* for cell-based product has recently been reviewed by Kuroda *et al.*[82] Furthermore, the Committee for advanced therapies of EMA has released a reflection paper on genotoxicity in GTPs.[83] Taken together, it is still debated to which degree available *in vivo* and *in vitro* models are able to accurately predict tumorigenic potential of cell-based products (GTP and CTP) with regard to clinical application.[2]

3.9 Dose Finding

Non–clinical studies should provide a data basis to allow selection of a safe and effective dose for the clinical trials. With regard to toxicity, the study should use the effective dose (intended for clinical application) with a suitable safety margin.[84] Additionally, a maximum feasible dose may be used with the aim to estimate the No Observed Adverse Effect Level (NOAEL). Efficacy studies should include several dose levels to establish a dose-response relationship. However, it is unsure if the established methods for calculating human equivalent doses do apply for cell-based products.[85]

3.10 Conclusion

Advanced therapeutic products like CTPs and somatic cell-based GTPs are the most complex medicinal products ever devised. On one hand their complexity comprises multilayered therapeutic functionality and therefore allows effective intervention for diseases with intricate pathology. On the other hand, the complexity is a challenge with regard to product characterization and non-clinical development programs.

Various guidelines have been implemented by regulatory bodies (e.g., EMA or FDA) in terms of pre-clinical development programs for CTPs, and GTPs which are even more complex as they combine the intricacy of living cells with gene transfer vector systems in order to implement therapeutic functions in the modified cells. Nevertheless, it is impossible to cover all relevant aspects for complex therapeutic products like CTPs and GTPs within these guidelines. This is why claiming a scientific advice is recommended for case-by-case assessment, considering the design of preclinical studies, the intended indication as well as the clinical strategy prior to the planning of a non-clinical program.

The preclinical assessments of cell-based therapies comprise in particular the evaluation of the mode-of-action and the determination of proof-of-concept of the therapeutic product *in vitro* and *in vivo* (primary pharmacodynamics), the distribution of the therapeutic cells (PK) and the assessment of safe therapeutic doses and side effects (safety/toxicity). In this regard, additionally, the tumorigenic potential is of interest for cell-based products. These data are essential for defining starting conditions and potential limitations for a first clinical application.

Along with these therapy-related considerations, manufacturing-related issues have to be taken into account during early stages like the discovery stage and during non-clinical development. These aspects focus on the definition of product specifications, the planning of the manufacturing process, the feasibility of GMP-compliant production, and the change from lab to large scale manufacturing.

References

1. Guideline on the Non-clinical Studies Required before First Clinical use of Gene Therapy Medicinal Products. (ed. Agency, E.M.) (2012).
2. Guidance for Industry: Preclinical Assessment of Investigational Cellular and Gene Therapy Products. (ed. Administration, F.a.D.) (2012).
3. Reflection paper on design modifications of gene therapy medicinal products during development. (ed. therapies, C.f.a.) (2011).
4. Guideline on quality, non-clinical and clinical aspects of medicinal products containing genetically modified cells. (ed. Agency, E.M.) (2012).
5. Note for Guidance on the Quality, Preclinical and Clinical Aspects of Gene Transfer Medicinal Products. (ed. Agency, E.M.) (2001).
6. Non-clinical safety studies for the conduct of human clinical trials and marketing authorization for pharmaceuticals. In *ICH Topic M 3 (R2)*. (ed. Agency, E.M.) (2008).
7. Reflection paper on stem cell-based medicinal products. (ed. Agency, E.M.) (2010).

8. Nasis, R., Cunningham, J.J., Brandon, E.P., and Cavagnaro, J.A. Considerations in the development of pluripotent stem cell-based therapies. In *Non-clinical Development of Novel Biologics, Biosimilars, Vaccines and Specialty Biologics*. (eds. Plitnick, L.M., and Herzyk, D.J.). Academic Press, Waltham, MA, 373–408 (2013).

9. Mouiseddine, M., Francois, S., Souidi, M., and Chapel, A. Intravenous human mesenchymal stem cells transplantation in NOD/SCID mice preserve liver integrity of irradiation damage. *Methods Mol. Biol.* 826, 179–188 (2012).

10. Noort, W.A., *et al.* Mesenchymal stem cells promote engraftment of human umbilical cord blood-derived CD34 (+) cells in NOD/SCID mice. *Exp. Hematol.* 30, 870–878 (2002).

11. Kim, S.W., Zhang, H.Z., Guo, L., Kim, J.M., and Kim, M.H. Amniotic mesenchymal stem cells enhance wound healing in diabetic NOD/SCID mice through high angiogenic and engraftment capabilities. *PLoS ONE* 7, e41105 (2012).

12. Kowolik, C.M., *et al.* CD28 co stimulation provided through a CD19-specific chimeric antigen receptor enhances *in vivo* persistence and antitumor efficacy of adoptively transferred T cells. *Cancer Res.* 66, 10995–11004 (2006).

13. Nakazawa, Y., *et al.* PiggyBac-mediated cancer immunotherapy using EBV-specific cytotoxic T-cells expressing HER2-specific chimeric antigen receptor. *Mol. Ther.* 19, 2133–2143 (2011).

14. Craddock, J.A., *et al.* Enhanced tumor trafficking of GD2 chimeric antigen receptor T cells by expression of the chemokine receptor CCR2b. *J. Immunother.* 33, 780–788 (2010).

15. Kimpel, J., *et al.* Survival of the fittest: Positive selection of CD4+ T cells expressing a membrane-bound fusion inhibitor following HIV-1 infection. *PLoS ONE* 5, e12357 (2010).

16. Vilalta, M., *et al.* Biodistribution, long-term survival, and safety of human adipose tissue-derived mesenchymal stem cells transplanted in nude mice by high sensitivity non-invasive bioluminescence imaging. *Stem Cells Dev.* 17, 993–1003 (2008).

17. Allers, C., *et al.* Dynamic of distribution of human bone marrow-derived mesenchymal stem cells after transplantation into adult unconditioned mice. *Transplantation* 78, 503–508 (2004).

18. Meyerrose, T.E., *et al.* In vivo distribution of human adipose-derived mesenchymal stem cells in novel xenotransplantation models. *Stem Cells* 25, 220–227 (2007).

19. Ramot, Y., Meiron, M., Toren, A., Steiner, M., and Nyska, A. Safety and biodistribution profile of placental-derived mesenchymal stromal cells (PLX-PAD) following intramuscular delivery. *Toxicol. Pathol.* (2009).

20. Ra, J.C., *et al.* Safety of intravenous infusion of human adipose tissue-derived mesenchymal stem cells in animals and humans. *Stem Cells Dev.* 20, 1297–1308 (2011).

21. Shultz, L.D., Ishikawa, F., and Greiner, D.L. Humanized mice in translational biomedical research. *Nat. Rev. Immunol.* 7, 118–130 (2007).

22. Legrand, N., *et al.* Humanized mice for modeling human infectious disease: Challenges, progress, and outlook. *Cell Host Microbe* 6, 5–9 (2009).

23. Watanabe, Y., *et al.* The analysis of the functions of human B and T cells in humanized NOD/shi-scid/gammac (null) (NOG) mice (hu-HSC NOG mice). *Int. Immunol.* 21, 843–858 (2009).

24. Perez, E.E., *et al.* Establishment of HIV-1 resistance in CD4+ T cells by genome editing using zinc-finger nucleases. *Nat. Biotechnol.* 26, 808–816 (2008).
25. Guideline on Non-clinical studies required before first clinical use of gene therapy medicinal products. (ed. Agency, E.M.) (2008).
26. Montini, E., *et al.* Hematopoietic stem cell gene transfer in a tumor-prone mouse model uncovers low genotoxicity of lentiviral vector integration. *Nat. Biotechnol.* 24, 687–696 (2006).
27. Montini, E., *et al.* The genotoxic potential of retroviral vectors is strongly modulated by vector design and integration site selection in a mouse model of HSC gene therapy. *J. Clin. Invest.* 119, 964–975 (2009).
28. Biffi, A., *et al.* Lentiviral vector common integration sites in preclinical models and a clinical trial reflect a benign integration bias and not oncogenic selection. *Blood* 117, 5332–5339 (2011).
29. Modlich, U., *et al.* Leukemia induction after a single retroviral vector insertion in Evi1 or Prdm16. *Leukemia* 22, 1519–1528 (2008).
30. Modlich, U., *et al.* Insertional transformation of hematopoietic cells by self-inactivating lentiviral and gamma retroviral vectors. *Mol. Ther.* (2009).
31. Kustikova, O., *et al.* Clonal dominance of hematopoietic stem cells triggered by retroviral gene marking. *Science* 308, 1171–1174 (2005).
32. http://ec.europa.eu/environment/chemicals/lab_animals/home_en.htm.
33. Cibelli, J., *et al.* Strategies for improving animal models for regenerative medicine. *Cell Stem Cell* 12, 271–274.
34. Kuzmuk (ed.). Pigs a model for biomedical sciences. In *The Genetics of the Pig.* (2011).
35. http://www.ensembl.org/Sus_scrofa/Info/Index.
36. Schook, L., *et al.* Swine in biomedical research: Creating the building blocks of animal models. *Anim. Biotechnol.* 16, 183–190 (2005).
37. Lunney, J.K. Advances in swine biomedical model genomics. *Int. J. Biol. Sci.* 3, 179–184 (2007).
38. Suzuki, S., *et al.* Il2rg gene-targeted severe combined immunodeficiency pigs. *Cell Stem Cell* 10, 753–758 (2012).
39. Staunstrup, N.H. *et al.* Development of transgenic cloned pig models of skin inflammation by DNA transposon-directed ectopic expression of human beta1 and alpha 2 integrin. *PLoS ONE* 7, e36658 (2012).
40. Rogers, C.S., *et al.* Disruption of the CFTR gene produces a model of cystic fibrosis in newborn pigs. *Science* 321, 1837–1841 (2008).
41. Roberts, R.M., Telugu, B.P., and Ezashi, T. Induced pluripotent stem cells from swine (*Sus scrofa*): Why they may prove to be important? *Cell Cycle* 8, 3078–3081 (2009).
42. Matsunari, H., and Nagashima, H. Application of genetically modified and cloned pigs in translational research. *J. Reprod. Dev.* 55, 225–230 (2009).
43. Forster, R., Bode, G., Ellegaard, L., and van der Laan, J.W. The 'rethink' project on minipigs in the toxicity testing of new medicines and chemicals: Conclusions and recommendations. *J. Pharmacol. Toxicol. Methods* 62, 236–242 (2010).
44. Gandolfi, F., *et al.* Large animal models for cardiac stem cell therapies. *Theriogenology* 75, 1416–1425 (2011).

45. Hughes, G.C., Post, M.J., Simons, M., and Annex, B.H. Translational physiology: Porcine models of human coronary artery disease: Implications for preclinical trials of therapeutic angiogenesis. *J. Appl. Physiol.* 94, 1689–1701 (2003).

46. Weaver, M.E., Pantely, G.A., Bristow, J.D., and Ladley, H.D. A quantitative study of the anatomy and distribution of coronary arteries in swine in comparison with other animals and man. *Cardiovasc. Res.* 20, 907–917 (1986).

47. Hughes, H.C. Swine in cardiovascular research. *Lab. Anim. Sci.* 36, 348–350 (1986).

48. Abdel-Aleem, S., St Louis, J.D., Hughes, G.C., and Lowe, J.E. Metabolic changes in the normal and hypoxic neonatal myocardium. *Ann. N. Y. Acad. Sci.* 874, 254–261 (1999).

49. van der Spoel, T.I., *et al.* Human relevance of pre-clinical studies in stem cell therapy: Systematic review and meta-analysis of large animal models of ischaemic heart disease. *Cardiovasc. Res.* 91, 649–658 (2011).

50. Poh, K.K., *et al.* Repeated direct endomyocardial transplantation of allogeneic mesenchymal stem cells: Safety of a high dose, "off-the-shelf", cellular cardiomyoplasty strategy. *Int. J. Cardiol.* 117, 360–364 (2007).

51. Hutter, G., *et al.* Long-term control of HIV by CCR5 Delta32/Delta32 stem-cell transplantation. *N. Engl. J. Med.* 360, 692–698 (2009).

52. Trobridge, G.D., *et al.* Protection of stem cell-derived lymphocytes in a primate AIDS gene therapy model after *in vivo* selection. *PLoS ONE* 4, e7693 (2009).

53. Capitanio, J.P., and Emborg, M.E. Contributions of non-human primates to neuroscience research. *Lancet* 371, 1126–1135 (2008).

54. Kriks, S., *et al.* Dopamine neurons derived from human ES cells efficiently engraft in animal models of Parkinson's disease. *Nature* 480, 547–551 (2011).

55. Takagi, Y., *et al.* Dopaminergic neurons generated from monkey embryonic stem cells function in a Parkinson primate model. *J. Clin. Invest.* 115, 102–109 (2005).

56. Guercio, A., *et al.* Production of canine mesenchymal stem cells from adipose tissue and their application in dogs with chronic osteoarthritis of the humero-radial joints. *Cell Biol. Int.* 36, 189–194 (2012).

57. Murphy, J.M., Fink, D.J., Hunziker, E.B., and Barry, F.P. Stem cell therapy in a caprine model of osteoarthritis. *Arthritis Rheum.* 48, 3464–3474 (2003).

58. Grigolo, B., *et al.* Osteoarthritis treated with mesenchymal stem cells on hyaluronan-based scaffold in rabbit. *Tissue Eng. Part C Methods* 15, 647–658 (2009).

59. Vieira, N.M., *et al.* Human adipose-derived mesenchymal stromal cells injected systemically into GRMD dogs without immunosuppression are able to reach the host muscle and express human dystrophin. *Cell Transplant.* 21, 1407–1417 (2012).

60. Gao, P., Ding, Q., Wu, Z., Jiang, H., and Fang, Z. Therapeutic potential of human mesenchymal stem cells producing IL-12 in a mouse xenograft model of renal cell carcinoma. *Cancer Lett.* (2009).

61. You, M.H., *et al.* Cytosine deaminase-producing human mesenchymal stem cells mediate an antitumor effect in a mouse xenograft model. *J. Gastroenterol. Hepatol.* 24, 1393–1400 (2009).

62. Di, G.H., *et al.* Human umbilical cord mesenchymal stromal cells mitigate chemotherapy-associated tissue injury in a pre-clinical mouse model. *Cytotherapy* 14, 412–422 (2012).

63. Prather, W.R., *et al.* The role of placental-derived adherent stromal cell (PLX-PAD) in the treatment of critical limb ischemia. *Cytotherapy* 11, 427–434 (2009).

64. Mardiros, A., *et al.* T cells expressing CD123-specific chimeric antigen receptors exhibit specific cytolytic effector functions and antitumor effects against human acute myeloid leukemia. *Blood* 122, 3138–3148 (2013).

65. Wilkie, S., *et al.* Retargeting of human T cells to tumor-associated MUC1: The evolution of a chimeric antigen receptor. *J. Immunol.* 180, 4901–4909 (2008).

66. van Lunzen, J., *et al.* Transfer of autologous gene-modified T cells in HIV-infected patients with advanced immunodeficiency and drug-resistant virus. *Mol. Ther.* 15, 1024–1033 (2007).

67. Gross, S., and Piwnica-Worms, D. Spying on cancer: Molecular imaging *in vivo* with genetically encoded reporters. *Cancer Cell* 7, 5–15 (2005).

68. Stegman, L.D., *et al.* Non-invasive quantitation of cytosine deaminase transgene expression in human tumor xenografts with *in vivo* magnetic resonance spectroscopy. *Proc. Natl. Acad. Sci. U.S.A.* 96, 9821–9826 (1999).

69. Morin, K.W., *et al.* Cytotoxicity and cellular uptake of pyrimidine nucleosides for imaging herpes simplex type-1 thymidine kinase (HSV-1 TK) expression in mammalian cells. *Nucl. Med. Biol.* 31, 623–630 (2004).

70. Bulte, J.W., and Kraitchman, D.L. Monitoring cell therapy using iron oxide MR contrast agents. *Curr. Pharm. Biotechnol.* 5, 567–584 (2004).

71. Guideline on repeated dose toxicity. (ed. Agency, E.M.) (2010).

72. Note for Guidance on Repeated Dose Toxicity. In *CPMP/SWP/1042/99 corr.* (ed. Agency, E.M.) (2000).

73. Shih, C.C., Forman, S.J., Chu, P., and Slovak, M. Human embryonic stem cells are prone to generate primitive, undifferentiated tumors in engrafted human fetal tissues in severe combined immunodeficient mice. *Stem Cells Dev.* 16, 893–902 (2007).

74. Jeong, J.O., *et al.* Malignant tumor formation after transplantation of short-term cultured bone marrow mesenchymal stem cells in experimental myocardial infarction and diabetic neuropathy. *Circul. Res.* 108, 1340–1347 (2011).

75. Tolar, J., *et al.* Sarcoma derived from cultured mesenchymal stem cells. *Stem Cells* 25, 371–379 (2007).

76. Garcia, S., *et al.* Pitfalls in spontaneous *in vitro* transformation of human mesenchymal stem cells. *Exp. Cell Res.* 316, 1648–1650.

77. Ben-David, U., and Benvenisty, N. The tumorigenicity of human embryonic and induced pluripotent stem cells. *Nat. Rev. Cancer* 11, 268–277 (2011).

78. Stein, S., *et al.* Genomic instability and myelodysplasia with monosomy 7 consequent to EVI1 activation after gene therapy for chronic granulomatous disease. *Nat. Med.* 16, 198–204 (2010).

79. Hacein-Bey-Abina, S., *et al.* Insertional oncogenesis in 4 patients after retrovirus-mediated gene therapy of SCID-X1. *J. Clin. Invest.* 118, 3132–3142 (2008).

80. Braun, C.J., *et al.* Gene therapy for Wiskott-Aldrich syndrome — long-term efficacy and genotoxicity. *Sci. Transl. Med.* 6, 227–233 (2014).

81. Kanemura, H., *et al.* Tumorigenicity studies of induced pluripotent stem cell (iPSC)-derived retinal pigment epithelium (RPE) for the treatment of age-related macular degeneration. *PLoS ONE* 9, e85336 (2014).

82. Kuroda, T., Yasuda, S., and Sato, Y. Tumorigenicity studies for human pluripotent stem cell-derived products. *Biol. Pharm. Bull.* 36, 189–192 (2013).

83. Aiuti, A., *et al.* The committee for advanced therapies of the European Medicines Agency: Reflection paper on management of clinical risks deriving from insertional mutagenesis. *Hum. Gene Ther. Clin. Dev.* 24, 47–54 (2013).
84. Reflection paper on stem cell-based medicinal products. (ed. Agency, E.M.) (2010).
85. Guidance for Industry Estimating the Maximum Safe Starting Dose in Initial Clinical Trials for Therapeutics in Adult Healthy Volunteers. (ed. Administration, F.a.D.) (2005).

Quality Management **4**

Andrea Hauser and Christoph Peter

4.1 Introduction

'The holder of a Manufacturing Authorization must manufacture medicinal products so as to ensure that they are fit for their intended use, comply with the requirements of the Marketing Authorization or Clinical Trial Authorization, as appropriate and do not place patients at risk due to inadequate safety, quality or efficacy. [. . .]. To achieve this quality objective reliably, there must be a comprehensively designed and correctly implemented Pharmaceutical Quality System incorporating Good Manufacturing Practice and Quality Risk Management' [EU GMP Guidelines].[1]

Medicinal products are very special goods and their quality is essential to assure patient safety and product efficacy. To achieve this goal, the principles of GMP were developed decades ago. These are compulsory guidelines for the manufacture of medicinal products in almost all countries around the world. Depending on the country or the region, GMP regulations or guidelines might slightly differ but in general they are comparable. Big industrial nations like the USA, Japan, Canada and Australia have all developed their own GMP rules. In Europe, the European Union (EU) Guidelines to GMP have been implemented to harmonize the requirements in all European member states and members of the European Economic Area (EEA). Apart from special GMP guidelines of certain countries or regions, the World Health Organization (WHO) publishes a version of GMP[2] that is used by pharmaceutical regulators and pharmaceutical industries in countries that have not developed their own guidelines. They are used primarily in the developing countries. For further details on GMP principles, see Section 4.2.

But GMP is only a part of the overall quality measures that have to be established and implemented for the manufacture of medicinal products. A more comprehensive system among the following is required: Quality Management (QM), Quality Assurance (QA) or Pharmaceutical Quality System (PQS). None of these terms is officially defined and often they are used interchangeably. Sometimes QA is interpreted as the system with the more narrow focus on the actual manufacturing process and the quality tools directly related to it, whereas QM is interpreted as the system with a wider view on the collectivity of all quality tools. The term PQS is used in the EU GMP Guidelines in order to achieve consistency with the International Conference on Harmonisation (ICH) Q10 terminology.[1,3] But other European regulatory documents such as, Directive 2003/94/EC, laying down the principles and guidelines of GMP,[4] use the term Quality Assurance System (QAS). Therefore, both terms can indeed be considered interchangeable.

Quality and QM are of course not restricted to medicinal products and pharmaceutical industry. High and reliable quality standards are equally important in other industrial branches, as for example, airline or aviation industry to assure the safety of crew and passengers. The same holds true for motor vehicles. QM, meanwhile, is common in many different sectors of industries and companies, regardless of their field of activity. The priority objective, thereby need not always be patient or customer safety. Other goals can be more business related as QM can also reduce costs by minimizing errors, lowering return rates and increasing productivity.

Outside pharmaceutical industry, very often QM is established according to ISO standards. ISO is the short term for the International Organization for Standardization, a non-governmental membership organization that develops voluntary international standards. ISO 9001: 2008[5] for example, sets out the criteria for a quality management system (QMS) and is a standard that can be certified to. It can be implemented in any company regardless of its size or field of action. Companies that operate internationally often use the ISO 9001 standard (in many cases together with the corresponding ISO certification), to demonstrate to customers and partners that an internationally known and widely accepted quality standard is implemented. Also various pharmaceutical manufacturers therefore implement the ISO standards in their company along with the GMP principles, although this would not be required to achieve a manufacturing license. Further details on ISO standards and certification are provided on the organization's web page (http://www.iso.org).

4.2　Principles of GMP

In Europe Commission Directive 2003/94/EC laying down the principles and guidelines of GMP in respect to medicinal products and investigational medicinal products (IMPs) for human use[4] mandates that all medicinal products including IMPs (even in early stages of clinical trials) have to be manufactured in accordance with the GMP principles and guidelines. Detailed guidelines in accordance with those principles are published in the Guide to GMP[6] which is regularly revised in order to reflect continual improvement. Drafts of new versions as well as revisions of existing chapters and annexes are made publicly available on the website of the EC (http://ec.europa.eu/health/documents/eudralex/vol-4/index_en.htm). The European GMP Guidelines serve competent authorities as a basis for inspection of pharmaceutical manufacturers and are used for the assessment of applications for manufacturing authorizations. The EU GMP Guidelines consist of three parts: Part I covers GMP principles for the manufacture of medicinal products; Part II covers GMP for active substances used as starting materials; Part III contains GMP related documents, which clarify regulatory expectations. Annexes to Part I reflect additional requirements for specific kinds of medicinal products (e.g., Annex 2 on the manufacture of biological medicinal products including cell-based medicinal products[7] or Annex 13 on the manufacture of IMPs).[8] In addition to the EU GMP Guidelines, the EC publishes EU directives that are primarily not binding on the individual EU or EEA member states but have to be implemented in national law within a certain time period. The European Medicines Agency (EMA), central authority for the approval of certain medicinal products (e.g., biological and cell-based medicinal products), publishes supplementary and explanatory guidelines that define requirements for MA.

　　In the United States, the Federal Food, Drug, and Cosmetic Act (FD&C Act) is a set of laws that is binding for the manufacture of food, drugs and cosmetics and gives authority to the U.S. Food and Drug Administration (FDA) to supervise the safety of these products. The FD&C Act defines certain standards known as current Good Manufacturing Practices (cGMPs) which must be complied by the manufacturers. In addition, the Code of Federal Regulations (CFR), a compilation of general and permanent rules and regulations, defines in title 21, parts 210 and 211, the regulations that govern food and drugs in the US. They are very similar to the European GMP Guidelines. 21 CFR 210/211 is also the basis for the inspections of the US FDA.

As already mentioned in the introduction, the principles of GMP have to be implemented together with an overarching PQS, in order to consistently manufacture high quality medicinal product batches (that is, batch to batch consistency). This assures efficacy of the product as well as product and patient safety. The GMP regulations, as for any type of medicinal product, also apply to cell-based medicinal products, at least as far as advanced therapies are concerned. In most countries, blood products, tissues and cells with non-significant manipulations are not considered as medicinal products and therefore do not have to be manufactured as per the GMP principles. In cases of doubt, it is important to discuss with the competent authority how a specific product is classified. In Europe, the EMA deals with such requests.

The key determinant for the quality of a medicinal product batch is of course the manufacturing process. The actual quality of a single product batch is determined by QC, but it is one of the central statements of GMP that quality must be built into the design process and cannot be achieved only by testing. This means that the manufacturing process must be properly designed, developed, and validated that it reproducibly achieves the quality specifications that are laid down in the MA or CTA and that QC is just a measure to confirm that. Nevertheless QC methods need to be equally well designed, developed, and validated in order to achieve reliable test results. But implementation and initial validation are not sufficient. Continuous QM is necessary to maintain the high standards. This task is fulfilled by the various tools of QM that are depicted in Figure 4.1.

The illustration depicts all essential parts of a QMS that follows the GMP principles as defined by the EU GMP Guidelines. The core process (dark grey) are production & QC together with product release and subsequent sale, supply or export. Around this core process the various QM tools have to be implemented in order to control each individual step as thoroughly as possible and in order to deal with deviations, non-conformances and complaints, whenever necessary.

In the following sections, we describe the key QM tools and further requirements together with necessary documents in more detail. However, this chapter can only provide an overview as each of the different GMP and QM requirements needs detailed implementation considering the specificities of the company or center, where they shall be used. We therefore recommend further reading of specialized literature on QM and GMP, since the basic principles are identical for all different kinds of products including cell-based medicinal products. The GMP MANUAL,[9] for example, is a comprehensive database that combines theory and practice of GMP and provides valuable hints and information for implementation. In a supplement to this chapter (see Section 4.10), we furthermore provide a list of required documents that have to be implemented in a Pharmaceutical Quality (PQ) or QMS to receive a manufacturing license from the competent authority.

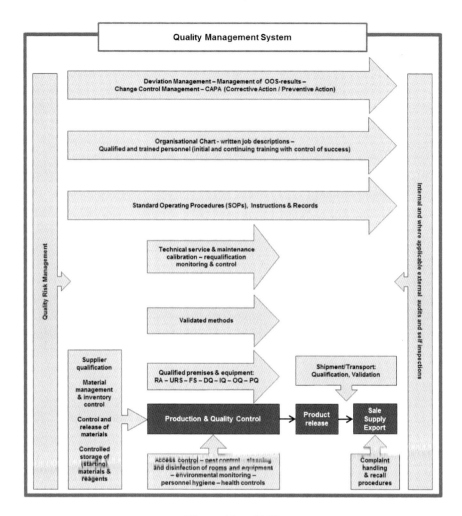

Figure 4.1: QMS.

Note: DQ: Design Qualification; FS: Functional Specification: IQ: Installation Qualification; OQ: Operational Qualification; PQ: Performance Qualification; QC: Quality Control; RA: Risk Analysis; SOP: Standard Operating Procedure; URS; User Requirement Specification.

The content of the following sections as well as the list of documents provided in the supplement are based on the requirements of the EU GMP Guidelines, but as GMP guidelines of different origin generally are quite comparable, the information should be equally valid in other parts of the world.

4.3 Pharmaceutical Quality System (PQS)

4.3.1 *Quality manual*

The Quality Manual is a compulsory document for each PQS. Chapter 1 of the EU GMP Guidelines[1] demands: '*The Pharmaceutical Quality System should be defined and documented. A Quality Manual or equivalent documentation should be established and should contain a description of the QMS including management responsibilities.*'

The Quality Manual usually describes basic elements of the Quality System and lays down the overall quality strategy of the company. The Quality Manual must be authorized by the senior management as '*senior management has the ultimate responsibility to ensure that an effective PQS is in place, adequately resourced and that roles, responsibilities, and authorities are defined, communicated and implemented throughout the organization*'.[1] As only the senior management is able to provide necessary human and financial resources, its active participation in the PQS is essential, even though Head of Production, Head of QC and Qualified Person (QP) are the key personnel for manufacturing and finished product batch release of a medicinal product and thus responsible for overall GMP compliance. The senior management on the other hand must establish a quality policy that describes the overall intentions and directions related to quality and this should be reflected in the Quality Manual (also compare Chapter 2 of the EU GMP Guidelines on personnel).[10]

Many QMSs are designed in different levels with the Quality Manual reflecting the first level or head document, standard operating procedures (SOPs) reflecting the second level and detailed work instructions for specific production or QC operations reflecting the third level. It is important to know that the Quality Manual has a mere describing character whereas SOPs and work instructions are of regulative nature. Different levels or layers of documents are not requested by the GMP guidelines but might be useful dependent on the overall design of the Quality System. In some QMSs, apart from the Quality Manual, a separate Quality Policy is established which then forms the first level of documents and describes in detail the actions that have to be taken and measures that are established to achieve the required level of quality.

Apart from authorization of the Quality Manual, the senior management should further be involved in the operation of the PQS to identify opportunities for continual improvement of products, processes and the system itself. This is implemented by preparation of periodic management reviews that have to be authorized by the senior management, too.

Table 4.1: SMF.

Chapter		Details
1. General Information of the Manufacturer	1.1. Contact information of the manufacturer	— Name and official address of the manufacturer. — Names and street addresses of the site, buildings and production units located on the site. — Contact information of the manufacturer including 24 hrs telephone number of the contact personnel in the case of product defects or recalls. — Identification number of the site, e.g., GPS details, or any other geographic location system, D-U-N-S (Data Universal Numbering System) Number (a unique identification number provided by Dun & Bradstreet) of the site.
	1.2. Authorized pharmaceutical manufacturing activities of the site	— Copy of the valid manufacturing authorization issued by the relevant Competent Authority in Appendix 1; or when applicable, reference to the EudraGMP database. If the Competent Authority does not issue manufacturing authorizations, this should be stated. — Brief description of manufacture, import, export, distribution and other activities as authorized by the relevant Competent Authorities including foreign authorities with authorized dosage forms/activities, respectively; where not covered by the manufacturing authorization. — Type of products currently manufactured on-site (list in Appendix 2); where not covered by Appendix 1 or EudraGMP entry.

(*Continued*)

Table 4.1: (*Continued*).

Chapter		Details
		— List of GMP inspections of the site within the last five years; including dates and name/country of the Competent Authority having performed the inspection. A copy of current GMP certificate (Appendix 3) or reference to the EudraGMP database, should be included, if available.
	1.3. Any other manufacturing activities carried out on the site	Description of non-pharmaceutical activities on-site, if any.
2. QMS of the Manufacturer	2.1. The QMS of the manufacturer	— Brief description of the QMS run by the company and reference to the standards used. — Responsibilities related to the maintaining of quality system including the senior management. — Information of activities for which the site is accredited and certified, including dates and contents of accreditations, names of accrediting bodies.
	2.2. Release procedure of finished products	— Detailed description of qualification requirements (education and work experience) of the Authorized Person(s) [AP(s)] / [QP(s)] responsible for batch certification and releasing procedures. — General description of batch certification and releasing procedure. — Role of AP/QP in quarantine and release of finished products and in assessment of compliance with the MA. — The arrangements between APs/QPs when several APs/QPs are involved.

(*Continued*)

Table 4.1: (*Continued*).

Chapter	Details
	— Statement on whether the control strategy employs Process Analytical Technology (PAT) and/or Real Time Release or Parametric Release.
2.3. Management of suppliers and contractors	— A brief summary of the establishment/knowledge of supply chain and the external audit program.
	— Brief description of the qualification system of contractors, manufacturers of active pharmaceutical ingredients (APIs) and other critical materials suppliers.
	— Measures taken to ensure that products manufactured are compliant with TSE (Transmitting animal spongiform encephalopathy) guidelines.
	— Measures adopted where counterfeit/falsified products, bulk products (i.e., unpacked tablets), APIs or excipients are suspected or identified.
	— Use of outside scientific, analytical or other technical assistance in relation to manufacture and analysis.
	— List of contract manufacturers and laboratories including the addresses and contact information and flow charts of supply-chains for outsourced manufacturing and QC activities; e.g., sterilization of primary packaging material for aseptic processes, testing of starting raw-materials etc., should be presented in Appendix 4.
	— Brief overview of the responsibility sharing between the contract giver and acceptor with respect to compliance with the MA (where not included under 2.2).

(*Continued*)

Table 4.1: (*Continued*).

Chapter		Details
	2.4. QRM	— Brief description of QRM methodologies used by the manufacturer. — Scope and focus of QRM including brief description of any activities which are performed at corporate level, and those which are performed locally. Any application of the QRM system to assess continuity of supply should be mentioned.
	2.5. Product Quality Reviews (PQRs)	Brief description of methodologies used.
3. Person-nel	—	— Organization chart showing the arrangements for QM, production and QC positions/titles in Appendix 5, including the senior management and QP(s). — Number of employees engaged in the QM, production, QC, storage and distribution, respectively.
4. Premise and Equip-ment	4.1. Premises	— Short description of plant, size of the site and list of buildings. If the production for different markets, i.e., for local, EU, USA, etc. takes place in different buildings on the site, the buildings should be listed with destined markets identified (if not identified under 1.1). — Simple plan or description of manufacturing areas with indication of scale (architectural or engineering drawings are not required). — Lay outs and flow charts of the production areas (in Appendix 6) showing the room classification and pressure differentials between adjoining areas and indicating the production activities (i.e., compounding, filling, storage, packaging, etc.) in the rooms. — Lay outs of warehouses and storage areas, with special areas for the storage and handling of highly toxic, hazardous and sensitizing materials indicated, if applicable.

(*Continued*)

Table 4.1: *(Continued)*.

Chapter	Details
	— Brief description of specific storage conditions if applicable, but not indicated on the lay outs.
	1. Brief description of heating, ventilation and air-conditioning (HVAC) systems: Principles for defining the air supply, temperature, humidity, pressure differentials, and air change rates, policy of air recirculation (%).
	2. Brief description of water systems.
	— Quality references of water produced.
	— Schematic drawings of the systems in Appendix 7.
	4.1.3. Brief description of other relevant utilities, such as steam, compressed air, nitrogen, etc.
4.2. Equipment	1. Listing of major production and control laboratory equipment with critical pieces of equipment identified should be provided in Appendix 8.
	2. Cleaning and sanitation: Brief description of cleaning and sanitation methods of product contact surfaces (i.e., manual cleaning, automatic Clean-in-Place, etc.).
	3. GMP critical computerized systems: Description of GMP critical computerized systems (excluding equipment specific Programmable Logic Controllers (PLCs).
5. Documentation	— Description of documentation system (i.e., electronic, manual).
	— When documents and records are stored or archived off-site (including pharmacovigilance data, when applicable): List of types of documents/records; Name and address of storage site and an estimate of time required retrieving documents from the off-site archive.

(Continued)

Table 4.1: (*Continued*).

Chapter		Details
6. Production	6.1. Type of products (References to Appendix 1 or 2 can be made)	— Type of products manufactured including • List of dosage forms of both human and veterinary products which are manufactured on the site. • List of dosage forms of IMPs manufactured for any clinical trial on the site, and when different from the commercial manufacturing, information of production areas and personnel. — Toxic or hazardous substances handled (e.g., with high pharmacological activity and/or with sensitizing properties). — Product types manufactured in a dedicated facility or on a campaign basis, if applicable. — Process Analytical Technology (PAT) applications, if applicable: general statement of the relevant technology, and associated computerized systems.
	6.2. Process validation	— Brief description of general policy for process validation. — Policy for reprocessing or reworking.
	6.3. Material management and warehousing	— Arrangements for the handling of starting materials, packaging materials, bulk and finished products including sampling, quarantine, release, and storage. — Arrangements for the handling of rejected materials and products.
7. QC	—	Description of the QC activities carried out on the site in terms of physical, chemical, microbiological, and biological testing.

(*Continued*)

Table 4.1: *(Continued).*

Chapter		Details
8. Distribution, Complaints, Product Defects & Recalls	8.1. Distribution (to the part under the responsibility of the manufacturer)	— Types (wholesale license holders, manufacturing license holders, etc.) and locations (EU/EEA, USA, etc.) of the companies to which the products are shipped from the site. — Description of the system used to verify that each customer/recipient is legally entitled to receive medicinal products from the manufacturer. — Brief description of the system to ensure appropriate environmental conditions during transit, e.g., temperature monitoring/control. — Arrangements for product distribution and methods by which product traceability is maintained. — Measures taken to prevent manufacturers' products to fall in the illegal supply chain.
	8.2. Complaints, product defects and recalls	Brief description of the system for handling complaints, product defects and recalls.
9. Self-inspections	—	Short description of the self inspection system with focus on criteria used for selection of the areas to be covered during planned inspections, practical arrangements and follow-up activities.

Note: Required information for the preparation of a SMF as defined in Part III of the EU GMP Guidelines.[12]

4.3.2 *Site master file (SMF)*

The SMF is a compulsory document for all pharmaceutical manufacturers, since the revised Chapter 4 of the EU GMP Guidelines was implemented in 2011.[11] Part III of the EU GMP Guidelines "GMP-related documents" provides detailed information on the required content of a SMF.[12]

    The SMF reflects a kind of dossier that is thought to present a pharmaceutical manufacturer to external partners and authorities (in contrast to the above mentioned Quality Manual that is an internal document). The SMF should contain specific information about the QM policies and activities of a specific site, the production and/or QC operations and any closely integrated operations at adjacent and nearby buildings. It is furthermore the basis for authorities to prepare for a GMP inspection and therefore should be updated regularly. Table 4.1 summarizes the requirements for the preparation of a SMF as laid down in Part III of the EU GMP Guidelines.[12]

4.3.3 *Quality Risk Management (QRM)*

QRM is one of the key elements of QM. Details are provided in part III of the EU GMP Guidelines,[12] where the ICH guideline Q9 on QRM[13] has been implemented. Since processes as well as systems, instruments, and equipments are highly complex in pharmaceutical industry, it is essential to identify potential risks and to evaluate their influence on the corresponding process and/or product. For risks that have been identified, mechanisms of control can be implemented to reduce the probability of occurrence or to increase the likelihood of discovery.

Risk management process usually contains the following elements:

⇨ Risk assessment.
⇨ Risk control.
⇨ Risk review.

Figure 4.2 provides an overview of a typical QRM process as defined in ICH guideline Q9 "Quality Risk Management".[13]

For the preparation of a risk analysis, several risk management facilitation methods do exist with a slightly different approach. The GMP Guidelines do not request to use a special type of method. The most well-known is the FMEA (Failure Mode Effects Analysis) which is primarily used throughout pharmaceutical industry. Several varieties of the classic FMEA do exist that might be advantageous under certain circumstances. Other examples are the FTA (Fault Tree Analysis) or the HACCP (Hazard Analysis and Critical Control Points). ICH Q9 provides further details and potential areas of use for each individual method.

As QRM is such an important tool, its principles have to be implemented and considered for various operations and activities. Examples are:

⇨ QM (e.g., for the evaluation of quality defects or for execution of change control procedures).
⇨ Facility, equipment and utilities (e.g., for the design of facilities and equipment, for qualification or for definition of preventive maintenance activities).

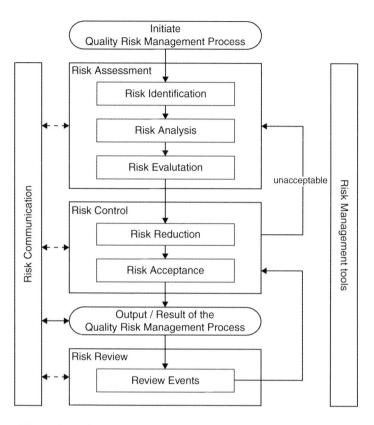

Figure 4.2: Overview of a typical QRM process as defined in ICH Q9.

↪ Materials management (e.g., for assessment and evaluation of suppliers and contract manufacturers).

↪ Production (e.g., for process validation or in-process testing).

↪ Laboratory control and stability testing [e.g., for evaluation of Out-of-Specification (OOS) results].

The so called risk-based approach offers the opportunity to adapt the GMP and regulatory framework, if it is required and justified by a detailed risk analysis. However, this does not obviate the obligation to comply with regulatory requirements. But effective QRM can facilitate better and more informed decisions and can provide regulators with greater assurance of a company's ability to deal with potential risks.[13]

4.3.4 *Deviation management*

During manufacturing, QC or QM operations deviations from the predefined procedures can occur. The reason for these deviations can be manifold. There could be operator mistakes, failures of equipment, and errors in (computerized) systems or force majeure. In these cases, it is important to first document the deviation in detail and then evaluate its potential influence on product quality. To achieve this, a comprehensive system of deviation management has to be implemented. Details of the system and individual steps that have to be taken must be described in a written procedure.

Deviation management should contain at least the following elements:

⇨ Detailed documentation of the deviation.
⇨ If applicable, immediate actions to reduce or eliminate the influence of the deviation on product quality. These actions have to be documented by the operator who performed them.
⇨ Notification of authorised persons (APs) (e.g., head of production, head of QC).
⇨ Root cause analysis and further investigation of the deviation.
⇨ If applicable, definition and execution of appropriate corrective and preventive actions. (See also Section 4.3.6 on CAPA management).
⇨ Classification of the deviation's influence on product quality.
⇨ Final evaluation and conclusion.

If corrective and/or preventive actions have been defined they have to be followed-up closely. It is important to make the QP aware of any kind of deviation, as she/he has to certify the product batch and thus needs to evaluate the deviation's influence on product quality in this respect. For further details, see Chapter 8 on product release.

OOS results are a special kind of deviation. They belong to QC and are therefore described in detail in Chapter 6 on QC.

4.3.5 *Change control management*

'*Change Control: A formal system by which qualified representatives of appropriate disciplines review proposed or actual changes that might affect a validated status of facilities, systems, equipment or processes. The intent is to determine the need for action that would ensure that the system is maintained in a validated state*'. [EU GMP Guidelines, Annex 15].[14]

Changes are usually planned actions (in contrast to deviations that occur unplanned). The reason for a change is commonly the potential for improvement of a certain process, procedure or product. As any change might impact on product quality, it is mandatory that changes are thoroughly evaluated before they are implemented. A comprehensive Change Control Management is necessary to achieve this goal. Required steps have to be defined and described in a written procedure.

The first step of a change control procedure is the change request. It should be possible for everyone in the company to file such an application. In a second step, a team of responsible persons has to evaluate the change request. In contrast to deviation management where it might be sufficient that only the head of the affected department evaluates the deviation, for change control procedures this evaluation should be facilitated by a group of people (change control team) that represents different departments of the company. This is necessary to reveal possible influences and impacts on product quality and to define required follow-up actions as thoroughly as possible. Change requests of course need not be accepted. The change control team can refuse applications if they are considered to negatively affect product quality or if the potential for improvement is not big enough or uncertain. If a change request is accepted then follow-up activities have to be defined. It has to be considered if SOPs, work instructions, protocols or plans have to be changed, if an amendment of the MA or CTA is necessary, if contract givers or contract acceptors have to be informed and asked for approval or if requalification, revalidation or calibration activities are required. As changes can also turn out to be disadvantageous, it is necessary that their influence is followed-up after implementation. This can be done with the help of the annual product quality review.

For cell-based medicinal products, changes of the manufacturing process are quite common, particularly for IMPs, as starting material as well as the manufacturing process itself underlies much higher varieties than is the case for conventional medicinal products. In addition, the possible impact of a change might be much more difficult to evaluate.

4.3.6 *Corrective action/preventive action (CAPA)*

'*A systematic approach that includes actions needed to correct (correction), prevent recurrence (corrective action), and eliminate the cause of potential non-conforming product and other quality problems (preventive action)*'.[29]

Deviations, non-conformances, negative findings or unexpected results do occur even if QM is implemented thoroughly. In these cases, it is important that immediate action is taken (if appropriate) and that CAPA is defined. Therefore, individual steps of a CAPA management have to be defined in a written procedure and implemented along with other QM tools.

Initiation of a CAPA procedure might be required because of one of the following flashpoints:

⇨ Deviations.
⇨ Complaints.
⇨ OOS results.
⇨ Negative trends.
⇨ Findings in self inspections.
⇨ Findings in audits or inspections.
⇨ Findings in supplier qualifications.
⇨ Findings, deviations or unexpected results in qualification, validation, calibration or maintenance activities.

In the first step of a CAPA procedure the potential impact of the deviation, non-conformance or negative trend on product quality has to be evaluated with a formal risk assessment. It is important to define if immediate actions have to be taken. In a second step, a root cause analysis has to be performed to identify the reason or source. This is the basis for the definition of reasonable and effective actions to correct the occurred error, fault or defect and/or to prevent their reoccurrence or the reoccurrence of related errors, faults or defects. The defined measures have to be followed up and their effectiveness has to be evaluated after implementation. All steps of a CAPA procedure have to be documented thoroughly and a report on the results is required.

4.3.7 *Product Quality Review (PQR)*

The (annual) PQR is an important and useful tool '*with the objective of verifying the consistency of the existing process, the appropriateness of current specifications for both the starting materials and the finished product, to highlight any trends and to identify product and process improvements*'.[1]

Actually PQRs are only mandatory for authorized medicinal products, but a similar kind of annual report might also be useful for IMPs, since only the synopsis of different batches produced over a longer time period might reveal trends and the necessity for improvements.

Chapter 1 of the EU GMP Guidelines[1] defines the minimal requirements for a PQR. According to Chapter 1, it should contain at least the following issues:

1. A review of starting materials including packaging materials used in the product, especially those from new sources and in particular the review of supply chain traceability of active substances.

2. A review of critical in-process controls and finished product results.

3. A review of all batches that failed to meet established specification(s) and their investigation.

4. A review of all significant deviations or non-conformances, their related investigations, and the effectiveness of resultant corrective and preventive actions taken.

5. A review of all changes carried out in the processes or the analytical methods.

6. A review of MA variations: Submitted, granted or refused, including those for third country (export only) dossiers.

7. A review of the results of the stability monitoring program and any adverse trend.

8. A review of all quality-related returns, complaints and recalls, and the investigations performed at the time.

9. A review of adequacy of any other previous product process or equipment corrective actions.

10. For new MAs and variations to MAs, a review of post-marketing commitments.

11. The qualification status of relevant equipments and utilities, e.g., HVAC, water, compressed gases, etc.

12. A review of any contractual arrangements as defined in Chapter 7 [*Note*: Chapter 7 of the EU GMP Guidelines on Outsourced Activities],[16] to ensure that they are up to date.

The pharmaceutical manufacturer and, where different, the MA holder have to evaluate the results of the review. It has to be concluded whether any corrective and preventive action has to be initiated or any revalidation is required.

4.4 Personnel

4.4.1 *Human resources, organization, and responsibilities*

As quality always relies upon people, one key issue of the GMP Guidelines (apart from training; see subsequent Section 4.4.2) is the definition and delineation of responsibilities. Requirements are defined in Chapter 2 of the EU GMP Guidelines "Personnel".[10] An organization chart that depicts at least the key personnel is one of the compulsory documents defined there. Authorities usually request that the organization chart is authorized by senior management, since it is senior management's ultimate responsibility to ensure that roles, responsibilities, and authorities are defined, communicated and implemented throughout the organization. But not only key personnel are important, individual responsibilities should be clearly understood by anybody who's job might directly or indirectly impact on any aspect of quality of the medicinal products that are manufactured.

The European GMP Guidelines request three key functions for the manufacture of medicinal products: Head of Production, Head of QC and QP. A Head of QA or Quality Unit is mentioned in Chapter 2 of the EU GMP Guidelines,[10] but this position is not mandatory. It is important that Head of Production and Head of QC are independent from each other, while it is possible that the QP acts simultaneously as either Head of Production or Head of QC. Smaller companies or academic centers might have difficulties in filling these jobs, at least in a case of absence of the actual job owner. Apart from the two head positions in production and QC, it is also important that there are no unexplained overlaps in the staff of both departments and that both are operating independently. The reason for this is, of course, that one and the same person may not check what she/he has produced. Generally, it is requested that the organization chart clearly shows the relationships between the Heads of Production, QC and QA (where applicable) and the position of the QP(s) in managerial hierarchy.

In addition to an organization chart, it is required that specific duties of people in responsible positions are recorded in 'written job descriptions'. Job descriptions must clearly define the rights and duties of the individual job owner and assign adequate authority to the job owner so that she/he can carry out her/his responsibilities. 'Written job descriptions' have to be signed by the job owner (and a deputy, if applicable) as well as by the senior management.

4.4.2 *Training*

Well-trained and qualified personnel are a key requirement for GMP compliant manufacturing. Initial and ongoing training is therefore mandatory for everybody whose operations might directly or indirectly impact on product quality. This includes cleaning personnel as well as technical staff.

Training objectives are:

⇨ To acquire new knowledge and skills, either to train new personnel or to extend the range of processes of existing personnel.
⇨ To maintain present knowledge.
⇨ To standardize processes between individual operators or different sites.
⇨ To update knowledge and skills of operators to the state of the art.

Several training methods do exist. Examples are:

⇨ Reading of SOPs.
⇨ Hands-on training of processes or analytical methods.
⇨ Class room training.
⇨ E-Learning.

Training objectives as well as training methods have to be described in a written procedure. Annual training programs are requested by the authorities. These training programs have to be followed up and individual trainings need to be documented.

During recent years, regulators pay more and more attention not only to the training itself, but also to the evaluation of training effectiveness. Trained personnel have to prove that the training was successful and that relevant information has been understood or technical skills have been acquired. There are various possibilities for the evaluation of training effectiveness such as written multiple choice tests, oral questioning or practical performance tests (e.g., gowning qualification for clean room operators). It might be reasonable to use different methods in parallel, as depending on the type of training, one or another method might be advantageous.

4.5 Documentation

4.5.1 *Required GMP documentation*

'*Good documentation constitutes an essential part of the Quality Assurance System and is the key for operating in compliance with GMP requirements*'. This quotation is derived from Chapter 4 of the EU GMP Guidelines[11] that deals with all different requirements on documentation in the GMP surrounding. The following types of documents are defined.

⇨ **SMF**.
⇨ **Instructions** (directions or requirements).
⇨ **Records and reports**.

All three types of documents have to be implemented in one or another way in the QMS of a pharmaceutical manufacturer. In Table 4.2, we provide further details on different sub-types, together with definitions and examples.

All documents must have unambiguous contents. SOPs and work instructions have to be written in an imperative mandatory style. They should not contain formulations as "use for example, instrument xy", "add approximately xy ml" or "use suitable equipment".

Table 4.2: Required types of GMP documentation.

Document Type	Document Sub-Type	Definition and Further Details
SMF	n/a	The SMF is a document that describes the GMP related activities of the manufacturer. Details are provided in Part III of the EU GMP Guidelines[12] and in section 4.3.2 of this chapter "Site Master File".
Instructions, Directions or Requirements	Specifications	*'Specifications describe in detail the requirements with which the products or materials used or obtained during manufacture have to conform. They serve as a basis for quality evaluation'.*[11] Specifications for starting and packaging material, intermediate and bulk products and the finished products are defined in the MA or CTA. These specifications (and additional specifications, if applicable) have to be implemented in the PQS [e.g., in testing or processing instructions or the Certificate of Analysis (CoA)]. The Product Specification File (PSF) as defined in Annex 13 to the EU GMP Guidelines[8] *'is a special reference file containing, or referring to files containing, all the information necessary to draft the detailed written instructions on processing, packaging, QC testing, batch release and shipping of an investigational medicinal product'.* The PSF is often the key document for written agreements with contract manufacturers.
	Manufacturing Formulae, Processing, Packaging and Testing Instructions	These documents *'provide details of all the starting materials, equipments and computerized systems (if any) to be used and specify all processing, packaging, sampling and testing instructions. In-process controls and process analytical technologies to be employed should be specified where relevant, together with acceptance criteria'.*[11]

(Continued)

Table 4.2: (*Continued*).

Document Type	Document Sub-Type	Definition and Further Details
		Prime examples are processing and testing instructions that form the basis for all manufacturing and QC operations. They must be in line with the definitions and specifications, as laid down in the MA or CTA and the PSF (where relevant). In contrast to the MA or CTA, these documents have to be much more detailed, as they must enable the relevant personnel to perform the described operations correctly.
	Procedures (SOPs)	'*Procedures (otherwise known as Standard Operating Procedures, or SOPs), give directions for performing certain operations*'.[11]
		As the name implies, SOPs describe standard procedures such as the general handling of basic QA tools (e.g., change control and deviation management, or handling of complaints). Specific procedures such as manufacturing and testing operations are usually not described in SOPs, but in instructions.
	Protocols	'*Give instructions for performing and recording certain discreet operations*'.[11]
		The term protocol is also used for a document that describes the objective(s), design, methodology, statistical considerations and organization of a clinical trial.[17]
	Technical Agreements	'*Are agreed between contract givers and acceptors for outsourced activities*'.[11]
		Chapter 7 of the EU GMP Guidelines on Outsourced Activities,[16] as well as Section 4.6 of this chapter provide more details on outsourced activities in general, and requirements for technical agreements and written contracts.

(*Continued*)

Table 4.2: (*Continued*).

Document Type	Document Sub-Type	Definition and Further Details
Records and reports	Records (including raw data)	'*Provide evidence of various actions taken to demonstrate compliance with instructions, e.g., activities, events, investigations, and in the case of manufactured batches, a history of each batch of product, including its distribution. Records include the raw data which is used to generate other records. For electronic records, regulated users should define which data are to be used as raw data. At least, all data on which quality decisions are based should be defined as raw data*'.[11] Prime example of a record is the batch record that usually consists of numerous different documents from production and QC. Batch Record Review is one of the prerequisites for the QP for certification and finished product batch release (further details are provided in Chapter 8 on Product Release). Summaries of records are usually termed reviews. One example is the PQR (compare Section 4.3.7 of this chapter). Logbooks should be kept to record in chronological order, e.g., calibrations, maintenance, cleaning or repair operations for major or critical analytical testing and production equipments, and areas where product is processed.
	Certificate of Analysis (CoA)	'*CoAs provide a summary of testing results on samples of products or materials together with the evaluation for compliance to a stated specification*'.[11] CoAs are either provided by suppliers for all different kinds of materials, products or reagents and form the basis for release of incoming goods or they are issued by the QC department for intermediate or finished products. Chapter 6 "QC" provides relevant details on CoAs, which are issued by the QC department of a pharmaceutical manufacturer.

(*Continued*)

Table 4.2: *(Continued).*

Document Type	Document Sub-Type	Definition and Further Details
	Reports	*'Reports document the conduct of particular exercise, project or investigation, together with results, conclusions and recommendations'.*[11] Examples for reports in the GMP surrounding are validation/qualification reports, stability reports, reports on OOS results or other non-compliances, or audit reports.

Note: Table modified based on Chapter 4 of the EU GMP Guidelines.[11]

4.5.2 *Generation and control of documentation*

'Documents should be designed, prepared, reviewed, and distributed with care'.[11] Not only products and processes, but also documents have a life cycle. Following the GMP principles, this document lifecycle has to be clearly defined and implemented. Usually the following steps are required and thus have to be managed:

1. Document preparation.
2. Document review.
3. Document approval by AP(s).
4. Training of personnel.
5. Document implementation (effective date).
6. Document distribution (if required).
7. Document invalidation and archiving.

Documents can either be handled manually as paper-based documents or with IT based, electronic document management systems. Also hybrid forms can exist. For IT based systems, it is important that the requirements of Annex 11 to the EU GMP Guidelines on Computerised Systems[18] are met. Irrespective of the system that is used, documents have to be uniquely identifiable. Therefore, they often do not only have a unique title but also a code or reference number. An inventory of all documents within the QMS has to be maintained.

Generally all documents in the PQS, irrespective of the type of document, have to be approved, signed, and dated by appropriate and APs. Instructions (SOPs, work instructions, etc.) are usually dated and signed by the author(s) who prepared the document, by the reviewer(s) and finally they are approved through date and signature of one or more responsible persons. Processing instructions, for example, have to be approved at least by the Head of production, testing instructions at least by the Head of QC, a SOP on Batch Record Review and product release at least by the QP.

It has to be considered that the date of approval is not equivalent to the effective date, since relevant personnel have to be trained before a document is implemented. As all documents of the QMS have to be kept up-to-date, a period of validity has to be defined, that can vary for different types of documents. The expiration date of the document marks the latest time point when either a new version has to be implemented or the document has to be invalidated and archived, in case it is no longer required.

Records and reports have to be dated and signed after they have been generated electronically or after all handwritten entries have been completed. As especially production and QC operations have to be traceable, associated records have to be signed by the operators who performed the work before they are reviewed and approved by an AP (head of production or QC).

Work instructions and SOPs are usually required at the location where a specific action has to be taken. Copies of the original documents are required in these cases. These copies have to be controlled, meaning that they are registered, dated, and signed by persons who are authorized to distribute documents (usually QA/QM staff). The registration of controlled copies is necessary so that they can be retrieved, in case a new version of the document is implemented or the original document is no longer required and therefore invalidated. It is also possible to generate uncontrolled copies but these have to be clearly marked as such. Usually uncontrolled copies are only valid on the day of printing/distribution as they are not followed-up. Also the reproduction of working documents from master documents has to be managed with care, in order not to allow any error to be introduced through the reproduction process.

But not only generation, approval and distribution are important, also archiving of documents has to be clearly defined and managed. '*All documents have to be stored for pre-defined periods of time in a way that they are for the whole time accessible, complete, and correct. Special care has to be taken for the storage of raw data to prevent modification, mix-up or losses*'.[11] Raw data which, for example, belong to a certain product validation, must be retained for a period at least as long as the records for all batches whose release has been supported on the basis of that validation. Specific requirements are defined for the retention period of batch documentation which must be kept for one year after expiry of the batch or at least five years after certification of the batch by the QP, whichever is the longer. For IMPs, the batch documentation must be kept for at least five years after the completion or formal discontinuation of the last clinical trial in which the batch was used.[11] For specific types of products, deviating retention periods might be required. Regulation (EC) No 1394/2007 on Advanced Therapy Medicinal Products (ATMPs),[19] for example, defines documents that serve traceability and hence must be kept for a minimum of 30 years after the expiry date of the product, or longer, if required by the Commission as a term of the MA.

Figure 4.3 provides an overview on the various steps of a document life cycle.

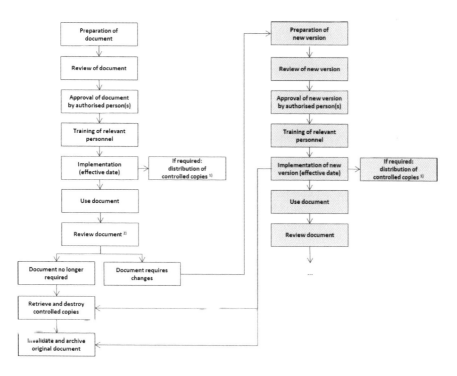

Figure 4.3: Document life cycle.

Note:

1) Controlled copies have to be registered in order to be able to retrieve them, when a new version is implemented. Generally, also uncontrolled copies can be generated, but these are not registered and are therefore not followed-up. They are only valid on the day of printing/distribution.

2) A document is reviewed because either it is known that changes are required or that they are about to expire (the document lifetime has to be predefined to assure that it is kept up-to-date).

4.5.3 *Good documentation practice*

Documentation of relevant actions (e.g., production or QC operations) is a key issue of GMP. A basic principle is: "What has not been documented has not been performed". Apart from recording various processes, documentation also serves investigation and evaluation of any observation. But not only the content, also the way of documentation is important. Attributes such as clear, legible, indelible, truthful, and traceable have to be followed. The EU GMP Guidelines define, in Chapter 4, "Documentation",[11] the principles of Good Documentation Practice. In Table 4.3, we summarize relevant do's and don'ts of GMP compliant documentation that should be considered and implemented in a written standard procedure.

GMP compliant documentation is relevant for anyone documenting actions that might directly or indirectly impact on the quality of the medicinal product. This

Table 4.3: Good Documentation practices — dos and don'ts.

Good Documentation Practice-Dos:	Good Documentation Practice-Don'ts:
Document in a clear way (unequivocally, self-explanatory).	Do not use pencils or pens whose writing can be removed or will fade.
Document in a legible way: This refers to the individual handwriting as well to documents where handwritten entries are required as they must provide enough space for the required information.	Do not use sticky notes or scrap sheets for the documentation of relevant information. Sticky notes are only allowed for marking certain pages or spots. If scrap sheets have been used, they must become part of the documentation and must therefore be referenced, dated and signed.
Document in an indelible way: Use permanent ink.[(1)]	Do not cancel or correct wrong entries in a way that does not allow reading the initial information (e.g., do not use correction fluids/white-outs, do not cross or scratch out an entry several times, and do not cut-out).
Document real time (at the time each action is taken) as relevant information will start being lost shortly after operations have been performed.	Do not add further information at a later time point without clearly marking the addition or amendment as such (together with date and signature).
Document truthfully (actual values).	Do not backdate or date ahead.
Be exact.	Do not generate "new originals" (e.g., when realizing that wrong entries have been made).

(Continued)

Table 4.3: (*Continued*).

Good Documentation Practice-Dos:	Good Documentation Practice-Don'ts:
Document in a traceable way: The documentation of significant activities must be dated and signed.	Do not generate additional "unofficial" documents.
If alterations to original entries are necessary they must be signed and dated and have to permit the reading of the initial entry. Wrong entries or empty fields that have not been used for documentation usually have to be cancelled with one straight line.	Do not delegate documentation of specific activities to others. The person who performed a certain operation must document it. An exception is only aseptic processing in a clean room environment, where usually the operator does not record himself/herself, in order not to contaminate the sterile gloves.
Document the reason for an alteration whenever it is not self-explanatory.	
More information is better than less: Write down abnormalities or peculiarities as they can, e.g., indicate problems or negative trends and might provide further valuable information.	
Calculations must be comprehensible: Add the calculation method (if it is not a part of the protocol).	

Note: [1] Some companies define to use solely blue ink in order to be able to differentiate originals from copies more easily. However, this is no request of the EU GMP Guidelines.

also includes cleaning and maintenance personnel. Initial and continuing training is important for everybody who has to relate to Good Documentation Practices.

4.6 Outsourced Activities

Outsourced activities need to be clearly defined and controlled. Chapter 7 of the EU GMP Guidelines "Outsourced Activities"[16] provides the relevant details. It is important to know that Chapter 7 formerly was termed "Contract Manufacture and Analysis" with a more narrow focus on outsourced production and QC operations. This has been changed in 2013 and the Chapter was renamed to point out that all outsourced activities which might have a potential impact on quality issues are now underlying the requirements of Chapter 7. Examples are cleaning/disinfection operations of the production or QC area or technical service and maintenance of production or QC equipment.

In principle, one can differentiate between contractors who have their own manufacturing license and those who perform operations that do not require a manufacturing license. In the first case, at least in the European system, a QP is responsible for product release of intermediate products or analytical test results. These are generally all contract manufacturers, as they are obliged to have a manufacturing license for each medicinal product they produce or for each type of production process, even if only small sub-processes are performed. Contract manufacturers therefore must employ a QP, as this is one of the prerequisites for obtaining a manufacturing license in Europe. Also some bigger contract laboratories might have a manufacturing license, when they are performing finished product release testing. Whenever a QP is involved at the Contract Acceptor, the QP who is responsible for certification and release of the finished product batch can rely on these intermediate release steps, but it is mandatory that a written agreement exactly defines for which operations the Contract Acceptor's QP is responsible and it should be clearly identified which matters are confirmed by the Contract Acceptor's QP. Specific details for contract manufacturing and the role and responsibilities of various QPs on different stages of manufacturing are provided in Annex 16 to the EU GMP Guidelines on Certification by a QP and Batch release[20] (also compare Chapter 8 "Product Release").

Outsourced activities such as cleaning/disinfection or technical service and maintenance do not require a manufacturing license, and typically those contractors do not perform their operations exclusively for companies or centers that have to follow the GMP requirements. Full responsibility in these cases has to be taken by the Contract Giver who has to assure that quality standards are implemented and followed by the Contract Acceptor.

In any case, written agreements have to define clearly the rights and duties of both parties: The Contract Giver's and the Contract Acceptor's. In principal, it is the Contract Giver's responsibility to exactly define the activities that have to be performed by the Contract Acceptor. As far as production or QC procedures are concerned, the relevant details are laid down in the CTA or MA. The PSF is often used as a summary of relevant information for production and/or QC operations and is therefore usually part of the written agreement. It might also be useful to agree on SOPs or more detailed instructions. It is important that both parties strictly adhere to change control principles (see Section 4.3.5 on Change Control Management) and that relevant changes are not implemented without the other party's approval. Contract Acceptors must further report relevant deviations,

OOS-results and other non-conformances. It should be determined that the Contract Acceptor is not allowed to subcontract to a third party any of the work entrusted to him under the Contract, without the Contract Giver's prior evaluation and approval. Finally the Contract Giver must have the right to initially and further audit relevant sites and documents of the Contract Giver.

4.7 Complaints and Product Recall

'*In order to protect public and animal health, a system and appropriate procedures should be in place to record, assess, investigate, and review complaints including potential quality defects, and if necessary, to effectively and promptly recall medicinal products for human or veterinary use and investigational medicinal products from the distribution network. Quality Risk Management principles should be applied to the investigation and assessment of quality defects and to the decision-making process in relation to product recalls, corrective and preventative actions and other risk-reducing actions*' [EU GMP Guidelines, Chapter 8].[21]

Chapter 8 of the EU GMP Guidelines[21] provides details on complaint handling and execution of product recalls. The chapter has been extensively revised recently to implement the principles of QRM for the investigation of quality defects or complaints and for making decisions in relation to product recalls or other risk-mitigating actions. Furthermore, the importance of a root cause analysis for the investigation and determination of possible reasons is emphasized together with the definition of appropriate preventative actions to guard against a recurrence of the issue.

The most important element of complaint handling is the obligation to document and follow up on every single notification, as it might reveal a quality defect. Documentation and follow-up are required, even if on first sight a complaint seems to be insignificant. Everybody in the company who has contact to customers (be it personal, *via* e-mail, conventional mail or phone), therefore has to be trained on complaint handling. This includes reception and front desk personnel. A written procedure describing the actions to be taken upon receipt of a complaint is mandatory.

After documentation, experienced and trained personnel have to initiate a formal investigation and perform a thorough root cause analysis. It is important to find out whether a complaint is indeed related to a quality defect. In this case, it has to be decided if the implementation of risk-reducing actions (including product recall) is required. For root cause analysis, it might be necessary to retest reference or retention samples or to review batch or distribution records. Special attention should be given to establishing whether a complaint or suspected quality defect relates to falsification (even if this is rather unlikely for cell-based medicinal products as they are often personalized). The QP who was responsible for the certification of the concerned product batch must be made formally aware of any investigations, any risk-reducing actions, and any recall operations, in a timely manner. In addition to the QP, quality defects have to be reported to the MA holder or sponsor of a clinical trial and all concerned competent authorities in cases where the quality defect may result in the recall of the product or in an abnormal restriction in the supply of the product.

In response to a quality defect, appropriate CAPAs have to be identified and taken. The effectiveness of such actions has to be monitored and assessed. Quality defect records have to be reviewed regularly and trend analyses should be performed for any indication of specific or recurring problems requiring attention.

In case recall operations are required, a system has to be defined and implemented that enables their initiation promptly and at any time. To protect public health it might be necessary to initiate recall operations before the full extent of the quality defect is understood and before a root cause is revealed. In the case of IMPs, all trial sites have to be identified. Recall procedures in any case have to be initiated and followed up together with the competent authorities. The contact point for reporting suspected quality defects to the competent authority must therefore be clear.

As many cell-based medicinal products have a very short shelf-life, the likelihood for the requirement of recall procedures is rather low, but it has to be considered nevertheless, that in these cases the competent authorities have to be informed.

We strongly recommend reading Chapter 8 of the EU GMP Guidelines[21] in more detail as a lot of additional information is provided there. In addition, it might be useful to read the so called "Compilation of Community Procedures on Inspections and Exchange of Information"[22] which is published by the EC. In the section "Procedures related to Rapid Alerts", the European Rapid Alert System (RAS) is defined together with the classification of product defects according to RAS. Even if the procedures described there are primarily intended for the use within and amongst competent authorities in Europe, the document helps to better understand the procedures for complaint handling and product recall on the whole, and facilitates the interaction with the competent authority.

4.8 Self-Inspections (SIs)

SIs are valuable tools to identify deficits, deviations, and non-conformances, to evaluate the efficacy of the QAS and to verify overall GMP compliance.

The EU GMP Guidelines request in Chapter 9 "Self Inspection",[23] the performance of SIs in all areas that might directly or indirectly influence the quality of a medicinal product. This also includes the QA department or Quality Unit. There must be a written procedure in place that precisely defines which departments/divisions have to be inspected and how regular SIs have to be performed. The compilation of annual SI programs is mandatory in this respect. Apart from these basic requirements, it has to be defined that all findings and deficits are thoroughly documented and followed up. Where necessary, CAPA procedures have to be initiated. The leader of a SI has to be independent of the department/division that she/he inspects, but of course enough expertise is required to be able to evaluate findings correctly. This might be difficult in smaller companies or academic centers with a limited number of personnel. Independent audits by external experts may also be useful. Responsible personnel of the inspected department/division should be involved to explain details.

Apart from the above mentioned routine inspections that are performed based on the annual SI program, SIs can additionally be initiated on purpose (e.g., as part of a CAPA procedure or a negative trend) or in preparation of an audit or inspection.

Competent authorities usually do not review SI reports in detail during inspections as they want to keep SIs as an internal tool where findings can be documented honestly, as otherwise SIs would lose their power.

4.9 Qualification and Validation

'It is a requirement of GMP that manufacturers identify what validation work is needed to prove control of the critical aspects of their particular operations. Significant changes to the facilities, the equipment and the processes, which may affect the quality of the product, should be validated. A risk assessment approach should be used to determine the scope and extent of validation'. [EU GMP Guidelines, Annex 15].[14]

Qualification and validation are one of the most important GMP tools for manufacture of medicinal products. Details for both activities are provided in Annex 15 to the EU GMP Guidelines.[14]

4.9.1 *Qualification*

'*Qualification*: Action of proving that any equipment works correctly and actually leads to the expected results. The word validation is sometimes widened to incorporate the concept of qualification'. [EU GMP Guidelines, Glossary].

The purpose of qualification is to ensure that facilities, equipment, instruments, and devices are fit for their intended purpose. As only the pharmaceutical manufacturer knows what the intended purpose is, which requirements have to be fulfilled and which specifications have to be met, qualification activities can never be outsourced completely. It is the responsibility of the head of production or QC to authorize at least qualification documents for premise and equipments in their departments.

A qualification usually has to cover the following four steps (compare Annex 15)[14]:

⇨ **Design Qualification (DQ)** — the documented verification that the proposed design of the facilities, systems and equipments is suitable for the intended purpose. A DQ has to include

- A detailed risk analysis.
- The definition of user requirement specifications (URS).
- The evaluation of functional specifications (FSs) provided by the supplier.

The DQ generally has to be closed with ordering.

⇨ **Installation Qualification (IQ)** — The documented verification that the facilities, systems, and equipments, as installed or modified, comply with the approved design and the manufacturer's recommendations. An IQ can range from quite short (e.g., for plug-in equipment with only a small number of functions) to rather extensive (e.g., for huge custom-made facilities).
⇨ **Operational Qualification (OQ)** — The documented verification that the facilities, systems, and equipments, as installed or modified, perform as intended throughout the anticipated operating ranges. The tests have to include upper and lower operating limits (worst case scenarios).
⇨ **Performance Qualification (PQ)** — The documented verification that the facilities, systems, and equipments, as connected together, can perform effectively and reproducibly, based on the approved process method and product specification. For PQ tests, it is required to use production materials, qualified substitutes or simulated product. Again, upper and lower operating limits (worst case scenarios) have to be included.

It is important that each qualification phase is completed before the succeeding step can commence. All qualification results have to be summarized in a qualification report that has to be authorized by responsible personnel. Successful qualification is the prerequisite for the release of facilities, equipments, instruments, and devices for GMP compliant use. For validation procedures (see Section 4.9.2), all facilities, equipments and instruments that are used within the validation procedure have to be successfully qualified.

Qualifications have to be performed at least initially before qualification objects can be released for use. Revalidations might be required whenever changes are made (either to the construction or software) or when specifications or acceptance criteria are altered. Re-qualification activities have to be as clearly defined as those for initial qualification. The extent of re-qualification has to be defined with a risk-based approach (detailed risk analysis).

Special re-qualification requirements are defined for HVAC-systems that supply the production area. Annex 1 to the EU GMP Guidelines on the manufacture of sterile medicinal products together with the ISO 14644: [Cleanrooms and associated controlled environments][30] request that some re-qualification activities (e.g., clean room classification by particle measurement) have to be performed annually, for A and B clean room grade, even twice a year. Further details on clean room qualification are provided in Chapter 5 "Process Development and Production".

4.9.2 *Validation*

'*Action of proving, in accordance with the principles of GMP, that any procedure, process, equipment, material, activity or system actually leads to the expected results*'. [EU GMP Guidelines, Glossary].

In contrast to qualification operations that are applied to premise and equipment, processes have to be validated. Validation is required at least for the following types of processes:

⇨ **Validation of production processes (process validation)** — Process validation usually has to be performed in a prospective way. The production of at least three validation batches is usually requested by the authorities. In case of starting materials of human origin, concurrent validation might be possible at least for IMPs. This should be discussed with the competent authority. It is accepted by most authorities that process validation of IMPs cannot be as complete as it has to be for authorized medicinal products. Further guidance on process validation is provided by the EMA[24] and the US FDA.[25] The validation of aseptic processes (also known as media fill) is a special kind of process validation. Media fills should demonstrate that personnel together with qualified facilities and equipments are able to achieve sterile products. The production process therefore has to be simulated as closely as possible and API, raw materials and excipients have to be substituted with growth medium. The Pharmaceutical Inspection Co-operation Scheme (PIC/S) provides valuable recommendations on the validation of aseptic processes in document PI 007-6.[26] Also compare Chapter 5 on process development and manufacturing.

⇨ **Validation of analytical methods** — The principles for validation of analytical methods are defined in ICH guideline Q2 (R1) "Validation of analytical procedures- text and methodology".[27] Details are provided in Chapter 6 "QC".

⇨ **Transport validation** — The methods for transportation of a medicinal product have to be validated to demonstrate that defined specifications, especially temperature, are maintained throughout the whole transportation process. Worst case scenarios for outdoor temperatures (summer and winter setting) as well as for the length of the transportation process have to be considered.

⇨ **Cleaning validation** — Cleaning validation is primarily required for equipment that is reused in the production process. For advanced cell-based medicinal products, this kind of validation mostly is of less significance as batches tend to be very small, and disposable, single-use equipment is used, wherever possible. Even smaller bioreactors are meanwhile available as disposable equipment. Apart from equipments, cleaning validation is important for clean rooms, as it has to be demonstrated that cleaning and disinfection procedures are able to achieve the required clean room status. A special kind of cleaning validation is required for *ex vivo* gene therapy medicinal products that are produced with the help of virus. Authorities usually request to demonstrate that spilled virus can be efficiently removed in order to prevent cross contamination (also compare Chapter 5 on process development and manufacturing).

⇨ **Computer validation** — Details for this special type of validation — that is rather the validation of systems than computers — are provided in Annex 11 to the EU GMP Guidelines[18] "Computerised Systems". In the US, 21 CFR 11 (also known as "part 11") defines requirements on computer validation. The Good Automated Manufacturing Practice (GAMP) guidelines are a well-known industry standard in this field, which is not compulsory but provides further details on the topic and reflects current good practices.[28] Further information is available on the homepage of the International Society for Pharmaceutical Engineering (ISPE) (http://www.ispe.org/gamp-5).

As for qualification, also for validation a detailed risk analysis is required as the basis for the validation activities that are necessary. An authorized validation plan that defines all activities that have to be taken is compulsory before the validation can commence. Results have to be documented in a corresponding report that has to be authorized by responsible personnel.

Re-validation is required whenever substantial changes are made. In the change control procedure, it has to be evaluated on a risk-based approach, whether a revalidation is required and if yes, which tests have to be performed. For production processes, it can, for example, be sufficient to revalidate only a part of the whole process.

4.10 Supplement on Required Documentation

In this supplement, we provide a list of documents that reflect the minimal requirements necessary for the QAS of a pharmaceutical manufacturer as defined by the EU GMP Guidelines (Table 4.4). Special documents for cell-based medicinal products are only included in so far as Annex 2 to the EU GMP Guidelines for the manufacture of biological active substances and medicinal products[7] is considered. Please note that no product or process specific documents (such as instructions for handling of machines and equipments or instructions for production or QC procedures) are included here as these are highly specific for each individual manufacturer, product and process. Depending on the company or structure of the QAS it might be advantageous to combine some of the documents listed in Table 4.4 in one single SOP or to establish individual documents for topics that are combined here.

Table 4.4:   List of Mandatory Documents for a PQS.

	Document Title
EU GMP Guidelines, Part I	
Chapter 1: PQS	Quality Manual (including responsibility of the senior management).
	How to write, supervise, approve, implement, change, and archive an SOP.
	QRM (also compare Part III of the EU GMP Guidelines).
	Change Control Management.
	Deviation Management.
	CAPA – Corrective Action & Preventive Action.
	Supplier Qualification (including specifications to perform audits).
	Inspection of incoming goods.
	Validation Master Plan (also compare Annex 15).
	PQR.
Chapter 2: Personnel	Organization Chart.
	Responsibilities of Key Personnel (including written job descriptions).
	Initial and continuing Training (including assessment of training effectiveness).
	Personnel Hygiene including periodic health controls (also compare Annex 1).
	Selection of consultants.

(Continued)

Table 4.4: (*Continued*).

	Document Title
Chapter 3: Premise and Equipment	Environmental monitoring (also compare Annex 1).
	Pest control.
	Access control.
	Hygiene, cleaning and sanitation.
	Service, maintenance, calibration, and repair of equipments and facilities.
	Qualification and periodic re-qualification of equipment and facilities (also compare Annex 15).
	Storage areas and warehousing (including monitoring of temperature, and where applicable, humidity).
Chapter 4: Documentation	Good Documentation Practices.
	Paper work, logbooks and laboratory journals.
	Specifications and PSF.
	Data evaluation and reporting.
	Signatures and Signature Authorization.
	Archiving.
Chapter 5: Production	Manufacturing instructions and records (individual documents for each product).
	Aseptic Processing.
	Process Validation (also compare Annex 15).
	Transport validation (also compare Annex 15).
	Inventory Management.
	Packaging and Labeling (including reconciliation of labels and line clearance).
	Re-processing (including re-packaging and re-labeling).
	Transport and Shipment.
Chapter 6: QC	Validation of analytical procedures and method transfer.
	Handling of samples, reagents and reference standards (including identification and labeling).
	Sampling procedures.
	Testing instructions and records for starting material, in-process controls and release testing (individual documents for each product).
	Handling OOS results.
	Stability program (including ongoing stability).
Chapter 7: Outsourced Activities	How to control and review GMP relevant outsourced activities (including template for written contracts and technical agreements).

(*Continued*)

Table 4.4:   (*Continued*).

	Document Title
Chapter 8: Complaints and Product Recall	Complaint handling (including handling of potentially falsified medicinal products).
	Handling Recalls and Returns.
Chapter 9: Self Inspection	Self-inspections: How to plan, conduct, report, and follow up on internal audits.
Annex 1: Manufacture of Sterile Medicinal Products	Validation of aseptic processing (Media fills).
	Operational process environmental clean room monitoring.
	Classification (Qualification) of clean rooms (also compare Chapter 3 and Annex 15).
	Sterilization (if applicable).
	Personnel hygiene and gowning (also compare Chapter 2).
Annex 2: Manufacture of Biological active substances and Medicinal Products for Human Use	Annex 2 contains specific guidance for manufacture and QC of cell-based medicinal products. The defined requirements have to be considered for the development of different SOPs listed in this table, as well as for manufacturing and QC instructions.
Annex 11: Computerised Systems	Validation of computerized systems [including validation of process and QC related software such as laboratory information systems (LIMS) and software for management of QA documents].
Annex 13: Manufacture of IMPs	Special considerations for labeling of IMPs (compare Chapter 5).
	Special considerations for final product release of IMPs (compare Annex 16).
	Special considerations for blinding and randomization (if applicable).
	Responsibilities of the Sponsor (to be followed for the preparation of a written contract, compare Chapter 7).
Annex 15: Qualification and Validation	Validation Master Plan (also compare Chapter 1).
	Qualification of equipment used in manufacturing and QC including re-qualification (also compare Chapters 5 and 6).
	Process validation (also compare Chapter 5).
	Validation of analytical procedures (also compare Chapter 6).
	Cleaning Validation.

(*Continued*)

Table 4.4: (*Continued*).

	Document Title
Annex 16: Certification by a QP and Batch Release	Batch Record Review and Product Release (also compare Chapter 1).
Annex 19: Reference and Retention Samples	Reference and Retention Samples.
EU GMP Guidelines, Part II	
Basic Requirements for Active Substances used as Starting Materials	Special documents related to Part II of the EU-GMP-guidelines might be required, if part of the manufacturing process of the cell-based medicinal product is classified as manufacture of an active substance (also compare Part I, Annex 2 that gives advice in which cases Part I and Part II of the EU GMP Guidelines are applicable).
EU GMP Guidelines, Part III	
SMF	SMF
ICH guideline Q9 on QRM	QRM (compare Chapter 1).
ICH guideline Q10 on PQS	Compare Chapter 1.
MRA Batch Certificate	Compare Annex 16.

References

1. EudraLex- The Rules Governing Medicinal Products in the European Union, Volume 4: Good manufacturing practice (GMP) Guidelines, Part I, Chapter 1: Pharmaceutical Quality System.
2. WHO Technical Report Series No. 986, Annex 2: WHO good manufacturing practices for pharmaceutical products. World Health Organization (WHO), 2014.
3. ICH Q10: Pharmaceutical Quality System, ICH Harmonised Tripartite Guideline. International Conference on Harmonisation of Technical Requirements for Registration of Pharmaceuticals for Human Use.
4. Directive 2003/94/EC laying down the principles and guidelines of good manufacturing practice in respect of medicinal products for human use and investigational medicinal products for human use. European Parliament and Council, October 8, 2003.
5. ISO 9001: 2008 Quality management systems — Requirements. International Organization for Standardization.
6. EudraLex — The Rules Governing Medicinal Products in the European Union, Volume 4: Good manufacturing practice (GMP) Guidelines.
7. EudraLex — The Rules Governing Medicinal Products in the European Union, Volume 4: Good manufacturing practice (GMP) Guidelines, Part I, Annex 2: Manufacture of Biological active substances and Medicinal Products for Human Use.

8. EudraLex- The Rules Governing Medicinal Products in the European Union, Volume 4: Good manufacturing practice (GMP) Guidelines, Part I, Annex 13: Manufacture of Investigational Medicinal Products.

9. The GMP Manual. Maas & Peither GMP. ISBN-13: 978-3934971233.

10. EudraLex- The Rules Governing Medicinal Products in the European Union, Volume 4: Good manufacturing practice (GMP) Guidelines, Part I, Chapter 2: Personnel.

11. EudraLex- The Rules Governing Medicinal Products in the European Union, Volume 4: Good manufacturing practice (GMP) Guidelines, Part I, Chapter 4: Documentation.

12. EudraLex- The Rules Governing Medicinal Products in the European Union, Volume 4: Good manufacturing practice (GMP) Guidelines, Part III: GMP-related documents.

13. ICH Q9 Quality Risk Management: Text and Methodology, ICH Harmonised Tripartite Guideline. International Conference on Harmonisation of Technical Requirements for Registration of Pharmaceuticals for Human Use.

14. EudraLex- The Rules Governing Medicinal Products in the European Union, Volume 4: Good manufacturing practice (GMP) Guidelines, Part I, Annex 15: Qualification and Validation.

15. CFR- Code of Federal Regulations Title 21, Part 820 Quality System Regulation. US Department of Health and Human Services, Food and Drug Administration (FDA).

16. EudraLex- The Rules Governing Medicinal Products in the European Union, Volume 4: Good manufacturing practice (GMP) Guidelines, Part I, Chapter 7: Outsourced Activities.

17. Directive 2001/20/EC on the approximation of the laws, regulations and administrative provisions of the Member States relating to the implementation of good clinical practice in the conduct of clinical trials on medicinal products for human use. European Parliament and Council, April 4, 2001.

18. EudraLex- The Rules Governing Medicinal Products in the European Union, Volume 4: Good manufacturing practice (GMP) Guidelines, Part I, Annex 11: Computerised Systems.

19. Regulation (EC) No 1394/2007 of the European Parliament and of the Council of November 13, 2007 on advanced therapy medicinal products and amending Directive 2001/83/EC and Regulation (EC) No 726/2004.

20. EudraLex- The Rules Governing Medicinal Products in the European Union, Volume 4: Good manufacturing practice (GMP) Guidelines, Part I, Annex 16: Certification by a Qualified Person and Batch Release.

21. EudraLex- The Rules Governing Medicinal Products in the European Union, Volume 4: Good manufacturing practice (GMP) Guidelines, Part I, Chapter 8: Complaints and Product Recall.

22. Compilation of Community Procedures on Inspections and Exchange of Information, EMA/572454/2014 Rev 17. European Commission, October 3, 2014.

23. EudraLex- The Rules Governing Medicinal Products in the European Union, Volume 4: Good manufacturing practice (GMP) Guidelines, Part I, Chapter 9: Self Inspection.

24. Guideline on process validation for finished products — information and data to be provided in regulatory submissions, EMA/CHMP/CVMP/QWP/BWP/70278/2012-Rev1.

25. Guidance for Industry Process Validation: General Principles and Practices, January 2011, US Department of Health and Human Services Food and Drug Administration (FDA), January 2011.
26. PI 007-6: Recommendation on the validation of aseptic processes. Pharmaceutical Inspection Convention, Pharmaceutical Inspection Co-operation Scheme (PIC/S), January 1, 2011.
27. ICH Q2(R1): Validation of Analytical Procedures: Text and Methodology, ICH Harmonised Tripartite Guideline. International Conference on Harmonisation of Technical Requirements for Registration of Pharmaceuticals for Human Use.
28. GAMP®5: A Risk-Based Approach to Compliant GxP Computerized Systems. International Society for Pharmaceutical Engineering (ISPE), http://www.ispe.org/gamp-5.
29. Guidance for Industry: Quality Systems Approach to Pharmaceutical CGMP Regulations. U.S. Department of Health and Human Services. September 2006.
30. ISO 14644: Cleanrooms and associated controlled environments. International Organization for Standardization.

Process Development and Manufacturing **5**

Carolin Hermann, Felix Hermann, Andrea Hauser, and Christine Günther

5.1 Introduction

Cell-based medicinal products are highly innovative drugs made from biologic materials of human or animal origin that offer great hope for a variety of diseases for which there are only limited or no other therapeutic options. In Europe, the term Advanced Therapy Medicinal Products (ATMPs) summarizes three different categories of cell-based medicinal products: gene therapy medicinal products, somatic cell therapy medicinal products, and tissue engineered products. The main focus of this chapter is on somatic cell therapy medicinal products (including genetically modified cells used as *ex vivo* gene therapy tools). Neither *in vivo* gene therapy nor tissue engineered products are covered in full detail here. Furthermore, xeno geneic products where cells or tissue of animal origin are used to produce medicinal products for human use are not within the scope of this book.

Somatic cell therapy medicinal products (sCTMP) are defined as medicinal products '*containing or consisting of cells or tissues that have been subjected to substantial manipulation so that biological characteristics [. . .] have been altered, or of cells or tissues that are not intended to be used for the same essential function(s) in the recipient and the donor*'. Additionally they '*have properties for, or are used in or administered to human beings with a view to treating, preventing or diagnosing a disease through the pharmacological, immunological or metabolic action of its cells or tissues*'.[1,2] In this context, the meaning of the term "substantial manipulation" is of great importance. Annex I to regulation (EC) No. 1394/2007 lists manipulations that are not regarded as being substantial (e.g., cutting, grinding, and centrifugation) and if no such steps of substantial manipulation are used in the manufacturing process, the products are not considered as ATMPs in the European legislation and are then regulated as conventional blood, tissue, or cell products. The complete regulatory maze is challenging. In order to establish regulatory harmonization on the European level, the European Regulation (EC) 1394/2007 on ATMPs has entered into force in December 2008. It requires that manufacturing of these products shall be authorized by the competent authority of the member state. Besides, the regulation claims that ATMPs are manufactured as per GMP (good manufacturing practice) compliant[3] and that they underlie a centralized authorization procedure *via* the European Medicines Agency (EMA). The GMP standards are enlisted in the corresponding EU Guidelines to GMP, *EudraLex Volume 4, Part I*, with special guidance given in Annex 1 on 'Manufacture of Sterile Medicinal Products' and Annex 2 on 'Manufacture of Biological active substances and Medicinal Products for Human Use'. The ATMP regulation was developed for helping to control and improve patient access to novel medicinal products, as well as to ensure the safety and quality of these products. Additionally, it should clarify the regulatory position and marketing authorization (MA) as well as pharmacovigilance aspects. Generally spoken, the ATMP regulation intends to safeguard public health, prevent the transmission of infectious organisms and facilitate the exchange of human tissues and cells by ensuring the same high quality and safety across the EU. Following the three-year transition period, as of December 2011, all above mentioned therapeutics in Europe must comply with the ATMP Regulation. In Germany, ATMPs were anchored in the German drug law (AMG) with the 15th Amendment (Section 4 miscellaneous terminology,[9] where ATMP are linked to (EC) 1394/2007). The Committee for Advanced Therapies (CAT), a committee at the EMA, is amongst other issues responsible for the classification of medicinal products as ATMP or non-ATMP with regard to their MA. As long as a cell-based medicinal product is used as an investigational medicinal product (IMP) within a clinical trial, the individual European member state is responsible for its classification. Nevertheless classification through the CAT can be initiated on a voluntary basis as early as for phase I clinical trials, to gain timely knowledge about the required regulatory processes for later marketing procedures. In 2012, the CAT published a reflection paper on classification of ATMPs (EMA/CAT/600280/2010) in order to introduce the ATMP classification procedure by means of providing information on the procedure itself, on necessary data that have to be submitted by applicants and by communicating the current status of discussion.[1]

Manufacturing of ATMP requires starting material derived from different human tissues, cells, blood, or blood components. Important European directives on the standards that must be met when carrying out any activity involving tissues and cells for human application (patient treatment) are regulated in the European Union Tissue and Cells Directives (EUTCD). The EUTCD embraces directive 2004/23/EC that sets standards of quality and safety for the donation, procurement, testing, processing, preservation, storage, and distribution of human tissues and cells, directive 2006/86/EC regarding the traceability requirements, notification of serious adverse reactions and events and certain technical requirements for the coding, processing, preservation, storage and distribution of human tissues and cells and directive 2006/17/EC regarding certain technical requirements for the donation, procurement, and testing of human tissue and cells. For blood-derived cell products directive 2004/33/EC regards certain technical requirements for blood and blood components and directive 2002/98/EC sets standards of quality and safety for the collection, testing, processing, storage and distribution of human blood, and blood components. Details in terms of donor selection and testing as well as traceability are provided in Chapter "Quality Control".

In Europe, the EMA offers helpful guidance for all different aspects of ATMP manufacturing [e.g., guideline on human cell-based medicinal products (EMEA/CHMP/410869/2006) or the reflection paper on stem cell-based medicinal products (EMA/CAT/571134/2009)].

In the US, the appropriate authority for ATMP is the FDA (US Food and Drug Administration within the US Department of Health and Human Services). Organized within the FDA is the Centre for Biologics Evaluation and Research (CBER) that regulates biological products for human use under applicable federal laws, including the Public Health Service Act and the Federal Food, Drug and Cosmetic Act (FD&C Act). It includes, amongst others, the Office of Cellular, Tissue, and Gene Therapies (OCTGT). The CBER is responsible for the collection of blood and blood components used for transfusion or for the manufacture of pharmaceuticals derived from blood and blood components. Its duty is to protect and advance the public health in the US by ensuring that biological products are safe and available to those who need them. Here, main codes of federal regulations (CFR) regarding cell-based medicinal products are 21 CFR part 1271: human cells, tissues, and cellular and tissue-based products, 21 CFR part 211: current GMP for finished pharmaceuticals and 21 CFR part 600 on biological products.

For historical reasons, the regulatory landscape in Europe was and for certain topics still is highly diverse, therefore a harmonization in standards applied for generating safe and efficient medicinal products within Europe is important, necessary, and one of the main objectives of the EU, but of course it can initially complicate things in some cases. Before the European Regulation (EC) No. 1394/2007 of the European Parliament and the Council on ATMPs came into force, the regulatory scenario in Europe was quite heterogeneous. In some countries, blood and blood products and cell-based products were not defined as medicinal products but, e.g., in Germany, blood and blood products (including peripheral blood stem cells) were already embraced by the term medicinal product and thus their manufacture had to follow the strict GMP rules including manufacture under A in B clean room conditions, as soon as open manufacturing steps had been applied. In other European member states, haematopoietic stem-cells (HSCs) and other cell-based therapies were manufactured without application of the GMP rules and outside qualified and classified clean rooms. After the ATMP regulation came into law, it was just not possible in these European countries (especially for most of the academic institutions) to cope with the high GMP standards required, especially for setting up A in B clean room conditions (see Section 5.3 for 'Premises and Equipment'). Due to this, the manufacture and application of some cell-based products had to be terminated, although they were used with success and without any negative reporting.

GMP facilities and especially clean rooms are very costly in terms of installation and maintenance. The manufacturing license and the firm quality assurance systems (QASs) are prerequisites for the successful development and manufacturing of cell-based medicinal products, as they are for all kinds of medicinal products. Therefore, a careful design of the production and quality control system (QCS) with the earliest possible introduction of GMP standards is as much fundamental for successful development of cell-based therapies as extensive scientific and regulatory know-how and a close and early cooperation with the competent authorities.

5.2 Process Development

Besides the high GMP requirements for the manufacture of ATMPs, their development is accompanied with additional difficulties as for many of the applied production processes no extensive GMP experience exists and required premises and instruments are often not available for installation in clean rooms. Besides, the need for early scale-up in the production process represents an additional challenge. This makes the way toward a clinically implemented cell-based therapeutics even longer.

Due to the great variety of cell-based products, their potential risk for the individual patient, the involved personnel and even the general population [e.g., with respect to the release of genetically modified organisms (GMOs) to the environment] should be addressed in a thorough risk analysis to generate a complete development plan.[45] This should be performed early and in detail, as later changes might have severe implications on future development and on the validity or significance of clinical and pre-clinical data obtained before the change. The potential risk of an ATMP highly depends on the applied biologics as well as on the non-biologic components, the manufacturing process and on the specific therapeutic use. Any risk factor associated with the quality and safety of the product has to be identified and great efforts have to be put into determining the extent has and focus of data collected during non-clinical and clinical development. When manufacturing cell-based medicinal products the risk estimation of the products should deal with the type of cells (e.g., self-renewing stem cell or progenitor cell), their source (tissue or blood), their origin (autologous or allogeneic), and their ability to initiate an immune response as well as their proliferation and/or differentiation potential. Other general points might include the extent of cell manipulation during manufacturing (e.g., expansion, activation, or genetic modification), the mode of administration (e.g., local or systemic) and the duration of exposure. For evaluation of the overall risk, it is very helpful to have clinical data on similar products. Early on from research phase, it is very important to check whether all the inserted materials are available in GMP grade quality and to prepare lists which material is needed for which process step and whether or how all steps can be performed under clean room conditions. The development includes all kind of aspects regarding the manufacturing of high quality and safe medicinal products. It embraces research phase, development of the cultivation method and other critical manufacturing steps, development of characterization assays [e.g., Fluorescence-activated cell sorting (FACS), differentiation], establishment of coherence between Quality and Specification (for details, compare chapter 'Quality Control'), technology transfer from R&D to production and process validation.

5.2.1 *Scale-up*

Up-scaling can be particularly challenging for process development of cell-based medicinal products. Scale-up generally means that companies increase their productivity in manufacturing. In terms of manufacturing of ATMPs this can involve increasing the efficacy of a single unit by increasing its volume or area, e.g., from a 75 cm^2 cell culture flask to a multilayer cell factory stack (for more details, see Section 5.4.3 on cell culture). Another classical case of up-scaling is seen when the research process needs to be adapted to the extent of the clinical application. Increasing, e.g., cell numbers in a certain preparation step by the factor 10 can easily lead to unmanageable volumes in the liter range, if up-scaling would be performed in a linear way. Where linear up-scaling is not feasible, a number of test runs might be required, especially when the providers of raw materials and premises do not offer a validated protocol for the manufacturing process, and experience with clinical-scale production is missing. Up-scaling of antibody-dependent processes is also often problematic as the suitable concentration is not always determined easily. Generally, test runs for cell-based products are often difficult to realize as starting material of human origin is not readily available and voluntary donors may not be put at the risk of the procurement procedure for the mere purpose of data collection. Any significant change of manufacturing has impact on the dossier provided to the competent authorities and amendments might be necessary. Also the need for eventual comparability runs/comparability exercises should be kept in mind. Scale-up is one of the major challenges in pharmaceutical manufacturing of ATMPs.

5.2.2 *Scale-out*

Manufacturing of substantially manipulated autologous cell-based medicinal products presents a number of specific challenges regarding the need to scale-out production (increasing the number of batches) to multiple manufacturing sites or to sites near the patient within hospital settings. Compared to highly profitable mass production of scalable allogeneic therapies, small-scale autologous therapies (as well as donor-patient-directed allogeneic products) must follow alternative manufacturing and distribution approaches, dependent on the product (indication and prevalence), the method of preservation of the product, and the compatibility with the systems at the final destination in the clinic. The existing regulatory structure in Europe (Note for guidance on biotechnological/biological products subject to changes in their manufacturing process: CPMP/ICH/5721/03) and the United States impose a requirement to demonstrate product equivalence between sites. With small lot sizes, short shelf-life and the clinically limited time available for product and lot release testing, this is a very cost and labor intensive process as comparability is achieved through a combination of *in vitro* studies, analytical testing, and biological assays.[6]

5.3 Premises and Equipments

The guidelines that regulate operation and maintenance of a clean room facility are quite clear and written down in detail in the EU GMP Guidelines (Part I, Chapter 3) and Annexes 1 and 2.[7–9] In general, for the manufacturing of ATMPs the guidelines included in Annex 1 have to be followed but can be adapted after thorough risk assessment according to Annex 2. If and to what extent a deviation from the clean room and environmental requirements of Annex 1 is possible is dependent on the type of product and the manufacturing process. Almost closed systems might allow for a downgrade of clean room grades, whereas many open steps in connection with long culture periods will request grade A in B clean room condition as defined for all conventional aseptically manufactured medicinal products. Deviations from Annex 1 should be discussed with the competent authorities early enough.

This section on premises and equipment is further divided in production area and clean rooms (Section 5.3.1), equipment and instrumentation (Section 5.3.2), and storage rooms and warehouses equipment (Section 5.3.3). This section is then accompanied by short sections on the qualification of clean rooms and equipment and the application of isolators (5.3.4–5.3.6).

In principle, the European GMP guideline (Part I, Chapter 3) states that the facility must be located, designed, constructed, adapted, and maintained to suit the operations to be carried out. Their layout and design must aim to minimize the risk of errors and permit effective cleaning and maintenance in order to avoid cross-contamination, build-up of dust or dirt and, in general, avoiding any adverse effect on the quality of products.

Nevertheless, when it comes to manufacturing cell therapy products, the manufacturer has to face a variety of difficulties that arise because, in contrast to a typical industry facility for parenteral dosage forms, there are less standardized available furnishings and equipment, even if the situation is about to change with the increase of promising therapies in the field of ATMPs with more companies entering the field, and thus with the rising request for specialized equipment.

5.3.1 Production area and clean rooms

General requirements for a clean room for manufacturing of sterile medicinal products are listed in detail in EU GMP Guidelines Annex 1 (Section 'Premises').[7] The rooms have to be built and equipped in a way that allows for maintenance of the specified cleanliness level (see Section 5.3.1.2). Generally, all surfaces as well as all instruments and devices installed in a clean room have to be smooth, impervious, and unbroken in order to reduce particle shedding or accumulation and to facilitate repeated applications of cleaning agents and disinfectants. This implies that no porous or fibrous material like wood or wall paint can be used for the inner surface of a clean room. Generally, material that is not susceptible for damages should be used. Dust accumulation can also be reduced by minimizing projecting ledges and shelves, cupboards, and equipments. Recesses have to be avoided when installing ducts or pipes, etc. as they are difficult to clean. Drains should be equipped with trapped gullies, opened channels should be avoided and if not possible, they should be shallow.[9] No sinks are allowed in grade A/B areas, in lower areas these sinks have to be fitted with seals to prevent backflow as remaining water is always associated with the growing of micro–organisms. Production areas should be effectively ventilated with air control units (temperature, humidity, and filtration, where necessary). Changing rooms should be designed as airlocks and provide physical separation of the different stages of changing. Another main topic in manufacturing of ATMPs is the avoidance of contamination and cross-contamination. The rooms should be constructed and maintained in a way that sustains the high standards of cleanliness level demanded. The product should be protected from contamination, but also the environment should be protected from any potential level of contamination coming from the product. Water sources, water treatment equipments, and treated water should be monitored regularly for chemical and biological contamination and, as appropriate, for endotoxins. Records should be maintained for the results of the monitoring and of any action taken.

Working with ATMPs often includes open systems handling (addition of buffers, media, etc.) and thus requires control measures like engineering and environmental controls on basis of Quality Risk Management (QRM) principles. Air handling units should be designed, constructed, and maintained to minimize the risk of cross-contamination between different areas. Where negative pressure areas or safety cabinets are used for aseptic processing of materials with particular risks (e.g., pathogens or genetically modified cells), they should be surrounded by a positive pressure clean zone. Primary containment should prevent escape of biological agents. The design, construction, and maintenance of units between different areas (considering single pass air systems) should minimize the risk of cross-contamination. Pressure cascades should be clearly defined and monitored. For the manufacturing of cell products, clean rooms classified as grade B with abundant areas for aseptic manipulations under grade A conditions are needed. Removal and inactivation of waste have to comply with local regulations.

A clean room is an environment that offers low levels of environmental pollutants such as dust, airborne micro–organisms, aerosol particles, and chemical vapors. More accurately, a clean room maintains a certain controlled level of contamination that is specified by the number of particles per area at a specified particle size (see Section 5.3.1.2 on Clean room grades). These settings provide a controlled and defined environment for the manufacturing of highly delicate products, as well as for medicines that are intended for parenteral applications in humans. This is especially important for cell-based medicinal products that can neither be sterilized by heat or irradiation nor by sterile filtration.

Working in a clean room setting requires a high level of discipline, patience, a special training, and the commitment to adhere stringently to the demanded requirements. Therefore, it is of great importance that the personnel is instructed extensively and repeatedly and is aware of the importance of the demanded requirements. The potential harmful consequences for patients have to be emphasized. This is not only important for the manufacturing personnel but for every person who is allowed to enter the clean rooms including cleaning personnel. In order to facilitate the work routine in a clean room setting, measures should be applied to enable undisturbed and safe operational procedures. Everyone who has ever worked in a clean room is aware how time consuming and frustrating it is during working process inside clean room grade B area in full garment, if the material stock has not been refilled or equipment was not introduced *via* the material airlock and is missing. Connecting to personnel outside the manufacturing cabinets and demanding the missing material is time consuming and can easily ruin a whole manufacturing process, when time limits are exceeded.

5.3.1.1 *Clean room design*

Designing a clean room should always start with definition of the medicinal products that should be produced, the manufacturing processes that should be executed in it and a risk assessment that covers all manufacturing steps as well as the clean room and the required instruments.

It is important to answer the following questions early in the planning phase:

- Which medicinal products should be produced, how are they regulated and which guidelines, rules and regulations have to be followed?
- Which clean room grade is necessary for the individual production processes and are there additional biosafety requirements (e.g., for genetically modified cell products)?
- How many batches should be produced per week/month and how big is one batch?
- What kind of starting material is used and which potential risks are emanating from it?
- Which raw materials are necessary and how do they have to be handled?
- Which devices and instruments are required in the clean room (laminar air flow bench, incubator, refrigerator, centrifuge, microscope, instruments for separation/enrichment of cells, etc.)?

- What kind of medium supply and connections are needed for each individual instrument (water connection, connection for power supply, connection to carbon dioxide, etc.)?
- What kind of operating and mounting conditions are required for each individual instrument (e.g., laminar air flow benches have to be installed in a way that room conditions do not interfere with the laminarity of the air flow; some instruments need a minimum distance to walls and neighboring instruments or furniture)?
- How can instruments and equipments be maintained, serviced, and repaired?
- What are the special handling necessities for the processed materials and the required equipments (e.g., temperature, humidity, and exposure to light)?
- How is material supposed to enter the clean room? Is a pass-through autoclave required?
- How much production staff is needed for each individual production step and how many persons have to be present in the clean room for each individual step?
- How do personnel enter the clean rooms?
- What are the gowning requirements for each clean room grade and how many air locks are needed to enter the highest clean room grade?
- What kind of gowning procedures do take place in each air lock and what kind of materials and furniture is required (sit over bench, lockers, storage racks, clothes hooks, etc.)?

With precise definition of the above mentioned user requirement specifications, a clean room expert should be able to find a solution for a suitable clean room design. The design of a certain clean room area will depend very much on the application that will be performed. No general design exists for a clean room that will suit all kind of different processes and products. A clean room should only be as big as necessary for the desired processes because the larger the clean room, the more air is needed to ventilate it and the more effort has to be put on cleaning procedures, which will finally rise maintaining costs.

5.3.1.2　*Clean room grades*

Contaminants are continually emitted into the environment by equipments, processes and facilities, but personnel are the main source of contamination. A motionless person sheds up to 500,000 particles of 0.3 μm size or larger per minute. When the person is active, this level can reach up to 45,000,000 particles per minute.[10] Therefore, clean room requirements prohibit certain items and activities, including wearing make-up or jewelry and moving fast. According to Annex 1 of the European GMP Guidelines, special requirements have to be fulfilled in order to minimize risks of microbiological, particulate, and pyrogenic contamination whenever sterile medicinal products are manufactured, especially when they have to be manufactured aseptically. It is essential that all personnel involved in the process (including cleaning and service personnel) are specially trained and that preparations and procedures are well defined and where necessary, validated. Sterile products should be manufactured in clean rooms which can only be entered *via* airlocks and which are maintained to an appropriate cleanliness standard including air supply through specialized filter systems (HEPA-filters of class H14 with a filtration efficiency of 99.995%, at least for grade A and B clean rooms). For different manufacturing operations, different classified characteristics of the environment may be required. Four different clean room grades can be distinguished according to Annex 1 of the European GMP Guidelines with grade D having the lowest requirements and grade A having the highest ones. Table 5.1 gives an overview of maximum permissible limits for particles.

Requirements for running clean rooms with regard to particle count, air pressure, air stream, clean room grades, humidity, temperature, filter systems and filter area, etc., are defined in EN ISO 14644-1 (14644-8 defines classification of airborne molecular contamination), VDI 2083, IES-RP-C C-006.2 and Eurovent 4/8.EN ISO 14644-2 provides additional guidance for clean room classification and regular re-qualification procedures.

Classically two different terms describe the operational state of a clean room: 'at rest' and 'in operation' (personnel present). In order to reach the required 'in

Table 5.1: Maximum permitted airborne particle concentration for each clean room grade (modified after EU GMP Guidelines Annex 1).[7]

Clean Room Grade		At Rest		Clean Room Grade		In Operation	
Annex 1	ISO	$\geq 0.5\,\mu$ m	$\geq 5.0\,\mu$ m	Annex 1	ISO	$\geq 0.5\,\mu$m	$\geq 5.0\mu$ m
Maximum Permitted Number of Particles per m³ Equal to or Greater than the Tabulated Size							
A	5/4.8[1]	3,520	20	A	5/4.8	3,520	20
B	5	3,520	29	B	7	352,000	2,900
C	7	352,000	2,900	C	8	3,520,000	29,000
D	8	3,520,000	29,000	D	—	Not defined	Not defined

Note: [1] Annex 1 to the EU GMP Guidelines defines the maximum permitted number of particles equal to or greater than 5.0 μm per m³ as 20, corresponding to an ISO classification of 4.8. ISO class 5 would permit 29 particles equal to or greater than 5.0 μm per m³. ISO = EN ISO 14644.

operation' conditions, dedicated clean room grade areas have to fulfill special air cleanliness levels already in the 'at rest' state. According to Annex 1 of the EUGMP Guidelines 'at rest' means the installation is installed and operating, complete with production equipments but with no operating personnel present. 'In operation' means that the installation is functioning in the defined operating mode with the specified number of personnel working. The according states should be defined for each clean room grade or clean room suite. 'In operation' classification can be demonstrated during normal operations, process simulations or during media fills as so called worst case scenarios. The European GMP Guidelines demand classification after EN ISO 14644-1 (for further details on classification, compare Section 5.3.4 'Qualification of clean rooms').

During service and maintenance, the clean room status has to be annulled and manufacturing processes are prohibited during that time. Before the manufacturing processes can commence after a clean room shut-down, defined re-qualification measurements are required. Independent of planned service and maintenance, it has to be defined which measures have to be taken after an unplanned break-down of the HVAC (Heating, Ventilation, and Air Conditioning) system or other disturbances of the air supply or differential pressure cascade.

In order to be able to monitor the cleanliness of a room, it is necessary that appropriate equipment is available. Particle counters are mandatory, installed as well as portable ones are used routinely. It is important to determine a zero measure point for the portable particle counter in order to ensure valid values. The frequency of measuring and the places where measuring is performed is determined *via* a risk based approach. Guidance is given in GMP Guidelines Annex 1 and the EN ISO 14644. In clean room class A, particle monitoring has to be performed continuously whereas this is not required for grade B, where it should be comparably frequent as in A, but not necessarily continuous. Finally in grade C, the frequency can be further reduced and drops down in clean room grade D. Particle monitoring in air locks has to be performed only in the 'at rest' status. After locking in of personnel, one can differentiate between an actual clean up phase (until the 'at rest' status is reached) and a defined clean up phase of 20 minutes, during which the 'at rest' status should be reached. Annex 1 to the EU GMP Guidelines requests an additional particle measurement after a short "clean up" period of 15–20 minutes (guidance value) in an unmanned state after completion of operations.

Certain rules of conduct are required in order to enable compliance of the guidance values for particles in dedicated clean room areas. Activities in clean areas and especially when aseptic operations are in progress should be kept to a minimum and movement of personnel should be controlled and methodical, to avoid excessive shedding of particles and organisms due to over-vigorous activity. No wristwatches, make-up or jewelry must be worn during manufacturing of sterile products. Which grade of clean room has to be used for a specific preparation clearly depends on whether the product can be finally sterilized or not. In case of cell products for human use this is obviously not possible (neither by heat or gas nor by filtration). In the case of manufacturing of cell-based medicinal products, aseptic handling of the product is mandatory from the first productions step onward. According to Annex 1 of the EU GMP Guidelines, handling of sterile starting materials and components (unless subjected to sterilization), and handling and filling of aseptically prepared products has to be performed in a clean room grade A environment with a grade B background. Normally such conditions are provided by a laminar airflow workstation. Laminar airflow systems should provide a homogenous air speed of 0.36 to 0.54 m/s at the working position (a velocity not normally reached by many of the standard laminar air flow benches used in research labs and offered by most of the providers). Grade B generally represents the background environment for a grade A area and any exemption from Annex 1 (e.g., A in D) have to be risk-based assessed and approved. Whereas in grade C and D, less critical stages in the manufacture of sterile products are carried out (such as preparation of buffers or solutions that can be sterilized prior to use).[7]

5.3.1.3 *Personnel and material flow*

Personnel and material flow should rely on the basis of quality risk management principles and where possible an unidirectional flow should be implemented. Separate air locks for entering and leaving the clean room often cannot be realized due to limited space, but it is mandatory that material and personnel enter the clean rooms independent of each other. Access of personnel (including all manufacturing or quality control staff working in the area, handling or taking samples, storage and testing as well as maintenance and service personnel) should be considered carefully to avoid any contamination or carry over.[8]

When building up clean room areas, it is very important to put special thoughts on how the areas are designed and where to place airlocks for material and personnel. The manufacturing process should be well known and defined in order to be able to conveniently plan the flow of incoming material and personnel and of the outgoing (in-process) quality control samples, the final product as well as the removal of waste. Only when personnel and material flow are well organized and coordinated, sterile manufacturing is made possible. Special considerations are necessary for working with GMO (genetically modified organisms). If no unidirectional workflow is possible, efforts should be undertaken to timely separate importing and exporting of materials. It should also be avoided that personnel entering and leaving designated clean room areas do have contact, in order to avoid cross contamination between areas containing different GMOs and areas where non-GMOs are handled. To avoid unnecessary locking in and out of personnel (in-process), control samples should leave the clean room *via* airlocks that reach to areas where quality control personnel can directly pick them up.

5.3.1.4 *Clothing*

Depending on the clean room class, workers have to wear special clothing and suit up in a gowning room before entering the clean room through an interlocking door. The clothing worn and its quality should be appropriate for the process and the grade of the working area. It should be worn in such a way as to protect the product from contamination. The higher the cleanliness grades of the clean room, the higher the requirements on clean room clothing. Production of cell-based medicinal products involves aseptic manufacturing due to the impossibility of sterilization of the final product. In the European understanding of clean room zones, grade A zones are not entered by personnel. This might be different to the US system, where personnel are working in grade 100 clean room areas. The gowning requirements for the European clean room classification are described below.

Grades A/B: Headgear should totally enclose the hair and, where relevant, beard and moustache. A single or two-piece trouser suit, gathered at the wrists and with a high neck, should be worn. The headgear should be tucked into the neck of the suit. A face mask should be worn to prevent the shedding of droplets. Appropriate, sterilized, non-powdered rubber or plastic gloves and sterilized or disinfected footwear should be worn. Trouser-bottoms should be tucked inside the footwear and garment sleeves into the gloves. The protective clothing should shed virtually no fibers or particulate matter and should retain particles shed by the body.

Outdoor clothing has to be changed before entering changing rooms that lead to C or B grade working area. This has to follow written protocols and should be documented carefully. Great importance has to be put on hygiene and basic elements of microbiology from the first air lock onwards.

It is of great importance to have a written instruction on how often gloves and face masks have to be changed during a manufacturing process or how many times the clean room worker has to disinfect the gloves. In many clean room facilities, commonly two pairs of gloves are worn one upon the other in the class A (and even class B) areas. The nether pair of gloves is often used in distinct colours (indicator glove) in order to detect holes in the upper sterile glove more easily. Sterile gowning (overall, boots, headgear, face mask, and gloves) must not be reused after leaving the clean room. All the preparation that is necessary for the personnel to enter the clean room of the desired classification is time consuming and should be carefully planned in advance in order to avoid unnecessary exits and re-entries. One has to mention that the gowning procedure and working in the clean room setting (especially A/B) in full garment is very challenging for the personnel and needs to be specially addressed and trained.[7]

5.3.1.5 *Gowning procedures and qualification of gowning*

According to EU GMP Guidelines Annex 1, changing and washing should follow a written protocol which was designed to minimize contamination of clean room clothes and avoid dissemination of contaminants to clean areas. For maintaining the requirements for clean room standards, it is of great importance that only a limited number of personnel should be present in clean areas. All personnel working in the clean room (including cleaning personnel) must be trained on how to behave in the clean room areas, what to wear and how to put these special clothes on. Clean room clothes have to be appropriate for the process and the grade of the working area. The clean room clothing should be handled very carefully in order not to damage fibers and thus increasing the risk of particle shedding. Sterile clothes (apart from boots) must not touch the ground during the gowning procedure (especially challenging for overalls) and should not be touched on the outside. It is also recommended that clean room clothing (where not one way) is cleaned in specialized facilities. When external providers are commissioned, technical agreements should be concluded. Gowning procedures have to be trained extensively and entrance should be restricted only to qualified personnel. For qualification purposes, it is common practice that personnel has to execute the gowning procedure three times with subsequent microbiological sampling of defined critical sampling points on the outside of the sterile clothing. Only if it is demonstrated that the gowning procedure was performed successfully three times (meaning the specifications of the microbiological samples are within the defined specifications), personnel is allowed to enter the clean rooms. Personnel should be trained and re-qualified at least once a year.

5.3.1.6 *Cleaning and disinfection*

A qualified and appropriately monitored clean room environment is the prerequisite to high quality GMP compliant manufacturing and crucial for guaranteeing the product's quality and patient's safety. Inadequate cleanliness or sterility of items and persons entering the clean room can compromise the environmental conditions during manufacturing. Keeping an area clean will always start with controlling what and how contaminants enter the facility because logically, when nothing is entering its presence does not have to be addressed. This involves both entering personnel and goods. Stationary equipment that is permanently installed in the clean room does, of course, not generate micro-organisms, but can be contaminated during usage or waiting and storage times or even shed particles and therefore nevertheless must be included in regular disinfection procedures. All cleaning and disinfection procedures (those for floors, walls, ceilings, and furniture as well as those for incoming goods and materials) need to be well defined and validated. A good alternative for disinfection of materials that are locked into the clean room is the use of double or even triple wrapped materials, where the outer packaging material simply has to be drawn off with a sterile cover beneath. This is a time-saving and secure method, but unfortunately most of the specialized cell-processing materials are not available with multiple wrappings.

It might be useful to differentiate between different levels of access authorization and the according qualification necessities for the personnel: (1) Access to all areas for maintenance or repair during clean room shut-down (followed by subsequent cleaning procedure), (2) Access authorization only for grade C and D areas for monitoring or cleaning tasks, and (3) Full access authorization to grade A and B areas that has to be renewed once a year are useful examples for graduated access permissions. Unauthorized entrance or entrance of untrained or unqualified personnel can result in exceedance of guidance values, and thus can result in a close down of the clean room and halt of manufacturing.

The whole clean room area needs to be cleaned in an effective and low particle shedding process. Cleaning and disinfection efforts can be minimized when entry of potential contaminants is controlled. It is necessary that validation protocols for sanitizers and disinfectants are available, that the environment is monitored regularly and that these data are used to determine trends. Microbiological monitoring should be performed frequently. According to GMP Guidelines Annex 1, personnel and surfaces should be monitored after critical steps and additionally after cleaning, sanitization, and validation/qualification processes. Limits are shown in Table 5.2. As regards GMP Guidelines Annex 2, environmental control of particulate and microbiological contamination of the production premises should be adapted to the active substance, intermediate or finished product. Methods to detect the presence of specific micro-organisms should be included. Product contamination should as well be avoided as contamination of the environment, whereas prevention is always regarded to be better than detection and removal.[8] An environmental monitoring

Table 5.2: Recommended limits for microbiological contamination depending on the test method.

Grade	Air Sample cfu/m^3	Settle Plates (Diameter 90 mm) cfu/4 Hours (b)	Contact Plates (Diameter 55 mm) cfu/Plate	Glove Print 5 Fingers cfu/Glove
	Recommended limits for microbial contamination (a)			
A	<1	<1	<1	<1
B	10	5	5	5
C	100	50	25	/
D	200	100	50	/

Note: (a) Values are average, (b) Individual settle plates may be exposed for less than four hours.
Source: EU GMP Guidelines Annex 1.[7]

program should be supplemented by the inclusion of methods to detect the presence of special micro-organisms. Annex 1 also contains information about minimizing particulate contamination during manufacturing and of the end product, avoidance of recontamination, performance of bio-burden assays, and validation of newly introduced procedures.[7]

Table 5.2 summarizes the different ways of sampling performed in clean rooms for the manufacturing of sterile medicinal products and the allowed levels of micro-organism growth on culture plates. The three mentioned sampling methods- active air sampling, passive air sampling (*via* settle plates), and contact sampling of personnel or surfaces are meant to be examples. 'Which method is used where' has to be defined by the manufacturer and is dependent on the clean room class as well as on the procedures that should be monitored. EN ISO 14698-1: 2003 'Biocontamination control' provides help on where and when sampling should be performed and what frequency is recommended.

The mechanical cleaning and the methodologies of applying disinfectants are crucial and therefore have to be validated. Not all disinfectants can be used for all surfaces. Some disinfectants (e.g., hydrogen peroxide) are too aggressive for some tubes (e.g., welding device). Disinfectants are available in GMP compliant quality and for practical reasons one way pre-soaked wipes and mops can be utilized. Finally the cleaning personnel working in the dedicated clean room areas needs to be extensively trained and supervised in order to avoid careless contamination. Training measures should not only cover gowning procedures but also correct cleaning procedures (which cleaning cloth to use where, how often swabs have to be changed, how disinfecting solutions are prepared correctly, how often and when disinfectants are changed and how cleaning procedures are documented after work). This applies for internal cleaning routine that is executed by production personnel as well as for external cleaning personnel. The disinfectants chosen must be able to maintain the low levels of microbial contamination pre-defined for each class of clean room, according to EU standards (see Table 5.2). According to GMP Guidelines Annex 1 section 'Sanitation', there should be a written program how the clean room areas should be cleaned. When disinfectants are used there should be at least two different types (with different modes of action) and a thorough monitoring in order to detect any resistant strains. Disinfectants and detergents should be monitored for microbial contamination; and dilutions should only be stored for defined time periods. For use in grade B and A clean rooms, disinfectants have to be sterile prior to use. All cleaning processes should be carefully documented. Following listed are some best practice measures on sampling procedures:

- Samples have to be collected before final disinfectant cleaning.
- The order of sampling is important for the generation of representative results.
- When air samples are taken in an airlock, the values for the higher grade class count.
- Air locks only need to be monitored when in 'at rest' conditions.
- When working under a laminar flow work bench, samples should be taken after production in order not to disturb the flow.
- Passive air sampling should be performed only during manufacture not when locking-in or -out or during relocation processes.
- The settle plates should be changed at least after four hours, their labeling is very important as more plates per sampling point are possible.
- In class 'A', settle plates should be changed at least every two hours or when a change of product occurs.
- Validating how long settle plates can stay open without drying out is necessary.
- The room samples should be taken from frequently used places like handles or switches.
- If any microbial growth occurs on sample plates taken in class A or B zones, their identification *via* an external lab might be helpful to identify the source.
- Morphology and appearance of detected micro-organisms should be documented.
- Additionally, every six month the resident/environmental spectrum of micro-organisms should be monitored.

5.3.1.7 *Personnel hygiene and health control of personnel*

People entering a clean room should apply high standards of personal hygiene and cleanliness. Any health condition with a risk of shedding an abnormal number of particles (e.g., cough, flu, influenza, but also skin diseases like atopic dermatitis), should be reported and personnel have to be trained on health conditions which put the manufactured products at risk. Periodic health checks for such conditions are desirable, but independent of these everybody entering the clean room is obligated to give notice of critical health conditions to a responsible person (e.g., the Head of Production) who decides if working in the clean area is possible or not. Personnel with potential to introduce undue microbiological hazard (e.g., after traveling to exotic countries but also after suffering from infectious diseases like abdominal influenza, diarrhea, pneumonia, or viral hepatitis) should be extra checked before working in the clean room areas again. Generally, health conditions that in principle or temporarily prohibit working in the clean room have to be pre-defined. Company physicians (who are bound to medical confidentiality) should perform initial health checks on personnel who are designated to work in the clean rooms. Whenever it is unclear whether working in the clean area is permissible, they should be consulted as well. As consultation of a company physician is not possible for external staff (e.g., service technicians), these persons should at least be advised of critical health conditions that would prevent their entry to the clean rooms and they should be asked to confirm that no such health conditions currently do exist. This should be documented and be part of the contract.

Personnel can have substantial impact on the quality of the environment in which the sterile product is processed, thus he should be trained in detail how to minimize pollution of the clean room areas by complying with the required measures like hand washing, disinfection of hands and gloves in defined clean room areas. A hygiene master plan is necessary to coordinate all different kinds of hygienic procedures. A vigilant and responsive personnel monitoring program should be established. Monitoring should be accomplished by obtaining surface samples of each aseptic processing operator's gloves, accompanied by an appropriate sampling frequency for other strategically selected locations of the gown (e.g., arm, waist) that might give additional information. A 10-finger touch plate should be taken from personnel working in grade A and/or B areas after finishing the production process. The quality control unit should establish a more comprehensive monitoring program for personnel involved in especially labor intensive operations. Maintenance of contamination-free gloves throughout operations is crucial for manufacturing personnel involved in the aseptic processing. When operators exceed established levels or show an adverse trend, an investigation should be conducted promptly. Follow-up actions may include increased sampling frequency, increased observation, retraining of personnel, gowning re-qualification, and if necessary, reassignment of the operator to processes outside of the aseptic manufacturing area. Microbiological monitoring of personnel is performed regularly *via* touch plates after finishing processes. The education of personnel is of great importance because only when it is clear how important these high standards are, especially in regard to patient safety, the standards will be followed rigorously. The involved personnel must be highly qualified, continuously trained and GMP proficient.[7]

5.3.2 *Equipments and premises*

As already mentioned above, all surfaces as well as all instruments and devices installed in a clean room have to be smooth, impervious, and unbroken in order to reduce particle shedding or accumulation and to facilitate repeated applications of cleaning agents and disinfectants. According to EU GMP Guidelines Annex 1, conveyor belts should not connect A/B grade areas with areas of lower air cleanliness, except when the belt is sterilized continuously. Operation, maintenance, and repair of equipments should be carried out outside the clean area where possible. Special requirements for water of appropriate quality should be fulfilled and every system or equipment used should be validated and routinely maintained and only used after approval. Production should take place in areas connected in a logical order. Equipments and materials should be positioned orderly and logical to avoid confusion between different medicinal products, cross-contamination and to minimize the risk of omission or wrong application.[9]

Shedding of particles is an issue whenever instruments have condensers and air coolers as they not only are known to generate particles but also might interfere with the clean room's airflow. Custom-made housing or water cooled instruments might help in these cases, if available (e.g., refrigerators, centrifuges). As housed instruments might need a connection to the HVAC system and water cooled instruments need water connection, their installation has to be planned as early as possible, and retrofitting in many cases is not possible or involves considerable costs and effort. Apart from the principle suitability of operating instruments in a clean room environment, critical parameters have to be monitored independently (e.g., temperature of refrigerators or incubators), since standard laboratory instruments are not equipped with such additional sensors. Often it is especially difficult to find adequate cell culture incubators as they not only have to fulfill the above mentioned requirements, but in addition carry an inherent risk of microbial contamination since they are thought to provide warm and humid conditions — an ideal environment for micro–organisms. There exist numerous examples of cell culture incubators of different types with all different features, but it is almost impossible to find one that fulfills the necessary demands for clean room equipments. One solution with respect to particle shedding is to encase an incubator into a custom made containment and thus decrease the amount of shed particles.

Another general problem is the lack of qualified providers as most companies in the cell therapy field equip and supply research labs with significantly lower demands. The manufacturer of the cell therapy product thus has to work together closely with the provider in order to establish all required qualification documents. Risk analysis and documentation of 'user requirement specifications' that precisely define all necessary details of the requested equipment, play a pivotal role and might be even more important for inexperienced vendors as they are for specialized pharma suppliers. Offer and functional specification of potential suppliers have to be checked carefully. Whenever custom-made equipment or adaptions, and adjustments of standard equipment are necessary, there is an increased risk since prototypes are generated in this way. Mock-up and factory acceptance tests might be required in these cases together with full scale qualification procedures including an extensive process qualification phase. Coming back to the above mentioned example of cell culture incubators, acquisition and initiation of a housed, self-autoclaving, low particulate incubator with independent monitoring of carbon dioxide and temperature, operated with sterile water together with a high monitoring frequency for contamination control, require extensive planning and documentation.

5.3.3 Storage rooms and warehouses

Chapter 3 of the GMP Guidelines contains general principles for storage areas, whereas the WHO Guide to good storage practices for pharmaceuticals gives more special guidance on the topic. Additional helpful advice can be found in the question and answer document mentioned in Section 5.4.10 (Transport and Shipping).

Storage areas should be of sufficient capacity to allow orderly storage of the various categories of materials and products: Starting and packaging materials, intermediate, bulk and finished products, products in quarantine, and released, rejected, returned or recalled items. Storage areas should be designed or adapted to ensure good storage conditions. In particular, they should be clean and dry and maintained within acceptable temperature limits. Where special storage conditions are required (e.g., temperature, humidity), these should be provided, checked, and monitored. Records should be maintained of these conditions, if they are critical for the maintenance of material characteristics. This monitoring is a very important task and has to be performed after careful consideration of possible influences on the system, like weather conditions or power failures. In order to find critical points like this, a so called mapping of rooms and cooling devices has to be performed including a possibly complete list of worst case scenarios. Large refrigerators and walk-in cold rooms should be monitored with a temperature-recording in one or more locations, depending on the size of the unit. Records should be checked daily and the system should include alarms that are triggered when critical temperatures are reached. Upon installation of a cooling device, the internal air temperature distribution should be mapped in the empty and full state, and afterwards under conditions of normal use. The opening of doors in order to remove items from an appropriate device should be simulated, too. Products should not be stored in areas shown by temperature mapping to present a risk (e.g., in the airflow from the cooling unit). All warehouses should be temperature mapped to determine the temperature distribution under extremes of external temperature (winter or summer). Mapping should be repeated regularly and after any significant modification to the premises or the HVAC system.

Receiving and dispatch bays should protect materials and products from the weather. Reception areas should be designed and equipped to allow containers of incoming materials to be cleaned, where necessary before storage. Where quarantine status is ensured by storage in separate areas, the physical quarantine should give equivalent security. There should normally be a separate sampling area for starting materials. If sampling is performed in the storage area, it should be conducted in such a way as to prevent contamination or cross-contamination. Segregated areas should be provided for the storage of rejected, recalled or returned materials or products. Highly active materials or products should be stored in safe and secure areas. Printed packaging materials are considered critical to the conformity of the medicinal product and hence special attention should be paid to the safe and secure storage of these materials.[9]

Detailed written instructions that define the route of materials and records should be available, which document all activities in the storage areas including the handling of expired stock. Permanent information should exist for each stored material or product indicating recommended storage conditions, any precautions to be observed and retest dates. Description of the goods, quality, quantity, supplier, supplier's batch number, the date of receipt, assigned batch number and the expiry date, pharmacopoeial requirements, and current national regulations concerning labels and containers should be respected at all times. Requirements for containers and adequate and sufficient labeling are also addressed. Inspection of incoming containers for possible contamination, tampering and damage, and if necessary, quarantine for further investigation, as well as the sampling for testing and quarantine storage until release by appropriate person, and also measures to ensure that rejected materials cannot be used, should be instructed and documented. Stock rotation and control of obsolete and outdated products, return regulations for goods, product recall and dispatch and transport are also addressed.[11] Unless there is an alternative system to prevent the unintentional or unauthorized use of quarantined, rejected, returned, or recalled materials, separate storage areas should be assigned for their temporary storage until the decision as to their future use has been taken.[12]

When working with cell-based products, apart from the final product, also media components like platelet lysate, growth factors, certain antibiotics, etc. have to be stored in frozen conditions (-20, $-80°C$ or lower than $-140°C$). For the activity at room temperature, it is of great importance that these items are stored according to the requested storage conditions. The freezers have to be strictly monitored and any deviation in the temperature profile detected should be discussed for further usability of the dedicated product. In case of a cell-based product, the final containment has to be suitable for those temperatures and the product itself must maintain its viability after freeze–thawing. Storage of cell products needs to be organized in a way to avoid any mistaken of identities. Starting material derived from living species needs to be handled at appropriate temperatures and the storage should be at room temperature or at $4°C$, until processing is validated, as this can have great impact on the product quality.

The authorities ask for accurate and durable labeling of the medicinal product (see Section 5.4.9 'Labeling'). With standard infusion bags this is easily manageable as they are provided with an extra labeling bag, but for smaller samples frozen in vials one has to prove by validation that the labeling is permanent under the storage conditions. Readily validated labeling tags are available from different providers.[13]

5.3.4 *Qualification of clean rooms*

General information on how qualification is performed including user requirement specification, risk analysis, design qualification (DQ), installation qualification (IQ), operational qualification (OQ), performance qualification (PQ), and risk quantification (RQ) can be found in the Quality Management (QM) chapter. For the qualification of a clean room, it might not be very practicable to strictly separate each of the elements of a qualification process, but according to Annex 15 of the EU GMP Guidelines, it is required that after each qualification step, at least a formal decision is taken whether the next qualification phase can commence.[14] Documentation has to occur in the right order and if one stage does not fulfill the required tasks,

Table 5.3: Tests performed for clean room qualification and required time intervals for their performance according to EN ISO 14644-1.

Type of Test	Requirement	Maximum Time Interval
Clean room classification (particle measurement)	mandatory	Six months for grade A and B ($\leq$ISO 5.0)
		12 months for grade C and D ($>$ISO 5.0)
Airflow volume or airflow velocity	mandatory	12 months
Air pressure difference	mandatory	12 months
Installed filter leakage	optional	24 months for all terminal filters
Airflow visualization	optional	24 months for all classes
Recovery	optional	24 months for all classes
Containment leakage	optional	24 months for all classes

the following element cannot be assessed. The qualification of a clean room is a very important issue because it is a prerequisite to GMP compatible manufacturing (Table 5.3). It includes classification measurements, recovery tests (particle counter), flow measurements, differential pressure measurements, filter tests, tightness and leakage air in air ventilation ducts, flow visualization, visual inspection, determining air change rate, recovery time, and microbiological monitoring. Qualification can be performed on a daily basis, weekly, monthly or per year, dependent on the potential risk associated with deviations of a certain parameter. The frequency is thus part of the risk assessment. Test measures are explained in EN ISO 14644-3 which defines, for example, the places where samples have to be taken and which volume of air has to be analyzed.

For classification purposes of grade A clean room zones, a sample volume of at least $1\,\text{m}^3$ per sampling point has to be chosen. Extrapolating values obtained from smaller sample volumes is not permitted. The minimum sample volume for the other clean room grades has to be calculated according to EN ISO 14644-1 by the means of the following equation:

$$V_s = \frac{20}{C_{n,m}} \times 1,000$$

V_s is the minimum single sample volume per location, expressed in litres. $C_{n,m}$ is the class limit (number of particles per cubic meter) for the largest considered particle size specified for the relevant class (for grade A the largest particle size to be considered is $\geq 5.0\mu\text{m}$ with a class limit of 20). 20 is the defined number of samples that could be counted if the particle concentration were at the class limit.

The higher the class limit (maximum permitted number of particles of the largest considered size), the lower is the required sample volume per location. But independent of the above mentioned equation, EN ISO 14644 defines that the volume sampled at each location has to be at least two liters, with a minimum sampling time of one minute at each location.

In Europe, the consideration of particle sizes equal to or greater than 0.5 and 5.0 μm is sufficient also for classification (qualification) purposes. In addition to the required sample volumes, EN ISO 14644-1 defines the methodology for classification including the minimum number of sampling points per room that depends on the size (area) of the room and has to be calculated according to the following equation:

$$N_L = \sqrt{A}$$

NL is the minimum number of sampling locations (rounded up to a whole number).

A is the area of the clean room in square metres.

EN ISO 14644-1 furthermore gives advice for the assessment of the collected data. Defined by the limit value for particles $\geq 5.0\ \mu$m, GMP clean room grade A complies with a classification of ISO 4.8, whereas the limit for particles $\geq 0.5\ \mu$m corresponds to ISO 5.0. Limit values for all other clean room grades (B, C, and D) each correspond with the limit values defined by one of the EN ISO 14644 classes. As Annex 1 to the EU GMP Guidelines differentiates between 'in operation' and 'at rest' conditions and sets different limit values, clean room grades B, C, and D correspond to different ISO classes, depending on the defined condition. For both particle sizes in grade B, the 'at rest' condition corresponds to ISO 5.0, whereas the 'in operation' condition corresponds to ISO 7.0. Grade C clean rooms correspond to ISO 7.0 for the 'at rest' condition and ISO 8.0 for the 'in operation' condition. Finally grade D corresponds to ISO 8.0 for the 'at rest' condition, whereas an 'in operation' condition (at least for airborne particles) is not defined.

5.3.5 *Qualification of equipments*

General information on how qualification is performed including user requirement specification, risk analysis, DQ, IQ, OQ, PQ, and RQ can be found in the QM chapter.

The requirements for the qualification of equipments used in a clean room depend on the influence of the relevant device/machine on the manufactured product. According to its influence on the manufacturing process, the qualification procedure can be adapted and be more or less extensive. For example, the qualification of a welding device would not have the same qualification scope as for the qualification of a FACS machine. Therefore, it is almost impossible to give general advice on how instruments have to be qualified. It is often helpful to use documents offered by the manufacturers of the equipments, but these documents have to be checked carefully and it should be stipulated that corrections and amendments are possible before the qualification starts, as the head of production is responsible and thus has to sign the qualification plan. Furthermore, a qualification must be based on a thorough risk analysis that in most cases is not offered along with the qualification documents. A further weak point in commercially available qualification documents is that acceptance criteria are often insufficiently or not at all defined and that it is therefore unclear when the qualification is successful. This is especially difficult when acceptable ranges for measured values are missing. Some providers offer qualification documents that for financial reasons should fit all different types of instruments and cover all possible options offered by the provider. In these cases, it often is not clear which tests actually have to be performed and which are not applicable to the equipment that should be qualified. This is not acceptable for a GMP compliant qualification plan. Also documentation of the executed qualification work is sometimes an issue, as not all providers have equally well trained personnel, and documentation therefore does not always follow the GMP rules. How the work has to be documented and how raw data have to be handled should therefore be part of the qualification plan. Additionally, it is strongly recommended to accompany the work or at least review the documents before the qualification personnel leaves.

Altogether commercially available pre-defined qualification documents can be an option — and are sometimes even compulsory, since highly engineered instruments cannot be qualified without the assistance of the instrument's provider and his specialized service technicians, but a thorough survey is mandatory.

5.3.6   *Isolator technique for ATMP manufacturing*

As mentioned above, the running costs for maintenance of a grade A/B clean room facility are very high and are a limiting factor, especially for smaller companies and academic centers. Additionally, working under A in B clean room conditions is challenging for the personnel due to the constricting clothing and the time consuming processes of locking in and out. Using isolator technology, the surrounding clean room area can be downgraded to class D (ISO 8.0) leading to reduction of costs and working time. Additionally, it could decrease human interventions in processing areas and thus microbiological contaminations could be minimized.

Different models of isolators exist, ranging from single use isolators to half-suit isolators. Parts of the isolator are prone to puncture and represent a risk for sterile manufacturing. For dedicated handlings, the inserted gloves can be too unhandy and the radius one can reach around is limited, too. Isolators are often purpose-built items that are constructed for one individual process and thus are not flexible for process changes. Starting an isolator for a process is time consuming and normally becomes economical only when high numbers of a well-defined product are manufactured, which is normally not the case for cell-based medicines. Isolators are well established tools in the production of chemotherapeutic drugs.[15] and manufacture of total parenteral nutrition. To establish an isolator in a clean room D environment is possible and might reduce costs, but when working with cellular components, one has to face the problem that jumping from D to A environment means skipping two clean room classes. This can only be made possible by sterilizing entering goods or at least undergo thorough disinfection which is not or hardly possible for cellular products. Validating the presence of zero surface micro-organisms seems to be very difficult when working with cells. Another difficulty when working with isolators in the ATMP surrounding is the incoming product. A gas permissible transfusion bag containing the patient material should not be wiped with alcohol and thus cannot be transferred as GMP compliant into the grade A working zone of the isolator.

Currently Isolators are not fully established in ATMP manufacturing for human use.

5.4 Manufacturing/Production

According to the German Drug Law (AMG Sec. 4 Paragraph 14), Manufacturing is defined as producing, preparing, formulating, treating or processing, filling as well as decanting, packaging, labeling, and release of medicinal products.[16]

The basic requirement for the manufacturing of ATMPs is a manufacturing license from the competent authority, independent of the fact whether the product is an IMP used within a clinical trial or an approved medicinal product with MA. In Germany, this permission is granted by the regional authority responsible for GMP licensing in collaboration with the national authority [Paul Ehrlich Institute (PEI), Federal Institute for Vaccines and biomedicines]. The conduction of the manufacturing process not only has to follow the requirements given by the GMP Guidelines but has also to be in accordance with the details given in the MA (where existing) or in the IMP dossier (IMPD). For manufacturing and application of an IMP, an independent body (review board or ethic committee), constituted of medical professionals and non-medical members is mandatory. It is their responsibility to ensure the protection of the rights, safety and well-being of human subjects involved in a trial and to provide public assurance of that protection. Furthermore, the principles and guidelines of good clinical practice (GCP) should be adhered to when conducting clinical trials on IMPs (Directive 2005/28/EC).

ATMP differ significantly from conventional medicinal products due to their complexity and diverse structural and biological properties. Thus their handling and their testing needs to be adapted to this fact. Aspects like cell heterogeneity, stability, identity, purity, viability, potency, persistence and integration into the recipient organism, absence of microbiological contaminants and potential tumorigenicity in the product itself have to be considered and addressed when manufacturing ATMP (compare also chapter 'Quality Control').

Autologous *versus* allogeneic products: Two scenarios for clinical applications can be differentiated: The patient receives a cell product originating from his own cells or tissue (autologous) and in the second case; the patient receives a cell product derived from another person (allogeneic). Allogeneic products can be either directed, originating from a donor who is human leukocyte antigen (HLA)-matched to the recipient (as established for HSC-based medicinal products) or non-directed (third party), where donor and recipient do not have to be matched and products can be prepared in advance (off the shelf products). In the manufacturing of autologous and directed allogeneic cell therapy products, each product batch represents a unique donor with a unique health status. Additionally to the individual donor characteristics, differences between tissue sources and in the isolation techniques may create significant product variability, especially in the autologous setting. This fact makes the following manufacturing process not completely predictable in terms of cell growth or final yield and requires a very stable and robust production process including critical in-process controls to ensure batch to batch consistency. Autologous and directed allogeneic cell products require a well-defined coordination of the concerned patient and clinicians, donation of starting material, the manufacturing process and eventually the application. Very important is the availability of manufacturing slots at any time a patient is in need for a cell product. Usually one batch will be manufactured per patient and cost of goods including individual release testing can be very high. With the use of allogeneic third party cell products that can be cryopreserved and therefore stored over longer time periods, manufacturing will get more projectable, as the processing of starting material can be precisely scheduled and is independent of the recipient. Cost of goods may be considerably lower, as usually a higher number of doses for several patients can be manufactured within a batch and release testing is done per batch.

The nature of cell products precludes terminal sterilization. Therefore, the highest standards of aseptic manufacturing need to be maintained throughout the entire manufacturing process, especially where manipulations are performed in open systems. Cell-based therapies gain more and more importance within the market of biopharmaceutical products. Among these therapies, stem cell-based therapies are investigated elaborately.[17]

Mesenchymal stem cells (MSCs) are one of the widely used and well-characterized cells in the field of ATMP. They can be isolated from different sources as bone marrow, adipose tissue or cord blood and can be cultivated and expanded *in vitro*. They exert anti-proliferative, immunomodulatory, and anti-inflammatory effects and have the capacity to differentiate into several tissues (chondrocytes, adipocytes, and osteocytes, etc.) with the latter being a property that becomes very important in regard to their ability for tissue repair. Additionally they promote hematopoietic cell expansion and differentiation through secretion of growth factors and cytokines. MSC additionally have the nature to migrate to sites of injured or inflamed tissue. Therefore, mesenchymal stromal/stem cells exhibit great potential for cell therapies with around 350 registered clinical trials on MSC-based products found in the ClinicalTrials.gov database (as of May 2014). Many completed trials demonstrated the safety and efficacy of MSC-based cell therapies. A recommended minimal therapeutic dose of MSC applied in clinical trials is approximately 1×10^6 MSC/kg of the recipient's body weight. In an autologous setting for individual patient doses, this is a manageable amount of cells for a standard laboratory scale but when translating to allogeneic multiple doses, the process has to be scaled up to an effective and robust process.[18−20]

EU GMP Guidelines Annex 2 gives detailed guidance on the manufacture of biological active substances and medicinal products for human use. In case the ATMP is intended to be used in clinical trials, Annex 13 of the EU GMP Guidelines and in Germany, the Sixth part of the German drug law (AMG), regarding the safety of the patient participating in the trial becomes relevant (Sections 40–42 AMG, GCP Art. 1 Paragraph 3 of guideline 2001/20/EG). Clinical trials in Europe are regulated nationally by each individual member state. In Germany, clinical trials can only be conducted with permission from the national competent authority, the local authorities responsible for the manufacturing authorization and a positive vote of the responsible ethics committee. Finally, for MA, a centralized MA is needed by the EMA.

Manufacturing of cell-based medicinal products always starts with the procurement of starting material. In the following sub-sections, the workflow from the isolation and enrichment of the target cells to their culturing and/or genetic modification is described. This chapter also provides information on final cryopreservation and storage as well as labeling, transport and finally on site preparation and administration to the patient. Furthermore, examples of approved ATMP (one of each class) and their manufacturing are listed.

In all cases, the primary material has to be released for further use in the manufacturing process and infectious diseases of the donor must be excluded, according to the applicable guidelines. The donation center may form part of the manufacturing license of the manufacturing unit or dispose of an own license covering the requirements (qualification of the operating room) for tissue or blood-derived products.

5.4.1 *Primary human cells as starting material for ATMP production*

Manufacturing of ATMPs must be fully GMP-compliant with a rigorous GMP quality control. This already starts with the selection of a donor and the procurement of starting materials and continues to the release of the final product by a Qualified Person (QP) or Quality Unit (QU) in the US. The GMP Guidelines claim that when available only authorized medicinal products or CE marked (European Conformity) medicinal devices should be used for manufacturing of ATMPs. Human cells or animal cells (used for virus production) imply a potential risk of contamination with adventitious agents. The control and test measures for such starting material should be based on Quality Risk Management (QRM) principles. Also other impurities and the potential cross-contamination dependent on the type of cells or viral vectors should be addressed to minimise risk during manufacturing, cleaning, and packaging. Local or when possible international safety measures should be applied and controls implemented according to the biological hazard class to guarantee recipients' and staff's safety.[8]

While GMP grade virus supernatant can be received from selected providers, the situation for fresh primary cells and tissues is more complicated. The access to starting material which is processed as a clinical grade pharmaceutical product according to GMP principles is one of the most pivotal and crucial parts of the entire manufacturing process and is usually embedded in the required manufacturing license issued by the responsible competent authorities. Tissues and cells are complex and delicate active substances. They are dependent on the environment they are exposed to and might even be reactive to it. Individual donor characteristics are responsible for significant differences in the properties of the starting material, for example the cell count of nucleated cells in bone marrow with a range of $5 \times 10^3/\mu$ l–$30 \times 10^3/\mu$ l.

Human tissues and cells that are used as starting material for a cell-based medicinal product must comply with the quality and safety requirements of the EUTCD including directives 2004/23/EC, 2006/17/EC, and 2006/86/EC [see Introduction (Section 5.1) and chapter 'Quality Control') with respect to their donation, procurement, and testing. In the case human blood or blood components are used as starting material for cell-based medicinal products, European Directives 2002/98/EC and 2004/33/EC are defining standards of quality and safety for the collection, testing, processing, storage and distribution. Further details for the procurement and testing of material of human origin are given in chapter 'Quality Control'.

Manufacturing and authorization of an ATMP involves a variety of different legislations. For cell-based medicinal products, the cell-containing starting material originates from a donor or patient and additional regulations are involved. The required quality standards in Europe are mainly defined by the above mentioned directives that had to be transferred into national legislation leading to slightly different rules and regulations in each individual European member state. The German regulatory landscape for blood, tissues and cells is particularly complex as blood, blood components, and certain types of cells (including peripheral blood stem cells) are regulated as conventional medicinal products that have to fully comply with the GMP Guidelines, whereas tissues (including bone marrow) can be handled under facilitated conditions [so called Good Professional Practice (GFP) instead of GMP] that allow the performance of open steps under A in D clean room conditions and other alleviations. Following this differentiation, facilities collecting blood, blood components, and certain types of cells require a conventional manufacturing authorization in Germany, whereas procurement of tissues requires a special type of tissue authorization. It has to be emphasized that the relieved GFP conditions for tissue procurement and processing in Germany are only applicable as long as the tissues are not processed using industrial procedures and the essential processing procedures are sufficiently well known in the European Union. Otherwise a company would have to apply for a conventional manufacturing authorization with the obligation to strictly follow the GMP rules. How exactly blood, blood components, tissues and cells have to be handled and which regulations have to be followed in different European member states should be evaluated carefully during process development, especially when the provider of the starting material is located in a different European member state than the manufacturer of the cellular product.

As soon as cells and tissues that serve as starting material arrive at the manufacturer of the cell-based medicinal product for all subsequent processing steps a manufacturing authorization is required and the GMP Guidelines have to be followed strictly as according to Regulation (EC) No 1394/2007 on ATMPs, since GMP principles are binding for the manufacture of ATMPs in whole Europe.

Regarding the starting material for producing an ATMP, it has to be considered that often the desired type of cells and/or tissues is not readily available in GMP grade or otherwise sufficient quality. If a facility specialized in the procurement of tissues and/or cells with the respective manufacturing license exists, the manufacturer of the cell-based medicinal product might be able to receive GMP grade cells or tissues released by a QP of the donation facility and can proceed from there with the starting material. If this is not the case, the availability of starting material in sufficient and defined quality is more difficult. In these cases, technical agreements and audits are essential to guarantee the desired level of quality. This agreement or contract should contain details on the type of tissue, procurement procedure, blood samples for donor testing, documentation, storage (e.g., container, labeling, and quarantine), transport (validated conditions), hand-out to the manufacturer, and audits and notification requirements. In such a case, the procurement facility has to commit to the defined quality standards and is supervised by the manufacturer and the competent authorities. The manufacturer of the cell-based medicinal product has to apply for the procurement authorization and in this special case the site at which the material is procured is included in his manufacturing license. The manufacturer is responsible for training of the personnel and all required documentation at the procurement site. In this scenario, it is of great importance that the QM system of the manufacturer sufficiently involves the donation site and the relevant laboratory responsible for donor testing. For the procurement of starting materials like, e.g., bone marrow or adipose tissue, the according operating rooms cannot offer clean room grades as defined in Annex 1 to the EU GMP Guidelines, therefore it is of great importance that the according standard specifications (e.g., DIN standard1946-4 "Ventilation in buildings and rooms of health care" amongst others in Germany) are met and controlled and that the necessary hygiene instructions (e.g., thorough local disinfection and disinfection of hands) are fulfilled. Detailed risk assessments, especially at the interface of manufacturer, procurement facility and laboratory, are mandatory. All documents have to be taught and it is necessary that change control and deviation procedures cover all contract partners.

5.4.2 *Isolation and selection of target cells for ATMP manufacturing*

5.4.2.1 *Procurement of starting material*

When using material of human origin in order to generate a desired type of cells, different sources may be used. The sources of starting material are as diverse as the multiplicity of products generated from them. Among cell-based therapies those using MSCs gain more and more attention. These cells can be collected and expanded from different sources like adipose tissue, umbilical cords, placentas, or bone marrow.[21] The methods to receive the desired material range from simple clipping it off (e.g., umbilical cord after birth), to puncturing a bone with a syringe (bone marrow extraction), and to suction of hypoderm adipose tissue up to the point of minor surgery procedures (e.g., cartilage extraction). A typical method to receive a broad variety of blood cells and blood components is the so called apheresis, which is described in more detail here due to its large field of applications.

Blood derived cells can be easily obtained *via* apheresis, an extracorporeal, medical technology in which a person's blood is lead into an apparatus that separates the different blood components by centrifugal forces. It removes the desired components and then returns the remaining blood back into the donor's blood circulation. The blood can be separated into plasma, leukocytes, platelets, and erythrocytes and the technique is widely used for the production of erythrocyte and platelet concentrates used in transfusion medicine. Leukapheresis is a specific type of apheresis where white blood cells are separated from whole blood. Depending on what kind of cells should be isolated, the underlying protocol of the apheresis and also the specific apheresis device is of great importance. Some cell types are more susceptible to sheer stress during centrifugation than others and often a couple of test runs have to be performed in order to find the most suitable program for the intended cell type. A special case is the mobilized apheresis for the procurement of enriched HSC products. The donor needs pretreatment by a granulocyte colony-stimulating factor (G-CSF) administration. After three to five days of treatment, the leucocyte number is significantly augmented and the hematopoietic progenitor cells (surrogate marker CD34+ fraction) are enriched in the peripheral blood. Both products (non-mobilized and mobilized peripheral blood) are currently used as starting material. Enrichment for mononuclear cells or "buffy-coat" is also applied. Apheresis machines as well as the necessary equipments for cell collection (apheresis set and transfusion bags) are licensed medicinal devices (CE-certified in Europe). Apheresis sets are available as sterile, disposable plastic material in high quality.

Disinfection of the skin following defined and validated procedures is mandatory to prevent microbial contamination of the apheresis product. The introduction of pre-collection sampling, where the first few milliliters of the blood donation are separated in an extra bag, helped to further reduce contamination rates. For the isolation of HSCs from peripheral blood (PBSC), donors need to be mobilized with G-CSF or other drugs that facilitate production and migration of HSCs from the bone marrow to the PBSC. From an ethical point of view mobilization procedures are critical, as they put the donor to an additional risk regarding potential adverse events caused by the mobilization drug. In these cases, a reduced process validation program might be accepted by the competent authorities, as it would be highly unethical to put voluntary donors at risk for the mere reason of data collection. This should be discussed with the authorities early in process development.

It should be mentioned that the composition of the starting material is not standardized and homogenous due to donor's characteristics, but also due to different protocols and devices used. This is relevant when manufacturing involving one qualified donor facility is extended to multiple donor sites. The diversity of the starting material may pose the process at risk and it should be considered that donor centers apply to the standards applicable for patient care, which do not necessarily reflect the needs of a pharmaceutical grade starting material. As an example for HSC collection, only the minimum required dose of progenitors is defined but the composition of most of the other cellular components is determined.

5.4.2.2 *Processing of starting material*

As soon as the starting material is further processed, a manufacturing license becomes mandatory. The mostly heterogeneic starting material is treated in order to receive a more or less pure population of a certain type of cells. These isolated cells can then be directly used or further processed. Processing can range from mere expansion, to differentiation or even genetic modification (see Section 5.4.3). Certain types of cells (e.g., MSC) can be simply isolated with high purity due to their property to adhere to cell culture vessels. Cells growing non-adherently can be removed easily *via* consecutive steps of medium exchange. If no such simple isolation or selection steps are possible, there are a number of other possibilities that can be used. The most common ones are described below.

5.4.2.2.1 Density gradient centrifugation

A standard procedure for separating blood into its main components is density gradient centrifugation *via* high molecular weight polysaccharide solutions such as Ficoll® (a trademark of GE Healthcare). Ficoll® is part of Ficoll-Paque® that is designed to prepare human mononuclear cells from peripheral blood, bone marrow, or umbilical cord blood *via* density gradient centrifugation. It is commonly used and available in GMP grade quality. Ficoll-Paque® is placed at the bottom of a centrifuge tube and topped with the collected blood. After centrifugation different layers are visible in the conical tube. Erythrocytes and granulocytes are centrifuged to the bottom of the tube to form a pellet, above which the Ficoll-Paque® layer is located. On top of the Ficoll® layer, resides a thin layer of mono–nuclear cells (MNCs) or peripheral blood mononuclear cells (PBMCs) called 'buffy coat'. The MNC-layer is covered with plasma and other blood constituents. The separation *via* Ficoll® allows an easy harvest of PBMCs, as the desired layer can be taken off with a pipette or syringe. As the procedure takes place in an open system, A in B clean-room conditions are required.

5.4.2.2.2 Mechanical break-up

Cells which are part of a more solid tissue will first need to be separated from other cells and connective tissues. Sometimes this can be performed chemically by simply chelating the environment (removing Ca^{2+}- and/or Mg^{2+}-ions), but in most instances the cells will need to be enzymatically (e.g., by collagenase or trypsin) or mechanically disaggregated. Proteases can be used for the disruption of the extracellular matrix to release cells from tissues which can then be seeded for primary cell culture. Another possibility is the mechanical disruption of the tissues with the use of blenders, mortars and pestles, so called bead mill homogenization or *via* mere mincing and sieving. These procedures often result in changes to the cells and commonly cell–cell communication *via*, e.g., tight junctions will be disrupted. The shear force must be controlled carefully in order not to destroy the whole fraction of cells. These procedures have to be standardized which becomes almost impossible when they are performed manually. After homogenizing mechanically or enzymatically, cells can be further isolated or enriched by different antibody-dependent methods (see examples below).

5.4.2.2.3 Magnetic-activated cell sorting (MACS)

This method was originally developed by MiltenyiBiotec for research-based cell isolation. The desired type of cells is labeled with an antibody linked to a non-toxic, biodegradable magnetic micro bead. Cells are then applied to a column containing a ferromagnetic matrix. The column is situated in front of a magnet. The flow-through fraction that is depleted of the labeled cells that remained in the column can be collected. After that the column is removed from the magnet and the retained cells can be eluted as the enriched, positively selected cell fraction. This research type separator was further developed for clinical applications with an almost closed system (CliniMACS® instrument) and reagents in GMP-grade quality. Labeling, centrifugation and washing steps are performed in blood bags that can be connected to waste bags or buffer bags by sterile connections generated with a sterile tubing welder that remains a functionally closed system during the connecting procedure. Washing buffers are removed manually after centrifugation steps with the help of plasma extractors. As centrifugation of bags has to be performed without using the centrifuge brakes in order not to disrupt the pellet and as the Clini-MACS® programs use more intensive washing as well as repeated removal and reapplication steps to the separation column, the whole procedure lasts significantly longer compared to the research protocol. This has to be kept in mind especially if two subsequent enrichment or depletion protocols or a combination of both should be used. As the standard CliniMACS® procedures use phosphate buffered saline containing EDTA, the obtained cell preparation is not suitable for clinical application. Complete exchange of buffer is mandatory for the final formulation in these cases.

Cells isolated, (pre-) enriched or depleted with MACS technology are generally not considered to be substantially manipulated and therefore in the European system are not defined as ATMPs, as long as no other manufacturing steps are applied that are thought to be substantial manipulations, such as activation steps.

MiltenyiBiotec along with the reagents, tubing set and the CliniMACS® instrument offers certified and pre-validated enrichment and depletion procedures and protocols for different types of target cells that do not need extensive process validation runs. But whenever new reagents are used or production processes are changed these steps need full process validation. If new production processes are developed in small scale research batches, linear scale-up might be difficult or even impossible as this would lead to overall volumes of several litres that cannot be processed anymore. Although the CliniMACS® system is considered to be almost completely closed using sterile docking for most production steps, there are some open steps remaining (such as injection of reagent to the cell preparation bag or connection of the buffer bag to the CliniMACS® set) that require clean room environment.

MiltenyiBiotec recently further developed the CliniMACS® instrument in order to reduce remaining open steps and therefore allow for a usage outside the clean room or at least in lower clean room grades. Thorough risk analysis together with media fill procedures will be necessary, in any case. Additionally, it will depend on the individual production steps of the used protocols and the question if they indeed do not contain any open steps. As broad experiences with the new instrument are currently still missing in line with the application for a manufacturing license, it should be discussed with the competent authorities which clean room conditions are required.

Apart from a potential down grade of the clean room environment, the new instrument is thought to additionally reduce manual handling steps due to an integrated centrifuge leading to a decrease in necessary manpower as well as to an increase in consistency. Exchange of EDTA-containing buffer can be performed as the last step of the enrichment- or depletion procedure leading to a finished product that could be used for application right away. Moreover, the centrifuge chamber (that is part of the set and therefore single use with no risk of cross-contamination) allows for additional options such as cell culture, since it can be tempered and connected to carbon dioxide.

One issue occasionally raised by the authorities is remaining antibodies and magnetic beads on the target cells of positively selected cell populations, because of possible adverse reactions when administered to the patient. Also an effect on the function of the enriched cells is conceivable due to the binding of the antibody-bead-complex. In addition, the epitopes used for selection are blocked for further processing steps or for quality control analysis. To prevent this, major histocompatibility complex (MHC) I molecules and Fab fragments have been developed to form complexes with magnetic beads that bind reversibly to the cell surface markers of interest and can be dissociated completely after the selection process.

5.4.2.2.4   FACS

FACS^{TM}, a trade mark of BD Biosciences, subsequently used as abbreviation for the technique of FACS, is an isolation technique based on fluorescence labeled antibodies. The target cell fraction can be characterized by several antigens in parallel, for which the cells are either positive or negative. This allows for the isolation of very distinct sub-populations as even discrimination between high and intermediate expression of the targeted antigen is possible. The technique provides purities of the target cell fraction of considerably over 95%. This might not be necessary for all cell-based medicinal products, but whenever it is known that non-target cells in minimal amounts would exert negative effects on the recipient, FACS is currently the only method to obtain sufficient purity for certain cell types. Also expansion of particular cell populations requires high purities whenever it is known that contaminating cells from the starting material would predominantly expand with the applied culture conditions leading to unacceptably high contamination rates in the finished product.

While FACS is a well-established method in research labs since many years, this method is so far not extensively used for manufacture of medicinal products (at least not in Europe), as fully GMP compliant instruments are currently missing. FACS is a procedure that contains open steps and therefore in Europe, grade A in B clean room conditions are required as soon as for phase I clinical trials. Furthermore, most of the instruments do not have exchangeable fluidics leading to a potential risk of cross-contamination. Since in the United States, full compliance to the GMP rules is not required for early stages of clinical trials, research instruments have been used there for phase I/II clinical trials (e.g., for sorting regulatory T-cells).[22,23] These instruments did not always use exchangeable fluidics and none of them was operated under grade A in B clean room conditions. In contrast to the US, in Europe full GMP compliance is necessary, irrespective of the stage of the clinical trial. Therefore, FACS machines for manufacture of medicinal products have to be housed to create an appropriate clean room environment together with the required particulate and microbiological monitoring. Single use fluidics kits (including all parts in immediate contact with the cells) have to be used. Extensive instrument qualification is required to prove that the manufacturing process is robust and consistent. This leads to the fact that clinical trials using FACS-sorted cells as IMP in Europe are absolutely rare to date with few exceptions.[24]

5.4.3 *Cell culture*

Cultivating cells always requires a good understanding of the biology of the cell type and its requirements with regard to their cultivation conditions. For ATMP manufacturing, the regulatory framework as well as the requirements regarding the process environment as well as the difficulties arising by that special environment should be assessed early and in great detail. Generally one can distinguish between cells growing adherently (anchorage dependent) and those growing in suspension (anchorage independent). If not working in small scale manufacturing of cell-based medicinal products (one batch, one patient), mainly in the autologous setting, manufacturing has a great need for maximization of the production lot. Adherent cells need surfaces to grow on and this normally means occupying area/space. A classical scale-up procedure for adherent cells is using cell stacks instead of conventional cell culture flasks, but of course their amount and size is limited to the available incubator space and can only be handled manually up to a certain amount.

Some primary cells require close cell to cell or cell to stimulus contact at the beginning of the cell culture; together with small overall volume of cell culture medium and thus it might be difficult to start in stacks or bags. To enable such conditions, it might be necessary to use large amounts of small compartments (e.g., well plates) in order to start the initial culture. This is labor intensive and thus not desirable, but can be essential for certain delicate cell types.

Apart from the cell culture method most regulatory authorities request antibiotic-free culture media, as antibiotics could mask microbial contamination and subsequently interfere with the method for microbiological control of the cell product or the cell culture supernatant. Therefore, culture methods in closed systems or at least with reduced steps of manual manipulation are preferable, if GMP conditions have to be met.

5.4.3.1 Adherent (anchorage dependent) cell culture and its scale-up potential

For adherent cells generally two different cultivation approaches can be differentiated:

1. Classical two-dimensional (2D), and
2. Carrier based (agitated or packed-bed) systems.

Whenever an ATMP is based on adherent cells and it comes to an up-scaling of the production lot, the difficulties will grow comparable with the desired lot size. In autologous setting or in the scale of a Phase I/Phase II trial, the manufacturing process of a 'one batch, one patient' way, is relatively easy to calculate. A typical dose of e.g., 1–2 Mio cells/kg body weight would occupy approximately 6×5 layer cell culture stacks ($19,080\,cm^2$) in one big incubator for a time period of maybe three to four weeks. Switching to one of the more advanced cell culture systems like the HYPERstack, one 36 layer stack ($18,000\,cm^2$) would be sufficient to manufacture the same amount of cells, but saving space in the incubator and man power in the lab, allowing for more units to be produced in parallel. Of course this system is further scalable but manual processing time and resources are limiting. Also a linear increase of cell harvest in direct correlation to the seeding surface is not realistic and culture conditions may have to be adapted (medium exchange, gas supply). But as soon as larger number of patients (e.g., Phase III trial) will be included, autologous 'one batch, one patient' manufacturing will become more and more unmanageable (time and space consuming) and the manufacturer has to think of switching to an allogeneic manufacturing process. By doing so, the culturing platform of a classical 2D system has to be most surely be replaced by a more efficient carrier-based bioreactor system where one harvest generates enough cells not only for one but for a couple of patients. Or, when sticking to the 2D system the whole manufacturing facility, quality control personnel and/or the timeline for the clinical trial have to be expanded. Unfortunately, the way toward such a carrier-based system is long and rough. Titrating the perfect culture parameters like the carrier material, the perfusion rate, nutrition supply, seeding concentration, etc., is a time consuming and challenging process and up to now only a couple of ventures have the experience with that. Besides, a carrier-based system makes at least one additional quality control assay necessary — the proof that the final product is free of any carrier or carrier fragment material. A very important factor that is not easy to be accomplished. The need for an up-scaling of a cell-based therapeutic where adherent cells are applied is a very tricky and substantial process and thus needs early planning and testing in order to allow the manufacturer to keep up with the increasing batch numbers of up-coming clinical trials.

5.4.3.1.1   Classical two-dimensional cell culture

Already in the early 1920, Alexis Carrel (1873–1944) and members of his laboratory at the Rockefeller Hospital including Lillian E. Baker pioneered methods for culturing cells in glass dishes.[25] The traditional 2D culture methods to grow anchorage-dependent cell types since then have developed intensively. Nowadays there are many different suppliers available who offer a wide variety of flasks in different sizes and with different coatings that are suitable for a wide variety of cells. These culture models are well established and easy to handle but problems arise when larger amounts of cells have to be processed. The procedure is labor intensive and shows limited scale-up potential due to the restricted available growth surface area. In early 2000, scaling up of 2D cell culture systems improved a lot by introduction of cell stack technology.[26] A special space-saving version of cell culture stacks are the so called HYPERStacks® from Corning. They utilize a gas-permeable film technology and consume less space than conventional stacks. Conventional 2D systems always occupy a lot of surface area which can only partially be reduced by the utilization of cell culture stacks. Maximizing the total area and the density of the cells at harvest are the main parameters to increase lot size of planar cell culture systems. For the scale up of these 2D systems, the following applies: The larger the total surface area of the unit that has to be handled during the manufacturing process (number of layers and size of each layer), the larger the possible harvest. For scale out, one would have to use multiple of these units, but it has to be considered that the overall handling time is as short as possible in order to achieve constant and comparable results.

To make such huge cell culture approaches manageable, a number of companies developed bioreactor controls for these planar culture systems. The cells are cultured in a classical 2D way, but these systems allow continuous medium as well as oxygen and nutrient supply without manual intervention. Culture parameters like oxygen partial pressure, carbon dioxide level and pH can thus be continuously monitored. Another planar system enabling adherent cell growth under the same conditions and surfaces as in standard tissue flasks is the multilayer Xpansion® system from ATMI, but in contrary to the systems mentioned above, in this case there are multiple layers of disc shaped culture surfaces in an individually controlled compartment that regulates medium supply and can measure different culture parameters.

Closed systems are very much appreciated, whenever GMP requirements have to be fulfilled in order to minimize the risk of microbial contamination. Examples for such systems are VueLife® Cell Culture Bags which additionally allow incubation of cells without any water loss. Due to this, there is no need to use humidified incubators, a possible source for microbiological contamination.

5.4.3.1.2 Carrier-based systems

Mechanically agitated micro carrier systems are the most common devices applied as bioreactors. They are used for all kind of cell types but with different agitator designs and air sparging schemes dependent on the sensitivity to shear stress of the applied cell types. These systems are another possible scale-up solution for adherent cells. The cells are offered a huge surface area to grow on by micro carriers and thus the culture does not occupy extensive planar layers of cell culture space. The surface-area-to-volume ratio is greatly increased over traditional static culture processes. To find a suitable carrier for your special type of cells is challenging and for some types of cells these carrier system might just not work. Similar to packed-bed systems, medium supply and culture conditions can be externally controlled and as a closed system the risk of contamination is also reduced.

One important factor of such agitated carrier-based bioreactors is the shear stress caused by the traditionally used impellers that have to be controlled closely because some cells (e.g., stem cells) are susceptible to spontaneous differentiation under such conditions.[27] Alternatives to traditional impeller-based stirred tank systems are air wheel driven systems with reduced shear forces, or the use of so called wave bioreactors (GE Healthcare) that use rocking motion to agitate the cell suspension in a single-use bag.[28] Another drawback of these systems is the lack of a reliable scheme to separate cells from medium during medium exchange. With a carrier-based system, it has to be guaranteed that the cells are efficiently removed from the carrier for harvesting and that no carrier fragments remain in the final product. Realizing this is a very challenging step but a prerequisite for possible clinical applications.

Packed-bed culture systems contain more or less porous carrier substrate e.g., glass or ceramic beads or polyester fibre with polypropylene disk Fibra-Cel® (available in GMP compliant quality) in a so called packed bed with a supply compartment that enables recirculation of the culture medium through the bed. Packed-bed bioreactors (PBRs) are suitable for adherent as well as for non-adherent cells. The cells are immobilized on, or even in the substrate and thus an extremely high surface area to volume ratio can be achieved resulting in high densities of cells per volume. The cells can be grown post confluence. Packed beds can be supplied with external or internal recirculation of nutrient medium. To find a suitable matrix for the cell of interest that allows for proliferation and productivity is a challenging and often time consuming process. All other operational parameters like the height and volume of the packed bed; medium perfusion rate and linear velocity of the medium across the packed bed have to be tested extensively at laboratory-scale before up-scaling is possible. The set up allows for real-time control of diverse cell culture parameters like pH and oxygen saturation.[29] Packed-bed systems so far are primarily used for the production of secreted products like proteins and antibodies. The cultivated cells secret their product into the medium, from where it can be easily harvested *via* a syringe. But cultivating adherent cells in PBR for maximizing cell numbers for large scale products becomes more and more customary. Nevertheless, the data available for growth of some cell types (e.g., MSCs) still remain very rare. Only very few companies have extensive practical experience with large scale manufacturing of adherent cells in perfusion systems like packed-bed cultures.

Compared to micro carrier and aggregate stirred-culture systems, the PBRs exhibit low shear stress forces to the cells. Similar to other cell culture methods, culturing adherent cells in a PBR includes three main stages: Cell seeding, cell culture, and cell harvest. Each step must be optimized based on cell type, carrier properties (porousness, surface charge) and packed-bed volume to achieve an effective process and optimal cell number and quality.[30] For example, Mizukami *et al.* cultivated 3×10^8 human cord blood MSC in a 500 ml volume packed-bed system. For the same amount of cells, it would have been necessary to use $120 \times 75 \, cm^2$ culture flasks.[31] One crucial step when culturing cells in packed-bed systems is the removal of cells from their carriers for harvesting. This is normally performed with proteolytic enzymes and becomes especially challenging because the more efficiently the cells could be initially seeded onto the bed, the higher the final cell number at harvest is. PBR systems exhibit a great potential for scaling up adherent cell culturing due to their capacity for high cell densities and controllable culture parameters. A direct determination of the cell concentration is not feasible. Setting up the system can be very time consuming, especially in regard to constant nutrient supply throughout the bed. Oxygen is the most critical substrate in terms of gradient formation across the packed bed due to its poor solubility in cell culture medium. The oxygen concentration is of major importance to keep the high density of immobilized cells viable and productive throughout the whole duration of the culture.[32] Packed-bed systems present many advantages and represent an attractive platform technology for a highly controlled and efficient large-scale culture of therapeutic adherent cells. A steady provision of nutrients through the whole packed bed is only possible for certain packed bed heights and thus till now only relatively small PBRs are available for cell production (~40 liters).

5.4.3.2　*Suspension cell culture and its scale-up potential*

Working with suspension cells, the scale up of the production process is easier than with adherent cells. A typical way of maximizing cell yield would be the transfer of the cell suspension into a fermenter, where simply the overall volume of the culture has to be increased. Of course this is not as simple and probably some adjustments have to be performed, but when looking at adherent cell culture, it becomes evident how much less challenging the scale up of suspension culture is. Numerous cell lines are already adapted to grow in smaller or bigger spinner bottles as well as in bioreactors. The biopharmaceutical industry routinely uses suspension cell cultures in bioreactors to manufacture clinically approved products (e.g., Genzyme's Lumizyme®), so vendors produce such systems in sizes that range from bench top models all the way up to industrial units. Many of these bioreactors now use disposable growth chambers to eliminate the difficulties of sterilization and reduce the risk of cross-contamination.[33–34]

5.4.3.3　*Cell culture media and media components*

According to EU GMP Guidelines Annex 2, the source, origin and suitability of biological starting and raw materials (e.g., cryoprotectants, feeder cells, reagents, culture media, buffers, serum, enzymes, cytokines, and growth factors) should be clearly defined. Additionally, the guideline on human cell-based medicinal products.[4] states that the quality of biologically active additives in culture media such as growth factors, cytokines, and antibodies, should be documented with respect to identity, purity, sterility, biological activity, and absence of adventitious agents. In order to minimize the risk of immune reactions against animal proteins and for potential infections with animal microbes, the GMP compliant manufacturing of medicinal products for human use should follow a so called animal-derived-component-free policy. It is possible to apply GMP to animal components if no better options are available, but animal- (and also human-) derived material is only accepted if it is safe, compliant with TSE (transmissible spongiforme encephalopathy) guidelines and does not represent a health hazard.[35] For example, using porcine trypsin to remove adherent cells from tissue flasks is such a case where alternatives are available but are either less active or not available in GMP grade quality (e.g., recombinant bacterial or plant-derived trypsin, enzymes from invertebrates, and TrypLE select®). The EMA Guideline on the use of porcine trypsin used in the manufacture of human biological medicinal products.[36] does not give general recommendation to replace porcine trypsin, considering that the alternatives need a careful assessment of suitability, quality, sterility, and performance characteristics as well as associated risks such as other adventitious agents. Nevertheless, the guideline which came into effect in September 2014, demands tightened testing and controls when porcine trypsin shall still be used.

Manufacturing of ATMPs often involves cultivation steps that have to be handled under aseptic clean room conditions. When the cells have to be expanded before application to the patient, it is necessary to find a suitable culture medium together with the required additives. For a couple of cells there exist standardized GMP grade culture media, but for some special cells more sophisticated media are needed. Because of the risk of TSE transmission and potential immunologic reactions, animal derived products like fetal bovine serum (FBS) should be avoided whenever possible. As alternatives for serum components in culture media, xenofree media or human derived serum has to be tested. When human derived serum is used as cell culture additive, some authorities (e.g., the German Paul-Ehrlich-Institute) request human serum manufactured under a manufacturing license, being produced under GMP conditions and tested in accordance with the relevant guidelines for procurement and testing of blood products in addition with national laws such as the German Transfusion Law. Serum manufactured and tested in this way is rare and manufacturers should check availability early in process development. Platelet lysates could be an alternative with better availability. Pooling of several donors (for serum as well as for platelet lysates) can equalize variations of a single donor and provides a better standardized manufacturing process. Autologous serum or plasma derived from the donor of the starting material could be an alternative source, as it is collected in many apheresis procedures anyway, but it has to be kept in mind that these substances can hardly be standardized due to donor dependent variability. Therefore, the use of autologous serum or plasma should be evaluated carefully as it is in many cases unclear if or to what extent the patient's health condition influences the quality of the serum or plasma.

In the culturing of human embryonic stem cells (hESC), the medium commonly contained FBS. In order to avoid animal derived products, the use of human serum instead of FBS in hESC culture media was described and even serum replacement efforts were realized, allowing for more standardized culture conditions, but were still not completely free of animal-derived components. The need for more human adaptation was additionally pushing the development of human feeder cells for hESC growth. Before, generally murine embryonic fibroblast feeder cells were applied. For most hESC lines, appropriately screened and GMP-grade, human feeder cells represent the best possible support for clinical-grade hESC lines.[37] Butler *et al.* created an artificial antigen-presenting cell (aAPC) that generates *ex vivo* long-lived HLA-A2-restricted CD8+ cytotoxic T-lymphocytes (CTLs). They successfully generated a clinical version of this aAPC and conducted a clinical trial where large numbers of anti-tumor CTLs are re-infused to cancer patients.[38]

Any additives to the culture medium like cytokines, antibodies, peptides or anticoagulants have to be of GMP compliant quality and are at best licensed medicinal products. Generally, the quality of raw or ancillary materials used for the manufacture of cell-based medicinal products is currently insufficiently defined (compare also chapter "Quality Control"). In Europe, there are so far no compendial texts available on raw materials in general or on specific substances (for further details on raw materials and their current status in Europe and USA, compare chapter 'Quality Control'). Some European authorities refer to the European Pharmacopoeia (Ph. Eur.) general monograph "Monoclonal Antibodies for Human Use" for antibodies used as raw materials, although the monograph clearly states that it is not applicable to antibodies used as reagents for the manufacture of medicinal products and most of the available antibodies used as raw materials will not meet these quality requirements, unless the rare events, when licensed medicinal products are available for this purpose. More guidance does exist for viral safety issues of biotechnological products, e.g. the "Guideline on Virus Safety Evaluation of Biotechnological IMPs" (Ref. EMEA/CHMP/BWP/398498/2005) which defines required viral safety data for authorization of a clinical trial of a human biotechnological medicinal product and ICH Topic Q5A (R1) "Quality of Biotechnological Products: Viral Safety Evaluation of Biotechnology Products Derived from Cell Lines of Human or Animal Origin" (Ref. CPMP/ICH/295/95) which defines data requirements for MA applications (MAA). Both documents summarize the required assays for viral detection and identification, as well as for virus reduction and viral clearance.

In the Ph. Eur., the Chapter 2.6.16 on tests for extraneous agents in viral vaccines for human use gives closer information on the necessary tests to detect adventitious viruses in vaccines. Additionally, Chapter 2.6.16 is also applicable for extraneous agents in master and working seed lots for the production of viral vectors, either for direct use as *in vivo* gene therapy medicinal product or for genetic modification of cells as *ex vivo* gene therapy medicinal products (also compare Ph. Eur. Chapter 5.14. Gene transfer medicinal products for human use). The revised text mainly covers viral vaccines for human use, but also takes account of novel production substrates based on insect cell systems.

In the US, the United States Pharmacopoeia (USP) contains Chapter ⟨1043⟩ on 'Ancillary Materials for Cell, Gene and Tissue-Engineered Products' that provides information on how to determine the safety, purity and quality of ancillary materials. But due to the broad nature of cell-based medicinal products and the corresponding ancillary materials, no detailed information on the kind of assays that should be performed and no specific tests are recommended. The USP further contains specific monographs on a very limited number of substances. These are the chapters ⟨1024⟩ Bovine Serum, ⟨90⟩ FBS Quality Attributes and Functionality Tests, ⟨92⟩ Growth Factors & Cytokines Used in Cell Therapy Manufacturing and ⟨123⟩ Protein A Quality Attributes.

5.4.4 *Activation and stimulation*

Some cell types such as T-cells require a stimulus to divide and expand. In research labs, APCs or feeder cells are frequently used in co-culture with the T-cells for this purpose. For cells that should be used as medicinal products, use of a feeder cell line or other cell types such as APCs for stimulation is critical as these cells would have to be removed thoroughly before administration of the cell-based medicinal product leading to extensive purification steps. Therefore, expansion beads with magnetic properties and covalently linked to anti-CD3 and anti-CD28 monoclonal antibodies had been developed that offer a simple method for *ex vivo* stimulation and expansion of human T cells. These beads are available in GMP-grade quality and have already been used in a number of clinical trials. Due to their magnetic properties, the beads can be removed relatively easily by magnetic forces (e.g., by CliniMACS® depletion procedure). After harvesting and removal of the beads, it is mandatory to determine the residual amount of beads. An appropriate threshold for residual beads has to be defined for the finished product. The depletion capacity of the removal process has to be validated.

An example for the generation of a certain cell population by stimulation are dendritic cells (DCs) manufactured from monocytes *via* a cytokine cocktail. In this study presented by Babatz *et al.*, they tested the generation and clinical applicability of DC from monocyte preparations (produced by immunomagnetic CD14+

selection) using a semi-automated clinical scale approach. PBMCs were used to obtain a cell suspension of high CD14+ purity with a high monocyte yield. Differentiation of CD14+ cells into mature monocyte-derived DC was induced by incubation with a cytokine mixture containing IL-4, granulocyte–macrophage colony-stimulating factor (GM-CSF), TNF-α, PGE2, IL-1 β, and IL-6.[40]

Also tumor specific cells can be manufactured according to the high standards required for the use in clinical trials. For example, in an immunotherapy approach against human melanoma, CD8+ CTLs were applied. The group developed a system to generate large numbers of long-lived antigen-specific CD8+ T-cells with a memory phenotype. The patient's immune cells were stimulated *ex vivo* with aAPCs, genetically modified to express tumor specific antigens. This *in vitro* culture system utilizes IL-15 and a standardized, renewable aAPC which was produced by transducing CD80, CD83, and HLA-A*0201 to the human cell line, K562. The melanoma antigen MART1 was chosen as a target antigen, since MART1-specific HLA-A*0201+-restricted precursor CTLs are detectable in some melanoma patients. This aAPC can uniquely support the priming and prolonged expansion of large numbers of antigen-specific CD8+ CTLs. Autologous CD8+ T cells were stimulated weekly with peptide-pulsed human cell-based aAPC and expanded with low dose IL-2 and IL-15. After three weeks, polyclonal MART1 CTLs were re-infused to the patients.[41]

Stimulation of cells is required for some separation strategies, e.g., antigen specific T-cells. Examples are EBV- or CMV specific T-cells that are isolated due to the property of T-cells to produce IFN-gamma upon stimulation. Antigen-specific peptides are required for the stimulation of the starting material (commonly a leukapheresis) and stimulated T-cells in the starting material are then isolated with anti-IFN-gamma-antibodies linked to magnetic beads by MACS separation. Due to the activation step, antigen specific T-cells generated with this method are currently considered to be an ATMP in Europe, as classified by the EMA. This is not the case when antigen-specific T-cells are isolated with specific MHC complexes as no stimulation step is required then.

Sipuleucel-T (Dendreon) is another example for the activation of certain cells for use in humans. Sipuleucel-T consists of autologous PBMCs; including APCs that have been activated *ex vivo* with a recombinant fusion protein (PA2024); see Section 5.4.6.2.

For all mentioned procedures, the used peptides, proteins, cytokines, growth factors, and other potent substances that provide the required activity have to be of GMP-grade or equivalent quality. For newly developed protocols, these substances might be difficult to find. This should be considered early in process development.

A further issue is in regard to the residual amounts of these substances in the finished product and their potential effect on the recipient. Most authorities will request to address this question, either by validating the manufacturing process in order to demonstrate robust removal or to analyze residual amounts in the finished product together with adequate acceptance criteria.

5.4.5 Genetic modification using viral vector systems

5.4.5.1 Introduction

Viral vectors are currently the most advanced gene transfer systems for cell-based *ex vivo* gene therapy. These systems take advantage of the intrinsic ability of viruses to effectively deliver their genomic information into target cells as part of their life-cycles and exploit the cellular biochemical machinery to translate their genomic information. The general approach to transform viruses into safe vector systems is to exchange viral genes, completely or in part, for therapeutic genes of interest, while retaining regulatory sequences in the viral genome as far as they are necessary (e.g., to allow encapsidation of the genome into particles or for vector expression in the target cell). Due to these modifications, viral vectors are replication-incompetent: The vectors allow delivery of genetic information to the target cell, but do not produce new viral progeny in the target cell. For production of the vector particles, the vector genome is introduced into a packaging cell line. As the vector genome is lacking viral genes to generate particles, the missing genetic information has to be substituted in *trans* using so called helper-constructs. These constructs provide the essential viral genes for regulation and structural genes necessary for the generation of the particles. Two types of packaging cell lines exist: Cell lines into which the necessary helper constructs and viral vectors have to be introduced for each production run, are called transient producer cells. Stable producer cell lines have the helper constructs and therapeutic vector stably inserted into their genome.

The three most widely used systems for gene therapy applications are retroviral, adenoviral, and adeno–associated viral vectors. Acceptable transfer efficiencies have been demonstrated in various clinical trials. General approaches with regard to GMP-compliant vector manufacturing and transduction processes will be described for all three systems here. Although recently various interesting developments have taken place in the field of non–viral gene transfer (e.g., sleeping beauty, Zink-finger nucleases, TAL-nucleases.[42]), non-viral systems will not be discussed here, as they are clinically still of lesser importance compared to viral vectors. Where animal derived materials are used during manufacture, the ATMPs must comply with the guidance to minimize the risk of transmitting TSE.

5.4.5.2 *General consideration with regard to producer cell lines*

5.4.5.2.1 Qualification of producer cell lines

Manufacture of viral vectors relies on cells, which provide the entire biochemical machinery necessary for the generation of vector particles. Due to this central position in the production process of viral vectors, these producer cells are one of the most critical starting materials. To achieve GMP-compliance for a producer cell line, a thorough qualification program is necessary. The aim of the qualification is to ensure the safety and production-specific suitability of the cells. Requirements for safety are defined in the relevant guideline for producer cells (e.g., Ph. Eur.,[43] FDA Guidance for Industry,[44] and ICH-guidelines[45]), while production-specific needs have to be defined by the manufacturer for each cell. Production specific-requirements define the suitability of the cell in question to generate the vector of choice. The ability of the cell to produce high vector titer in relation to the number of passages should be assessed. Furthermore, it should be ensured that the cell will function under the intended production process (e.g., adherent *vs.* non-adherent, serum-free *vs.* serum containing medium). To ensure safety, various properties of the cells should be analyzed, as listed below. The previous mentioned guidelines offer accepted testing methods that should be used to characterize the cell line.

Complete history of the cell line: To allow the regulatory agencies to thoroughly asses the risks that may be associated with a specific producer cell, a complete history of the cell line is necessary. This should include the species and the tissue of origin. Also, the entire history of culture conditions including the used medium batches should be available. The complete history is in many cases not documented, if cells have been obtained from cell line collections or academic research labs. In this case a starting point should be defined, from which on the cell line is documented. The extent of necessary characterization should be determined on a risk–based approach and should be discussed as early as possible with the regulatory authorities.

Identity of the cells: Markers should be defined which allow unambiguous identification of the cells. Accepted assays to verify the identity of cells are isoenzyme screening and DNA-finger printing. Cell line specific polymerase chain reaction (PCR)-based assays may also be used.

Absence of biological contaminants: The cell line should be free of bacterial (including mycoplasma) and fungal contaminants. Absence of adventitious viruses should be shown. The risk of viral contamination is dependent on the origin of the cell line and the used culture supplements (animal derived products). An appropriate test panel should be compiled and discussed with the competent regulatory agencies. If bovine supplements have been used to culture the cells, the risk of TSE should be assessed and appropriate measures should be taken depending on the origin of the used supplement.

Tumorigenicity: The producer cells have the potential risk that they release oncogenic factors (e.g., Large T antigen in 293T cells) which may lead to the formation of tumors in the patient after application. Regulatory agencies are concerned if the cell line has been transformed with oncogenes[46] Nevertheless, such a cell line may be acceptable for GMP if the safety has been demonstrated. An example would be the tumorigenic HT1080 cell line which is used for the production of commercial therapeutic proteins [Dynepo® (epoietin delta), Replagal® (agalsidase alpha), and Elaprase® (recombinant human idursulfase)]. It should therefore be shown that neither host cell genome nor cellular extract pose a risk of transformation of target cells.

Genetic stability: The genetic stability of the cells over the intended cultivation period during the production runs should be assessed.

The aim of the process is the generation of a fully qualified cell bank consisting of master (MCB) and working cell bank (WCB). The MCB consists of several (up to hundred) units of cells. A single unit of the MCB serves as starting point for the generation of the WCB, which again may consist of several hundred units. A single unit of the WCB is used in each manufacturing run to produce a single vector batch. It is important to keep in mind that the MCB has to support the manufacture of the viral vectors for the whole product life-cycle starting with the first clinical trial to MA, until the end of product marketing. To estimate the required numbers of units per MCB/WCB and the unit size, the following factors should be taken into account: Productivity of the manufacturing process (i.e., number of particles per batch), the dose per patient and the market size (to estimate the number of patients). Creating a new MCB at any point may require extensive (clinical) studies to show comparability between the old and the new MCB.

The generation and qualification of a GMP-compliant cell bank is extremely time consuming and may take up to a year. In many cases various cell lines are available for vector production; the choice is dependent on product specific requirements (envisioned production process, required yield). It is therefore reasonable to compare potential cell line candidates with regard to desired features like history and documentation supporting absence of contamination.

5.4.5.2.2   Serum-free vs. serum containing cell culture systems

For most packaging cell lines animal serum is still commonly used in the cultivation process ranging generally in concentration from 5–10%. From a commercial point of view serum is likely to be the major cost driver for large scale production runs. With regard to GMP-compliance, serum is an undesirable supplement for several reasons. As it is an animal derived product, a considerable risk concerning bovine adventitious viruses is associated with it. Also, it is a potential source for TSE. Furthermore, serum is poorly defined with regard to its components, has a high batch-to-batch variability and residues can cause allergic reactions to the patient. Therefore, considerable effort for release testing is required to use a certain serum batch for GMP manufacturing. Nevertheless, the most current early stage clinical trials still rely on production processes for viral vectors, which require animal serum. It is questionable if serum containing production process may be acceptable once a product reaches the market. It is therefore advisable to invest into the development of serum-free processes at an early development stage.

5.4.5.2.3   Inadvertent generation of replication competent viruses

The approach to generate replication defective viral vectors is identical for viruses and based on the separation of *cis* acting and *trans* acting elements. This means that the viral genes are deleted from a virus as far as possible. Only necessary regulatory sequences are retained in the vector genome and the therapeutic gene of interest (GOI) is added into the vector. The required proteins for vector production are provided on separate transcriptional units (helper constructs) *in trans* in the packaging cell line. Therefore, the possibility exists that replication competent viruses (RCVs) will be generated in the packaging cell as a result of recombination events between the vector and the helper constructs. Generation of RCVs is a considerable concern with regard to safety. Several measures can be taken to reduce the risk of RCV generation: Homology between the helper constructs and the vector should be avoided. Furthermore, helper functions should be divided on several independent transcriptional units to reduce the likelihood of productive recombination. Additionally, vector preparations should be tested for the presence of RCVs.

5.4.5.3   *Integrating vector systems: The retroviral family*

5.4.5.3.1   Retroviral biology and vector design

With regard to their use as gene transfer vectors, the most important members in the retroviral family are gamma-retroviruses and lentiviruses. The most widely used gamma-retroviral vectors are derived from the murine leukemia virus (MLV), while the clinically most relevant lentiviral vectors are derived from the human immunodeficiency virus (HIV). Retroviral vectors are attractive gene transfer vessels due to their ability to stably integrate genomic information into the target cell, which ensures long-term expression of the vector. Lentiviral vectors have the additional advantage that they are able to transduce non–dividing cells.

Retroviruses are single stranded $+/-$ RNA viruses enveloped with a diameter of approximately 100 nm. The name of the virus family refers to their ability to reverse-transcribe their RNA genome into double-stranded DNA. This pro-viral DNA is integrated into the genome of the host cell after infection. The genomic architecture of lentiviruses and gamma-retrovirus types is very similar.

As integrated provirus, Long Terminal Repeat (LTR) sequences are found at either end of the viral genome. The sequences contain regulatory elements necessary for reverse transcription and integration. Furthermore, the promoter is located here, which allows transcription of the genome for the generation of new viral progeny. Downstream of the 5'-LTR, the packaging signal (Psi) is located. This sequence facilitates encapsidation of viral RNA genomes into new particles. The genome encodes only two genes, 'gagpol' and 'env'. 'Gagpol' provides the genetic information for all enzymatic functions (pol) and also all structural proteins (gag). The 'gagpol' proteins assemble at the inner leaflet of the cellular plasma membrane from which viral particles bud. 'Env' encodes the envelope protein, which is inserted into the lipid membrane of the viral particles. In contrast to gamma-retroviruses, lentiviruses are so called complex retroviruses and encode several additional accessory proteins, which are dispensable for the generation of viral particles, but increase virulence of the wild-type virus.

To derive vectors from retroviruses, viral genes are removed, retaining only the LTRs and the packaging signal. The available space (app. 9–10 kb) can then be filled with genes of interest and internal promoters to drive expression. The LTRs at both ends of the retroviruses carry viral promoter sequences. In several clinical trials, the presence of these promoters in gamma-retroviral vectors leads to the transactivation of oncogenes in the cellular genome (insertional mutagenesis) and to (pre-)leukemic events[47] The latest retroviral vector generations have a modified 3'-LTR, in which the promoter activity has been deleted [self-inactivating (SIN)-LTR]. During the reverse transcription, this inactivated 3'-sequence replaces the promoter in the 5'-LTR. When SIN-LTRs are used, no active viral promoter sequences remain in either LTR after integration of the vector. It has been shown that these SIN-vectors have a significantly improved safety profile with regard to insertional mutagenesis. In SIN vector, the transgene transcription is driven by internal promoters.

To produce retroviral vectors, a split-genome packaging system is used. The transfer vector carrying the therapeutic construct is introduced in a producer cell. Separate non-overlapping helper constructs encode 'gagpol' and 'env' driven by heterologous promoters. These constructs provide the necessary viral proteins for particle formation. In the case of lentiviral vectors, the addition of a construct encoding the accessory protein 'Rev' is also required to allow production of high titer vector preparations. To broaden the tropism of the vectors and to transduce various target cells, the wildtype envelope gene may be replaced with an envelope from a different virus. This process is called pseudo typing. For retroviruses, several envelope glycoproteins have been used including MLV's amphotropic 4070A and 10A1,[48] GaLV's (gibbon leukemia virus)[49] and RD114 from cat endogenous virus.[50] Lentiviral vectors are generally pseudo typed with VSV-g that allows for a broad spectrum of target cells and increases their stability.

5.4.5.3.2 Production of gamma-retroviral vectors

For therapeutic applications, gamma-retroviral vectors are produced using stable producer cell lines. Stable producer cell lines have several advantages with regard to GMP compliance and pharmaceutical development. Production processes based on these cell lines are generally consistent and show only a small degree of variability. Furthermore, stable producer represent a good platform technology to implement fully scalable processes. The downside of this stable system is that they require cumbersome and time consuming establishing and selection of stable producer clones, which may take up to one year.

The latest generation of retroviral packaging cell lines use recombinase-mediated cassette exchange (RMCE) technology, which accelerates the identification of highly productive packaging cell line clones. Generation of the packaging cell line requires multiple steps of transfection. In the first two steps, the helper constructs are introduced into the cell and stable clones are selected, which show acceptable protein expression. In the third step, a so called tagging construct is transfected into the packaging cell line. This construct consists of a retroviral vector, which only encodes selectable markers for easy detection and titration of vector particles. Furthermore, the construct is flanked by recombinase target sites. After the construct has been integrated into the genome, clones are selected and screened for their ability to produce the retroviral tagging vector with a high titer. Once a highly productive producer clone has been identified, the tagging vector can be replaced with a therapeutic vector of interest using the corresponding recombinase. A tagged producer cell line is a convenient platform to generate relatively quickly efficient packaging cells for multiple different therapeutic vectors. Several RCME systems have been described which are either 293 or PG13-based.[51-53]

5.4.5.3.3   Production of lentiviral vectors

In contrast to gamma-retroviral vectors, the generation of stable packaging cell lines for lentiviral vectors has proven to be extremely difficult due to the toxicity of the lentiviral protease (encoded in the 'gagpol' gene) and the VSV-g envelope protein, which is most commonly used to pseudo type lentiviral vectors. Although a limited number of stable producer cells have been developed where the expression of the toxic gene products is regulated by inducible promoters (tet system), none of the stable packaging cell lines has ever been used to produce vectors for clinical trials. The reason might be that inducible promoters often show some basal background expression (leakiness). It can be assumed that the currently available producer cell lines do not have a sufficient long-term stability to allow the generation of a GMP compliant MCB and WCB system.[54–56]

Currently, the state of the art production method for lentiviral vectors used in clinical application is transient transfection of producer cells. 293T or HEK293 cells (both Human Embryonic Kidney cells) are transiently transfected with the therapeutic lentiviral vector and the corresponding helper constructs, as outlined above. The production method is highly dependent on manual processing, which hinders the scalability of the process. Although the current protocols used in clinical trials of different companies allow generation of high-titer vector preparations, the transient transfection method shows a considerable degree of batch-to-batch variability. The transient transfection process also requires large amounts of high quality plasmid DNA, which makes the process expensive. Also extensive downstream processing is necessary to purify the lentiviral vectors and to deplete plasmid DNA from the preparations. In general, current down-stream processing uses a benzonase treatment step to digest DNA. Furthermore, ion-exchange chromatography steps are included in the current protocols followed by a concentration/diafiltration and sterilization step before vialing. If 293T cells are used for production, the down-stream processing has to deplete the Large T antigen to achieve regulatory acceptability of the preparations.[57–59] Currently, it remains unclear if a scalable process that could fulfill the requirements for a commercial production process can be implemented for lentiviral vectors in the long-run.

5.4.5.4   *Non-integrating systems*

5.4.5.4.1   Adenovirus biology and vector design

Adenovirus is a non-enveloped, icosahedral virus of 70–90 nm in diameter with a linear, double-stranded DNA genome of 30–40 kb. All the human adenovirus serotypes[51] have been classified into six groups (A–F) based on their ability to agglutinate blood and sequence homologies. This review focuses on the serotype 2 (Ad2) and 5 (Ad5) viruses of group C, as most clinically relevant adenoviral vectors have been derived from these viruses.

Adenoviruses consist of an icosahedral outer shell, which surrounds an inner nucleoprotein core. The fiber proteins with a terminal knob protein are anchored to the vertices of the outer shell. Infection starts with the attachment of the virus to the Coxsackie virus B and Adenovirus Receptor (CAR) *via* binding of the fiber knob. CAR is present in many human tissues and physiologically functions as a cell-to-cell adhesion molecule.

The genome is flanked by inverted terminal repeats (ITRs) of around 100–140 bp to which the terminal protein is covalently linked. Genes are encoded on both strands in a series of overlapping transcription units. The packaging signal is located down-stream of the 5' ITR. The adenovirus life cycle is bisected. Shortly after infection, the expression of the early genes (E1–E4) is initiated. The function of the early genes is to modify the cellular metabolism in order to support viral replication. The first expression unit to be activated is E1 (consisting of E1A and E1B), which has multiple functions. It *trans*-activates the other early and late transcription units and is therefore the key regulator in the viral life cycle.[60] Furthermore, it induces the cell to enter S-phase to enhance viral replication. Furthermore, apoptosis *via* p53 activation is suppressed to prolong cell survival for viral replication.

Although E1 genes are able to immortalize primary cells in culture, they have not been found to be associated with human cancers. E2 encodes proteins necessary for viral DNA replication: DNA polymerase, pre-terminal protein and a single stranded DNA binding protein. Products of the viral E3 region function to subvert the host immune response and allow persistence of infected cells by interfering with the MHC class I pathway, inhibition of apoptosis and inhibition of secretion of inflammatory mediators. Finally, the E4 proteins are engaged in cell cycle control. Most of the proteins have anti-apoptotic effects. Expression of the early genes enables viral DNA replication, followed by the second half of the viral life cycle: The expression of the five adenovirus late genes (L1–L5). These transcripts primarily encode structural proteins and proteins involved in assembly. After assembly and encapsidation of viral DNA, the viral protease cleaves a subset of the structural proteins into their mature form and with that fully infectious virions are produced. Approximately 30 hours after infection, the cells are lysed and the virions are released.

5.4.5.4.2 Production of first generation vectors

The simplest approach to generate adenoviral vector is the removal of the major transactivator E1 from the genome, as this results in replication incompetent vectors. To produce these vectors, the necessary functions are provided in *trans* by an E1 expressing cell line. With the deletion of the E1 region, approximately 5 kb are available for insertion of therapeutic genes. Many of the first generation Ad-viruses also contain a deletion in the E3 region. E3 is dispensable for replication of viruses *in vitro* and its deletion increases the available space for therapeutic genes to around 8 kb. To prevent recombination between the E1 region and the viral vector, which may lead to the formation of a replication competent adenovirus, the GMP compliant cell line PER.C6 has been developed. Here, sequence overlap between the E1 region and the viral vector were removed. The cell lines allow scalable and serum-free processes for the production of adenovectors (reviewed[61]).

As the production of vectors requires the lysis of the producer cells, a major contaminant in the vector preparations is cellular genomic DNA. Elaborate downstream processing is necessary to purify the vector particles. GMP compliant downstream processing generally involves the application of Benzonase to break down DNA contaminations. This treatment is combined with chromatography steps (size exclusion and ion exchange) to generate a purified product. Diafiltration steps are included for buffer exchange and/or concentration of the vector preparation.[62]

5.4.5.4.3 Production of second generation vectors

In the second generation of Ad-viruses, additional genes (mainly E2 and E4) are removed compared to the first generation. This generates more loading capacity for therapeutic genes. For the production of these vectors more complex packaging cell lines are needed, which provide the missing genes in *trans*. The advantage of these vectors is that the risk of replication competent adenovirus (RCA) generation is further reduced. Production of the vector is comparable to the process described for the first generation vectors (Section 5.4.5.4.2). The cell line 293-ORF6 has been used in GMP productions.[63]

5.4.5.4.4 Production of helper dependent vectors

A promising approach for long term gene expression was introduced with the so called helper dependent or 'gutless' adenoviral vectors. Here, all of the viral structural genes are removed, leaving only the LTR and the packaging signal, allowing for introducing therapeutic genes of up to 37 kb. However, two major obstacles currently hinder progress of this promising technology: (1) The difficulty of large-scale vector production, and (2) Helper virus contamination. Production of gutless vectors relies on the use of replication competent helper viruses to provide necessary gene functions. Therefore, the contamination with helper virus currently seems to be still at unacceptable levels with regard to GMP compliance.[64–65] Nevertheless there are reports that an Israeli group uses helper-dependent adenoviral vectors expressing erythropoietin (EPO) in a clinical trial with the so called EPODURE BioPump treatment.[66]

5.4.5.4.5 Adeno-associated viral vector biology

The adeno-associated virus (AAV) is a small ($\sim$25 nm), non-enveloped virus with a single-stranded DNA genome. It can only replicate in the presence of helper virus (either Adeno- or Herpes virus) and has therefore been placed into the genus of dependoviruses. AAV has very simple genome architecture. The genome is flanked by ITRs. It consists of only two genes 'Rep' and 'Cap'. 'Rep' encodes enzymatic functions (Rep 78, Rep 68, Rep 52, and Rep 40) needed in the viral life cycle, while 'Cap' encodes structural proteins necessary for the capsid (VP1, VP2, and VP3).[67] The obligatory co-infection with helper virus modulates the target cell to provide the necessary metabolic environment to support AAV replication. The respective adenoviral genes that provide the necessary helper functions to AAV have been identified and include E1a, E1b, E2a, and E4. Herpes virus supports AAV gene expression with the DNA polymerase and helicase functions as well as early phase genes.

5.4.5.4.6 Production of AAV

To generate AAV-vectors, Rep and Cap genes are deleted from the genome, keeping only the ITRs. The available space can then be used for the GOI including a promoter. The packaging limit of AAV is app. 4.7 kb. Rep and Cap genes are provided in *trans* on separated transcription units. The additional helper functions (e.g., Adenoviral genes) to provide a permissive cellular milieu for AAV propagation have to be provided in parallel. Two production platforms have emerged that have gained broad support for producing both research and clinical grade vectors. Production of AAV-vectors is mostly based on the use of adherent cell lines cultivated on 10–15 cm plates. For mid to large-scale productions, generally 20–50 of these plates are used or production is performed in cell factories or roller bottles. The main drawbacks of these approaches [see Section 5.4.3.1 'Adherent (anchorage dependent) cell culture and its scale-up potential'] include the need of manual manufacturing and space requirements. Slowly, the various production methods are being adapted to address these issues and bioreactors have been introduced, either traditional stainless steel reactors or disposable bag-type cultivation systems, are being used.[68]

HEK 293-based production: Adherent growing 293 cells are transfected with GOI vector, together with 'Rep' and 'Cap' encoding plasmids. Adeno–helper genes are provided on additional plasmids. Polyethyleneimine (PEI) is the most widely used transfection reagent for the production of AAV-vectors. The process has been used for clinical trials, but suffers from scalability problems due to the labor intensive transfection method. The absence of cell-to-cell transmission limits AAV-vectors production to those cells which are initially transfected with plasmid DNA and perhaps retained in sufficient copy number in daughter cells.[69] Therefore, this system is not suitable for large-scale productions with regard to manufacturing of a marketing authorized medicinal product (see also Section 5.4.6.3 'Glybera').

Sf9 cell-based production: The invertebrate cell line Sf9 supports generation of AAV-vectors. Similarly to the 293 system, *cis* and *trans* acting elements have to be provided to allow vector formation. These factors are provided by three replication competent baculovirus constructs including 'Bac-VP' (Cap functions), 'Bac-Rep' and 'Bac-GOI' (therapeutic vectors). Furthermore, the baculovirus itself provides the helper functions necessary and sufficient for rAAV genome replication in Sf9 insect cells. Sf9 cells have the advantage that they can be cultured and infected in suspension allowing for scalability of the system (see also Section 5.5.4.6.3 'Glybera©'). Although clinical material has been successfully produced with this system, problems are encountered with regard to GMP compliance; the need for three different high-quality baculovirus preparations (VP, Rep, GOI) apart from the cell line, as starting material requires considerable qualification efforts since the producer cells have a central position in the production process of viral vectors.

5.4.5.4.7 Down-stream processing of AAV

At the end of the replication process, the cells are lysed and the viruses are released. In general, the down-stream processing for AVV can be divided in the following steps: Release of the vectors from the producer cells, separation of the vector from the biomass, concentration of the vector, and vialing of the product. AAV in comparison to other viruses is very stable. Therefore, the down-stream processing may include harsh conditions which would be detrimental to other vectors. This may include repeated freeze–thaw cycles, elevated temperatures and treatment with organic solvents.

The release of the vector from the producer cells is achieved by treatment with surfactants (e.g., Triton) and/or mechanical disruption. The biomass is treated with nucleases to breakdown DNA, which would otherwise interfere with subsequent filtration and chromatography steps. A series of filters with decreasing pore sizes is used to separate the vectors from cell debris. This preparation is further purified using ion-exchange and size exclusion chromatography. Finally, tangential flow filtration is employed to concentrate the product or to exchange buffers.

5.4.6 *Examples for GMP manufacture of ATMPs*

5.4.6.1 *Tissue-engineered ATMP*

ChondroCelect® (TiGenix) was the first ATMP to be approved by the EMA in October 2009, and it is the first ATMP to have its MA renewed. ChondroCelect® is an autologous cell- based product indicated for the repair of single symptomatic cartilage defects of the femoral condyle of the knee in adults to restore the functionality of the joint's cartilage. The manufacturing of ChondroCelect® starts with a cartilage autopsy (with a special biopsy kit) that is obtained by arthroscopy from non-affected articular cartilage of the patient's knee. The cells are expanded *ex vivo* (substantial manipulation) with the main focus on maintaining the cells pre-culture phenotype and cartilage-forming capacity. The biopsy specimen are transferred aseptically in sterile Hanks' Balanced Salt solution (HBBS) containing penicillin, streptomycin, and amphotericin B and are minced into smaller pieces, and any bone fragments present are removed. The cartilage fragments are transferred to allow for dissociation of the cartilage tissue and release of chondrocytes from the tissue matrix. This step is normally performed in spinner bottles and in the presence of collagenase containing medium. This medium and the cultivation medium contain 10% FBS and the above mentioned antibiotic/antimycotic mix. After that the cells are filtered, washed, counted and diluted in culture medium and seeded into cell culture flasks. Regular medium changes are performed and the cells are split and reseeded. After a maximum of three passages, the cells are harvested. Used medium is pooled and tested for microbiological contamination. At the end of the cultivation phase the cells are collected by trypsinization, washed, and pelleted. Their ability to form stable hyaline cartilage *in vivo* was predicted by a quantitative gene expression profile. The cell pellet is regarded as the active substance (living human autologous cartilage forming cells). The dosage per patient is $0.8 - 1 \times 10^6$ cells per cm^2 defect size. This pellet is then immediately resuspended in the excipient medium (DMEM + Glucose) and filled in a maximum of three glass vials with 4 Mio cells/vial, which are then packed for shipment. A maximum lesion of 15 cm^2 can be treated with the lower dose of 0.8 Mio cells/cm^2. Similar to manufacturing of other ATMPs, expected challenges occurred due to the complex starting material and the biological variety with regard to cell growth, characteristics and differentiation pattern. All steps were standardized precisely starting from the biopsy (surgeon training, surgery protocol, and biopsy tool) to the digest, from cell density and confluency to cell viability.[70–73]

5.4.6.2 *Somatic cell therapy/tumor vaccine products*

On April 29, 2010, the FDA approved the drug Sipuleucel-T (PROVENGE®, manufactured by Dendreon Corporation) for the treatment of asymptomatic or minimally symptomatic metastatic castrate-resistant (hormone refractory) prostate cancer.

Sipuleucel-T is an active cellular immunotherapy (therapeutic cancer vaccine) consisting of autologous PBMCs, including APCs that have been activated *ex vivo* with a recombinant fusion protein (PA2024). This protein consists of a prostate antigen, prostatic acid phosphate (PAP) that is fused to a GM-CSF, an immune-cell activator.

Due to the increasing demand, the coordination of patient supply with PROVENGE® is a very precisely planned and organized process including patient scheduling, appointments, and shipment of the cells. The time interval from blood donation of the patient in an apheresis center to manufacturing and the final infusion is only three to four days. The process of manufacturing Sipuleucel-T starts in an apheresis center, where the patient donates blood. The patient's blood cells are collected by standard leukapheresis. The leukapheresis bag is immediately provided with a barcode and shipped to Dendreon's manufacturing facility for processing. When arriving at the manufacturing facility, the bag with the cells is directed to the receiving area (lower cleanliness level), verified by scanning the barcode and is then transferred *via* pass through windows to the product corridor (higher cleanliness level) and from there *via* pass through window in the manufacturing room with the biosafety cabinet (highest cleanliness level). There, the cells undergo two density gradient separations. After centrifugation, the APCs are collected and measured. Afterwards PAP–GM-CSF, a recombinant protein which consists of human PAP linked to human GM-CSF, is added to the cells and culture medium. DCs are usually cultivated in cell differentiation bags which offer significant practical and regulatory advantages for the generation of clinical-grade DCs in a completely closed system.[74] The GM-CSF portion of the protein helps to target the PAP protein to APCs and activate those cells. PAP provides the tumor-specific antigen that is intended to direct the immune system to target prostate cancer. The cells are cultured in the presence of PAP–GM-CSF for 36–44 hours. After culture, the cells are washed and suspended in Lactated Ringer's solution with a total volume of 250 ml and filled in a sealed, patient-specific infusion bag. Sipuleucel-T contains a minimum of 50 million autologous activated CD54+ cells. Minimal residual levels of the intact PAP–GM-CSF are detectable in the final product. The course of therapy is three doses, given at approximately two week intervals. Each leukapheresis produces one dose; therefore the patient undergoes three separate leukapheresis procedures. Each leukapheresis product passes through the identical manufacturing process to produce a unique lot of Sipuleucel-T. If a lot fails to meet requirements for quality, the patient must undergo an additional leukapheresis to manufacture a new lot of product. Each dose is shipped and administered fresh (without cryopreservation) within 18 hours of manufacture. Due to the autologous nature of the product, specifically patient-to-patient variability in the cellular composition and total cell number of the leukapheresis, the product has high inherent variability. Product lot release specifications were based on a statistical analysis of historical manufacturing data and set around three standard deviations from the mean.[75]

5.4.6.3 Gene therapy products

Although this book is concentrating on cell-based therapies, Glybera® (UniQure) is mentioned here as it is the very first gene therapy product approved in the EU. In October 2012, the European Commission (EC) granted MA for Glybera® (alipogene tiparvovec). Glybera® is a gene therapy that is designed to restore the lipoprotein lipase (LPL) enzyme activity required to enable the processing, or clearance, of fat-carrying chylomicron particles formed in the intestine after a fat-containing meal. Lipoprotein lipase deficiency (LPLD) is a rare genetic disease affecting one or two per million people. With a normal diet, patients lacking sufficient levels of lipoprotein lipase have abnormally high serum triglycerides causing recurrent and life threatening pancreatitis.[76] The product consists of an engineered copy of the human LPL gene packaged with a tissue-specific promoter in a non-replicating AAV1 vector, which has a particular affinity for muscle cells. The company produces Glybera® using its insect cell-based (Sf9) manufacturing process. Earlier mammalian cells (HEK 293) for AAV production were used, but this system was too cost effective for a high yield vector production due to the adherent growth of the cells and the difficulty to scale up this system (see Section 5.4.3.1). Due to the change in the manufacturing process for the commercial product the company had to perform extensive additional experiments to show overall consistency in product quality including non-clinical studies. Comparability does not necessarily mean that the quality attributes of the pre-change and post-change product are identical, but that they are highly similar and that the existing knowledge is sufficiently predictive to ensure that any differences in quality attributes have no adverse impact upon safety or efficacy of the drug product.[77] This change to the insect cell/baculovirus system did reduce the manufacturing process from 10 to one week. The manufacturing of Glybera® involves a MCB and a WCB, and master and working viral seed stock. Sf9 cells, that can be cultivated in serum-free medium, are infected in suspension with the baculovirus expression vector system. The Sf9 cells are transduced with three different replicating baculovirus vectors either expressing the recombinant AAV vector genome with the LPL cassette or the 'rep' gene or the 'cap' gene (see also Section 5.4.5.4.6). These baculoviruses then replicate in the insect cells and produce recombinant AAV particles. The baculovirus infected AAV1–LPL particles producing cells are seeded in 2×25 l bioreactor and are allowed to expand. At the end of this cultivation, the AAV particles are released by incubation with cell lysis buffer. The product is further processed by depth filtration for clarification followed by a viral inactivation step and then an immunoaffinity chromatography is performed. This chromatography specifically binds AAV serotypes which can be eluted after washing of the column. The eluted viral particles are then concentrated *via* tangential flow filtration (TFF) using hollow fibre modules and are finally filled. Glybera® drug product is a sterile injection solution in single use vials. Each vial contains 3×10^{12} genomic copies of alipogene tiparvovec in 1 ml of phosphate-based buffer containing glucose. Clinicians administer Glybera® in a one-time series of up to 60 intramuscular injections in the legs. The dose is 1×10^{12} genomic copies/kg body weight. The patient is administered spinal anaesthesia or deep sedation during the procedure. In addition, an immunosuppressive regimen is recommended from three days prior to and for 12 weeks following Glybera® administration.[67,78–81]

5.4.7 *Formulation of finished product*

The down-stream processing is elaborate and includes two main bottlenecks: Volume reduction and filling of the final product. Volume reduction can be achieved by centrifugation steps, but larger volumes cannot be handled in laboratory centrifuges. When filling large batches of cells, the influence of a present cryopreservant [e.g., dimethylsulfoxide (DMSO)] on the viability of the cell product will dictate process timing and might be unmanageable for filling of multiple small aliquots (compare section 'cryopreservation').

At the end of the manufacturing process, the main focus lies on generating a defined product with a maximum of purity. Therefore, culture medium including serum, proteins, and metabolic excretion products as well as buffers shall be eliminated as thoroughly as possible. After cell culture, the cells have to be harvested and medium is removed after centrifugation. Washing steps can be applied if necessary. After removal of the supernatant post centrifugation, the cell pellet remains as almost pure active substance. For determination of the cell number, the cells are counted and by adding a certain volume of infusion buffer (for immediate use) or cryo-medium (for further storage), the desired cell concentration is adjusted. The specifications documented in the IMPD or MA with regard to total volume, total amount of (target) cells and minimum/maximum concentration have to be fulfilled. The final concentration of the cells in the cryo-medium is a very crucial point and has to be adopted to and validated for each type of cells, not only in order to enable the appropriate dosage, but rather to maintain cell viability after freeze–thawing. The cryo-medium should contain enough protein [e.g., human serum albumin (HSA)]. Also see Section 5.4.8 'cryopreservation' to guarantee product stability. Validation of stability is essential for non-cryopreserved products as well as for cryopreserved ones (compare chapter 'Quality Control').

Also for final formulation and filling, systems like the CliniMACS® instrument can be used, for example, if the removal of magnetic expansion beads is the final manufacturing step. The target cell fraction is eluted by the CliniMACS® instrument in a blood bag. The bag is welded off the tubing set and weighed in order to determine the mass of the finished product corresponding to its volume. Samples are drawn from the bag for final release testing. After determination of the cell concentration (e.g., by manual counting with a haemocytometer), the total amount of cells is calculated and it is determined if or rather how many cells have to be removed from the bag to adjust the defined cell dose. If a certain cell concentration is required, buffer would have to be added to the bag.

In use, shelf life is another important point to consider. For products that cannot be cryopreserved, shelf life must be long enough to allow distribution from the manufacturer to the point of use. Shipment logistics and coordination of manufacturing and clinics will be more challenging if the shelf life is shorter. A shelf life of at least 48 hours should be pursued, if the cell product is intended to be distributed outside the proximity of the manufacturer.

5.4.8 *Cryopreservation*

Careful attention should be paid to specific requirements at any cryopreservation stage, e.g., the rate or temperature change during freezing or thawing. The type of storage chamber, placement and retrieval process should minimize the risk of cross-contamination, maintain the quality of the products and facilitate their accurate retrieval. Documented procedures should be in place for the secure handling and storage of products with positive serological markers[8]

Cryopreservation is the use of low temperatures to preserve living cells. Cryopreservation is based on the principle that chemical, biological, and physical processes are sufficiently decreased at temperatures below $-140°C$. Besides, at these temperatures there is insufficient thermal energy to allow for chemical and metabolic processes to proceed at biochemical relevant rates. This is made possible by storage in liquid nitrogen (which under GMP conditions has to occur in the vapor phase). The cells are first cooled under controlled conditions to $-100°C$ in a freezing chamber and then they are transferred into the liquid nitrogen storage tank. For successful cryopreservation of cells, a standardized and reproducible protocol has to be followed. Each protocol may require optimization for a given cell type or cell line, in order to achieve maximum viability after thawing. A very critical point during cryopreservation is the utilization of an appropriate freezing program. The cooling rate is essential and has to be carefully controlled. When the cooling rate is too slow, the cells can die of osmotic stress. On the other hand when the cooling rate is too high, cells can die because of formation of intracellular ice crystals. The cryopreservation of higher volumes (as in bags) is critical as the whole volume needs to be frozen homogenously. Temperature rises at the crystallization point, as the formation of crystals generates an increase of temperature, which causes a slight rise in the solution's temperature. The cooling rate must be increased at this point to prevent warming of the cell product. This is the most critical part of the procedure.

Due to reasons of product release testing and determination of viability after thawing, additional pilot vials normally have to be frozen from the final product. If the finished product is cryopreserved in cryo–bags, it is necessary to prove that the product frozen in the bag and the pilot sample frozen in a vial show the same characteristics after thawing. Comparative studies thus have to be performed. For assessment of viability after thawing, see also chapter 'Quality Control'.

Figure 5.1 shows a typical example of a freezing curve of a cell-based medicinal product. After the freezing process is completed, the product can be transferred to storage in the vapor phase of liquid nitrogen. For larger cell numbers, the product is frozen in a cryo–bag; nevertheless the pilot samples, as well as the retention samples, are mostly frozen in standard cryo–vials. In the depicted curve, the freezing curves for both reference vessels bag and cryo–vial are shown (red and blue line). The rapid temperature change after around 16 minutes (green and pink line) is necessary in order to grade the temperature rise occurring during crystallization and thus avoiding a temperature increase in the product.

Formation of ice crystals and osmotic stress can damage cells during freezing procedures. Therefore, cryoprotectants have to be added. Typically DMSO or

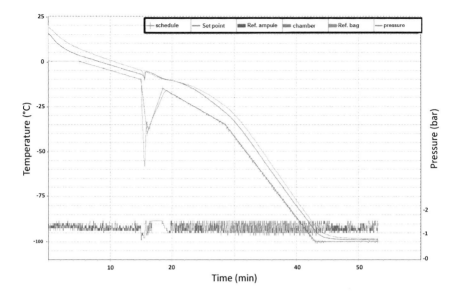

Figure 5.1: Example of a typical freezing curve of a cell-based medicinal product.

glycerol is used, with DMSO prevalently applied. Classically 10% of DMSO is added. An ideal cryoprotective solution should be non-toxic for cells and patients, non-antigenic and chemically inert providing high cell surviving rates after thawing. DMSO penetrates cell membranes and prevents cell rupture, but is potentially cyto-toxic. Therefore, options were searched to reduce the amount of DMSO. It has been shown that addition of hydroxyethyl starch (HES), a less effective cryoprotectant than DMSO, can reduce the inset of DMSO to 5%.[82] The use of human serum or FBS might bear the potential risk of an infection with prions or other unidentified pathogens. Besides, these products could induce an allergic response. Serum-free cryo-media are therefore increasingly being developed. If serum protein is required, HSA would be an alternative, as it is available as licensed medicinal product that is tested extensively and is of lower risk for adventitious agents as virus removing steps can be applied during production.

Frozen cell products can be kept over a long time. This allows for comple-tion of all analytics and final release testing. Long term storage in liquid nitrogen should guarantee that the product is only exposed to the vapor phase in order to avoid cross-contamination through the liquid phase. Potentially infected material should be stored separately. Shipment distances and times are then less an issue. However, other challenges arise. Transportation of liquid nitrogen containing dry shippers or dry ice packages together with the need of temperature logs requires specialized couriers and validation. Storage of the frozen cell products, reproducible thawing procedures at the point of use, in use shelf life of the thawed product and possibly reconstitution with a stabilizing buffer still need to be developed carefully to match the capabilities of the intended users like hospitals or specialized general practitioners. Great efforts will be needed for the training, and procedures should be designed as easy and practicable as possible.

5.4.9 *Labeling*

Labeling of intermediates, bulk and finished products (primary as well as secondary packaging materials, where appropriate) is an important part of the manufacturing process as correct labeling is the prerequisite for correct identification of a medicinal product during the manufacturing process and after packaging. Labeling thus has to follow the GMP rules in order to ensure that the information defined by the MA or the Clinical Trials Authorization (CTA) is covered, precise and able to prevent mix-ups that are especially dangerous for autologous cell preparations or those therapies which have to be applied in a directed way. Guidance for medicinal products as well as for APIs is given in several chapters of the EU GMP Guidelines. These are Part I Chapter 4 'Documentation' (section Packaging instructions), Chapter 5 'Production' (sections General, Starting Materials, Packaging Materials and Packaging Operations) and Annex 2 (section Operating Principles). Chapter 6 'Quality Control' points out, that it is the Quality Control Department's duty to ensure the correct labeling of containers of materials and products. Annex 8 provides additional guidance on sampling of packaging materials. Special considerations for labeling of IMP is defined in Annex 13. For APIs, part II of the EU GMP Guidelines provides information in section 6.3 (Records of Raw Materials, Intermediates, API Labeling and Packaging Materials) and in section 9 [Packaging and Identification, Labeling of Active Pharmaceutical Ingredient (APIs) and Intermediates].

Entrance to areas where labels (especially when they are pre-printed) and also packaging materials are stored, should be restricted. The printers used for label printing should be controlled and the printed labels should be checked for proper identity and conformity to specifications as defined in the MA or CTA. These controls have to be properly documented. Written procedures designed to ensure that correct labels are used should exist.

Line clearance is an important measure to avoid errors: Packaging and labeling facilities should be inspected immediately before and after each packaging/

labeling operation to ensure that all materials not needed for the next packaging/labeling operation have been removed. This examination should be documented. It is further important that there are procedures in place to reconcile the quantities of labels issued, used, and returned. Any discrepancies found should be investigated and evaluated by a responsible person. Any excess labels bearing batch numbers and/or other batch-specific information should be destroyed. One of the batch labels should be included in the batch record for documentation purposes. This is particularly important for autologous and directed products, where it is not possible to keep retention samples. Packaged and labeled intermediates, bulk products, and finished medicinal products should be examined to ensure that they are labeled correctly. Results of these examinations should be documented in the batch record, and at least for finished medicinal products, this should be double checked by the Quality Control (QC) Department and documented in the control records.

Special consideration has to be given to labels that are used for deep freeze storage (either at −80°C or in the vapor phase of liquid nitrogen at temperatures below −140°C). These labels should be validated for the intended purpose with respect to their adhesiveness at cold temperature over longer time periods and their readability. As many authorities request the validation to be followed up as long as the labeled product is maintained, these validation procedures have to be initiated as early as possible in order not to lose valuable time. Readily validated labeling tags are available from different providers, but it has to be evaluated if the validation of the label itself is applicable to the container, box or vial used for storage.

Not only the process of labeling as such is important, but also the content of the labels is essential for identification at the site of manufacture and within the supply chain, as well as for physicians and patients who apply the medicinal products. Therefore, the minimum content of labels for finished medicinal products is defined precisely by several European Guidance documents. Basic information on product labeling and patient information leaflets are set out in Title V of Council Directive 2001/83/EC, Article 55 (2) and (3), which was amended by Council Directive 2004/27/EC and Council Directive 2010/84/EU. Besides, EMA published the Guideline on the readability of the labeling and package leaflet of medicinal products for human use (ENTR/F/2/SF/jr (2009) D/869) and the Guideline on Excipients in the label and package leaflet of medicinal products for human use. Additional national regulations might exist (e.g., German Drug Law, Section 10 on labeling) and have to be followed. Furthermore, special requirements for IMPs have to be considered as already mentioned above (EU GMP Guidelines Annex 13, sub-item 26). Their labeling should also comply with directive 2003/94/EC. Generally, labeling of IMPs is often more complex and error-prone than labeling of authorized medicinal products, and mislabeling is harder to detect, especially when blinded products with similar appearance are used.

Labels used on containers of intermediates, bulk products or medicinal products/drugs should indicate the name or identifying code, the batch number of the product, and storage conditions, when such information is critical to assure the quality of the object. If the intermediate, bulk product or medicinal product/drug is intended to be transferred outside the control of the manufacturer's material management system, the name and address of the manufacturer, quantity of contents, and special transport conditions and any special legal requirements should also be included on the label. If an expiry date exists, the expiry date should be indicated on the label and Certificate of Analysis (CoA). Where retests are necessary, the retest date should be indicated on the label and/or CoA.

Table 5.4 shows an example of a label with all information required for a conventional IMP, according to Annex 13 of the EU GMP Guidelines.

In addition to the particulars mentioned in Directive 2001/83/EC (related to the medicinal products for human use in general), special requirements on the labeling of blood products, tissues, and cell-based medicinal products are given in various guidance documents. Regulation 1394/2007 on ATMPs gives detailed information on the labeling of ATMPs in Annex III. Apart from general information, it is requested to denote that the medicinal product contains cells of human or animal origin (as appropriate) together with a short description of these cells or tissues and of their specific origin. In the case of ATMPs for autologous use, the unique patient identifier and the statement 'For autologous use only' have to be added.

Directive 2006/86/EC which is applicable to human tissues and cells defines requirements for final labeling for distribution in Annex II. Similar to the ATMP regulation, it also points out that products for autologous use have to be specified as such and that the donor/recipient has to be identified. In the case of directed donations, the label must identify the intended recipient. When tissues and cells are known to be positive for a relevant infectious disease marker, they must be marked as 'BIOLOGICAL HAZARD'. Apart from the labeling of the medicinal product itself, further requirements are defined for the external labeling of the shipping container. In addition to the identification of the originating tissue establishment and the organization responsible for the application of the product, a statement has to be added that the container should be handled with care and must not be irradiated ('DO NOT IRRADIATE') in order to keep the cells or tissue viable.

Table 5.4: Guideline of labeling of IMPs according to GMP guidelines annex 13, 26–30.

(a) name, address and telephone number of the sponsor, contract research organisation or investigator (the main contact for information on the product, clinical trial and emergency unblinding);	**GENERAL CASE** For both the primary and secondary packaging (§26) Particulars a[4] to k
(b) pharmaceutical dosage form, route of administration, quantity of dosage units, and in the case of open trials, the name/identifier and strength/potency;	
(c) the batch and/or code number to identify the contents and packaging operation;	
(d) a trial reference code allowing identification of the trial, site, investigator and sponsor if not given elsewhere;	**PRIMARY PACKAGE** Where primary and secondary packaging remain together throughout (§29)[5] a[6] b[7] c d e
(e) the trial subject identification number/treatment number and where relevant, the visit number;	
(f) the name of the investigator (if not included in (a) or (d));	
(g) directions for use (reference may be made to a leaflet or other explanatory document intended for the trial subject or person administering the product	**PRIMARY PACKAGE** Blisters or small packaging units (§30)[5] a[6] b[7,8] c d e
(h) "for clinical trial use only" or similar wording;	
(i) the storage conditions;	
(j) period of use (use-by date, expiry date or re-test date as applicable), in month/year format and in a manner that avoids any ambiguity.	
(k) "keep out of reach of children" except when the product is for use in trials where the product is not taken home by subjects.	

Source: EU GMP Guidelines.[83]

In the US, guidance with respect to labeling is provided by USP chapter ⟨1046⟩ Cell and Gene Therapy Products, and by the US FDA in 21 CFR 610 sub-part G and 21 CFR part 801. Further valuable information is provided by the Circular of Information for the Use of Cellular Therapy Products, a document prepared by the Circular of Information for Cellular Therapy Products Task Force, consisting of representatives from the American Society for Blood and Marrow Transplantation (ASBMT), the International Society for Cellular Therapy (ISCT), the National Marrow Donor Program (NMDP), and the Joint Accreditation Committee of ISCT and European Society for Blood and Marrow Transplantation (EBMT), the JACIE, to name only a few. Important information (either on the affixed product label, or on an attached label or in accompanying documentation) might be that the product must not be administered through a filter designed to remove leukocytes, that the product should be mixed thoroughly before use, that the product (despite donor selection and testing) might transmit infectious diseases and that (in case of autologous or directed products) the recipient has to be properly identified prior to use.

Finally, a special coding system- Information Standard for Blood and Transplant (ISBT) 128 has to be mentioned, which is an international standard for the nomenclature and labeling of human blood, tissue, and cellular therapy products. This coding system allows information about biological products to be transferred from one computer system to another in a way that is unambiguous and accurate for the highest levels of accuracy, safety, and efficiency for the benefit of donors and patients. The acronym ISBT was originally derived from the important role played by the International Society of Blood Transfusion (ISBT) in the development of the standard. Today it expands as Information Standard for Blood and Transplant. The number 128 reflects the 128 characters of the ISO/IEC 646 7-bit character set that the standard uses. Featuring a unique, highly flexible, and comprehensive coding method for every collected product, the standard provides international consistency to support the transfer, transfusion, or transplantation of medical products of human origin.

ISBT 128 was developed to increase the level of standardization in transfusion medicine and to support traceability through the combined use of a globally unique Donation Identification Number (DIN) and a product code. The DIN includes an assigned facility identification number (FIN), the collection year, a serial number, and an internal check digit to prevent bar code misreads. Because all products from a single donation will have the same DIN, uniqueness of each product is achieved through a combination of the DIN and the product code. Specific products and blood treatment processes receive the same coding every time this system is used. The ISBT 128 bar code allows for more information to be coded into a small space.

Further information is available *via* the International Council for Commonality in Blood Banking Automation (ICCBBA) which was established and given the responsibility for implementation and management of ISBT 128.[84–85]

5.4.10 *Transport and shipping*

The EC states that 'the wholesale distribution of medicinal products is an important activity in the integrated supply chain management. The quality and the integrity of medicinal products can be affected by a lack of adequate control'. Therefore, the

Commission has published guidelines on Good Distribution Practice of medicinal products for human use in the form of a Commission guideline 2013/C 343/01. The present guidelines are based on Articles 84 and 85b (3) of Directive 2001/83/EC of the European Parliament and of the Council of November 6, 2001 on the Community code relating to medicinal products for human use (Directive 2001/83/EC). Additionally, a 'Question and Answer' document (version 1.0 March 2014) responds to frequently asked questions in relation to the guidelines on Good Distribution Practice of medicinal products for human use.[86-87]

Shipping, as well as storage should generally provide optimal conditions for the appropriate product. This is especially important for blood, tissues, cells and all cell-based materials as they are easily affected by temperatures that are too high as well as temperatures that are below $0°C$ (at least as far as they are not cryopreserved). Therefore, special attention has to be paid to the transport of both, the starting material as well as the finished product. Depending on the kind of starting material used (fresh tissue, blood or bone marrow aspirates), different recommendations on how the material should be shipped or stored before processing exist. These range from keeping it at room temperature or on ice to $4°C$ in the fridge. This pre-treatment often has great impact on the following quality of the biologic material (e.g., vitality of cells). Freezing of cells and deep cold storage are explained in more detail in Section 5.4.8. Independent of whether short term storage or long term storage or transport over shorter or longer distances is required, all these conditions have to be carefully tested and validated in order to guarantee the quality and comparability of the product. Besides the correct handling of the starting material and of the final product, all the way during processing and after thawing, controlled, monitored, and optimized conditions necessary to maintain the safety, stability, identity, and potency of the products have to be applied. Transport validation includes a risk assessment and all possible influences (e.g., time delays) and is performed with temperature loggers in validated and adequate containers.

Intermediates, bulk products and medicinal products/drugs should be transported in a manner that does not adversely affect their quality. Special transport or storage conditions should be stated on the labels. The manufacturer should ensure that the contract acceptor (contractor) for transportation of the Intermediate, bulk product or medicinal product/drug knows and follows the appropriate transport and storage conditions. A system should be in place by which the distribution of each batch of intermediate, bulk product and/or medicinal product/drug can be readily determined to permit its recall.[12] As transportation of temperature sensitive materials can have significant influence on their quality, a technical agreement with the transport company is necessary that defines transport conditions, training of personnel and other duties of the contract acceptor.

5.4.11 *On-Site preparation and administration*

For ATMPs, on-site preparation of the final product is in many cases part of the manufacturing process; therefore validated procedures have to be applied. It has to be checked whether on-site preparation procedures have to be covered by a manufacturing license. If an IMP is reconstituted only before administration, no manufacturing permission is necessary for the hospital and the involved physicians.

Reconstitutions are to be understood as processes, like dissolving or dispensing finished and released (investigational) medicinal products for ensuring immediate application or mixing (investigational) medicinal products with other substances, if this is necessary for the application. It is clarified that this reconstitution does not require a manufacturing authorization. Reconstitution is distinguished from blending a substance with an active ingredient to produce an IMP. The latter equals manufacture and requires a corresponding authorization. If this step has to be performed prior to application in the hospital or clinic, it might be necessary that a hospital pharmacy or another facility with the required authorization execute these manufacturing steps. Special attention has to be paid whenever the finished product is cryopreserved and has to be thawed for application, as handling errors can result in a complete loss of viable cells. When thawing, filtration or dilution steps have to be performed outside the manufacturing facility; a laminar flow work bench might become necessary for products where aseptic handling is required. It is absolutely mandatory that personnel performing these steps (manufacturer and clinical personnel) are thoroughly trained.[83]

5.5 Validation

5.5.1 *Process validation*

Identical to conventional medicinal products, the entire GMP compliant manufacturing process of cell-based medicinal products from initial selection/enrichment, cell seeding, cell harvesting and reseeding, any manipulations performed on the cells (e.g., genetic transformation), final harvesting, and filling of the final product and, where appropriate, storage of the final product, has to be validated. According to Annex 15 EU GMP Guidelines,[14] process validation has to be done prospectively and a minimum of three batches is common practice to prove consistency of the manufacturing process, but process validation of cell-based medicinal products has several challenges and difficulties.

Depending on the kind of starting material, it might be ethically not justifiable to put donors at risk of the procurement procedure (e.g., when donors would have to be mobilized or undergo a surgical procedure). In these cases, it has to be discussed with the authorities if process validation can be done concomitantly with the first patient batches. This is often the case in phase I/II clinical trials. A higher number of batches might be necessary in these cases. In an autologous or allogeneic directed setting, an additional bottleneck often is the limited number of cells that does not allow for extensive testing and that can prolong the validation process drastically. Limited cell numbers also do not allow for the validation of the maximum admissible amount of starting material– a worst case scenario that normally is mandatory to validate. Due to the heterogeneous nature of the starting material for ATMP manufacturing, it is important to consider the variability of the validation process. It might be difficult to define suitable specifications and acceptance criteria that are tight enough to identify changes in the manufacturing process, but at the same time are wide enough to cover donor variability. Therefore, it is all the more important that the analytical procedures used for quality control of the product are well established and validated before production of the first process validation batches starts.

Discussions with the competent authorities might be necessary to clarify the approach and the extent of process validation that is needed for a certain cell-based product. For phase I/II clinical trials, it is generally recognized that the production process is not yet fully validated at the beginning of the trial. GMP Guidelines Annex 13 (Paragraph 17) IMPs[83] says: Production processes for IMPs are not expected to be validated to the extent necessary for routine production, but premises and equipments are expected to be qualified.

In contrast to Europe, in the United States, IMPs for phase I/II clinical trials generally need not be produced under full GMP conditions, as the grade of GMP that has to be adhered to increases gradually from phase I to phase III. Additional alleviations might be possible there.

5.5.2 *Validation of aseptic handling via media fills*

For conventional medicinal products, filling of a sterile product is the only aseptic manufacturing step. Therefore the term "media fill" was invented for the validation of aseptic processing and is suitable in these cases. For cell-based medicinal products, the whole manufacturing process needs to be performed aseptically and therefore needs to be simulated with nutrient medium — this is no longer just the simulation of the filling process. As manufacturing processes for cell-therapy products often take several days to weeks and some authorities do not allow to split the process in separate parts, process simulation is a mature issue that is cost, time and labor extensive and a sincere obstacle, particularly for small companies and academic centers. Media fills are thought to be critical microbiological tests that should simulate the normal manufacturing conditions by replacing the pharmaceutical product with culture media. Personnel have to perform media fills in order to qualify for the aseptic handling of the actual work processes. As the manufacturing process needs to be simulated as closely as possible, it is important to include occurring hold steps in the risk assessment and define the time that certain preparation steps consume. Only personnel trained to recognize a certain turbidity level are allowed to analyze the media fill vessels with the culture medium after incubation.

In Annex 1 of the EU GMP Guidelines[7] on manufacturing of sterile medicinal products, the requirements for media fills are explained in paragraph 66. It says that validation of aseptic processing should include a process simulation test using a nutrient medium (media fill). Selection of the nutrient medium should be made based on dosage form of the product and selectivity, clarity, concentration and suitability for sterilization of the nutrient medium. The process simulation test should mimic as closely as possible the routine aseptic manufacturing process and include all the critical subsequent manufacturing steps. It should also take into account various interventions known to occur during normal production as well as worst-case scenarios. Media fills should be performed as initial validation with three consecutive satisfactory simulation tests per shift, and repeated at defined intervals and after any significant modification to the HVAC system, equipments, process and number of shifts. Normally process simulation tests should be repeated twice a year per shift and process. For small batches, the number of containers for media fills should at least equal the size of the product batch. The qualification limits are the following:

---

1. When filling fewer than 5,000 units: no contaminated units should be detected
2. When filling 5,000 to 10,000 units: (a) One contaminated unit should result in an investigation, including consideration of a repeat media fill;
(b) Two contaminated units are considered as cause for revalidation, following investigation.
When filling more than 10,000 units: (a) One contaminated unit should result in an investigation;
(b) Two contaminated units are considered cause for revalidation, following investigation.

Intermittent incidents of microbial contamination may be indicative of low-level contamination that should be investigated. Investigation of gross failures should include the potential impact on the sterility assurance of batches manufactured since the last successful media fill. Care should be taken that any validation does not compromise the processes.

The Pharmaceutical Inspection Convention and Pharmaceutical Inspection Co-operation Scheme (jointly referred to as PIC/S) offer a guideline document PIC/S: PI 007-6 'Recommendation on the Validation of Aseptic Processes'. This document offers information on process simulation test procedures (for different dosage forms, clinical trials materials and biological and biotechnology products), process simulation test conditions (incubation temperatures, selection of the medium, validated culture conditions, and frequencies), environmental and personnel monitoring, help on data interpretation and information on staff training.[88]

5.5.3 Cleaning validation after employment of viral particles for ATMP production

As for cell-based medicinal products, almost all materials in immediate contact with the cells are sterile and disposable in contrast to conventional medicinal products, and cleaning validation is generally not an issue. Cleaning validation often plays only a role in connection with the clean room environment, as it has to be demonstrated that cleaning and disinfection procedures are adequate to obtain the defined microbial specifications.

The objectives of GMP include prevention of possible contamination and cross-contamination. Viral removal and viral inactivation steps are critical processes and should be validated. General information on avoidance of cross-contamination is found in GMP Guidelines Part I on Basic requirements for medicinal products.[89] In order to minimize the risk of cross-contamination, the production of certain additional products should not be conducted in the same facilities. For those products, in exceptional cases, the principle of campaign working in the same facility can be accepted, provided that specific precautions are taken into account and that necessary precautions are made. Apart from certain antibiotics or hormones, special requirements do exist for gene therapy medicinal products. Measures to remove organisms before subsequent manufacturing should be performed and validated. Special cleaning and decontamination methods required for the range of micro-organisms handled should be considered. Measures for accidental spills or other release of viable organisms should be in place including for containments, personal protection, cleaning, and decontamination. Facilities where viruses are handled should be separated from other areas and the use of closed systems wherever possible is highly demanded. Any addition or removal of samples should prevent the release of virus. Concurrent manufacture of different viral containing products is forbidden and change over procedures between campaigns should be proved to be effective. A detailed description from starting material (including plasmids, genes, and regulatory sequences, etc.) to the finished product is essential when manufacturing genetically modified cells or viral vectors[8]. Where replication limited vectors are used, measures should be in place to prevent the generation of wild type viruses which may lead to occurrence of replication competent viruses. It is of great importance to find a suitable system that allows for viral inactivation. Whenever viral supernatants are handled, it is of great importance to ensure that neither the personnel working in the clean room nor any following manufactured product can potentially be contaminated by residual virus particles. During development of the manufacturing process of a genetically modified cellular product, a cleaning method has to be developed and validated that ensures that the virus used for production is efficiently removed by cleaning and disinfection measures.

A variety of disinfectants effective against viruses are available like, for example, alcohols, aldehydes, hydrogen peroxides, or chlorine compounds. The disinfectant needs to be strong enough to eliminate the applied virus with the applied cleaning measures. The main risk is exposed by spills or drops of viral supernatant or culture medium. The validation should be performed with the applied virus, but in order not to pollute the clean room areas; it should be performed in a separate, suitable laboratory room. In order to mimic the process that is going to be performed in the clean room later, the same materials should be utilized for the validation process. For example, the interior of a laminar flow bench can be simulated by a smaller item made from the same material. A defined amount of viral supernatant can then be applied on the chosen surface and afterwards wiped away with the appropriate disinfectant. The time, the virus sample remains on the surface before it is wiped away should include a worst case scenario (e.g., an undetected spill that dried). Any remaining virus can then be collected with swab tests or is resuspended in the appropriate medium. Afterwards viral presence can be detected by PCR analysis or by reinfection of sensitive indicator cells.

Generally, for the handling of living micro–organisms in the manufacturing process of an ATMP, a thorough knowledge of the used organisms (live cells or adventitious agents, e.g., viruses), their potential pathogenicity, detectability, persistence, and possible inactivation are basic requirements. This should be accompanied with detailed knowledge about the donor's health status, the avoidance of open systems (e.g., use of tube filling systems) and single use components. In addition to the regulatory requirements for the manufacturing of ATMPs, the national demands in regard to bio-safety levels and like, e.g., in Germany, the Genetic engineering law (GenTG) lists requirements for the safety of the personnel working in such environments including their personal protective equipments (PPEs) and the constructional requirements for the facility.

References

1. CAT Committee for Advanced Therapies. Reflection paper on classification of advanced therapy medicinal products. In *EMA/CAT/600280/2010*. (ed. EMA). EMA-CAT (2012). (http://www.ema.europa.eu/docs/en_GB/document_library/Regulatory_and_procedural_guideline/2012/04/WC500126681.pdf).
2. Directives Commission. Directive 2009/120/EC of September 14, 2009 amending Directive 2001/83/EC of the European Parliament and of the Council on the Community code relating to medicinal products for human use as regards advanced therapy medicinal product. (ed. Union, O.J.o.t.E.) (2009).
3. EU Commission Directive 2003/94/EC laying down the principles and guidelines of good manufacturing practice in respect of medicinal products for human use and investigational medicinal products for human use. (ed. Communities, T.C.O.T.E.) (2003). (http://ec.europa.eu/health/files/eudralex/vol-1/dir_2003_94/dir_2003_94_en.pdf).
4. CHMP, C.f.m.p.f.h.u. Guideline on Human Cell-Based Medicinal Products. In *Doc. Ref. EMEA/CHMP/410869/2006* (ed. Agency, E.M.). EMA (2007). (http://www.ema.europa.eu/docs/en_GB/document_library/Scientific_guideline/2009/09/WC500003898.pdf).
5. Guideline on the risk based approach to annex I part IV of Dir. 2001/83/EC applied to ATMP (ed. ATMP, C.f.). EMA-CAT (2013). (http://www.ema.europa.eu/docs/en_GB/document_library/Scientific_guideline/2013/03/WC500139748.pdf)
6. Hourd, P., Ginty, P., Chandra, A., and Williams, D.J. Manufacturing models permitting roll out/scale out of clinically led autologous cell therapies: Regulatory and scientific challenges for comparability. *Cytotherapy* 16, 1033–1047 (2014).
7. GMP guideline Annex 1, Manufacture of sterile medicinal products. (ed. pharmaceuticals, C.g.). Eudralex, European Comission Brussels (2009). (http://ec.europa.eu/health/documents/eudralex/vol-4/index_en.htm).
8. GMP Guideline Annex 2, Manufacture of biological active substances and medicinal products for human use. (ed. Products, M.). Eudralex, European Comission Brussels (2013). (http://ec.europa.eu/health/documents/eudralex/vol-4/index_en.htm).
9. GMP guideline Part I, Basic requirements for medicinal products, chapter 3 Premises and Equipment. (ed. Pharmceuticals, C.g.). Eudralex, European Commission Brussels. (http://ec.europa.eu/health/documents/eudralex/vol-4/index_en.htm).
10. Corporation, F. Evaluating Indoor Air Quality with the Fluke 983 Particle Counter. (ed. Fluke). Internet (2005).
11. WHO. Guide to good storage practices for pharmaceuticals. Technical Report Series, No. 908, 2003 Annex 9. WHO guideline, WHO (2003).

12. EMA. Part II. Basic requirements for active substances used as starting material: GMP Guideline. (ed. guidelines, G.). Eudralex (2010).
13. Harel, A. Cryopreservation and cell banking for autologous mesenchymal stem cell-based therapies. *Cell Tissue Transplant. Ther.* 5, 1–7 (2013).
14. GMP Guideline Annex 15, Qualification and Validation (New Version available from Oct 2014). (ed. Efficacy, M.P.Q.S.). Eudralex, European Comission Brussels (2001). (http://ec.europa.eu/health/documents/eudralex/vol-4/index_en.htm).
15. Crauste-Manciet, S., Sessink, P.J., Ferrari, S., Jomier, J.Y., and Brossard, D. Environmental contamination with cytotoxic drugs in healthcare using positive air pressure isolators. *Ann. Occup. Hyg.* 49, 619–628 (2005).
16. BGBl. Gesetz über den Verkehr mit Arzneimitteln (Arzneimittelgesetz) von 2005 zuletzt geändert 27.3.2014. (ed. Verbraucherschutz, B.d.J.u.f.). (Bundesministerium der Justiz und für Verbraucherschutz (2014). (http://www.gesetze-im-internet.de).
17. Oppermann, T., and Leber, J. hMSC production in disposable bioreactors in compliance with cGMP guidelines and PAT. *Am. Pharm. Rev.*, 1–9 (2014).
18. Le Blanc, K., and Ringden, O. Mesenchymal stem cells: Properties and role in clinical bone marrow transplantation. *Curr. Opin. Immunol.* 18, 586–591 (2006).
19. Kollar, K., Cook, M.M., Atkinson, K., and Brooke, G. Molecular mechanisms involved in mesenchymal stem cell migration to the site of acute myocardial infarction. *Int. J. Cell Biol.* 2009, 904682 (2009).
20. Wang, S., Qu, X., and Zhao, R.C. Clinical applications of mesenchymal stem cells. *J. Hematol. Oncol.* 5, 19 (2012).
21. Hass, R., Kasper, C., Bohm, S., and Jacobs, R. Different populations and sources of human mesenchymal stem cells (MSC): A comparison of adult and neonatal tissue-derived MSC. *Cell Commun. Signal.* 9, 12 (2011).
22. T1DM Immunotherapy using CD4+CD127lo/−CD25+ Polyclonal Tregs. In *University of California, San Francisco.* (ClinicalTrials.gov Identifier: NCT01210664). Clinical Trials.gov (2010). (http://clinicaltrials.gov/show/nct01210664).
23. Phase 1 Infused Donor T Regulatory Cells in Steroid Dependent/Refractory Chronic GVHD. (ClinicalTrials.gov Identifier: NCT01911039). Laura Johnston, Stanford University (2013). (http://clinicaltrials.gov/show/NCT01911039).
24. Universität-Regensburg. Treatment of steroid resistant severe acute gastrointestinal graft-versus-host disease with *in vitro* expanded donor-derived regulatory T cells. In *EudraCT Number: 2012-002685-12, Steroid Resistant Severe Acute Gastrointestinal Graft-versus-Host disease.* (ed. University-Hospital-Regensburg). Treg002 (2013). (https://www.clinicaltrialsregister.eu/ctr-search/search?query=eudract_number:2012-0026 85-12).
25. Growing mammalian cells and tissues in culture. Rockefeller University (2010). (http://centennial.rucares.org/index.php?page=Mammalian_Cells).
26. Berger, T.G., *et al.* Large-scale generation of mature monocyte-derived dendritic cells for clinical application in cell factories. *J. Immunol. Methods* 268, 131–140 (2002).
27. Santos, F., *et al.* Toward a clinical-grade expansion of mesenchymal stem cells from human sources: A microcarrier-based culture system under xeno-free conditions. *Tissue Eng. Part C Methods* 17, 1201–1210 (2011).
28. Hashimura, Y. *Comparison of the Novel PBS Air-Wheel TM Bioreactor against the Traditional Stirred-Tank Bioreactor in Microcarrier Applications.* PBS Biotech, IBET.

29. Meuwly, F., Ruffieux, P.A., Kadouri, A., and von Stockar, U. Packed-bed bioreactors for mammalian cell culture: Bioprocess and biomedical applications. *Biotechnol. Adv.* 25, 45–56 (2007).

30. Wendt, D., Riboldi, S.A., Cioffi, M., and Martin, I. Potential and bottlenecks of bioreactors in 3D cell culture and tissue manufacturing. *Adv. Mater.* 21, 3352–3367 (2009).

31. Mizukami, A., *et al.* Efficient expansion of mesenchymal stromal cells in a disposable fixed bed culture system. *Biotechnol. Prog.* 29, 568–572 (2013).

32. Meuwly, F., *et al.* Oxygen supply for CHO cells immobilized on a packed-bed of Fibra-Cel disks. *Biotechnol. Bioeng.* 93, 791–800 (2006).

33. Dove, A. *Living Large: Scaling up Cell Culture* (December 2013). (http://www.science mag.org/search?site_area=sciencejournals&fulltext=living%20large&journalcode=sci &journalcode=sigtrans&journalcode=scitransmed&submit=yes).

34. Ratner, M. Genzyme's Lumizyme clears bioequivalence hurdles. *Nat. Biotechnol.* 27, 685 (2009).

35. Note for guidance on minimising the risk of transmitting animal spongiform encephalopathy agents *via* human and veterinary medicinal products in *EMA/410/01 rev.3*, Vol. 2011/C73/01. (ed. EU). EU (2011). (http://www.ema.europa. eu/docs/en_GB/document_library/Scientific_guideline/2009/09/WC500003700.pdf).

36. EMA. Guideline on the use of porcine trypsin used in the manufacture of human biological medicinal product. (ed. CHMP, C.f.m.p.f.h.u.). EMA homepage (2014).

37. Unger, C., Skottman, H., Blomberg, P., Dilber, M.S., and Hovatta, O. Good manufacturing practice and clinical-grade human embryonic stem cell lines. *Hum. Mol. Genet.* 17, R48–53 (2008).

38. Butler, M.O., *et al.* A panel of human cell-based artificial APC enables the expansion of long-lived antigen-specific CD4+ T cells restricted by prevalent HLA-DR alleles. *Int. Immunol.* 22, 863–873 (2010).

39. Broichhausen, C. Regulatory macrophages as therapeutic targets and therapeutic agents in solid organ transplantation. *Curr. Opin. Transplant.* 17, (2012).

40. Babatz, J. Large-scale immunomagnetic selection of CD14+ monocytes to generate dendritic cells for cancer immunotherapy: A phase I study. *J. Hematother. Stem Cell Res.* (2003).

41. Butler, M. Establishing CD8+ T cell immunity by adoptive transfer of autologous, IL-15 expanded, anti-tumor CTL with a central/effector memory phenotype can induce objective clinical responses. In *ASH Annual Meeting Abstracts, Vol. Blood*, 114 (2009). (http://abstracts.hematologylibrary.org/content/vol114/issue22/).

42. Carlson, D.F., Fahrenkrug, S.C., and Hackett, P.B. Targeting DNA with fingers and TALENs. *Mol. Ther. Nucleic Acids* 1, e3 (2012).

43. 5.14 Gene Transfer Medicinal Products for Human Use. In *European Pharmacopoeia Vol. 8.0* (ed. Commission, E.). European Directorate for the Quality of Medicines & HealthCare, EDQM (2014). (https://www.edqm.eu/en/edqm-databases-10.html).

44. FDA. Guidance for Industry, FDA Guidance for Human Somatic Cell Therapy and Gene Therapy. (ed. Research, C.f.B.E.a.) (1998). (www.fda.gov).

45. ICH. Derivation and Characterisation of Cell Substrates used for Production of Biotechnological/biological Products. (ed. Use, I.F.R.o.P.f.H.) (1997). (www.ich.org).

46. Plattner, R., *et al.* Loss of oncogenic ras expression does not correlate with loss of tumorigenicity in human cells. *Proc. Natl. Acad. Sci. U.S.A.* 93, 6665–6670 (1996).

47. Maier, P., von Kalle, C., and Laufs, S. Retroviral vectors for gene therapy. *Future Microbiol.* 5, 1507–1523 (2010).

48. Miller, A.D., and Chen, F. Retrovirus packaging cells based on 10A1 murine leukemia virus for production of vectors that use multiple receptors for cell entry. *J. Virol.* 70, 5564–5571 (1996).

49. Miller, A.D., *et al.* Construction and properties of retrovirus packaging cells based on gibbon ape leukemia virus. *J. Virol.* 65, 2220–2224 (1991).

50. Takeuchi, Y., *et al.* Type C retrovirus inactivation by human complement is determined by both the viral genome and the producer cell. *J. Virol.* 68, 8001–8007 (1994).

51. Schucht, R., *et al.* A new generation of retroviral producer cells: Predictable and stable virus production by Flp-mediated site-specific integration of retroviral vectors. *Mol. Ther.* 14, 285–292 (2006).

52. Coroadinha, A.S., *et al.* The use of recombinase mediated cassette exchange in retroviral vector producer cell lines: Predictability and efficiency by transgene exchange. *J. Biotechnol.* 124, 457–468 (2006).

53. Loew, R., *et al.* A new PG13-based packaging cell line for stable production of clinical-grade self-inactivating gamma-retroviral vectors using targeted integration. *Gene Ther.* 17, 272–280 (2010).

54. Broussau, S., *et al.* Inducible packaging cells for large-scale production of lentiviral vectors in serum-free suspension culture. *Mol. Ther.* 16, 500–507 (2008).

55. Farson, D., *et al.* A new-generation stable inducible packaging cell line for lentiviral vectors. *Hum. Gene Ther.* 12, 981–997 (2001).

56. Ni, Y., *et al.* Generation of a packaging cell line for prolonged large-scale production of high-titer HIV-1-based lentiviral vector. *J. Gene Med.* 7, 818–834 (2005).

57. Merten, O.W., *et al.* Large-scale manufacture and characterization of a lentiviral vector produced for clinical *ex vivo* gene therapy application. *Hum. Gene Ther.* 22, 343–356 (2011).

58. Bellintani. ESGCT 2008 oral presentations. *Hum. Gene Ther.* 19, 1076–1097 (2008).

59. Schweizer, M., and Merten, O.W. Large-scale production means for the manufacturing of lentiviral vectors. *Curr. Gene Ther.* 10, 474–486 (2010).

60. Reach, M., Xu, L.X., and Young, C.S. Transcription from the adenovirus major late promoter uses redundant activating elements. *EMBO J.* 10, 3439–3446 (1991).

61. David Curiel, J.D. *Adenoviral Vectors for Gene Therapy.* Elsevier Inc., U.S.A. (2002).

62. Lusky, M. Good manufacturing practice production of adenoviral vectors for clinical trials. *Hum. Gene Ther.* 16, 281–291 (2005).

63. Kovesdi, I., and Hedley, S.J. Adenoviral producer cells. *Viruses* 2, 1681–1703 (2010).

64. McConnell, M.J., and Imperiale, M.J. Biology of adenovirus and its use as a vector for gene therapy. *Hum. Gene Ther.* 15, 1022–1033 (2004).

65. Palmer, D. Improved system for helper-dependent adenoviral vector production. *Mol. Ther.* 8, 846–852 (2003).

66. Stern B.S., *et al.* Erythropoeisis sustained 1 year by the EPODURE biopump in patients with chronic kidney disease: Further results of phase I/II proof of concept trial. *Mol. Ther.* 18, (2010).

67. Cecchini, S., Virag, T., and Kotin, R.M. Reproducible high yields of recombinant adeno-associated virus produced using invertebrate cells in 0.02- to 200-liter cultures. *Hum. Gene Ther.* 22, 1021–1030 (2011).

68. Aucoin, M.G., Perrier, M., and Kamen, A.A. Critical assessment of current adeno-associated viral vector production and quantification methods. *Biotechnol. Adv.* 26, 73–88 (2008).
69. Kotin, R.M. Large-scale recombinant adeno-associated virus production. *Hum. Mol. Genet.* 20, R2–R6 (2011).
70. Brittberg, M., *et al.* Treatment of deep cartilage defects in the knee with autologous chondrocyte transplantation. *N. Engl. J. Med.* 331, 889–895 (1994).
71. EMA. Assessment Report for ChondroCelect. In *EMEA/H/C/000878.* (ed. Use, E.o.M.f.H.) (2009). (http://www.ema.europa.eu).
72. Tigenix. Development course of an ATMP ChondroCelect case study. (ed. Bekker, G.d.) (2011). (http://www.gipso.org/documents/4ee0ae439734c_tigenixger tdebeckkerpdf.pdf).
73. TiGenix NV. Articular cartilage-derived cells (ChondroCelect®). In *All In Vitro Cells > Primary Cell Card.* (ed. discovery.lifemapsc.com). NV, TiGenix. (http://discovery.lifemapsc.com/stem-cell-differentiation/in-vitro-cells/cartilage-homo-sapiens-articular-cartilage-derived-cells-chondrocelect-tigenix-nv).
74. Rouas, R., *et al.* Dendritic cells generated in clinical grade bags strongly differ in immune functionality when compared with classical DCs generated in plates. *J. Immunother.* 33, 352–363 (2010).
75. FDA. Thomas Finn, P., Chair of the Review Committee. Provenge Summary Basis for Regulatory Action. (ed. Office of Cellular, T., and Gene Therapies). FDA (2010). (http://www.fda.gov/downloads/BiologicsBloodVaccines/CellularGeneTherapyProducts/ApprovedProducts/UCM213114.pdf).
76. Bryant, L.M., *et al.* Lessons learned from the clinical development and market authorization of Glybera. *Hum. Gene Ther. Clin. Dev.* 24, 55–64 (2013).
77. Petry, H. Glybera® & Platform Technology for Manufacturing of Clinical grade AAV. (2013). (http://www.a.pda.org/docs/default-source/attendee-presentations/europe/2013-pda-europe-conference-on-atmps/harald-petry-unique.pdf?sfvrsn=4).
78. EMA. Assessment report Glybera. *EMA EMEA/H/C/002145.* (2012). (http://www.ema.europa.eu/docs/en_GB/document_library/EPAR_ _Public_assessment_report/human/002145/WC500135470.pdf)
79. Llau, G. Lessons learned from the manufacture and clinical translation of gene and cell therapy products. In *ASGCT.* Salt lake city. (2013).
80. Kramer, S. Key element of the clinical scale-up manufacturing process used for Glybera® developed by the National Heart Lung and Blood Institute investigators at the National Institutes of Health in *ASGCT* (unknown).
81. UniQure. In http://www.uniqure.com/r-d/platform/).
82. Naaldijk, Y., Staude, M., Fedorova, V., and Stolzing, A. Effect of different freezing rates during cryopreservation of rat mesenchymal stem cells using combinations of hydroxyethyl starch and dimethylsulfoxide. *BMC Biotechnol.* 12, 49 (2012).
83. GMP Guidelines Annex 13, Investigational Medicinal Products. (ed. Pharmaceuticals, C.g.). Eudralex, European Commission Brussels (2010). (http://ec.europa.eu/health/documents/eudralex/vol-4/index_en.htm).
84. ICCBBA. ISBT 128- The Global Information Standard for Medical Products of Human Origin. International Council for Commonality in Blood Banking Automation (2014). (http://www.iccbba.org/).

85. Rice, B. Standard Terminology for Blood, Cellular Therapy and Tissue Product Descriptions. (ed. ICCBBA) (2014). (http://www.iccbba.org/uploads/a5/e4/a5e457eb943399fd4f5bb6237c5ec4a9/Standard-Terminology-for-Blood-Cellular-Therapy-and-Tissue-Product-Descriptions-v5.4.pdf).

86. Good Distribution Practice of medicinal products for human use. In *2013/C 343/01*. (ed. Union, O.J.o.t.E.). European Commission (2013). (http://ec.europa.eu/health/human-use/good_distribution_practice/index_en.htm).

87. EMA. Good Distribution Practice for Medicinal Products for Human Use, Questions and Answers. (ed. Directorate-General, E.C.H.A.C.) (2013).

88. PIC/S. Recommendation on the Validation of Aseptic Processes. (ed. SCHEME, P.S.P.I.C.P.I.C.-O.) (2011).

89. EMA. GMP Guideline Vol.4 Part I- Basic Requirements for Medicinal Products. (ed. Commission, E.). Eudralex.

Quality Control   6

Andrea Hauser, Elena Meurer, Nadja Noske, and Christine Günther

6.1 Introduction

The Quality Control (QC) department of a pharmaceutical manufacturer — independent of what kind of product is produced — plays a key role not only for final release of the manufactured products, but also for the ascertainment of quality throughout the whole process of manufacturing. Responsibilities of the QC department commence with testing and release of starting materials and active pharmaceutical ingredients (APIs), followed by in-process controls and ending with release testing. Apart from that, QC also analyzes and releases all critical raw materials and excipients used for production including primary packaging materials and labels. The EU Good Manufacturing Practice (GMP) Guidelines in Chapter 6 "Quality Control"[1] even go one step further in claiming that QC is not limited to laboratory operations, but must be involved in all decisions which may concern the quality of the product. Assessment of the finished product is not restricted to analytical procedures, but also has to consider all relevant factors including production conditions and review of manufacturing documentation. Complete independence of QC from Production is therefore mandatory to ensure reliable results.

This chapter provides an overview of all duties and responsibilities of a QC department in pharmaceutical manufacturing with special focus on QC of cellular products. However, it is important to read this chapter in conjunction with the chapter on Quality Management (QM) as some GMP prerequisites on qualification of equipment and facilities, initial and ongoing training of personnel and GMP compliant documentation are not repeated in detail here.

QC of cell therapy medicinal products (CTMPs) is for several reasons more challenging than QC of standard medicinal products:

- Very heterogeneous starting material due to donor-dependent variability.
- Up- and down-regulation of analytical targets [e.g., the cluster of differentiation (CD) markers].
- Short shelf life of many cell therapy products (CTPs) resulting in administration of the products before testing of the finished product can be completed.
- Limited cell numbers/test material does not allow complete control testing.
- Specific mechanism of action (MoA) is often hard to define.
- Limited availability of test reagents with sufficient quality.
- No compendial, WHO or other internationally accepted reference standards available.
- Adequate negative and positive controls are sometimes difficult to define — especially in flow cytometry.
- Evaluation of flow cytometry data is not automated and therefore highly susceptible to bias of the operator.

Apart from that many of the applicable rules and regulations were developed for conventional medicinal products and therefore do not fit the special requirements of cellular products. Altogether huge efforts are necessary to comply with the authorities' requests to receive either manufacturing or marketing authorization (MA) or approval of a clinical trial. As manufacturing processes in clinical trials — at least in early stages — tend to be not fully validated, QC of investigational medicinal products (IMPs) is of special significance there.

6.2 QC of Materials

6.2.1 *Terms and definitions*

As cell-based medicinal products (CBMPs) cannot be sterilized or undergo any virus reducing steps, quality of both the starting material and all materials and substances coming into contact with the cells during manufacture is of special significance and importance. Independent of the cell source, many different guidance documents exist that prescribe specifications and acceptance criteria for the starting material, whereas all other materials and substances used during the manufacturing process are regulated to a much lesser extent. Especially pharmacopoeial monographs for raw materials and excipients used in the cell therapy field are mostly missing and pharmaceutical grade substances are hard to find in contrast to conventional medicinal products, where the majority of raw materials and excipients are described in a Pharmacopoeia.

Since there are regulatory differences in relation to starting materials, raw materials/ancillary materials (AMs), and excipients, it is worth to have a closer look on terms and definitions first, even if they slightly differ depending on the source. Table 6.1 gives an overview on definitions used for the different materials in Europe, USA and the International Conference on Harmonisation (ICH)-region.

6.2.2 Starting material

6.2.2.1 Primary cells and tissues as starting material

Starting materials for CBMPs are mostly either blood (leukapheresis products, whole blood, cord blood, etc.) or tissue (bone marrow, fatty tissue, placenta, etc.) used in an autologous or allogeneic way. Allogeneic utilization can be either directed [defined donor and recipient as known from hematopoietic stem cell (HSC) transplantation] or without restriction of possible recipients (third party use, off-the-shelf products).

Independent of the type or source, all biological starting materials bear the risk of transmitting viral and microbial contamination together with the target cells as neither sterilization nor virus reducing steps are possible before or during cell processing. Donor selection, donor testing (compare Section 6.2.3. Donor Testing and Traceability), and analysis of the starting material are therefore mandatory to address these risks especially in the allogeneic setting where transmission of severe infectious diseases such as Human Immunodeficiency virus (HIV) or Hepatitis C virus (HCV) have to be prevented implicitly. Microbial contamination of the starting material cannot be fully excluded despite well-defined disinfection procedures of the skin prior to puncture but trained personnel and the separation of the first part of the donation (pre-donation sampling) helped to reduce contamination rates of blood products to rates considerably below 1%.[2–5] Pre-donation sampling with the separation of the first milliliters of the initial blood volume is therefore compulsory in many countries, e.g., Germany.[6] But also contamination rates for HSC donations of around 5% have been reported. Microbiological contamination rates of tissues such as adipose tissue, bone marrow, and cord blood tend to be even higher than those of conventional blood products or leukapheresis products as the procurement procedures are not minimally invasive (e.g., bone marrow harvest by percutaneous needle aspiration of the iliac crests) and cannot be executed in closed systems or under clean room conditions.[7–10]

Table 6.1: Terms and definitions: starting material, APIs, raw/AMs and excipients.

	EU	USA	ICH
(API) Starting material	**API starting material:** A general term used to denote starting materials, reagents, and solvents intended for use in the production of intermediates, APIs or medicinal products. (EU GMP Guidelines, Part II). For the purposes of this Annex [note: Annex I to Directive 2001/83/EC], **starting materials** shall mean all the materials from which the active substance is manufactured or extracted. For biological medicinal products, **starting material** shall mean any substance of biological origin such as micro-organisms, organs, and tissues of either plant or animal origin, cells or fluids (including blood or plasma) of human or animal origin, and biotechnological cell constructs (cell substrates, whether they are recombinant or not, including primary cells). (Part I of Annex I to Directive 2001/83/EC).	**Starting Material:** Materials that mark the beginning of the manufacturing process as described in an application [...]. The starting material for a drug substance obtained from a biological source is considered to consist of the (1) Cells; (2) Plants [...]; or (3) Animal tissues, organs, or body fluid from which the drug substance is derived (FDA Guidance for Industry, Drug Substance Chemistry, Manufacturing, and Controls Information).	**Starting material:** A material used in the synthesis of a new drug substance that is incorporated as an element into the structure of an intermediate and/or of the new drug substance. **Starting materials** are normally commercially available and of defined chemical and physical properties and structure (ICH Q3A). **API Starting Material:** A raw material, intermediate, or an API that is used in the production of an API and that is incorporated as a significant structural fragment into the structure of the API. An **API Starting Material** can be an article of commerce, a material purchased from one or more suppliers under contract or commercial agreement, or produced in-house. API Starting Materials are normally of defined chemical properties and structure (ICH Q7).

API or Drug substance	**Active substance:** An substance or mixture of substances intended to be used in the manufacture of a medicinal product and that, when used in its production, becomes an **active ingredient** of that product intended to exert a pharmacological, immunological or metabolic action with a view to restoring, correcting or modifying physiological functions or to make a medical diagnosis (Article 1(3a) of Directive 2001/83/EC).	**API = Drug Substance:** An active ingredient that is intended to furnish pharmacological activity or other direct effect in the diagnosis, cure, mitigation, treatment, or prevention of disease or to affect the structure or any function of the human body, but does not include intermediates used in the synthesis of such ingredient [21 CFR 314.3(b)].	**API (Drug Substance):** Any substance or mixture of substances intended to be used in the manufacture of a drug (medicinal) product and that, when used in the production of a drug, becomes an active ingredient of the drug product. Such substances are intended to furnish pharmacological activity or other direct effect in the diagnosis, cure, mitigation, treatment, or prevention of disease or to affect the structure and function of the body (ICH Q7)
Raw material or AM	**Raw material** shall be considered as materials used during the manufacture of the active substance (e.g., culture media, growth factors) and that are not intended to form part of the active substance (Directive 2009/120/EC). Any other substances used for	The defining property of **AMs** is that they are not intended to be present in the final product. They are materials used as processing and purification aids or agents that exert their effect on the therapeutic substance (USP <1043>). Synonym: Processing material means any material or substance that is used in, or to facilitate, processing, but which is not	**Raw material:** A general term used to denote starting materials, reagents, and solvents intended for use in the production of intermediates or APIs (ICH Q7).

(Continued)

Table 6.1: *(Continued)*

	EU	USA	ICH
	manufacturing or extracting the active substance(s) but from which this active substance is not directly derived, such as reagents, culture media, foetal calf serum, additives, and buffers involved in chromatography, etc. are known as **raw materials** (Part I of Annex I to Directive 2001/83/EC).	intended by the manufacturer to be included in the human cellular or tissue-based product when it is made available for distribution [21 CFR Part 1271, Federal Register 66 (5)]. **Raw Material:** any substance used in the production of a product excluding packaging materials (USP <1078>).	
Excipient	**Excipient:** Any constituent of a medicinal product other than the active substance and the packaging material (Article 1(3b) of Directive 2001/83/EC).	**Excipient:** Any substance, other than the active drug or product, that have been appropriately evaluated for safety and are included in a drug delivery system to either aid the processing of the drug delivery system during its manufacture, protect, support or enhance stability, bioavailability, or patient acceptability, assist in product identification, or enhance any other attribute of the overall safety and effectiveness of the drug delivery system during storage or use (USP <1078>).	**Excipient:** Anything other than the drug substance in the dosage form (ICH Q1A). **Excipient:** An ingredient added intentionally to the drug substance which should not have pharmacological properties in the quantity used (ICH Q6B).

Sources: USP <1043> "Ancillary Materials for cell, gene, and tissue engineered products".
USP <1078> "Good manufacturing practices for bulk pharmaceutical excipients".

Apart from the above mentioned viral and microbial safety aspects the starting material has to have a defined minimum quality in terms of overall and/or target cell number, cellular composition, cell concentration, and viability. Product-specific acceptance criteria for these parameters should be defined and the starting material should be tested for these parameters prior to use. Unlike chemical substances used for conventional medicinal products materials of human origin tend to be more variable, thus specifications have to be set carefully with respect to a much lower batch-to-batch consistency. This variability might be even greater in the autologous setting where blood, tissue, or cell donations are taken from the recipients of the CBMPs, hence the donors are often seriously affected by impaired health conditions. Optimal parameters for the donation and procurement procedure cannot be achieved in many cases and the diseases that are supposed to be treated with the cellular products often influence the quality of the blood, cell, or tissue donation. In any case ethical issues exacerbate the access to materials of human origin as it is not justifiable to put donors at risk for the mere purpose of gathering data and information with no benefit for the donor and/or recipient. Therefore, some questions with regard to the procurement procedure and the quality of the starting material cannot be sufficiently approached before the first clinical phases.

In addition to the above mentioned quality of the donated material itself, the presence of certain excipients in the starting material [e.g., anticoagulants such as heparin or Ethylenediaminetetraacetic acid (EDTA)] might be of special importance for the subsequent manufacturing as they might be necessary or could adversely affect production processes. In these cases, the absence of certain excipients or their presence in acceptable or required limits or concentrations has to be defined.

The EU GMP Guidelines, Annex 2,[11] acknowledges that the necessary tests for analysis of the starting material can take a long time where the shelf life of the starting material is reduced to some hours or days. "*In these cases, it may be permissible to process starting materials before the results of the tests are available, but the risk of using a potentially failed material and its potential impact on other batches should be clearly understood and assessed under the principles of quality risk management*".

If the donation of the starting material is not carried out under the responsibility of the manufacturer of the CBMP, it has to be clearly defined who is responsible for the examination and testing of the donor prior to donation, for analysis of the donation, for traceability and for preservation of look back or retention samples. In some countries (e.g., Germany) blood donations (including leukapheresis products) are medicinal products that have to be produced under a manufacturing license following the GMP guidelines and released by a Qualified Person (QP). In these cases, the QP of the CBMP can rely on the certification of the QP of the donation center. In most of the other European Member States as well as in the USA, blood and tissue is not regulated as medicinal product and the GMP rules are not applicable. In these cases, the QP of the manufacturer of the CBMP is fully responsible for the donation when used as starting material as there is no QP release and batch certification of the starting material. The Head of QC has to ensure that all defined quality standards and specifications are met. Technical agreements between the responsible parties might be necessary to assure that both sides are fulfilling their duties.

6.2.2.2 *Primary cell lines from banking systems as starting material*

Primary cells originating from autologous or allogeneic (matched) donors have the disadvantage of high batch-to-batch variability and availability in absolute limited quantities. However, if the quantities and characteristics of primary cells allow for their storage with subsequent manufacturing of multiples batches, they can be used as cell lines.

To ensure robust batch-to-batch quality, banking strategies in analogy to other biologic production processes are of interest, especially when it comes to larger batch numbers and advanced clinical development.

Where cell lines are used, an appropriately characterized Master Cell Bank (MCB) and Working Cell Bank (WCB) should be established, whenever possible. Cell banking and characterization, and testing of the established cell banks should comply with the ICH guideline Q5D.[12]

Cell bank system:

A cell bank is a collection of cells obtained from pooled cells or derived from a single cell clone or donor tissue that is stored in bags or vials under defined conditions that maintain genotypic and phenotypic stability. The cell bank system usually consists of a MCB and a WCB, although alternative approaches are possible. The MCB is produced in accordance with (c)GMP and preferably is obtained from a qualified source (one that is free from adventitious agents) with known and documented history. Human cells and tissues should be obtained by means of a licensed tissue acquisition vendor with a donor qualification program in accordance to e.g. 21 CFR 1271 on "Human Cells, Tissues, and Cellular and Tissue-based products". The WCB is produced or derived by expanding one or more vials of the MCB. The WCB, or MCB in early trials, becomes the source of cells for every batch produced for human use. Cell bank systems contribute greatly to production batch consistency because the starting cell material is always the same. However, it may not be possible or feasible to create a cell bank, so appropriately tested and qualified primary cells may be used *in lieu* of creation of cell banks. The MCB and WCB should be minimally tested for identity, sterility, purity, viability, and the presence of viruses and mycoplasma.

Cell bank qualification:

Cell bank safety testing and characterization are important steps toward obtaining a uniform final product with lot-to-lot consistency and freedom from adventitious agents. ICH Q5A (R1) "Viral Safety Evaluation of Biotechnology Products Derived from Cell Lines of Human or Animal Origin" gives specific recommendations for testing cell banks for viral agents. While this guideline is not specifically intended to cover cell or tissue-based products, the same tests are generally applicable. Additional virus testing may be needed depending on the prevalence of viral diseases endemic in the donor population. Testing to qualify the MCB is performed once and can be done on an aliquot of the banked material or on cell cultures derived from the cell bank. Specifications for qualification of the MCB should be prospectively established. It is important to document the MCB history, the methods and reagents used to produce the bank, and the storage conditions. All the AMs required for production of the banks, such as media, sera, cytokines, growth factors, and enzymes, should also be qualified, documented, and appropriately tested.

USP General Chapter <1046> "Cell and Gene Therapy Products" provides information on the characterization of cell banks.[13]

MCB- Safety testing to qualify the MCB includes testing to demonstrate freedom from adventitious agents and endogenous viruses. The testing for adventitious agents should include tests for bacteria, fungi, mycoplasma, and viruses. Freedom from adventitious viruses should be demonstrated using both *in vitro* and *in vivo* test systems and appropriate species-specific tests.

WCB- Safety testing of the WCB is less extensive and generally focuses on the potential for introduction of adventitious viruses or activation of latent virus during the additional culture required to create the WCB. End-of-production (EOP) safety testing should also be performed to ensure that the cells can be expanded to a known maximum number of generations while still producing an acceptable product. For information about which types of adventitious virus testing should be performed on the MCB, WCB, and the EOP cells, USP General Chapter <1050> "Viral Safety Evaluation of Biotechnology Products Derived from Cell Lines of Human or Animal Origin" provides further requirements.

Characterization of MCB and WCB:

Characterization of the MCB and WCB includes identity testing to establish species origin, e.g., isoenzyme analyses to confirm the human origin of the cells. However, cell bank characterization should encompass additional assessments such as the following:

- Growth kinetics and population doubling time.
- Morphological assessment.
- Percent confluence at passage.
- Cell counts.
- Viability (pre- and post-cryopreservation).
- Phenotypic expression of desired and undesired cell types (pre- and post-cryopreservation).
- Monitoring of unique biochemical markers (pre- and post-cryopreservation).
- Assessments of functional activity (pre- and post-cryopreservation).
- Gene and protein expression analysis (pre- and post-cryopreservation).
- Expression of immune histocompatibility antigens [human leukocyte antigen (HLA)/major histocompatibility complex (MHC)].
- Molecular fingerprinting.
- Chromosomal stability.

6.2.2.3 *Vectors and plasmids as starting material for CBMPs*

For gene therapy medicinal products (GTMPs) that contain genetically modified (GM) cells (stably transduced by viral vector systems), the European Directive 2009/120/EC[14] states that not only the cells but also the components used to obtain the GM cells (i.e., the starting material to produce the vector) are defined as starting materials. The principles of GMP therefore must apply for the bank system used to produce the vector onwards. In the case of products consisting of plasmids, non-viral vectors and GM microorganisms other than viruses or viral vectors, the starting materials are defined to be the components used to generate the producing cell, i.e., the plasmid, the host bacteria, and the MCB of recombinant microbial cells. Depending on the type of the CBMP and its classification as either somatic cell therapy medicinal product or *ex-vivo* gene transfer medicinal product, vectors, and plasmids can also be defined as raw materials (compare Section 6.2.4. Ancillary Materials/Raw Materials). It is important to discuss with the competent authorities what holds true for each individual product, raw or starting material.

Different viral vector systems, such as retro-, lenti-, adeno-, AAV, and herpes virus might be used for gene transfer into host cells, in terms of gene therapy applications. Lenti- and retroviral vector systems are already used for cell-based clinical applications with GM mesenchymal stem cells (MSCs), HSCs or immune cells. For GM cells in general, the "Note for Guidance on the quality, preclinical, and clinical aspects of gene transfer medicinal products"[15] and the "Guideline on quality, non-clinical, and clinical aspects of medicinal products containing GM cells"[16] are relevant European guidance documents that should be followed, giving details on the QC and characterization of gene transfer vectors.

Viral based gene transfer strategies lead to efficient gene expression of incorporated therapeutic genes. Native cells are treated by the viral units in the context of *ex vivo* transduction. These transducing units together with the receiving cells form the basis of the therapeutic product (drug substance). Vectors for the use of genetic modification as well as the receiving cells can be defined as starting materials. In this case and the one dependent on the selected gene transfer method, the production underlies strict regulatory manufacturing guidelines defining material safety, purity, function, and efficacy.

Production of viral vectors is performed by using producer cells from a MCB established under GMP compliant conditions. For assuring optimal quality, supernatants derived from a certain producer cell line must be tested in experimental scenarios prior to performing the therapeutic transduction. Cells producing viral particles have to be transfected (producer cell line) by plasmids containing DNA elements (including transfer plasmid), before they express viral proteins, package viral particles and, release non-replicative viral vectors. The establishment of the MCB is derived from a selective clone harboring the desired DNA elements. This characterized clone will be freshly cultivated for each single bulk production. The final clone is selected for high titer (amount of produced viral particles) production, which can be determined by immune assays mostly performed by flow cytometry analysis. Sterility (microbial and mycoplasma) and genomic stability (confirmation of genetic elements) have to be evaluated for the MCB before starting the viral vector bulk production. Concerning the amount and quality of the produced viral vectors, the MCB should produce the desired transfer elements. Adventitious combinations of packaged elements have to be strictly excluded and tested accordingly. This should be shown in specific designed assays, i.e., cellular assays or PCR-based assays. *In vivo* assays (suckling mouse, etc.) assure the contamination risks by adventitious existence of viruses that might induce pathogenicity in organism. Also in case bovine raw material has to be used in cultivation, adventitious bovine viral contaminants have to be excluded from the MCB before producing viral bulk. This can be achieved by specific cellular assays.

The viral vector batch is tested for the virus titer, quantifying the potent infectious viral particles (cellular assay with subsequent flow cytometry). A reference cell line might be used which has been transduced by the viral vector. If transferred and integrated elements are present and functional, and also the transgene is functional, the expressed amount of the transgene can also be measured by immune assays after transduction of cells and can also be included into titration assays. Specifications will be defined and selected for qualitative standards sufficient for its application, and may also be used as a release criterion. Sterility, the absence of mycoplasma and replication competent viral particles, as well as the absence of other viruses (bovine, human, and murine) should be ensured before using viral vectors for *ex vivo* cell therapy.

For the usage of viral vectors or DNA-containing vesicles for gene transfer into cells, various aspects concerning residual amounts of undesired contaminants have to be considered besides conventional sterility tests, detecting microbiological contaminations. Product and process related impurities may occur during the manufacturing of viral vectors. Assays for the determination of residuals of, e.g., host cell proteins and DNA as well as viruses should be performed. The European Pharmacopoeia (Ph. Eur.) defines requirements for gene transfer medicinal products in Chapter 5.14.[17]

Residues of DNA

The content of host cell DNA after production of the viral vector and harvesting of the supernatant has to be determined by using a predefined and suitable method. For the demonstration of clearance of DNA impurities, quantitative PCR technologies are recommended. In case plasmids are selected for transient production, residual amounts of plasmids must be quantified in contrast to stably used plasmids.

Residues of proteins

Due to the cellular source of the bulk supernatant, residual host-cell proteins have to be determined by a suitable method, for instance by sensitive immunochemical methods. This method might be performed separately or included into the production process of viral vectors. The content of residual host cell-DNA of producer cells should also be determined for purity, unless the process does not indicate validated clearance. Due to high sensitivity and specificity, PCR based technologies, such as quantitative PCR, are recommended, but can also be replaced by other sensitive methods.

Residues of replicative competent viral particles

The formation of replication competent viral particles (RCV-particles) has to be excluded. Usually these tests include the expansion of vector infected cells, followed by nucleic acid based detection technologies on specific viral genes or by immunochemical techniques for detection of virus specific antigens, such as p24 (for Retrovirus). For assuring the absence of RCVs, infectivity assays on sensitive detector cell lines not being able in complementing viral DNA genes in the vector or adequate tests have to be performed. Purity testing on the existence of RCV has to be carried out for viral harvest or bulk production before entering into an application, and therefore has to be an important release criterion. As a consequence, the absence of replicative active viral particles is absolutely required for releasing viral vectors as starting material for genetic modification of cells.

Testing of the starting material for functionality

The manufacturer should ensure safety and functionality prior to release of a viral batch for therapeutic transduction processes. The viral vector batch must be tested for its functional activity on indicator cells before release as starting material according to predefined specifications. The tests applied should reflect the production process of the medicinal product. The transduction of reference cells with single batches of viral vector indicates the functionality of the process. The testing of potency depends on the transgene introduced. The expression and the therapeutic activity of the translated protein might be tested. Safety assays shall be used to address potential risk factors due to potential insertional mutagenesis mediated by the transfer machinery (tested by, e.g., soft agar assay for excluding tumorigenicity).

6.2.3   *Donor testing and traceability*

6.2.3.1   *Rules and regulations for procurement and testing of blood, tissues and cells*

Irrespective of whether human blood, tissues or cells are used as starting or raw material for the production of a CBMP, their quality and safety is crucial for the quality and safety of the finished product. In order to prevent the transmission of diseases by human blood, tissues, and cells (especially in the allogeneic setting) and in order to assure their microbiological safety, a number of guidance documents exist that regulate donor selection and testing. Table 6.2 gives an overview on the relevant European guidelines, but it has to be stated that in individual European Member States, national rules and regulations do exist with more stringent protective measures [e.g., Germany, compare Table 6.3: Minimally Required Laboratory Tests on Infectious Disease Markers (IDMs) for blood, blood components, tissues and cells].

Apart from the directives and guidelines listed in Table 6.2 and apart from national laws and regulations, current announcements of the competent authorities regarding newly defined infectious diseases, current changes or amendments of

Table 6.2: Relevant European guidance documents for procurement, testing and traceability of blood, blood-components, tissues, and cells.

Document Reference Number	Document Title	Remarks
Directive 2002/98/EC	Setting standards of quality and safety for the collection, testing, processing, storage, and distribution of human blood and blood components, and amending Directive 2001/83/EC.	Relevant guideline if human blood or blood components are used as starting material, raw material, or excipient for cellular products. Defines the required extent of donor testing.
Directive 2004/23/EC	On setting standards of quality and safety for the donation, procurement, testing, processing, preservation, storage, and distribution of human tissues and cells.	Important guideline for procurement and testing of cells and tissue.
Directive 2004/33/EC	Implementing Directive 2002/98/EC of the European Parliament and of the Council as regards certain technical requirements for blood and blood components.	Defines amongst other things specific eligibility (acceptance and deferral) criteria for donors of whole blood and blood components as well as specific storage, transport, and distribution conditions for blood and blood components.
Directive 2005/61/EC	Implementing Directive 2002/98/EC of the European Parliament and of the Council as regards traceability requirements and notification of serious adverse reactions and events.	Relevant guideline for traceability and pharmacovigilance/ haemovigilance of human blood and blood components.
Directive 2006/17/EC	Implementing Directive 2004/23/EC of the European Parliament and of the Council as regards certain technical requirements for the donation, procurement, and testing of human tissues and cells.	Important guideline for procurement and testing of cells and tissues. Defines the required extent of donor testing.

(Continued)

Table 6.2: (*Continued*)

Document Reference Number	Document Title	Remarks
Directive 2006/86/EC	Implementing Directive 2004/23/EC of the European Parliament and of the Council as regards traceability requirements, notification of serious adverse reactions and events, and certain technical requirements for the coding, processing, preservation, storage, and distribution of human tissues and cells.	Directive applies to the coding, processing, preservation, storage, and distribution of human tissues and cells, and defines details for the traceability and the reporting of serious adverse reactions, and events to the donation, procurement, and testing of human tissues and cells.
EMA/CHMP/ BWP/ 706271/2010	Guideline on plasma-derived medicinal products.	Reagents of human origin (e.g., albumin, immunoglobulins) should be evaluated for their suitability in a manner identical to that employed for plasma-derived medicinal products.
ENTR/F/2/ SF/dn D(2009) 35810	Detailed guidelines on good clinical practice (GCP) specific to advanced therapy medicinal products (ATMPs).	Further information on traceability of ATMPs used as IMPs.
EMA/CHMP/ BWP/ 353632/2010	CHMP/CAT position statement on Creutzfeldt-Jakob disease and ATMPs	Short overview in which cases a risk-based approach concerning the risk of transmitting Creutzfeldt–Jakob disease (CJD) or Variant CJD (vCJD) is required.
Ph. Eur. 5.1.7.	Viral safety.	Provides general advice for risk assessment of medicinal products with respect to their viral safety.

exclusion criteria or other important information with respect to donor selection and testing have to be followed. As the regulatory landscape is diverse in individual countries and even within the EU, some authorities might request a retesting of IDMs and other relevant analytical parameters whenever blood, tissues or cells are imported from other countries with different requirements.

Table 6.3: Minimally required laboratory tests on IDMs for Blood, Blood Components, Tissues, and Cells.

Infectious Disease	German Haemotherapy Guideline[1] (Scope: Blood and Blood Products Including PBSC)	Directive 2006/17/EC (Scope: Tissue and Cells)	USP Chapter <1046> (Scope: Starting Material for CTPs and GTPs).
Hepatitis B	HBs-antigen Anti-HBc[2]	HBs-antigen Anti-HBc[3]	X[5]
Hepatitis C	Anti-HCV-antibodies HCV-genome (NAT)	Anti-HCV-antibodies —	X[5]
HIV	Anti-HIV-1/-2 antibodies HIV-1-genome (NAT)	Anti-HIV-1/-2 antibodies —	HIV-1, -2[5]
HTLV	—	HTLV-I antibodies	X[5]
Syphilis	Antibody against *Treponema pallidum*	Testing algorithm to exclude presence of active *Treponema pallidum* infection	*Treponema pallidum*[5]
CMV	—	—	X[5]

Notes: [1]German Haemotherapy Guideline published by the German Medical Association.[19] The document is binding for all German donor centers.

[2]In case the test result for anti-HBc is positive, the donation can be released only if further testing shows the following results: The titer of anti-HBs-antibody is ≥ 100 IU/L and the test for HBV-genome (NAT) is negative.

[3]When anti-HBc is positive and HBs Ag is negative, further investigations are necessary with a risk assessment to determine eligibility for clinical use.

[4]HTLV-I antibody testing must be performed for donors living in, or originating from high-incidence areas or with sexual partners originating from those areas or where the donor's parents originate from those areas.

[5]Unlike the Germen and European guidelines, the US Pharmacopoeia does not prescribe which test methods have to be used.

PBSC: Peripheral Blood Stem Cells; HBs: Hepatitis B surface, HBc: Hepatitis B core, HCV: Hepatitis C Virus, HIV: Human Immunodeficiency Virus; NAT: Nucleic-acid Amplification Technique.

6.2.3.2 *Donor selection and testing*

The main focus in testing of donated materials is placed on safety parameters. Thus, IDMs, such as HIV, HCV, and Hepatitis B virus (HBV) have to be analyzed obligatory. Further test parameters may differ between regulations of different countries and are dependent on the geographical distribution of particular diseases. In case of autologous donation, the serum tests for HIV, HBV, and HCV are usually sufficient. In allogeneic donation, validated nucleic acid tests (NATs) are obligatory in many countries. The time-point of IDM testing is not defined clearly for human-derived materials used as starting material for CBMPs. For practical reasons donor testing usually can be performed up to seven days prior to donation. This gives time to release the donor for the donation and to repeat the test in case of ambiguous results and avoids retesting on the day of donation.

Minimally required tests for the qualification of allogeneic donors are listed in Table 6.3. Depending on the risk evaluation of the starting material and the intended use of the CBMP, additional tests have to be included. The US regulation gives guidance on the risk-based approach.[18] As an example, the risk evaluation of the starting material includes the content of leucocytes and recommends to include testing for agents usually transmitted by leucocytes such as Cytomegalovirus or Parvovirus B19. In case of clinical application of a CBMP in patients who had received stem cell transplantation, and/or are under immunosuppression, usually the full set of donor testing defined for HSC transplantation is required by the clinicians. It is recommended to seek advice before implementing donor testing systems.

Donor suitability and eligibility has to be determined with questionnaires, interviews performed by qualified and trained healthcare professionals, medical examination of the donor, and donor testing. These steps are important not only for the safety of the recipients but also to protect the voluntary donors from potential negative impacts and side effects of the procurement procedure and to assure their medical and physical integrity.

A thorough donor selection with questionnaires and interviews is important to gain knowledge about the donor's medical and behavioral history as well as about the donor's origin from or longer stays in high-incidence areas for certain viruses or pathogens (e.g., WNV- West Nile Virus, HTLV- Human T-Lymphotropic Virus). Physical examination is crucial to ensure the absence of signs and symptoms of diseases that negatively influence the viral or microbiological safety of the donation and to assure that no exclusion criteria do exist such as presence, or previous history, of malignant diseases or systemic infections that are not controlled at the time of donation (including bacterial diseases, systemic viral, fungal or parasitic infections). Dependent on the type of exclusion criterion donors might be excluded from donation of blood, tissues or cells permanently or temporarily for defined time periods.

Apart from physical examination donors in an allogeneic setting have to be tested for several IDMs. Table 6.3 compares obligatory laboratory tests on IDMs in different guidance documents. In the autologous setting, it might be possible to use donations even if exclusion criteria exist or laboratory tests on IDMs are positive, but it has to be assured that no cross-contamination occurs during processing and storage of these materials. The decision to use contaminated material and the measures that have to be taken should in any case be risk based. Clear separation and labeling of contaminated material is mandatory in these cases.

Apart from the minimal requirements for laboratory tests, it has to be decided whether additional testing is necessary. These decisions must be based on a risk assessment taking into account the probability of disease occurrence, the donor's history and the characteristics of the tissue or cells donated. In Europe, for example, HTLV-I antibody testing must be performed for donors living in, or originating from, high-incidence areas or with sexual partners originating from those areas or where the donor's parents originate from those areas. For WNV, the situation is similar and currently donors have to be tested whenever they stayed in certain areas for a longer time. Additional testing can be required for malaria, Cytomegalovirus (CMV), toxoplasma, Epstein–Barr virus (EBV), and other viruses or pathogens.

Apart from testing on infectious diseases, analysis of blood group and Rhesus factor, HLA-typing, antibody screening, and other analytical tests might be necessary. Further safety tests, such as sterility and absence of mycoplasma contamination may also be required.

Some tissues that serve as starting or raw material for CBMPs can also be obtained from deceased donors. Special requirements for post-mortem examination have to be followed in these cases.

6.2.3.3 *Traceability*

'*Traceability*' means the ability to locate and identify the tissue/cell during any step from procurement, through processing, testing, and storage, to distribution to the recipient or disposal, which also implies the ability to identify the donor and the tissue establishment or the manufacturing facility receiving, processing or storing the tissue/cells, and the ability to identify the recipient(s) at the medical facility/facilities applying the tissue/cells to the recipient(s); traceability also covers the ability to locate and identify all relevant data related to products and materials coming into contact with those tissues/cells (Directive 2006/17/EC).[20]

Full traceability for all substances of human origin is necessary for several reasons:

- IDMs may not yet be detectable at the time of donation as the concentration of nucleic acid, antibodies or other markers is below the detection limit of the applied test method, but donations can already be infectious at that time.
- Initial laboratory tests can be false negative.
- Donors can be determined to be infected with transmissible pathogens or there are reasonable grounds to suspect an infection, and potential risk of transmission cannot be ruled out through previous donations.
- Recipients of materials of human origin can be found to be infected with HIV, HBV, HCV or other transmissible pathogens (including viral, microbial or parasitic transmissions) and there are reasonable grounds to suspect that the infection was caused by the donation of material of human origin.
- New infectious diseases may be discovered.

For blood and blood components as well as for tissues and cells, it is therefore mandatory that full traceability is guaranteed throughout collection, testing, processing, storage, release, and/or distribution until application. This traceability has to be guaranteed from donor to recipient and *vice versa* and must cover all substances coming into contact with the cells, no matter if they are used as starting material, raw material or excipient. All data needed to achieve this kind of traceability in the European Union have to be kept for at least 30 years.

Whenever donor or recipient health information becomes available after procurement or application, which affects product safety and quality, recall or look back procedures have to be initiated. Therefore, procurement centers as well as manufacturers of CBMPs must have in place well-defined and efficient withdrawal procedures. A notification at the competent authority that supervises look back and withdrawal procedures is required in many countries.

Annex 2 of the EU GMP Guidelines[11] summarizes the requirements and guidelines that have to be followed in Europe: *Where human cell or tissue donors are used, full traceability is required from starting and raw materials, including all substances coming into contact with the cells or tissues through to confirmation of the receipt of the products at the point of use whilst maintaining the privacy of individuals and confidentiality of health related information (Article 15 of Regulation 1394/2007). Traceability records [see ENTR/F/2/SF/dnD (2009) 35810, "Detailed guidelines on GCP specific to ATMPs" for further information on traceability of investigational ATMPs] must be retained for 30 years after the expiry date of the medicinal product. Particular care should be taken to maintain the traceability of medicinal products for special cases, such as donor-matched cells. Directives 2002/98/EC and Commission Directive 2005/61/EC of September 30, 2005 implementing Directive 2002/98/EC of the European Parliament and of the Council as regards traceability requirements and notification of serious adverse reactions and events apply to blood components when they are used as starting or raw materials in the manufacturing process of medicinal products. For ATMPs, traceability requirement regarding human cells including HSCs must comply with the principles laid down in Directives 2004/23/EC and 2006/86/EC. The arrangements necessary to achieve the traceability and retention period should be incorporated into technical agreements between the responsible parties.*

6.2.4 *Ancillary Materials (AMs)/Raw materials*

For the manufacture of CBMPs many different reagents and devices often with specific function and biological activity are needed on various steps of the production process. These reagents and devices are termed raw or AMs and are used, e.g., for cell separation and depletion, cell culture, stimulation, differentiation, genetic modification, dilution, and washing. As shown under terms and definitions, "raw materials" is the commonly used term in Europe, whereas in the United States the term "AMs" is predominantly used. In contrast to excipients, raw materials are not intended to be present in the final product but they nevertheless could become part of the final product, at least in traces. Table 6.4 shows common examples.

For the manufacture of conventional medicinal products, raw materials do not play a key role as normally the API or drug substance is mixed together with various excipients to form the finished drug product. Excipients for conventional medicinal products are usually covered by a pharmacopoeia and are available in pharmaceutical grade quality; hence specifications and acceptance criteria are pre-defined.

For the manufacture of CBMPs, apart from excipients that help forming the final product a variety of different raw materials is necessary for the production of the drug substance — the cells in their final state. These raw materials are in most cases not covered by a pharmacopoeia and raw materials for CTPs are quite often novel substances which are never before used for production of a licensed medicinal product. But as these materials are coming into contact with the cells during the manufacturing process and often have significant biological activity, they have to be classified as critical regarding the safety, purity, and potency of the final product. Therefore, in-house specifications have to be provided in cases where references to pharmacopoeial monographs cannot be made considering the potential risk of any raw material used.

The quality of raw materials varies from high quality licensed medicinal products such as therapeutic cytokines and HSA to research grade materials such as

Table 6.4: Common Examples of Raw/AMs for the Manufacture of CBMPs.

Reagents	Devices[1]
• Cell culture media. • Cytokines for stimulation or differentiation. • Growth factors. • Human (pool) serum and human serum albumin (HSA). • Platelet lysate used as cell culture additive. • Animal derived serum (e.g., fetal bovine serum) used as cell culture additive. • Antibodies used for selection or depletion of certain cell populations or for stimulation or differentiation in cell culture. • Density gradient media for (pre-) enrichment of certain cell populations. • Enzymes, e.g., for detaching adherent cells or digesting tissue. • Buffers for washing or dilution steps. • Antigens for stimulation. • Plasmids and vectors.[2]	• Pipettes and pipette tips. • (Transfer) bags. • Syringes. • Needles. • Separation devices (disposable plastic sets). • Cell culture flasks. • (Centrifugation) tubes. • Disposable bioreactors. • Connecting devices.

Notes: [1]Whereas in Europe devices are not considered in the draft of the European Pharmacopoeia Chapter 5.2.12. "Raw materials for the production of cell-based and gene therapy medicinal products", in the United States these materials are part of USP chapter <1043> "Ancillary Materials for Cell, Gene, and Tissue-Engineered Products".
[2]Depending on the classification of the CBMP and the type of nucleic acid used for genetic modification, plasmids and vectors can also be defined as starting material (compare Section 6.2.2.3. Vectors and Plasmids as Starting Material for CBMPs).

research use-only antibodies that are not well characterized in terms of purity and impurity profiles and often lack detailed information necessary for the application of a clinical trial or MA. Minimal requirements for QC of critical raw materials are identity, biological activity/potency, content, purity, sterility, and microbial safety (including mycoplasma, where applicable), viral safety/transmissible spongiform encephalopathy (TSE, where applicable), and stability.

To what extent raw materials have to be analyzed upon receipt and prior to use in the manufacturing process is dependent on their quality (including the extent of QC provided by the supplier), their specific biological activity, their potential toxicity, and the amount and time when they are used in the production process. The control strategy should be in any case risk-based. If high quality licensed medicinal products are used, it might be sufficient to rely on the provided quality documentation. For other substances identity testing and/or analysis of biological activity might be required to demonstrate at least lot-to-lot consistency. But generally efficiency or potency testing of raw materials is complex, since the test procedures are supposed to correlate with the intended use in terms of target cells, relative amount, and concentration, etc. Production conditions are often hard to mimic in smaller scales and test procedures that are based on cells are often underlying donor-dependant variations leading to many variables in the test systems. International or national reference standards are not readily available for most substances making it almost impossible to compare different analytical test procedures used by different suppliers.

Generally human derived materials need special consideration when used as raw materials as they are often associated with a high risk for disease transmission, at least as long as they cannot undergo effective virus or pathogen reducing steps during their manufacture. Therefore, materials and reagent of human origin have to be evaluated carefully with respect to their suitability. The use of synthetic alternatives or autologous materials (e.g., serum) should be investigated and preferred, whenever possible.

6.2.4.1 *Regulatory situation for raw materials in Europe*

In Europe, to date no specific regulations do exist for raw materials used for the manufacture of CBMPs. The European Pharmacopeia does not yet provide monographs or general chapters and reference standards for most of the substances used as raw materials. The European cells and tissue Directive 2004/23/EC and its technical directive 2006/17/EC for procurement and testing of tissues and cells is applicable only in so far as viral and microbial safety of starting and raw materials of human origin is concerned.

As there is an increasing interest of the cell therapy community for harmonization within Europe and for setting minimal standards and requirements for raw materials, the European Directorate for the Quality of Medicines and Healthcare (EDQM), a directorate of the Council of Europe responsible for the European Pharmacopoeia, entered this field in 2012, setting up a working party (RCG Working Party) to elaborate a text on raw materials for the production of cell-based products and GTPs. In October 2014, the EDQM published the first draft of the new Chapter 5.2.12 "Raw materials for the production of cell-based and gene therapy medicinal products", that is thought to apply to raw materials of biological origin including sera and serum replacements, proteins produced by recombinant DNA technology (e.g., growth factors, cytokines, enzymes, and monoclonal antibodies), proteins extracted from biological materials (e.g., polyclonal antibodies and enzymes), and vectors. It provides examples for critical quality attributes specific to each class of raw materials covered by the compendial text. Chemically synthesized raw materials, medical devices, and plastics are not thought to be within the scope of the new chapter. According to the compendial text, it is the raw material user's ultimate responsibility to ensure that only substances of suitable and sufficient quality are used for the production of CBMPs/GTMPs. The impact of each individual raw material on the quality, safety, and efficacy of the CBMP/GTMP has to be evaluated using a risk-based approach. As raw materials are used in order to consistently yield an active substance or medicinal product of a specified quality, it is necessary that they are evaluated in terms of their biological activity, purity/impurity profile, and the risk of adventitious agents' transmission. Further general requirements for raw materials are their origin (including traceability), the production methods, general quality requirements (e.g., identity, content, microbiological control, and biological activity), storage, and labeling. The compendial text points out that it is the responsibility of both the manufacturer and user of a raw material to qualify the raw material in accordance with the above mentioned considerations.

Apart from the new pharmacopoeial chapter, general requirements for raw materials are also provided by Annex 2 of the EU GMP Guidelines for the "manufacture of biological active substances and medicinal products for human use". Annex 2 points out that special consideration should be given on the source, origin, and suitability of raw materials. Raw materials may need '*additional documentation on the source, origin, distribution chain, method of manufacture, and controls applied, to assure an appropriate level of control including their microbiological quality*'. For biological medicinal products with a short shelf life where the final product has to be released before completion of all QC tests, according to Annex 2, a suitable control strategy must be in place taking into account the controls and attributes of raw materials. The controls required for the quality of raw materials, particularly for cell-based products, where final sterilization is generally not possible and the ability to remove microbial by-products is limited, assume greater importance.

Regulation (EC) No 1394/2007 on ATMPs points out in Article 15 "Traceability", that '*the holder of a MA for an ATMP shall establish and maintain a system ensuring that the individual product and its starting and raw materials, including all substances coming into contact with the cells or tissues it may contain, can be traced through the sourcing, manufacturing, packaging, storage, transport, and delivery to the hospital, institution or private practice where the product is used.*' Batch documentation of all raw materials used during cell processing is therefore mandatory (compare also Section 6.2.3. Donor Testing and Traceability).

A good understanding of raw material quality is not only required for MA purposes. Even at early stages of clinical trials, some authorities ask for detailed information on raw material quality, and safety as part of the IMP Dossier (IMPD). But as Clinical Trials in Europe are regulated nationally, it has to be stated, that the requirements are highly diverse between individual Member States.

Since the production of raw materials in Europe is not clearly regulated at the moment, different quality attributes are used such as "GMP compliant", "GMP-like", "GMP grade" or "Clinical grade". All these terms are not legally defined and it is difficult for the users to understand what kind of quality is provided by the raw material supplier. The principles of GMP are meant to be a quality system for medicinal products and APIs and do not apply for the manufacture of raw materials. Therefore, vendor audits might be the only way to gain sufficient information on the raw materials in terms of their quality (including batch-to-batch consistency), safety, and traceability.

There is an ongoing debate in Europe on whether to establish a Drug Master File (DMF) system comparable to the one in the USA. Particularly, raw material suppliers would be very much in favor of such a system as this would allow the manufacturer of a CBMP or sponsor of a clinical trial to refer to the DMF in the clinical trials or MA application (MAA) without forcing the raw material suppliers to reveal confidential information such as exact composition or production details. European authorities point out that the regulatory situation in Europe is quite different in this respect to that in the USA, as in Europe the applicant of a clinical trials and especially MA, is fully responsible for the quality of the medicinal product and this includes all raw materials used. Besides that the requirement for a certain raw material is always dependent on its intended use and can therefore vary for distinct CBMPs. A DMF may not cover all those potentially different specifications. Therefore, at the moment it seems unlikely that EU legislation will allow raw material suppliers to submit a DMF independent of a concrete medicinal product. Nevertheless for early stages of clinical trials regulatory support files from raw material suppliers might be helpful for the applicant.

6.2.4.2   *Regulatory situation for AMs in the USA*

Compared to Europe, the regulatory situation in the USA is quite different as there is a DMF System established and the US Pharmacopoeia has already introduced chapters specific for AMs (USP Chapters <1043> "Ancillary Materials for Cell, Gene and Tissue-Engineered Products" and USP chapter <92> "Growth Factors and Cytokines Used in Cell Therapy Manufacturing").

Chapter <1043> gives advice on how to qualify AMs for use in CBMPs to ensure the traceability, consistency, suitability, purity, and safety of the AM and finally the CBMP. The following three sections on AM Qualification, AM Risk Classification, and AM Performance Testing give an overview of USP chapter <1043> summarizing its main issues.

AMs Qualification

Key elements for the qualification of AMs according to USP chapter <1043> are the following steps:

1. **Identification.** Listing of all AMs used in a given product manufacturing and indication where in the production process they are used. This includes the source and intended use of each AM as well as the necessary quantity or concentration. Alternate sources should be considered already in this first step.
2. **Selection and Suitability for use.** Establishment and documentation of selection criteria for each AM as well as establishment and documentation for qualification criteria for each vendor. Selection criteria for AMs should include assessment of microbiological and chemical purity, identity, and biological activity. AMs of human or animal origin should be selected with special care. To what extent the material qualification has to be performed in the following steps is dependent on a risk assessment for each AM. The AMs with a strong safety profile, used in minimal amounts in up-stream steps of the manufacturing process being thoroughly washed out from the system in following steps are, for example, low-risk and the extent of qualification activities can be reduced.
3. **Characterization.** Development and implementation of specific QC characterization tests including, for example, identity, purity, functionality, and freedom of microbial or viral contamination. The appropriate level of testing must be based on a risk-assessment profile for each raw material.
4. **Vendor Qualification.** This includes an audit of the manufacturing facility and testing program of the AM supplier as well as established GMP or quality assurance systems and programs.
5. **QC and Quality Assurance.** All actions taken for the qualification of raw materials should be in compliance with GMP and monitored by either QC or Quality Assurance. This might include the following systems:

   - Incoming receipt, segregation, inspection, and release of materials prior to use.
   - Vendor auditing.
   - Certificate of analysis verification (testing).

- Formal procedures and policies for materials that are tested to be out of specification.
- Stability testing.
- Archival sample storage.

AMs Risk Classification

A further important task of chapter <1043> is Risk Classification of an AM. Four different tiers of sample risk categories are introduced that are based on the source and manufacturing process of the AM and the overall quality that is provided by the supplier. These risk categories do not take into account the impact of quantity or stage of use of the AM.

AMs that are approved or licensed medicinal or therapeutic products with an established toxicological profile and manufactured according to controlled and documented procedures are in the lowest risk category (tier 1), whereas materials that are not produced in compliance with GMP and are not intended to be used in the manufacture of CBMPs are in the highest risk category (tier 4).

The following table gives an overview on the four different sample risk categories as presented in the chapter <1043> together with examples and activities that are necessary for the qualification of the AM in each category.

Table 6.5: AMs risk classification.

Risk Category	Definition	Examples	Qualification or Risk Reduction Activities
Tier 1	Low-risk, highly qualified materials that are well-suited for use in manufacturing. These are licensed biologics and medicinal/therapeutic products or approved drugs as well as medical devices.	HSA for injection, injectable monoclonal antibodies, IV bags, syringes, needles, etc.	• DMF cross-reference (when possible or practical). • Certificate of Analysis (CoA). • Assessment of lot-to-lot effect on process performance. • Assessment of removal from final product. • Assessment of stability of AM as stored for use in manufacturing.

(Continued)

Table 6.5: (*Continued*)

Risk category	Definition	Examples	Qualification or Risk Reduction Activities
Tier 2	Low-risk, well-characterized materials that are well-suited for use in manufacturing and produced in compliance with GMP. Their intended use is for drug, biologic or medical device manufacturing.	Recombinant growth factors and cytokines, immunomagnetic beads, monoclonal antibodies, tissue culture media, and sterile process buffers.	Same as for tier 1 plus: • When relevant: Confirmation of CoA test results critical to the product. • Vendor audit.
Tier 3	Moderate risk materials that will require higher level of qualification. These are materials used for *in vitro* diagnostics and are not intended for use in the production of cell or gene products.	Recombinant growth factors and cytokines, monoclonal antibodies (diagnostic grade), purified chemicals (reagent grade), and tissue culture media.	Same as for tier 2 plus: • Upgrade manufacturing process to GMP. • Development of stringent internal specifications. • Determination if lot-to-lot biocompatibility, cytotoxicity, or adventitious agents testing are needed.
Tier 4	Highest risk level. Extensive qualification is necessary prior to use in manufacturing. These materials are neither produced in compliance with GMP nor are they intended for use in manufacture of CBMPs. This level includes highly toxic substances and most complex, animal-derived fluid materials that are not subjected to adventitious viral removal or inactivation procedures.	Fetal bovine serum, animal-derived (including human) extracts, purified enzymes, animal or human cells used as feeder layers, and chemical entities with known toxicity.	Same as for tier 3 plus: • Verification of traceability to country of origin. • Assure country of origin is qualified as safe with respect to source-relevant animal diseases, including TSE. • Adventitious agent testing for animal source-relevant viruses.

Source: Modified after USP chapter <1043> "Ancillary Materials for Cell, Gene and Tissue-Engineered Products", tables 1 to 4.

AMs Performance Testing

According to USP Chapter <1043> performance testing is necessary whenever an AM provides a special biological activity that is crucial for the manufacturing process of the CBMP. This is the case when AMs have significant impact on product manufacturing yield, purity, or final product potency. Lot-to-lot variability of these AMs would be critical in these cases and needs to be addressed prior to use. Since these AMs do not have simple identity tests and cannot be characterized easily by physico–chemical assays, well-defined performance assays have to be developed to ensure process reproducibility and final product quality.

DMF

Apart from the guidance provided by the US Pharmacopoeia for qualification of AMs, the US Food and Drug Administration (FDA) offers suppliers the possibility to submit a DMF for these materials that might be referenced by manufacturers of cell therapeutics. In the guideline for DMFs, FDA defines DMF as

> "*a submission to the FDA that may be used to provide confidential detailed information about facilities, processes, or articles used in the manufacturing, processing, packaging, and storing of one or more human drugs. The submission of a DMF is not required by law or FDA regulation. A DMF is submitted solely at the discretion of the holder. The information contained in the DMF may be used to support an Investigational New Drug Application (IND), a New Drug Application (NDA), an Abbreviated New Drug Application (ANDA), another DMF, an Export Application, or amendments and supplements to any of these.*"

DMFs are not approved or disapproved and they are only reviewed in connection with one of the above mentioned applications. They are generally created to allow a party other than the owner of the DMF to reference material without disclosing to that party the contents of the file.

A DMF should contain a summary of all significant steps in the manufacturing and QCs of the related substance/material.

6.2.4.3 *Raw materials of animal origin*

Raw materials of animal origin are used for example as (fetal) bovine serum serving as cell culture additive or as supportive cells in the manufacturing process of CBMPs.

Similar to materials of human origin, also substances of animal origin bear the risk of disease transmission and have to be considered carefully when used as raw materials. Please note that xenogeneic medicinal products, where substances of animal origin are used as starting material for the production of CBMPs, are not within the scope of this chapter and potential additional guidelines and requirements are not considered here.

Apart from potentially harboring infectious agents, animal derived substances may also increase undesirable immunological responses in the recipient. Therefore, the use of animal reagents should be avoided and replaced by non-animal derived reagents of defined composition, whenever feasible.

If material of animal origin is used, a number of guidance documents exists that have to be followed. Table 6.6 summarizes the European guidelines that have to be followed.

Biological active substances and medicinal products must comply with the latest version of the Note for Guidance on Minimising the Risk of Transmitting

Table 6.6: European guidance documents for the use of animal-derived materials.

Document Reference Number	Document Title
CPMP/BWP/3354/99	Note for guidance on production and quality control of animal immunoglobulins and immunosera for human use.
CPMP/1199/02	Points to consider on Xenogeneic Cell Therapy Medicinal Products.
EMA/CVMP/IWP/206555/2010	Guideline on requirements for the production and control of immunological veterinary medicinal products.
2011/C 73/01	Note for guidance on minimising the risk of transmitting animal spongiform encephalopathy agents *via* human and veterinary medicinal products (EMA/410/01 rev.3).
EMA/CHMP/BWP/457920/2012 rev 1	Guideline on the use of bovine serum in the manufacture of human biological medicinal products. *Note*: This guideline replaces Note for Guidance on the use of bovine serum in the manufacture of human biological medicinal products (CPMP/BWP/1793/02).
Ph. Eur. 5.2.8.	Minimising the risk of transmitting animal spongiform encephalopathy agents *via* human and veterinary medicinal products.

Animal Spongiform Encephalopathy Agents *via* Human and Veterinary Medicinal Products.

6.2.5 *Excipients*

In contrast to raw materials or AMs, excipients are added intentionally to the final product and therefore are administered to the patient together with the cellular component in significant amounts.

For non-cryopreserved cellular products, excipients are in most cases physiologic salt solution together with HSA in concentrations varying from 1–10%. Salt solutions and HSA are available as authorized medicinal products in pharmaceutical grade quality and although HSA is of human origin and theoretically bears the risk of transmitting pathogens and micro-organisms, it will not be classified as substance of the highest risk category as the manufacturing process is highly standardized and includes virus reducing steps. Of course batch documentation of HSA is mandatory to guarantee traceability. As production of HSA is dependent on human donors (at least if it is not used as recombinant product) there is sometimes a bottleneck in supply. Depending on the required amounts, it might be advisable to purchase or at least reserve whole batches for security of supply.

Far more difficult to handle are novel excipients that are not commonly used for manufacture of medicinal products, and where no or only limited data exist on the interactions between the cells and the excipient. Intensive characterization has to be done by the manufacturer of the CBMP in these cases and data have to be collected as early as possible in product development.

Dimethyl sulfoxide (DMSO) is an essential cryoprotectant for preservation of cells in liquid nitrogen and is therefore a special excipient in cryopreserved cell-products. Although DMSO is known to exert toxic effects when administered to the patient together with the cell-product after thawing, there is currently hardly any alternative, as other substances with a significantly better risk–benefit profile are not available and washing the cells before administration is not possible in many cases. A reduction of DMSO concentrations from 10% down to 7.5% or even 5% (possibly in combination with hydroxyl ethyl starch) should be aimed for whenever the cells tolerate it. High quality DMSO produced under GMP conditions and/or registered as medical device should be used in any case.

6.2.6 *Reagents and materials for QC*

Even though reagents and materials used for QC are not coming into contact with the medicinal product their quality is of importance for the validity of the obtained analytical results for in-process controls and release testing. Therefore, vendor qualification and control of incoming materials and reagents is almost as important as it is for production materials.

Whenever possible for *in vitro* diagnostic use, certified test kits or reagents and medicinal devices should be used as they are extensively qualified by the providers and batch-to-batch consistency is guaranteed in most cases.

Problems can arise, when qualified reagents and materials are not available as it is often the case for highly innovative early phase IMPs. Sometimes reagents and materials in research-grade quality have to be used where characterization is missing and even CoA are not provided. Validation of an analytical procedure using these kinds of reagents can be difficult, for example when the specificity of an antibody is not defined well enough.

It is important that uncertified materials and reagents are intensively tested and qualified during assay development to address both, overall quality and batch-to-batch consistency. It might be necessary that these reagents are tested for their quality and activity prior to use. A side-by-side test of already released and new reagent batch can be suitable to assess quality and consistency. In any case, specifications for each reagent have to be set and all required test methods have to be defined on a risk-based approach.

6.2.7 *Quality agreement*

As raw materials and excipients can have significant influence on the quality of the drug product and as raw material and excipient suppliers are in most cases not inspected by governmental authorities, it is advisable for the manufacturers of the CDMPs to negotiate a Quality Agreement with the raw material/excipient suppliers, at least for those products that are not licensed medicinal products or devices. But also for reagents and materials used for QC, the conclusion of a Quality Agreement might be reasonable, especially when custom-made or special order reagents are used that are not readily available.

The International Pharmaceutical Excipients Council (IPEC) in 2008 published a document titled "Qualification of Excipients for Use in Pharmaceuticals" that amongst other issues gives advice on the content of a Quality Agreement. Although in the scope of this document are excipients for conventional medicinal products whereas special requirements for CBMPs are not considered, many of the given examples are applicable to excipients and raw materials for these special preparations as well. Therefore, a Quality Agreement may cover but is not limited to issues shown in Table 6.7.

Table 6.7: Points to consider for conclusion of a quality agreement.

	Quality Agreement
Specifications	Definition of excipient/raw material specifications, including for example, • Identity. • Purity and Impurities. • Content. • Potency assays and (additional) functional tests. • Microbiology/Sterility. • Levels of Bacterial Endotoxins and/or Pyrogens. • Mycoplasma. • Stability. • Batch-to-batch consistency. • Altered ranges of tests already in the suppliers' standard specification. • Alternative test methods either for parameters already in the manufacturers' specification or for additional parameters.
Sourcing	• Bovine spongiform encephalopathy (BSE)/TSE, genetically modified organisms (GMOs), allergens', etc. risk assessment. • Acceptability (as appropriate) of excipient/raw material from multiple manufacturing locations. • Restriction of contract operations such as manufacturing, packaging, and laboratory testing. • Identification of the country of origin and restriction to specified locations. • Importation restrictions.
Auditing	• The right of the customer to audit supplier's facilities and systems at a mutually agreeable time. • Confidentiality agreement as required. • Customer to issue a written report within a specified timeframe. • Supplier to respond to report with a specified timeframe.
Change control	• All changes have to follow change control procedures. • Handling of change notification according to written procedures. • Conformance to designated quality system. • Conformance to specified compendia such as United States Pharmacopeia–National Formulary (USP–NF), Ph. Eur., and Japanese Pharmacopoeia (JP), if applicable. • Disclosure of regulatory agency inspections and findings, if applicable.

(Continued)

Table 6.7: *(Continued)*

Quality Agreement	
Communication of non-conformance and other quality issues	• Out-of-Specification (OOS) test results to be investigated and documented according to written procedures and communication to the customer. • Significant process deviations to be investigated and documented according to written procedures and communication to the customer. • Investigation of complaints involving product quality according to written procedures and communication to the customer. • Promptly reporting complaints and provision of samples by the customer as appropriate and cooperation between both parties in the investigation.
Manufacturing, packaging and labeling	• Qualification of manufacturing and packaging processes. • Validation of cleaning methods, where appropriate. • Validation of analytical procedures. • Sample retention. • Special labeling requirements.
Documentation and records	• CoA to be supplied with each lot. • Content of the CoA and additional information to be included on the CoA, if applicable. • Retention period for applicable records.
Storage and distribution	• Documentation in support of recommended storage conditions and retest interval. • Recommended storage and transportation conditions. • Storage and shipment in conformance to recommendations.
Recalls	• Supplier must have a recall procedure that has been demonstrated as effective • Prompt notification to the customer by the supplier. • Cooperation of both parties in the recall.

Source: Modified after "Qualification of Excipients for Use in Pharmaceuticals", IPEC.[21]

6.3   Assay Development

Assay Development is the optimization process prior to validation in which assay parameters are defined and enhanced for the intended purpose.

Biological assays are usually designed for the characterization of biological or biotechnology products and are used for stability, in-process, and release testing. The accuracy, specificity, precision, and robustness requirements are differentially stated for each of the potential applications. Often the use of bioassays aims at the optimization of product manufacturing, including scale–up processes.[22] Generally, assay development takes place prior to the validation process and describes a phase of assay definition according to the product characteristics. Performance character-istics such as stability, accuracy, and precision have to be clearly implemented in an established assay. Robustness as well as reproducibility is recommended. The quality of reagents used in the assay is of high importance and must be defined (material qualification). Degradation products (i.e., stress and storage induced) and their influence on test results have to be considered. The process of optimizing an assay is a continuous procedure that directly starts after defining performance char-acteristics and continues until the performance metrics are established. The results obtained from an assay should be defined as confident. As soon as the manufac-turing process is feasible, the assay enters into the final step of development, the qualification phase. After completing the assay design and finalizing the definition of qualified parameters, the assay can be shifted to the validation process (see Sec-tion 6.11. Validation of Analytical Procedures). Validation includes the description of a protocol based on given data and predefined criteria arising from the develop-ing phase.[23] The developing phase of an assay still allows adaptation of the testing strategy. If an assay does not meet the predefined criteria at this stage, the assay can still be re-optimized or rejected, newly designed and tested for "fit for use" criteria.

The readout of an established assay might be of qualitative, semi or fully quan-titative nature. For quantification, an assay should usually include a standard or calibration curve within the intended and reasonable detection range. The statisti-cal methods applied should be evaluated in the concept of linearity with multiple samples tested in replicates. Development is completed with the preparation of the standard operating procedure (SOP) for the bioassay and at this stage accuracy, linearity, and reportable range are covered.[24]

Development of assays used for CBMPs usually involves different depart-ments according to the stage of development. Unlike conventional pharmaceuticals, advanced therapeutics differ due to their high biological and functional complexity, which often makes the implementation of an assay under GMP conditions dif-ficult. Assays that have been developed under R&D conditions cannot always be transferred successfully to routine testing. In the GMP context, the assay has to be cost- and time-efficient as well as robust and reproducible.

The R&D department usually selects the most suitable method and predefines critical aspects and parameters. The pharmaceutical development team prepares and defines the GMP-relevant parameters. Once detailed and accurate data are sufficiently collected, the validation of the method for implementation into the GMP unit takes place. The workflow follows the standards of a regulated technical method-transfer (compare section 6.11.4 "Method Transfer") including the consideration of the "state-of-the-art" working progress.

6.4 Analytical Methods for QC of CBMPs

Numerous different analytical procedures are required to analyze the quality of a CBMP. In most cases, the methods applied vary from those used for conventional medicinal products, where small molecules or proteins have to be analyzed and chromatography-based procedures are very common. Many of the analytical procedures used for cellular products are not described in a pharmacopoeia and usually for these methods no other guidance document is available. For some cellular products, research-based procedures have to be adopted to address certain questions and these assays have to be validated extensively in order to demonstrate their suitability.

Among all the methods used for analysis of CBMPs, flow cytometry is for sure the key technology that allows the analysis of a whole set of different parameters (often in one single stain) and is therefore suitable to answer numerous different questions. Flow cytometry is a highly sophisticated method that is evolving continuously and measuring principles that are developed to address new scientific questions today might become the QC procedures of tomorrow.

Table 6.8 provides an overview of analytical methods most commonly used for analysis of CBMPs. Of course, other methods than those listed might exist that are equally suitable or even better to address a specific question. As measuring principles of all the methods listed can be studied in detail in various scientific books and papers, we only provide a brief summary for every method.

Please note that methods applied for microbiological control and sterility testing (including Pyrogen and Endotoxin Testing) are described in Section 6.6.9 (Microbiology). Methods used for cytogenetic analysis are described in more detail in Section 6.7 (Genetic Stability and Tumorigenicity).

6.5 In-Process Controls

In-process controls (IPC) are particularly important for cellular products as starting material and production processes tend to be much more variable than chemical APIs or physico–chemical manufacturing processes.

The European guideline on human CBMPs[43] points out that the manufacturing process needs to be controlled by several in-process controls at the level of critical steps of intermediate products. Specifications of these products have to be

Table 6.8: Overview on analytical methods used for QC of CBMPs (selection of methods).

Methods	Measuring Principle	Read-out Parameter	Examples for Application
Flow Cytometry	Light scatter (forward and side scatter) is used to measure the intrinsic size and granularity of cells. Differentiation of different cell populations is thus possible even without fluorescence labeling. Fluorescence can be used to measure specific protein expression and nucleic acid content by adding reagents such as fluorescent stains and labeled antibodies. Fluorescence-labeled antibodies are used to stain specific antigens (e.g., CD markers) on the cell surface. After permeabilization and fixation, also intracellular and intranuclear structures can be analyzed. Production of mediators such as cytokines, chemokines and growth factors can be measured by intracellular staining (potentially after blocking the Golgi apparatus in order to prevent secretion) or by Cytometric Bead Array. Cell proliferation can for example be measured *via* CFSE. Fluorescent CFSE can covalently bind to intracellular structures and is therefore retained over long time periods. Fluorescence intensity diminishes with every cell division. Cell cycle analysis can be performed *via* DNA staining. Flow cytometry can be applied qualitatively (positive or negative for a certain marker) or quantitatively (high, low, and intermediate expression of certain markers).	• Size and granularity of particles. • Cell Surface markers. • Intracellular markers. • Intranuclear markers (e.g., transcription factors). • Production of different mediators such as cytokines, growth-factors, chemokines, cell signaling proteins, etc. • Cell membrane integrity (uptake of fluorescence dye). • Viability. • Cell cycle analysis. • Proliferation. • Number of particles (either as percentage among other particles or as direct number). • Enzymatic activity.	• Cellular purity (e.g., *via* cell surface markers). • Cellular Impurities (e.g., *via* cell surface markers). • Process-related Impurities (e.g., residual antibodies). • Identity (typical panel of surface markers, if necessary combined with intracellular markers). • Potency (e.g., cell surface and/or intracellular markers as surrogate parameters, transgene expression, bystander killing, cytokine production). • Viability (e.g., 7-AAD viability dye).

(Continued)

Table 6.8: (*Continued*)

Methods	Measuring principle	Read-out parameter	Examples for application
	Quantification of particles (cells) can be performed as single platform analysis using counting beads or as dual platform analysis where particle/cell concentration is measured with a second platform (e.g. haematology analyser). Flow cytometry is a compendial method (25) (26). In the Ph. Eur. flow cytometry is used for nucleated cell count and viability (27) and for numeration of CD34/CD45+ cells in haematopoietic products (28).	• Others (flow cytometry is a highly multifaceted method that can measure numerous other parameters).	• Content (e.g. numeration of cells that express certain cell surface markers) • Activation status of certain subpopulations
ELISA Enzyme Linked Immuno–sorbent Assay	Antigens present in a sample are specifically immobilized to a solid surface (e.g. 96–well plate) *via* capture antibodies. Then, enzyme-linked specific detection antibodies are applied to form a complex with the antigen. Finally, the enzyme's substrate is added. The subsequent enzymatic reaction produces a detectable signal, most commonly a color change that is directly proportional to the amount of antigen. ELISA provides qualitative (antigen present yes/no) and quantitative (calculation of amounts *via* calibration with standard) information.	• Presence and quantification of a specific antigen structure.	• Potency (e.g. cytokine production). • Process-related Impurities (e.g. host cell proteins, residual cytokines, and residual antibodies).

(*Continued*)

Table 6.8: (*Continued*)

Methods	Measuring Principle	Read-out Parameter	Examples for Application
ELISpot Assay Enzyme Linked Immuno Spot Assay	Assay principle is comparable to ELISA. Cells are seeded onto a membrane that is pre-coated with a specific capture antibody. When cells are stimulated to produce a certain antigen (e.g., cytokine) that specifically binds to the capture antibody, this antigen is immobilized on the membrane in direct proximity to the secreting cell. Usually the stimulation of the cells is antigen-specific. Cells are then removed and captured antigens can be detected as distinct spots *via* an enzyme-linked detection antibody and subsequent enzymatic reaction. As every spot marks an antigen-secreting cell, the ELISpot assay shows high sensitivity and accuracy. It allows the detection of one antigen-specific cell among a greater cell pool (usually 200.000 to 400.000) and is therefore suitable to detect rare populations. ELISpot provides qualitative information (secreted antigen present yes/no) and quantitative information (frequency of responding cells).	• Direct measurement of a certain secreted antigen (e.g., cytokine). • Indirect measurement of specific cells (e.g., antigen-specific T- or B-cells) that were stimulated to produce a certain antigen (e.g., cytokine or antibody).	• Identity (e.g., of antigen-specific T-cells). • Potency (e.g., of antigen specific T-cells to produce cytokines upon stimulation). • Content (e.g., frequency of antigen specific T-cells). • Cellular Impurities (presence of immunogenic cells). • Monitoring of immune reactions in patients after administration of cellular products.

Mixed Lymphocyte Reaction (MLR)	Lymphocytes of one individual (stimulator) are inactivated (e.g., by irradiation) and mixed with lymphocytes of another individual (responder). If there is a HLA-mismatch between both individuals CD4+ T-cells of the responder are stimulated to proliferate, CD8+ T-cells are stimulated to mediate cytotoxicity. T-cell proliferation is usually measured by H^3-thymidine uptake, cytotoxicity can be measured, e.g., by chromium-release assay. Alternative methods are FACS-based (CFSE-assay) or MTT MLR represents an immunoassay that detects histoincompatibility and alloreactivity as well as cell-mediated cytotoxicity.	• Proliferation of CD4+ T-cells. • Cytotoxicity (cell lysis).	• Detection of alloreactivity between two or more individual lymphocyte subsets. • Safety (unwanted alloreactivity). • Potency (wanted alloreactivity). • Potency assay for suppressive function of regulatory cells.
Colony Forming Unit Assay (CFU)	Used to quantify lineage-restricted progenitors [e.g., hematopoietic progenitor cells (HPCs)] from various cell sources (e.g., peripheral blood, bone marrow). While culturing in semi-solid growth medium, colony forming cells are able to divide and to differentiate into colonies of more mature cells. These colonies can be counted by eye after staining or by optical microscopy. CFU assay is a compendial method in the Ph. Eur.[29]	• Amount of countable cell colonies. • Diversity of cell colonies.	• Potency (ability of certain cell populations to proliferate and/or to differentiate in several lineages).

(Continued)

Table 6.8: *(Continued)*

Methods	Measuring Principle	Read-out Parameter	Examples for Application
Soft Agar Colony Formation Assay	Analyzes anchorage independent growth of cells (in a soft agar gel) which normally grow anchorage dependant as a sign of transformation (e.g., after genetic modification).	• Proliferation via generation of spheroids.	• Tumorigenicity. • Surrogate for biologically relevant genetic aberration.
Vascular Tube Formation Assay	The assay determines the ability of cells, with appropriate extracellular matrix support, to form capillary-like structures (tubes). Tube formation is then quantified by measuring the number and length of these capillary-like structures under a microscope.	• Generation of vascular tubes.	• Potency (angiogenesis). • Safety (unwanted angiogenesis).
Determination of Cell Number and Blood Components	Usually Hematology Analyzers are used for this purpose. Instruments are available in various configurations offering various possibilities for detection of different parameters. They are able to discriminate and count Red Blood Cells (RBCs), platelets, and White Blood Cells (WBCs) by basic principles of flow cytometry and direct current detection with hydrodynamic focusing technology. Some instruments can also differentiate Reticulocytes and measure Hemoglobin and other hematologic parameters. Usually Hematology Analyzers cannot precisely differentiate viable from non-viable cells.	• Cell number (e.g., WBC count, RBC count, and platelet count) • Differentiation of mononuclear subsets (MNCs).	• Content (Cell number). • Purity. • Cellular impurities (contaminating cell populations). • Characterization of starting material.

Karyo-typing	The karyotype describes the number and appearance of chromosomes (e.g., under the light microscope after staining). For cytogenetic analysis, cells have to be arrested during cell division. Chromosomes are then stained with a suitable dye, e.g., Giemsa. After digestion of chromosomes with trypsin and subsequent Giemsa staining, a specific pattern of bands appears (G–banding) that can be analyzed for abnormalities (e.g., translocations). On a molecular basis, cytogenetic analysis can be performed by Fluorescence *in situ* Hybridization (FISH) or Comparative Genomic Hybridization (CGH).	• Numerical and qualitative analysis of chromosomes (loss, augmentation of genetic material, translocation, and aberration). • Appearance of chromosomes (e.g., length, position of centromer, and banding pattern). • Molecular-based techniques for detection of abnormalities beyond detection limit of karyotyping.
		• Genetic stability. • Clonal aberrations in starting material (bone marrow) associated with disease condition. Note: Biologic significance in end product analysis is not defined.
SDS-PAGE/Western Blot	Used to detect specific proteins in a sample of tissue or cell homogenate or extract. Proteins are separated on gels (usually polyacrylamide gels) by electrophoresis. Under non-denaturing conditions native proteins are separated by their structure and charge; under denaturing conditions proteins are separated by the length of their polypeptides/molecular mass. Proteins can either be analyzed directly on the gel (e.g., after Coomassie stain) or after transfer to a membrane (Western Blot) where	• Presence of a certain protein. • Amount of a certain protein. • Process-related Impurities (e.g., residual antibodies). • Potency (e.g., presence of specific proteins after genetic modification or stimulation).

(Continued)

Table 6.8: (*Continued*)

Methods	Measuring Principle	Read-out Parameter	Examples for Application
	they can be stained with antibodies specific to the target protein. SDS-PAGE and Western Blot can be evaluated qualitatively and quantitatively. Electrophoresis[30,31] and Isoelectric focusing[32,33] are compendial methods.		• Stability (e.g., monitoring of degradation process).
Polymerase Chain Reaction (PCR)/ Nucleic-acid Amplification Technique (NAT)	Amplification of a piece of nucleic acid sequence (genomic DNA, artificial DNA, e.g., from vectors, or RNA either from retroviruses or messenger RNA) across several orders of magnitude *via* cycles of repeated heating and cooling. Specific primers that mark the starting point and the end of the sequence to be copied are the prerequisite for a specific assay. PCR can also be used for sequence analysis. PCR products can either be analyzed *via* an agarose gel (detection of one or several bands after staining with DNA intercalating dyes) or real time *via* fluorescence-labeled probes or dyes that intercalate during the reaction. PCR/NAT can be applied qualitatively (signal yes/no) or quantitatively (real time PCR, analysis of relative copy number). NAT is a compendial method.[34–40]	• Presence of a specific nucleic acid sequence. • Amount of a specific nucleic acid sequence (e.g., normalized to a housekeeping gene or relative amount).	• Identity (e.g., of transgene). • Impurities (e.g., residual host cell DNA). • Potency (e.g., up-regulation of mRNA). • Vector Copy Number (Integrity of transgene in cells). • Mycoplasma DNA. • Microbiological Control (Rapid Microbiological Method). • Donor Testing (e.g., HIV, HCV, and HBV).

(*Continued*)

Table 6.8: (*Continued*)

Methods	Measuring principle	Read-out parameter	Examples for application
Optical Microscopy	Allows a magnified view of a sample (up to 40×; with oil immersion up to 100×) by passing visible light (either transmitted through or reflected from the sample) through a system of lenses (ocular and objective). Particles of approximately 1 μm in size or greater can be characterized by light microscopy. Samples can be stained with different dyes or observed unstained *via* phase contrast. Optical microscopy is a compendial method[41,42] that focuses on the characterization and limit testing of particles in medicinal products. Nucleated cell count and viability with the use of a hemocytometer are part of Ph. Eur. Chapter 2.7.29.[27]	• Appearance/Morphology of particles (cells). • Number of particles (cell number). • Discrimination viable/non-viable cells (either *via* their appearance and morphology or after staining with viability dyes). • Presence of conspicuous cells.	• Content (e.g., cell count with haemocytometer). • Viability (e.g., after staining with trypan blue). • Identity (Morphology, e.g., after Pappenheim stain of blood smears or tissue). • Cellular Impurities (e.g., morphology of cells after staining). • Analysis of primary cells as starting material (blood, apheresis, and bone marrow). • Analysis of end product (e.g, MSC).
MTT Assay	A colorimetric assay for assessing cell viability. Special cellular enzymes can reflect the number of viable cells present. These enzymes are capable of reducing the dye MTT to its insoluble product, which has a purple color.	• NAD(P)H-dependent cellular oxidoreductase enzymes.	• Cytotoxicity (loss of viable cells). • Cytostatic activity (shift from proliferation to quiescence). • Potency (e.g., sensitivity to ganciclovir).

Notes: CBMPs represent a very heterogeneous group of medicinal products and thus the applied analytical procedures and assays vary extremely. This table can therefore only be understood as a summary of methods most commonly used for QC of cellular products. CFSE: Carboxyfluorescein succinimidyl ester; 7-AAD: 7-Aminoactinomycin D; FISH: fluorescence *in situ* hybridization; CGH: Comparative Genomic Hybridization; MTT: 3-(4, 5-dimethylthiazol-2-yl)-2, 5-diphenyltetrazolium bromide; NADPH: Nicotinamide adenine dinucleotide phosphate.

established in order to assure the reproducibility of the process and the consistency of the final product. Tests and acceptance criteria have to be described.

The relevant section of Annex 2 of the EU GMP Guidelines[11] argues similarly: *In-process controls have a greater importance in ensuring the consistency of the quality of biological active substance and medicinal products than for conventional products. In-process control testing should be performed at appropriate stages of production to control those conditions that are important for the quality of the finished product.*

As not all cellular products can be cryopreserved or otherwise stored for longer time periods without negatively affecting their viability and/or potency microbiological in-process controls are of special importance for cellular products with short shelf life where testing of the finished product cannot be completed before product release or even administration to the patient. Test results of these microbiological in-process controls can then be used as release criteria to follow a negative-to-date concept (compare Section 6.6.9. Microbiology).

Annex 2 of the EU GMP Guidelines further points out that where end product tests are not available due to the short shelf life of the preparation, alternative methods of obtaining equivalent data to permit initial batch certification should be considered (e.g., rapid microbiological methods). The procedure for batch certification and release may be carried out in two or more stages with the first step being the assessment of batch processing records, results from environmental monitoring (where available) which should cover production conditions, all deviations from normal procedures, and the available analytical results for review, in preparation for the initial certification by the QP.

But as important as in-process controls might be, on the other hand it is essential that these controls do not compromise the products as sampling in many cases is associated with a risk for contamination or other types of negative impact (e.g., on cell culture conditions). Moreover, cellular material is often scarce and in-process controls should not endanger the achievement of a sufficient cell dose to treat the patient.

Chapter 6 of the EU GMP Guidelines prescribes that all in-process controls, including those made in the production area by production personnel have to be performed according to methods validated and approved by QC.

For any in-process control, irrespective of the method used, apart from validation, the following issues have to be considered and defined:

- When does the in-process control have to be performed?
- Who is responsible (production or QC)?
- How frequently does the in-process control have to be executed?
- What sampling method is used?

- What sample volume is needed?
- Which test procedure is used?
- Can samples be stored prior to analysis and if so for how long and under which storage conditions?
- What acceptance criteria are defined?

For CBMPs, the process of cell culture is one of the most variable manufacturing steps, especially for cellular products in early stages of clinical trials where practical experiences are scarce and culturing steps are not yet fully developed and validated. Culturing processes can range from very simple approaches with open steps using normal cell culture flasks to fully automated bioreactors. In any case, the maximal duration of the cell culture should be defined and it has to be validated that acceptance criteria are still met under these worst case conditions. Which in-process controls are performed, how frequently and which acceptance criteria are set is dependent on both the culturing process and the type of cells that is cultured. The control strategy must be in any case risk based.

For cell culture characterization the following in-process controls can be suitable to ensure optimal growth as well as preservation of integrity and function of the cells:

- **Viability** is an important in-process control for cell culture as suboptimal culture conditions can have significant influence on the viability of the cells. Viability can be analyzed microscopically, with help of automated cell counters or by flow cytometric analysis using vital dyes (e.g., trypan blue, 7-AAD, and DAPI).
- **Purity** is important as contaminating cell populations often grow under the same culture conditions as the target population (sometimes even better).
- **Confluence, expansion rate or population doublings** are measures for cell growth. If no continuous cell culture system is used it has to be defined when the culture has to be split. In these cases acceptance criteria are necessary upon which the decision for splitting is based. For suspension culture, a sample can be taken to define the expansion rate and/or maximal culture density, which can be set as numerical parameters. From adherent culture, a sample often cannot be taken and the decision about splitting has to be based on the microscopic analysis of the cell confluence. This is a more subjective parameter and is therefore more difficult to address. Microscopic pictures that define a certain status of confluence can help in this respect.
- **Metabolic activity** can be a measure for viability, cell growth or even purity when applied quantitatively. Metabolic activity can for example be addressed by analysis of the cell culture supernatant (e.g., by ELISA) or by flow cytometry

(e.g., intracellular staining and analysis for production of cytokines) or simply by macroscopic observation of the cell culture medium (especially when indicator dyes are used). Measuring major metabolites, such as glucose and lactate are also commonly used to address the determination of metabolic activity.

- **Expression of new markers and proteins after genetic modification.** It is necessary to measure the efficacy of a genetic modification. This can be done either on DNA level by use of PCR-based methods or on the protein level by flow cytometric analysis of the target protein. When a newly introduced protein has to provide a certain function (e.g., enzymatic activity), it is necessary to additionally address this functionality under culture conditions.

- **Morphology** is a useful parameter for adherent as well as suspension cells and can — together with other tests — prove identity as well as the general condition of the culture.

- **Microbiology/absence of adventitious microbial agents (e.g., bacteria, fungi, yeast, and mycoplasma):** If cell product is scarce, cell culture supernatant can be used as surrogate for analysis of microbial contamination or sterility testing. For the assessment of a potential contamination with mycoplasma, the analysis of cell culture supernatant would not be sufficient as mycoplasma are known to be intracellular micro-organisms.

- **Senescence and Genetic/Epigenetic Stability:** *In vitro* cultivation can result in the accumulation of genetic or epigenetic changes that may influence the safety and potency of the product. Prolonged cultivation may furthermore lead to cell ageing followed by the loss of function. Together with the control of population doublings, the analysis of senescence and (epi-) genetic stability provides a useful control to the status of cell culture.

Apart from assessing the status of cell culture, in-process controls can be necessary before and after crucial manufacturing steps, such as activation or stimulation of cell populations with cytokines or the step of genetic modification. Another example of a crucial manufacturing step is cryopreservation, a process known to have significant influence on cell viability and quality. Some antigens (e.g., some CD markers) are also known to be regulated by cryopreservation and it is important to know if this is also true for the relevant markers used for identification, assessment of purity or potency. This question has to be addressed at least during process validation, where in-process controls should be analyzed at numerous stages of the manufacturing process, and especially before and after cryopreservation in order to characterize this critical manufacturing step. It is furthermore important to define which analytical data are used as release criteria as in some cases not the full range of tests can be performed with the finished product, either because of the lack of sufficient material or because of an alteration of the cells through the process of cryopreservation that leads to a less significant result afterwards. If this applies, data obtained from analytical tests performed with the intermediate product have to serve as release criteria. Typically viability is a parameter that is known to be significantly affected by cryopreservation and is therefore usually analyzed before and afterwards, whereas parameters like identity are not altered and is therefore analyzed at only one stage, either before or after cryopreservation.

The information collected from the in-process-controls is utterly useful for more thorough understanding of the biology behind cell cultivation and modification steps and for defining the parameters and borders of the given manufacturing process.

6.6 Specifications and Release Criteria

6.6.1 *Terms and definitions*

6.6.1.1 *Acceptance criteria*

Numerical limits, ranges, or other suitable measures for acceptance of the results of analytical procedures which the drug substance or drug product or materials at other stages of their manufacture should meet (ICH Q6B).

Acceptance Criteria means numerical limits, ranges, or other suitable measures of test results necessary to determine acceptance of the drug substance, drug products, or materials at stages of their manufacture (Guidance for Industry, CGMP for Phase 1 Investigational Drugs, FDA).

6.6.1.2 *Specification*

A specification is defined as a list of tests, references to analytical procedures, and appropriate acceptance criteria which are numerical limits, ranges, or other criteria for the tests described. It establishes the set of criteria to which a drug substance, drug product or materials at other stages of its manufacture should conform to be considered acceptable for its intended use. "Conformance to specification" means that the drug substance and drug product, when tested according to the listed analytical procedures, will meet the acceptance criteria. Specifications are critical quality standards that are proposed and justified by the manufacturer and approved by regulatory authorities as conditions of approval (ICH Q6B).[44]

Specifications describe in detail the requirements with which the products or materials used or obtained during manufacture have to conform. They serve as a basis for quality evaluation.[45]

6.6.1.3 *Release specification*

The combination of physical, chemical, biological, and microbiological tests and acceptance criteria that determine the suitability of a drug product at the time of its release [ICH Q1A (R2)].

6.6.1.4 *Shelf life specification*

The combination of physical, chemical, biological, and microbiological tests and acceptance criteria that determine the suitability of a drug substance throughout its retest period, or that a drug product should meet throughout its shelf life [ICH Q1A (R2)].

6.6.2 *Choice and justification of specifications and acceptance criteria*

Every manufacturer of a medicinal product has to define specifications and acceptance criteria that assure the quality of the product and consistency of the manufacturing process including specifications for the starting and raw materials, for intermediates or in-process controls and for the finished product. These specifications are part of the authorization [either MA or clinical trials authorization (CTA)] and are the basis for batch certification and batch release by a QP.

Although the manufacturer together with the MA holder (MAH) or sponsor of the clinical trial, is fully responsible for the choice of specifications and definition of the corresponding acceptance criteria, there are basic and special guidelines, directives and regulations that have to be followed. These documents define the types of tests that have to be performed. In addition, there might be relevant pharmacopoeial monographs or general chapters that are applicable to the CBMP. In these cases, the relevant pharmacopoeia defines an analytical test procedure (sometimes with alternatives) together with the corresponding acceptance criteria. These test methods are considered to be validated and validation activities therefore can be reduced to matrix validation. Methods, other than the prescribed test methods can be used if they were shown to be equally suitable or even better. Apart from tests requested by guidance documents or pharmacopoeias, additional testing can be required for special cell types or manufacturing processes and it is important that all potential risks are addressed and additional testing is defined, wherever necessary.

If acceptance criteria are not defined by a guidance document or a pharmacopoeia, these limits have to be specified by the sponsor or MAH, together with the manufacturer. Defining these limits for novel therapeutics such as CBMPs can sometimes be difficult as worst case scenarios of many parameters are often still not studied sufficiently, to conclude about their impact on product quality. Furthermore, the probability of their occurrence due to biological variability of the process or the starting material is not clear from the beginning. Therefore, at early stages, acceptance criteria are often established with rather narrow ranges, if it is suspected that a broader range could compromise patient safety. For cryopreserved cells it has to be defined whether release criteria have to be obtained with the finished product or at the intermediate stage before cryopreservation has to be defined. Some parameters such as viability usually have to be addressed at both stages (also compare Section 6.5. In-Process Controls).

It is required that acceptance criteria are based on practical experiences with batches produced for preclinical or clinical development, during pharmaceutical development or scale-up, for demonstration of manufacturing consistency or for stability testing. As acceptance criteria for IMPs in early stages of clinical trials are often based on a limited number of batches, they might be adjusted during further development steps.

Table 6.9 provides a list of relevant quality documents for CTMPs in Europe (not exhaustive) that give advice or prescribe specifications (sometimes together with acceptance criteria). Please note that not all mentioned documents may be applicable to all types of cellular products and that there might be additional documents for special cell types.

All guidance documents acknowledge that batch consistency of cellular products due to variability of the starting material and manufacturing processes is significantly lower than those of conventional medicinal products. Therefore, Quality Risk Management (QRM) principles should be followed to develop a control strategy.

According to the European guideline on human CBMPs, extensive characterization of the cellular component has to be established in terms of identity, purity, viability, potency, and suitability for the intended use, unless justified.

For MA of ATMPs, European Directive 2009/120/EC defines the following for characterization and control strategy for somatic CTMPs:

- Relevant information shall be provided on the characterization of the cell population or cell mixture in terms of identity, purity (e.g., adventitious microbial

Table 6.9: List of relevant European guidance documents for quality aspects of CBMPs. In addition to the guidance documents listed in this table, several ICH Q documents might also be relevant for CBMPs or at least provide valuable advice on certain topics.

Document Reference Number	Document Title	Remarks
Relevant Pharmacopoeial Texts		
Ph. Eur. 2.6.1.	Sterility.	Monograph for sterility testing of conventional medicinal products. Defines the use of direct inoculation and membrane filtration method.
Ph. Eur. 2.6.7.	Mycoplasmas.	Culture method for Mycoplasma or PCR on mycoplasma-DNA.
Ph. Eur. 2.6.14.	Bacterial endotoxins.	Limulus amebocyte lysate (LAL) test (assessment of turbidity in presence of bacterial endotoxins).
Ph. Eur. 2.6.16.	Tests for extraneous agents in viral vaccines.	This chapter is not only applicable to viral vaccines but also to viral vectors used for gene therapy. Master and working seed lots have to comply with Chapter 2.6.16.
Ph. Eur. 2.6.21.	NAT	General chapter for NAT-based methods.
Ph. Eur. 2.6.27.	Microbiological control of cellular products.	Direct inoculation method for cellular products (blood culture test bottles and assessment of CO_2 release as read out parameter).
Ph. Eur. 2.6.30.	Monocyte-activation test (MAT).	Alternative test method to rabbit pyrogen test.
Ph. Eur. 2.7.23.	Numeration of CD34+/CD45+ cells in hematopoietic products.	Relevant for HSCs only. Introduces single platform measurement for flow cytometry.
Ph. Eur. 2.7.24.	Flow cytometry.	General chapter on the method of flow cytometry.
Ph. Eur. 2.7.28.	Colony-forming cell assay for human HPCs	Relevant to HSCs only. Defines assessment of clonality.
Ph. Eur. 2.7.29.	Nucleated cell count and viability.	Chapter on cell count with hemocytometer or automated methods and analysis of viability using manual methods and dye-exclusion or automated systems.
Ph. Eur. 5.1.7.	Viral safety.	The chapter provides general requirements concerning the viral safety of medicinal products whose manufacture has involved the use of materials of human or animal origin.

(*Continued*)

Table 6.9: *(Continued)*

Document Reference Number	Document Title	Remarks
Ph. Eur. 5.1.9.	Guidelines for using the test for sterility.	N/A
Ph. Eur. 5.1.10.	Guidelines for using the test for bacterial endotoxins.	N/A
Ph. Eur. 5.6.1.	Alternative methods for control of microbiological quality.	Chapter has no binding character. Introduces rapid methods in microbiology and gives advice on validation of these methods.
Ph. Eur. 5.14.	Gene transfer medicinal products for human use.	General chapter defines requirements for production and QC of GTMPs.

European Directives and Regulations

Directive 2003/63/EC.	Amending Directive 2001/83/EC of the European Parliament and of the Council on the Community code relating to medicinal products for human use.	Annex I "Analytical, pharmaco-toxicological and clinical standards and protocols in respect to the testing of medicinal products".
Directive 2009/120/EC.	Amending Directive 2001/83/EC of the European Parliament and of the Council on the Community Code relating to medicinal products for human use as regards ATMPs.	Special Regulation concerning MA application for ATMP (Common Technical Document modules 3, 4, and 5).
Regulation (EC) No. 726/2004.	Laying down Community procedures for the authorization and supervision of medicinal products for human and veterinary use and establishing a European Medicines Agency (EMA).	Medicinal Products centralized MA procedure (not specific for CBMPs or ATMPs).
Regulation (EC) No. 1394/2007.	On ATMPs and amending Directive 2001/83/EC and Regulation (EC) No. 726/2004.	Lays down centralized MA procedure for ATMPs.

(Continued)

Table 6.9: (*Continued*)

Document Reference Number	Document Title	Remarks
Regulation (EC) No. 668/2009.	Implementing Regulation (EC) No. 1394/2007 of the European Parliament and of the Council with regard to the evaluation and certification of quality and non-clinical data relating to advanced therapy medicinal products developed by micro, small and medium sized-enterprises (SMEs).	Special Regulation concerning SMEs.
EMA Guidelines		
CPMP/QWP/ 155/96.	Note for Guidance on Development Pharmaceutics.	Considerations for formulation development and establishment of parameters crucial for quality of finished product.
CPMP/BWP/ 41450/98.	Points to consider on the manufacture and quality control of human somatic cell therapy medicinal products.	Document is replaced by the Guideline on human CBMPs (EMEA/CHMP/ 410869/2006).
CPMP/BWP/ 3088/99.	Note for Guidance on the quality, preclinical and clinical aspects of gene transfer medicinal products.	Document is supplemented and updated by the "Guideline on quality, non-clinical, and clinical aspects of medicinal products containing genetically modified cells" (EMA/CAT/GTWP/ 671639/2008).
EMEA/CHMP/ BWP/398 498/05.	Guideline on virus safety evaluation of biotechnological investigational medicinal products.	The guideline provides advice on the viral safety data and documentation that should be submitted in a request for CTA of a human biotechnological medicinal product. The document actually applies to human biotechnological IMPs prepared from cells cultivated *in vitro* from characterized cell banks of human or animal origin as described in ICH Q5A, but basic principles are applicable also to other types of biotechnological products such as raw and starting materials used for the production of CBMPs.

Table 6.9: *(Continued)*

Document Reference Number	Document Title	Remarks
EMEA/CHMP/ 410869/2006.	Guideline on human cell based medicinal products. This guideline replaces the "Points to Consider on the Manufacture and Quality Control of Human Somatic Cell Therapy Medicinal Products" (CPMP/BWP/41450/98).	"Mother guideline" for CBMPs. Defines amongst other things specifications. QC of GTMPs is not in the scope of this document (for QC of these cells, compare EMA/CAT/GTWP/671639/2008). Document reflects all stages of CBMP including (pre-) clinical development and CBMPs in clinical trials.
EMEA/CHMP/ BWP/271475/ 2006.	Guideline on potency testing of cell based immunotherapy medicinal products for the treatment of cancer.	Although specifically developed for immunotherapy medicinal products, document provides valuable general information for potency testing.
EMEA/CHMP/ GTWP/ 587488/2007 Rev.1.	Reflection paper on quality, non-clinical, and clinical issues related to the development of recombinant adeno-associated viral vectors.	Guideline in revision (not effective).
EMA/CAT/ GTWP/ 671639/2008.	Guideline on quality, non-clinical, and clinical aspects of medicinal products containing genetically modified cells.	Defines amongst other issues in-process controls and QC testing of GM cells. Guideline is an integral part of the Note for Guidance on the quality, preclinical, and clinical aspects of GTMPs.
EMA/CHMP/ GTWP/ 212377/2008.	Questions and Answers on gene therapy.	N/A
EMEA/CAT/ 418458/2008.	Procedural advice on the certification of Quality and Non-clinical data for Small and Medium-sized Enterprises developing Advanced Therapy Medicinal Products.	The document gives guidance and describes the procedures, timelines and practical steps to be followed by the applicants and the EMA for the submission, evaluation of a certification application and if applicable, the issuing of the certificate.

(Continued)

Table 6.9: (*Continued*)

Document Reference Number	Document Title	Remarks
EMA/CAT/ 486831/ 2008/corr.	Guideline on the minimum quality and non-clinical data for certification of advanced therapy medicinal products.	Defines necessary scientific data for MA of ATMP (required scientific data for modules 2, 3, and 4).
EMA/CHMP/ GTWP/BWP/ 234523/2009.	Concept paper on the revision of the note for guidance on the quality, pre-clinical and clinical aspects of gene transfer medicinal products.	Document in revision (not effective).
EMA/CAT/ GTWP/ 44236/2009.	Reflection paper on design modifications of gene therapy medicinal products during development.	Document presents a collection of regulatory considerations given for specific GTMPs, where the characteristics have been changed at various stages during clinical development.
EMEA/CHMP/ ICH/449035/ 2009.	ICH Considerations: General Principles to Address Virus and Vector Shedding.	The document provides recommendations for designing non-clinical and clinical shedding studies, when appropriate. It focuses on the analytical assays used for detection, and considerations for the sampling profiles and schedules in both non-clinical and clinical studies.
EMA/CAT/ 571134/2009.	Reflection Paper on Stem-cell based medicinal products.	Document covers specific aspects related to Stem-CBMPs for MAA. Stem cell preparations that are not substantially manipulated or intended to be used for the same essential function in the recipient are not within the scope of this reflection paper.

agents and cellular contaminants), viability, potency, karyology, tumorigenicity, and suitability for the intended medicinal use. The genetic stability of the cells shall be demonstrated.

- Qualitative and, where possible, quantitative information on product- and process-related impurities, as well as on any material capable of introducing degradation products during production, shall be provided. The extent of the determination of impurities shall be justified.

In the United States, the US Pharmacopoeia in chapter <1046> "Cell and Gene Therapy Products"[13] provides an overview on possible analytical tests for Cell and Gene Therapy Biological Products (compare Table 6.10).

Cellular products often cannot be discriminated in drug substance and drug product as clearly as this is the case for conventional medicinal products with chemical APIs. The following sections on individual specifications therefore apply for both, drug substance and drug product.

Table 6.10: Overview on analytical tests for cell and gene therapy biological products according to USP Chapter <1046>.

Test	CTPs (somatic CTPs and GM cells)	Viral GTPs (used for *in vivo* gene therapy)
Identity of biological substance	• Surface marker determination. • Species. • Morphology. • Bioassay. • Biochemical marker.	• Restriction enzyme map. • PCR. • Immunoassay for expressed gene sequencing
Dose	• Viable cell number. • Enumeration of specific cell population. • Total DNA. • Total protein.	• Particle number. • Transducing units (DNA hybridization assay). • Total protein. • HPLC assay using authenticated reference standard.

(Continued)

Table 6.10: (*Continued*)

Test	CTPs (somatic CTPs and GM cells)	Viral GTPs (used for *in vivo* gene therapy)
Potency	Viable cell number (cells intended for structural repair). Bioassays: • Colony-formation assay. • Function of expressed gene. • Induction of secondary effect (e.g., HLA induction, secretion of cytokines, and up-regulation of surface marker).	Function of expressed gene (induction of secondary effect and other bioassays).
Purity	• Percentage of viable cells. • Percentage of transduced cells. • Percentage of cells with specific surface marker. • Process contaminants (e.g., serum).	• Residual host cell DNA. • Process contaminates (e.g., serum, and cesium chloride). • Residual helper virus. • Optical density ratio. • Residual host-cell proteins. • Viral protein profile (HPLC assay for defective or immature particles). • Residual RNA.
Safety	• Mycoplasma. • Sterility. • Endotoxins and Pyrogen. • Adventitious Viruses. • Residual virus (for transfected/ transduced cells). • Replication-competent vector virus (for transfected/transduced cells).	• General safety. • Mycoplasma. • Sterility. • Endotoxins and Pyrogen. • Adventitious Viruses. • Replication-competent virus.

Note: Table modified according to USP chapter <1046> "Cell and Gene Therapy Products".

6.6.3 *Identity*

Identity of the cellular component can be based on phenotypic and/or genotypic characterization. The identity assay used must be relevant for both the cell type as well as the specific manipulations applied to the cells during the manufacturing process.

The most common method used for phenotypic determination of identity of the cellular component is flow cytometry (Ph. Eur. 2.7.24[25] and USP <1027>[26]) where one or more different cell surface, intracellular and/or intra nuclear markers can be addressed in parallel to form a pattern of different characteristics. Concurrent assessment of several different markers is necessary in many cases as most cell types cannot be sufficiently distinguished from others by only just one single antigen, especially when the cell product consists of different cell populations. It has to be kept in mind that antigens can be up- and down-regulated under certain conditions (e.g., upon stimulation during cell culture), hence the suitability of a distinct marker has always to be considered in conjunction with the activation state of the cells to be analyzed.

For adherent cells morphology can be an additional characteristic addressing identity of the cells.

The EU guideline on human CBMPs furthermore proposes assessment of biochemical activity, response to exogenous stimuli and capability to produce biologically active or otherwise measurable molecules (cytokines, growth factors, etc.) as possible approaches for analysis of identity. These molecules could be measured, for example, by ELISA or intracellular flow cytometry. But since response to stimuli and production of active substances can be part of the MoA, these test methods can also be suitable as potency assays.

Genotypic profiling is often necessary for genetically engineered cells, where not only the identity of the cell type or population has to be demonstrated but also the genetic modification. Analysis of gene expression is usually done by nucleic acid amplification techniques (NAT; Ph. Eur. 2.6.21[34] and USP <1127>[37]) whereas expression of the newly acquired characteristic(s) can also be analyzed on protein level using flow cytometry or Western Blot analysis (being the far less sensitive method for protein analysis compared to flow cytometry).

For allogeneic preparations typing for polymorphisms (e.g., blood group antigens and major histocompatibility HLA classes I and II) may be necessary but this is usually part of donor testing and characterization of the starting material (compare Section 6.2. QC of Materials).

Irrespective of the analytical procedure used for determination of identity, it is essential that these methods are specific for the addressed marker or nucleic-acid sequence as otherwise the obtained test results are not significant and reliable (compare Section 6.11 "Validation of Analytical Procedures").

6.6.4 *Purity*

Determination of purity is crucial as usually only a defined type of cells or for GTMPs only efficiently transformed cells are able to administer the desired MoA. The target cell population may be a defined cell type or a mixture of several different cell types in a defined combination, potentially carrying an intended genetic modification for the therapeutic purpose. Since purity is affected by many different factors (see below), it has to be determined together with potentially contaminating components and impurities that can be of cellular, chemical or microbiological nature.

Purity might be affected by:

- Other cell populations and/or cells of different differentiation stage and/or not sufficiently genetically engineered cells, all of them originating from the starting material (compare product-related impurities),
- Impurities originating from manufacturing (compare process-related impurities),
- Non-viable cells (compare viability).

For allogeneic products purity can be of significant importance as contaminating cells with different properties than those aimed for might cause severe unwanted effects (e.g., donor lymphocytes in HLA–mismatched settings).

Same as for identity, flow cytometry is the most common method used for determination of cellular purity, at least if purity should be addressed as percentage of non-target and/or non-viable cells in the total product. Usually it is not possible to use the assay established for assessment of identity also for determination of cellular purity even if in most cases flow cytometry is the core technology employed for both purposes. If it is not possible to address different markers for identity compared to purity, the assessment of signal strength (high, intermediate, and low) could yield additional information. To avoid unspecific antibody binding, it is advisable to exclude non-viable cells first (compare section viability) and to perform further phenotypic analysis of the viable cell population. The purity of the target cell fraction will be expressed as percentage of cells amongst all viable cells.

The percentage of purity together with the percentage of viable cells and the total number of cells present in the finished product allow the calculation of total number of target cells present in the finished product.

For transiently GM cells where foreign nucleic acid sequences are removed for final formulation of the product, purity assays have to be applied that show the absence of cells carrying the foreign nucleic acid sequences.[16]

6.6.5 *Impurities*

According to ICH Q6B[44] an impurity is any component present in the drug substance or drug product which is not the desired product, a product-related substance, or excipient including buffer components. It may be either process- or product-related. In contrast contaminants are any adventitiously introduced materials (e.g., chemical, biochemical, or microbial species) not intended to be part of the manufacturing process of the drug substance or drug product.

No matter what kind of impurity is addressed, upper limits should be defined for all possible impurities on a risk-based approach. For certain impurities, testing of the finished product may not be necessary if efficient control or removal to acceptable levels can be demonstrated by either in-process controls or during process validation.

6.6.5.1 *Product-related impurities*

Product-related impurities are defined as molecular variants of the desired product (e.g., precursors, certain degradation products arising during manufacture and/or storage) which do not have properties comparable to those of the desired product with respect to activity, efficacy, and safety (ICH Q6B).

The ICH definition does not completely match product-related impurities of CBMPs as usually these are contaminating cells originating from the starting material that have either different characteristics or differentiation state than the target cell fraction.

Based on the composition of the starting material and the manufacturing process it is important to know which cell types could be present as contaminating cell populations in the finished product and what effect these cells could have on the recipient of the CBMP, keeping in mind the medical indication for administration of the product and the general health status of the patient. For example, it is known that more than 2.5×10^4 contaminating CD3+ lymphocytes per kg of the recipient's body weight in an HLA haploidentical setting can trigger graft-*versus*-host disease (GvHD). HSC based medicinal products for allogeneic use are therefore analyzed for the residual amounts of lymphocytes after lymphocyte–depletion or stem cell-enrichment procedures.

As manufacturing processes in cell therapy tend to be more variable than those for conventional pharmaceutical production and as these manufacturing processes are often not fully validated in early stages of clinical trials, analysis of contaminating cells in the finished product of every batch is almost always a release criterion requested by the authorities. Upper limits have to be set in these cases and the overall amount of contaminating cells (differentiated in sub-populations, if applicable) has to be indicated. In the majority of cases, flow cytometry will be the most appropriate analytical method as different cell surface and intracellular markers can be included in one single stain allowing the analysis of different cell populations in parallel.

If cellular purity as well as cellular impurities are analyzed in one single flow cytometric stain it has to be ensured that not only the target cell population but also the contaminating cell types are considered appropriately (i.e., MSCs are relatively big cells and one would not recognize other contaminating cells of smaller size, if the area with them is cut off as debris). As the acceptable limit for impurities is usually very low, unspecific antibody binding has to be avoided in order to prevent false positive staining results. Exclusion of non-viable cells is therefore especially important for flow cytometric analysis of impurities. Blocking of unspecific antibody binding to Fc-receptors might also be necessary depending on the cell type.

The required validation strategy for the relevant analytical methods is dependent on the type of analytical procedure: If these product-related impurities are determined with a limit test, it is sufficient to validate specificity and detection limit of the method. If the impurities should be determined quantitatively, a full validation including all analytical characteristics is necessary (compare Section 6.11. Validation of Analytical Procedures).

6.6.5.2 *Process-related impurities*

Process-related impurities are defined as impurities that are derived from the manufacturing process. They may be derived from cell substrates (e.g., host cell proteins, host cell DNA), cell culture (e.g., inducers, antibiotics, or media components), or down-stream processing (e.g., processing reagents or column leachables) (ICH Q6B).[44]

Process-related impurities of CBMPs are often originating from raw materials used for cell processing. Typical raw materials for manufacturing of cellular products are cytokines, antibodies, serum, culture media with different medium components, fine chemicals, enzymes, and nucleic acids for genetic modification (compare Section 6.2. QC of Materials).

There are two major issues related to impurities originating from raw materials used for production of cellular products:

1. In the emerging field of cell therapy very often novel substances have to be used as raw materials that are not of pharmaceutical grade or otherwise produced under quality assured conditions and therefore are not well characterized. Experiences with these substances when administered to the patient are in the majority of cases completely missing.
2. Raw materials used during manufacture of cellular products are often very potent substances in terms of activation or stimulation of cells — the reason why they are actually used. But when these substances are administered to the patient as process related impurities, even low quantities might have a significant unwanted effect.

Almost all cell therapy guidance documents therefore emphasize that residual amounts of process-related impurities have to be addressed carefully. It is important that all raw or AMs are evaluated on a risk-based approach. The medical indication of the CTP has to be considered as the health status of the recipient might have significant influence on the possible reaction caused by a certain substance (e.g., patients might be immune compromised or otherwise in poor general condition making them more susceptible to adverse reactions).

There are three basic approaches for the determination of process-related impurities:

1. Arithmetical approach: Calculation of residual amounts based on the initial amount used for processing and reduction by washing or dilution steps;
2. Analysis (quantitative or limit test) of impurity in the finished product during process validation;
3. Analysis (quantitative or limit test) of impurity in every batch.

The arithmetical approach can be suitable for impurities with low risk for the patients (e.g., cell culture media or media components of high quality or pharmaceutical grade). Analysis of a certain impurity for every finished batch can be necessary or even requested by the authorities when substances are suspected to bear a significant risk.

Residual Amounts of Antibodies

Unlike therapeutic antibodies that are produced as medicinal products and are therefore well characterized in terms of potential adverse reactions, antibodies used as raw materials for separation or depletion of certain cell populations (e.g., by magnetic cell separation such as MACS®-technology or by fluorescence-based cell-sorting such as FACS™-technology) or for stimulation (e.g., coated on magnetic beads to facilitate expansion of certain cell types in *in vitro* cell culture) are often of unknown effect and activity (at least if there are no therapeutic antibodies of the same clone directed against the same antigen or epitope). It can be necessary or requested by the authorities that these antibodies are further characterized, for example, with respect to their ability to stimulate cells *in vitro* (e.g., absence of super-agonistic properties).

Moreover antibodies used as raw materials very often are murine proteins that can trigger allergic reactions when administered to the patient. Apart from allergic reactions murine antibodies are known to induce production of human anti-murine antibodies (HAMA) as known from the first generation of therapeutic antibodies that still contained murine protein structure. Furthermore, antibodies can initiate antibody-dependent cellular cytotoxicity (ADCC), another unwanted reaction, at least for raw materials used for manufacture of CTMPs.

Since antibodies used for certain production processes in most cases specifically bind to the cell surface of the target cells (unless they are used for depletion of special cell populations and therefore should not be present in the final product), they cannot be washed away. Small amounts of antibodies will always stick to the surface of the cells.

As a conclusion, a residual amount of antibodies is an issue that has to be addressed very carefully. One possibility to analyze residual amounts of antibodies that contain murine protein structure is cell surface staining with anti-murine or anti-mouse antibodies and subsequent flow cytometric analysis. Western Blot analysis would also be possible but due to a much lower sensitivity of this method flow cytometry should be preferred.

To determine residual amounts of soluble antibodies in the finished product, ELISA-based techniques can be a suitable approach using capture and detection antibodies directed against murine protein structure or, if available, directed specifically against the antibody that should be detected.

The definition of suitable acceptance criteria for these tests is challenging as for most antibodies used as raw materials it is unclear what quantity is sufficient for triggering an adverse reaction. Of course it would be desirable to have negative results (meaning below detection limit of the applied analytical methods), but this may be hard to achieve. In addition, even the determination of the detection limit is not too easy, as the correlation between the percentage of marker-positive cells detected by flow cytometry and the actual amount of protein bound to the cell surface is difficult to address.

It might also be a helpful approach to calculate theoretical amounts of protein present in the final product (either considering that a certain amount of antibody is washed away during the production process or using the entire amount of protein introduced to the manufacturing process as a worst case scenario) and to compare these amounts with doses typically used for therapeutic application.

Residual Amounts of Cell Culture Media and Media Components

Residual amounts of cell culture media or even of certain components of the culture medium are difficult to address as medium composition is kept secret by almost all suppliers. One possible argument would be that the purpose of cell culture media is cell growth and that the media therefore may not have negative effects on the physiology of the cells, otherwise they would not be appropriate for their intended use. Indicator dyes could mark a problem as these substances in many cases are organic chemicals with benzene rings. Nevertheless in many cases it will be sufficient to calculate residual amounts theoretically instead of analyzing them practically. The same holds true for media components as serum that is added to the culture medium in quantities of around 5–10%.

The use of antibiotics as cell culture additives should be avoided and most authorities generally do not allow their use. If for special reasons antibiotics are used, nevertheless residual amounts in the finished product could be critical as they might interfere with sterility testing or could even adversely affect the recipient, at least if substances with high sensitization potential are used (e.g., β-lactam antibiotics). Requirements for analytical testing could therefore be strict.

Residual Amounts of Cytokines

Many cytokines are known to be potent substances that can facilitate biologic or immunologic action in the recipient even in small quantities. Therefore, it might be necessary to analyze residual amounts of cytokines in the final formulation, e.g., by ELISA technique. Certified test kits might be commercially available at least for cytokines that are frequently used in research or even therapeutically.

This applies, for example, to human Interleukin 2 (IL-2), a cytokine broadly used for *in vitro* culture of T-cells. IL-2 is also used as medicinal product for the treatment of renal cell cancer or melanoma where it is applied as human recombinant IL-2 variant with slight changes in the amino acid structure to enhance its therapeutic properties. If this GM protein is used as raw material, test methods — even if commercially available and certified — have to be validated in terms of accuracy and in order to demonstrate that also the GM protein can be analyzed equally well. Reference standards might be adjusted, if test kits use unmodified protein.

Residual Amounts of magnetic beads

Magnetic beads are used either for cell separation (enrichment or depletion procedures based on magnetic cell separation technology) or as artificial stimuli in cell culture (e.g., expansion beads coated with anti-CD3/anti-CD28 for T-cell cultivation). Bead size is variable dependent on the intended use or the provider and ranges from nanobeads (approximately 100 nm in size) to microbeads (several micrometers in size).

Using magnetic cell separation procedures, depletion and enrichment protocols have to be differentiated in terms of presence of beads in the final product: After depletion steps the labeled cells that carry the magnetic beads are in the negative fraction and therefore are not or only in traces present in the final product. For enrichment or selection steps the target cells are labeled with the bead-conjugated antibodies and magnetic beads (bound to the target cells) are present in the positive fraction and are therefore part of the finished product, — at least as long as beads cannot be efficiently removed from the cells after the enrichment procedure *via* predetermined cleavage points that facilitate the release of the antibody or antibody fragment from the magnetic bead.

CD34-selection of HSCs by MACS®-based enrichment procedure is meanwhile a widespread method and hundreds to thousands of these products have been administered to patients over the last years with no clear hints of negative effects caused by the magnetic beads that are infused together with the cells. Nevertheless, presence of magnetic beads in the final formulation is an issue raised by the authorities because of potential negative effects and also by researchers and pharmaceutical manufacturers because of difficulties in QC and/or further processing steps of these cells, as epitopes of the selection markers used for enrichment are blocked by the bead-antibody complex. The development of removable beads is a possible way out of this dilemma, but it has to be kept in mind that efficiency of the removal procedure has to be validated and the residual amount of beads in many cases has to be addressed nevertheless.

Removal of expansion beads used for activation of cells during cell culture is equally important in terms of their possible adverse reactions in the recipient as described for enrichment/depletion beads. Currently used expansion beads are typically magnetic and almost of the same size as WBCs since they should simulate antigen-presenting cells (APCs) and not only the mere presence of antibodies is important but also their steric configuration on the bead surface. Unlike enrichment and depletion procedures with nanobeads, where many bead-conjugated antibodies bind to one cell, the cell–bead-ratio of expansion beads is usually much lower (down to ratios of one bead per cell and even lower). Due to their magnetic properties, expansion beads can be removed by magnetic columns or placement on solid magnets. Both systems are working with use of blood bags and are therefore almost completely closed. But again, removal efficiency has to be demonstrated with validated analytical procedures. This can be done either microscopically (by manual or automated counting) or by flow cytometric analysis since beads represent particles that can be visualized *via* their scatter properties or they can even be stained in some cases with specific fluorescence-labeled antibodies. Discrimination between beads and cell debris is important in any case, particularly when the detection method is thought to provide quantitative data.

6.6.5.3 *Adventitious (microbial) agents*

Possible adventitious agents in CBMPs are viruses, mycoplasma, bacteria, or fungi. The contamination could originate from the starting or raw materials used for production, or it can be adventitiously introduced during the manufacturing process. At least, the finished product therefore has to be tested for the absence of bacteria, fungi, and mycoplasma. For further information, see Section 6.6.9 (Microbiology).

6.6.6 *Quantity*

As for any medicinal product also for CBMPs the quantity expressed as dose and/or content of the finished drug product has to be analyzed and indicated.

The cell dose is often expressed as number of target cells per kilogram of recipient's body weight. The content is the overall amount of either all viable cells, all nucleated cells or all target cells per unit of finished product (e.g., per bag or vial). Together with the overall volume of the finished product the cell concentration can be calculated. Authorities might ask for the definition of an acceptable range for the cell-concentration as cell concentrations that are either too high or too low can negatively influence viability of the finished product, either during shelf life or during cryopreservation procedures.

General guidance is provided by the European Pharmacopoeia in chapter 2.7.29 "Nucleated Cell Count and Viability" and by the US Pharmacopoeia in chapter <1046> "Cell and Gene Therapy Products", section dose-defining assay. Enumeration of cells may be performed manually using a hemocytometer or with an automated system such as particle counters or flow cytometers. The use of a hemocytometer or a flow cytometer both offer the possibility of including viability dyes such as trypan blue (most commonly used for manual counting) and 7–AAD or other substances (commonly used in flow cytometry), thus allowing not only enumeration of total cell numbers but also discrimination between dead and live cells (compare also section on viability). This is not the case for particle counters that solely measure particle size.

It has to be pointed out that enumeration of cells by flow cytometry is not readily available as most instruments are not able to determine overall cell numbers on their own since they lack the ability to measure the analyzed sample volume. The number of (target) cells can only be expressed as percentage of cells amongst other cells. To determine the total number of target cells the percentage of target cells has to be multiplied by the total cell number present in the product determined, either manually or by another automated system and therefore deriving from different analytical platforms (hence this approach is called dual platform analysis). As two different platforms analyze the cells in two different ways this approach might lead to analytical errors. Single platform methods have been established to circumvent this issue. For flow cytometric single platform analysis, it is either necessary to use an instrument that is able to measure the analyzed sample volume directly or to add counting beads or reference particles of defined size to the sample in a known concentration. The flow cytometer is able to count these beads and together with the known bead concentration it is possible to calculate the sample volume that has been analyzed. For single platform analysis where the accuracy of the method is dependent on the precise enumeration of counting beads, so called lyse–no–wash protocols are mandatory as otherwise it cannot be determined to what extent beads (and cells) are lost due to centrifugation and aspiration of the supernatant.

Single platform analysis is requested by the European pharmacopoeia for the numeration of CD34+ HPCs. Dual platform approaches for these cell products can only be used unless it has been demonstrated that they are equally suitable in terms of accuracy and precision (compare Ph. Eur. Chapter 2.7.23. "Numeration of CD34+/CD45+ cells in hematopoietic products").[28] It has to be disucssed with the authorities whether single platform analysis is also requested for other CBMPs. Generally it seems that single-platform analysis is advantageous mainly for heterogeneous cell-preparations, where there is not too much benefit for highly pure cell products.

USP Chapter <1046> provides further examples for dose–defining assays for GTPs such as determination of milligrams of plasmid, viral particle numbers, or level of expression of gene products. For virally transduced cells the infectious titer is commonly determined by measuring the number of transduced or infected cells expressing a selection marker or reporter gene. Transduction rates of vectors without a marker gene can be quantified using quantitative PCR.

6.6.7 *Viability*

For determination of cell viability, the Ph. Eur. Chapter 2.7.29 "Nucleated cell count and viability"[27] is the relevant guidance document in Europe. The two basic approaches for administration of cell viability introduced by the European Pharmacopoeia are cell staining with viability dyes and subsequent manual or automated counting by either using a hemocytometer or a flow cytometer (compare also Section 6.6.6. Quantity).

Both methods (manual *versus* automated counting) are based on the exclusion of certain dyes from viable cells and absorbance of these dyes by damaged or dead cells with altered membrane integrity.

For manual dye-exclusion methods, trypan blue is most commonly used to distinguish between viable and non-viable cells. All unstained (=viable) cells are counted under the light microscope as well as the total number of cells to determine the percentage of viable cells in a given sample. It is essential that incubation with the dye does not exceed a defined time period (not more than four minutes according to Ph. Eur. 2.7.29.) and cells are counted without delay after incubation as otherwise the number of dead cells may increase significantly afterwards leading to analytical errors. Care should be taken when recently trypsinized or thawed cells are stained as they might have leaky membranes leading to a positive staining result, although the cells are viable.

Automated methods based on flow cytometry rely on dyes that are able to cross damaged membranes and intercalate with the DNA, leading to fluorescence emission and a positive fluorescence signal. Most commonly used dyes are 7-AAD and propidium iodide (PI), but other dyes exist that have been demonstrated to be equally or even more suitable as they have more favorable fluorescence emission profiles with less spectral overlap to other fluorescent dyes that are used for simultaneous determination of distinct cell surface markers.

Compared to manual dye-exclusion methods where the cells can be regarded visually under the light microscope and cell debris can be excluded from counting easily, this is not the case in flow cytometry. The correct gating strategy is important to exclude debris without excluding dead cells that tend to be smaller than viable cells. For hematopoietic cells it is therefore advisable to include the common leukocyte marker CD45 allowing to define a side scatter/CD45+ gating region to achieve better separation of nucleated cells from debris and platelets (if these are still present in the sample). For definition of correct gating regions and for validation of a viability assay, stabilized (dead) cells can serve as positive control.

Determination of cell viability is of special importance after cryopreservation, as this is known to have significant influence on viability due to formation of ice crystals or osmotic stress. During process validation it has to be demonstrated that cell viability after cryopreservation does not fall under a defined minimum percentage. The cryopreservation process itself is crucial in this respect but thawing of the cells is almost equally important, since the most commonly used cryopreservative DMSO exerts toxic effects on cells and viability can be reduced significantly within minutes after thawing. Washing the cells to remove DMSO might not be permitted as washing steps can significantly influence the ratio between live and dead cells and therefore alter sample composition. To achieve a maximum recovery and viability after thawing, protein has to be added to the cells (HSA or serum ranging from 5–90%, compare USP chapter <1046>). Most European authorities require thawing and analysis of pilot vials that are cryopreserved together with the finished product for final product release. Viability in these vials must meet a defined acceptance criterion. Apart from determination of the percentage of viable cells, it might be required to determine the recovery rate of the target cells as the percentage of live cells is dependent on the gating strategy where smaller particles/cells and debris (potentially originating from formerly viable cells) are excluded from counting, resulting in a high percentage of viable cells but a compromised quantity of target cells.

6.6.8 *Potency*

Potency is defined as the measure of the biological activity using a suitably quantitative biological assay (also called potency assay or bioassay), based on the attribute of the product which is linked to the relevant biological properties. Biological Activity is defined as the specific ability or capacity of the product to achieve a defined biological effect (ICH Q6B).[44]

A potency assay for a CBMP is requested by almost all guidance documents and should be established as early as possible not only for characterization and product release, but also to evaluate changes that have been made in the manufacturing process. Potency assays are therefore stipulated by many authorities as early as for phase I clinical trials. In addition assessment of biological activity is an important issue for stability testing as it has to be demonstrated that cells even at the end of their shelf life are still potent to induce clinical response (compare Section 6.10. Stability). All guidance documents point out that potency assays have to be based on the MoA of the cell product, an issue especially difficult to address at early stages of clinical trials.

A specific guidance document in Europe is the "Guideline on Potency Testing of Cell Based Immunotherapy Medicinal Products for the Treatment of Cancer"[46] that is actually restricted to viable cell products for cancer-immunotherapy but can also provide valuable advice for other types of products. The European "Guideline on quality, non-clinical and clinical aspects of medicinal products containing genetically modified cells"[16] defines requirements for GTMPs requesting that for estimating potency of transduced cells, '*biological tests should be applied to determine the functional properties achieved by the genetic modification. Potency can be expressed as a combination of several parameters including, e.g., the number of genetically modified cells, the gene copy number, the expression level of the transgene and the product activity level, as shown to be efficacious in clinical studies. The potency test(s) should provide, as far as possible, quantitative information on the newly acquired characteristics. Wherever possible, a reference batch of cells with assigned potency should be established and used to calibrate tests.*'

In addition to tests that only monitor the expression level of a gene-product, assessment of the correct biological function of the encoded protein might be required. It depends on the desired therapeutic function of the gene-product which potency assay has to be selected. If for example, an enzymatic activity is the function of the protein, the *in vivo* or *in vitro* test should be designed in a way to reflect correct function of the enzyme.

In the USA, FDA Guidance for Industry "Potency Tests for Cellular and Gene Therapy Products" as well as US Pharmacopoeia USP chapter<1046> "Cell and Gene Therapy Products" are relevant guidance documents for potency assays.

USP chapter <1046> points out that potency often is assessed by *in vitro* and *in vivo* (animal-based) bioassays for which it is not uncommon to have coefficients of variation between 30–50%. '*These assays require a well-defined, representative reference material that can be used as a positive control for the assay. The positive control serves to qualify the performance of an individual assay. Potency assay development should focus on characterizing and controlling variability. For some cell-based products such as hematopoietic progenitor cells, assays for product potency have been correlated with clinical efficacy. In this case, a traditional colony-forming assay that quantifies committed progenitor cells such as colony-forming unit–granulocyte-macrophage (CFU–GM) has been correlated with clinical engraftment outcomes in some studies. For example, the ability to determine specific cell-surface identity markers by employing flow cytometry techniques or vital stains may be an acceptable measurement of potency if properly validated and correlated with clinical outcome.*'

The development of a validated potency assay at early stages of product development is often hampered by insufficient scientific insight in the product's MoA because a complex response is typical for cell therapeutics and cannot always be presented by measuring a single activity parameter. First measures of product potency /efficacy often come from *in vivo* assays in preclinical studies. These assays are too time-intensive and cost-intensive for a routine release test and cannot be performed on each batch but they can provide the linkage between the *in vivo* effect and its measure in the *in vitro* potency assay. As the clinical experience accumulates, better correlation of product characteristics and the observed clinical effect can be made, which facilitates the establishment of an appropriate potency assay. Both direct and surrogate potency assays are accepted if the read out parameters are shown to be clearly linked to the therapeutic activity of the product.

In 2013, International Society for Cellular Therapy (ISCT) Product and Process Development Subcommittee issued a review dedicated to strategies of potency assay development for cell therapeutic products. The authors discuss relevant guidelines and provide examples of known potency assays.[47]

6.6.9 *Microbiology*

The microbiological status of a CTMP is an important feature as sterilization of the finished product is not possible and starting materials (autologous or allogeneic cells or tissue in most cases) are on their own critical in terms of microbiological contamination (also compare Section 6.2.2. Starting Material). Complex and not fully automated or closed production processes put an additional risk of contamination to these products during manufacture. Furthermore due to a sometimes very short shelf life of only some hours or days, these products have to be applied to the patient before microbiological testing of the finished product is fully completed.

Sterility testing or microbiological control of the finished product is the most relevant microbiological analysis required from almost all authorities and for all cell types. In addition, bacterial endotoxins and/or pyrogens are requested by many authorities. For cultured cells testing of Mycoplasma is required in most cases, too.

Microbiological test procedures for CTMPs are therefore typically:

- Sterility Test or Microbiological Control.
- Test on Pyrogens and/or Bacterial Endotoxins.
- Mycoplasma Test (for cultured cells).

Further details are given in the subsequent sections.

6.6.9.1 *Sterility testing and microbiological control*

Microbiological control or sterility testing of cellular products is the most important of all microbiological tests and requested by all authorities and for every type of product, but compared to conventional medicinal products these tests have their pitfalls when applied to CBMPs.

What kind of term is used for the analysis — Sterility testing (resulting in sterile or non-sterile products) or microbiological control (resulting in low-germ/culture negative or culture positive products) — is more or less formality. The only possible impact in Europe is the fact that medicinal products termed as sterile have to fully comply with Annex 1 of the EU GMP Guidelines "Manufacture of Sterile Medicinal Products" whereas otherwise Annex 2 "Manufacture of Biological active substances and Medicinal Products for Human Use" is applicable, offering the opportunity to deviate on a risk-based approach from the strict demands of Annex 1 concerning clean room grades and particulate as well as microbial monitoring limits. Nevertheless, it is worth pointing out here that the definition of sterility proposed by the European and US Pharmacopoeia is the lack or complete absence of all viable micro–organisms, defined as a sterility assurance level (SAL) of 10^{-6} for all replicating micro–organisms (meaning assurance of less than one chance in one million that viable micro–organisms are present in a sterilized article). In pharmacopoeial as well as GMP definitions sterility cannot be defined by testing (because it is technically unfeasible to prove a negative absolute and it cannot be practically demonstrated without testing every article in a batch), but only by application of a validated sterilization process (steam, dry heat, ionizing radiation, or filtration through a $0.22\,\mu\mathrm{m}$ filter), none of which is feasible for CBMPs. Furthermore, viruses or other fastidious species that are occasionally present in cell cultures cannot be detected with the normal sterility test making it seem not justifiable to use the term "sterile" for cellular products, even if they have passed a sterility test.

Sterility testing per se is one of the test methods that is internationally harmonized, as the ICH Steering Committee recommends that the official pharmacopoeial texts from Europe, Japan and the USA (Ph. Eur. 2.6.1. Sterility, JP 4.06 Sterility Test, and USP <71> Sterility Tests) can be used as interchangeable in the ICH regions, subject to the conditions detailed in ICH guideline Q4B Annex 8 to note for evaluation and recommendation of pharmacopoeial texts for use in region on sterility test — general chapter.

The two methods described for sterility testing are membrane filtration and direct inoculation of the culture medium, with the technique of membrane filtration being the one that has to be used *"whenever the nature of the product permits"* (Ph. Eur. 2.6.1). For conventional medicinal products, it is quite clear that for release testing the finished product has to be analyzed. For cellular products the situation is far more difficult as cellular products, at least the ones that are not cryopreserved, often have a very short shelf life of only some hours or days and both methods need an incubation time of at least 14 days, making it impossible in those cases to complete the test before administering the product to the patient. Furthermore, batch sizes due to the autologous or directed use of most cellular products are very small, sometimes consisting of only one bag or vial, and cellular material is often rare. Therefore, the prescribed minimum quantities and minimum numbers of items to be tested per batch in most cases cannot be fulfilled. For this reason, the EDQM included an additional chapter to the European Pharmacopoeia on "Microbiological Control of Cellular Products" (Ph. Eur. Chapter 2.6.27). The method described there, basically a direct inoculation method, is thought to be more sensitive, with a broader range and which is more rapid for certain cellular products compared to the tests introduced in Chapter 2.6.1, at least if automated culture systems are used. But although the test method described in Chapter 2.6.27 reduces the incubation time to seven days (for automated systems) and the inoculum volume to less than 1 mL for preparations with very small overall volumes, even these requirements are hard to comply with in some cases. To address these ongoing challenges chapter 2.6.27 is currently under revision. One of the perspectives offered in the revision proposal is the possibility to use rapid microbiological methods (RMMs) as described in Ph. Eur. general Chapter 5.6.1 "Alternative methods for control of microbiological quality" as sole test method (also compare sections on RMMs). In addition, considerations and recommendations about "negative-to-date" results for product release are included; an approach already followed by many authorities. The negative-to-date concept means that either the results of in-process controls are used for product release or intermediate results of the finished product (or even intermediate results of an in-process control). In any case, the ongoing tests have to be followed up closely, after product release, to be able to inform investigators, physicians, or users as quickly as possible if microorganisms are detected. Identification of micro-organisms recovered from a sterility test is mandatory anyway and is especially important in these cases, helping to define the measures to be taken for treatment of the patient.

Which approach is acceptable if sterility testing cannot be finished before administration of the product to the patient and what kind of in-process controls are required in these cases, should in cases of doubt, be discussed with the competent authority.

Irrespective of the type of analysis used for microbiological control (conventional *versus* rapid method, growth-based *versus* direct measurement), it is important to know that all methods underlie a certain sampling error. This sampling error is greater when the initial number of microorganisms in the medicinal product to be tested is lower, leading to the fact that samples of a product can be tested negative (sterile/culture negative) while the product in fact is not. To keep the sampling error low, samples should be taken as late as possible (concept of "late sampling"), allowing small numbers of contaminating bacteria to multiply before sampling takes place, thus increasing the probability of detection.[48] Advantages for late sampling were observed mainly for platelet concentrates that have to be stored at 22.5°C. Unfortunately, this positive effect is minimized for products that have to be stored at cold temperatures (2–6°C) as this retards or even avoids bacterial growth. And late sampling of course is not feasible for cellular products that are cryopreserved as this takes place immediately after harvest and final formulation.[49]

General Requirements

There are some prerequisites for microbiological control and sterility testing that need to be fulfilled independent of the method that is used.

One of these basic requirements is aseptic handling of both the product/sample that is analyzed and the culture medium that is used (together with all necessary equipment, adaptors, needles, membranes, etc.), to prevent microbial contamination due to handling errors resulting in false positive results. To meet these requirements, the European Pharmacopoeia recommends A in B clean room conditions (corresponding to ISO 4.8 and ISO 5) or use of an isolator together with regular monitoring of the working conditions by carrying out appropriate controls and taking appropriate samples (compare Ph. Eur. 2.6.1, Ph. Eur. 5.1.9 and Annex 1 to EU GMP Guidelines for particulate and microbial environmental control and corresponding limits).

If evidence of microbial growth is found, the preparation to be tested does not comply with the specification sterile or culture negative, unless it can be proven that microbial growth is not related to the preparation to be tested. As for invalidation of any OOS result, also in case of false positive sterility tests, it has to be clearly demonstrated why the positive result is invalid. Ph. Eur. Monograph 2.6.1 lists the following four possible conditions for false positive results of which one or more have to be fulfilled for invalidation of the positive result:

1. The data of the microbiological monitoring of the sterility testing facility show a fault.
2. A review of the testing procedure used during the test in question reveals a fault.
3. Microbial growth is found in the negative controls.
4. After determination of the identity of the micro-organisms isolated from the test, the growth of this/these species may be ascribed unequivocally to faults with respect to the material and/or technique used in conducting the sterility test procedure.

If the test is declared to be invalid, it has to be repeated with the same number of units as in the original test. If no evidence of microbial growth is found in the repeat test the product examined complies with the test for sterility. For CTMPs, this approach in most cases will not be feasible as repetition of the test depends on sufficient test material that is scarce for finished product as well as for in-process controls.

Micro-organisms recovered from a sterility test have to be identified with either microbiological/biochemical techniques or more sensitive typing techniques (e.g., molecular typing with RNA/DNA homology), if the results are necessary to demonstrate false positive results (compare Ph. Eur. 2.6.1). Conventional medicinal products may not be released before completion of sterility testing. Therefore, identifying the micro-organisms found in a sterility test is solely important for root cause analysis. In contrast to that (as mentioned above) cellular products are sometimes administered to the patient before sterility testing of the finished product is completed. Hence identification of the detected contaminants to a suitable taxonomic level (Ph. Eur. 2.6.27) together with an antibiogram has to be established to gather valuable data for the medical treatment of the patient.

Validation Strategies

Validation of sterility testing or microbiological control can involve three individual validation procedures:

1. Validation of the culture medium (growth promotion test) if it differs from the formula prescribed by the relevant Pharmacopoeia. In these cases, defined strains of micro-organisms in defined quantities and under defined culture conditions have to be added to aliquots of the culture medium and evidence of microbial growth has to be detected in all preparations. The pharmacopoeias in most cases prescribe how many different strains of micro-organisms have to be used and in which quantity (number of CFU) they have to be added. Sometimes authorities provide information about pre-validated media as the German Paul-Ehrlich-Institut (PEI) does, for example, for blood culture media (compare institute webpage: www.pei.de).

2. Complete validation of the analytical procedure, whenever different methods are used than those prescribed by the relevant Pharmacopoeia. In these cases the methods have to be fully validated as described in ICH Q2 (R1) Validation of Analytical Procedures (compare Section 6.11).

3. Validation of the method in presence of the sample matrix used (so called matrix validation) to prove that the matrix itself has no negative influence on microbial growth. To prove this, a small number of different strains of micro-organisms (preferably 10–100 CFU) have to be spiked to the sterility test in presence of the preparation to be tested. Evidence of microbial growth has to be detected in all preparations. Problematic in this respect can be the presence of serum in the

formulation to be tested as serum is known to have bacteriostatic properties. Even more problematic is the presence of antibiotics (for example, in cell culture media that are used for microbiological in-process controls). Sensitive microbial strains will not grow in presence of antibiotics, at least if direct inoculation methods are used. Annex 2 of the EU GMP Guidelines requests that sterility tests should be conducted on antibiotic-free cultures of cells or cell banks to provide evidence for absence of bacterial and fungal contamination and consider the detection of fastidious organisms. Most authorities do not allow the use of antibiotics in cell culture media for their known potential to mask microbial contaminations.

Membrane Filtration

For membrane filtration methods, the preparation to be tested is filtered over a membrane with a nominal pore size not greater than 0.45 μm with sufficient effectiveness to retain micro-organisms. After this first filtration step, the membrane can be rinsed several times, e.g., to wash away antibiotics or other agents that might compromise bacterial growth. After that the membrane is either transferred to or covered with suitable growth media (at least one for aerobic and one for anaerobic culture conditions) and incubated at 30–35°C and/or 20–25°C for 14 days. The incubated membranes are checked daily and at the end of the incubation period for turbidity of the culture medium that indicates microbial growth. For further details, compare the relevant pharmacopoeial monographs (e.g., Ph. Eur. Chapter 2.6.1)

Several companies offer complete filtration devices including the necessary pump as well as closed filtration chambers with filters, filling lines, needles, all kinds of adapters, and even growth media and rinse fluids — everything being compliant with the relevant pharmacopoeial chapters. All parts of the device directly in contact with the preparation to be tested or with rinse fluids and growth media are sterile and for single use. The risk of false positive results is therefore significantly reduced. Most of these devices already include two individual filtration chambers, one for anaerobic and one for aerobic culture conditions. The membranes are covered with the growth media directly in the filtration chambers, hence the membranes do not have to be touched or otherwise handled manually. Some of the companies sell qualification packages of the equipment [Instrument Qualification (IQ) and Operational Qualification (OQ)] and even offer support with Performance Qualification (PQ) or matrix validation. See Table 6.11 for Pros and Cons of the method.

Direct Inoculation of the Culture Medium

Direct inoculation of the culture medium is a method applied for conventional sterility testing as defined by Ph. Eur. Chapter 2.6.1 as well as for microbiological control

Table 6.11:   Pros and cons of the membrane filtration method for microbiological control.

Membrane Filtration — Pros	Membrane Filtration — Cons
• Method works even in presence of antibiotics or other substances with bacteriostatic or fungistatic properties as membranes can be washed several times prior to incubation with the growth medium. That makes the use of antibiotics in cell culture media possible even if the supernatant has to be used for microbial in-process controls. • Commercially available sterile single use filtration chambers that reduce the risk of false positive results are commercially available. • High sample volumes can be examined (e.g., total volume of cell culture supernatant) leading to reliable and significant results.	• Relatively high sample volume is needed; at least if commercially available single use filtration chambers are used. Therefore, the method is hardly suitable for finished products with low overall volume. • Cells present in the test sample can clog the filter. • No automated culture and read out system compared to fully automated blood culture systems. Filtration chambers have to be checked for microbial growth by personnel regularly and turbidity as read out parameter is sometimes difficult and error-prone. • Method is more laborious than direct inoculation to blood culture test bottles with automated culture systems.

of cellular products as defined by Ph. Eur. Chapter 5.6.27. In the conventional setting the samples to be tested are inoculated into containers of culture medium, the containers are incubated at suitable temperatures and subsequently examined visually for macroscopic evidence of microbial growth (turbidity) at intervals during the incubation period and at its end (day 14). The compendial text on microbiological control of cellular products, besides the conventional culture method over 14 days and visual read out of turbidity of the culture medium, alternatively allows the use of automated culture systems with continuous agitation and permanent monitoring of the containers (blood culture bottles), thus reducing the required incubation time down to seven days. The read-out parameter in these automated systems is the production of carbon dioxide by micro–organisms when metabolizing nutrients of the culture medium. Carbon dioxide reacts with a dye present in the blood culture bottle leading to a change of fluorescence emission that is analyzed by a fluorescence detector. Due to this fluorescence-based detection system, turbidity of the samples to be tested (a common problem with cellular products) is no longer obstructive.

As automated systems are predominantly analyzing the increase in carbon dioxide emission rather than distinct levels, it is important that blood culture bottles that are inoculated with the test sample are loaded up into the blood culture instrument as soon as possible after inoculation in order not to miss the increase in carbon

Table 6.12:   Pros and cons of the direct inoculation method for microbiological control.

Direct Inoculation — Pros	Direct Inoculation — Cons
• Relatively low sample volumes are needed for this method (down to 1 mL or less for finished products with very low overall volume). • Fully automated culture and read out when automated blood culture systems are used. Test bottles are checked continuously during incubation time and positive results are reported immediately. • Inoculation of samples to blood culture test bottles is quick and easy and therefore reduces the risk of contamination and false positive results.	• Method does not work in presence of antibiotics or other substances with bacteriostatic or fungistatic properties. Even the presence of serum can interfere with microbial growth in the test bottles. • Only small overall sample volumes can be examined if blood culture bottles are used (maximum filling volume of blood culture bottles <10 mL). Therefore, testing of high volumes (e.g., cell culture supernatants) is not feasible with this method. • Equipment (automated blood culture system) is expensive.

dioxide emission, leading to a false negative result.[50] Whenever there is a known delay between inoculation and loading (e.g., because inoculated blood culture bottles have to be sent to a contract laboratory), maximum time periods have to be defined and validated. See Table 6.12 for the Pros and Cons of the method.

Another issue to consider for cell-based products is the fact that samples should be added to the culture medium as soon as possible after collection as certain types of cells (for example, neutrophils) are capable of phagocytosis of microorganisms. If samples cannot be added promptly after collection, they have to be stored at $5 \perp 3^\circ$C to avoid phagocytosis.

Rapid Microbiological Methods (RMMs)

The introduction of RMMs for in-process controls and release testing of CBMPs is intensively discussed since many years, as established compendial methods require at least seven days and cannot be completed before release of products with short shelf life. Some authorities (e.g., the US FDA) accept a Gram stain as rapid method for the release of cellular products with short shelf life but with a detection limit of around 10^5 CFU/mL (that is considerably higher than that of all compendial as well as alternative methods) only gross contamination can be detected.[51]

Both, the European and the US Pharmacopoeia acknowledge the necessity for alternative microbiological methods and therefore introduced Chapter 5.1.6 "Alternative methods for control of microbiological quality" to the European

Pharmacopoeia and Chapter <1223> "Validation of Alternative Microbiological Methods" to the US Pharmacopoeia. In addition, the US FDA published the Guidance for Industry on "Validation of Growth-Based Rapid Microbiological Methods for Sterility Testing of Cellular and Gene Therapy Products".[52]

In addition to official guidance documents, the Parenteral Drug Association (PDA) published in 2013, the revised PDA Technical Report No. 33 "Evaluation, Validation, and Implementation of Alternative and Rapid Microbiological Methods".[53] The document is intended to provide guidance for the successful evaluation, validation, and implementation of alternative and RRMs needed by the pharmaceutical, biotechnology, and medical device industries to assure product quality. The document is thought to help establish industry-wide criteria on what constitutes an acceptable alternative or rapid microbiology test to the compendial or classical method and advises how to prove it to the satisfaction of quality organizations and regulatory agencies.

However, RMMs are not widely used despite their potential advantages and the authorities supporting attitude. Table 6.13 summarized advantages of RMMs as well as possible obstacles for their implementation.

Table 6.13: RMMs: advances and potential barriers to change.

RMMs — Pros	RMMs — Potential Barriers to Change
• Rapid: Real-time analysis and time sensitive-outputs. • Reduction of product release cycle time. • Potential for automation and high throughput. • Small sample volumes. • Facilitating investigations by generating earlier results. • Improvement of manufacturing consistency by allowing faster implementation of corrective actions and fostering opportunities to improve the safety of the process. • Assessment of viable but non-culturable microorganisms.	• Regulatory agencies might request using the official compendial and the alternate method run in parallel. • Cost of validation (labor and/or money) may be too high and/or the return on investment (ROI) too low. • Limited support by management as the methods submitted and approved continue to work → no incentive to implement new assays. • Lack of microbiological expertise prevents development and execution of appropriate comparability protocols to establish equivalency to RMM with the official method. • Some methods show low sensitivity due to background signals.

The table opposes advances of RMMs and potential barriers for their implementation in pharmaceutical industry. Adopted after John Duguid *et al.*, Rapid Microbiological Methods: Where Are They Now?[54] and Störmer, M., *et al.*, Bacterial safety of cell-based therapeutic preparations, focusing on HPCs.[49]

The European Pharmacopoeia introduces several RMMs in Chapter 5.1.6 that can be classified in three different groups dependent on their basic principle of detection: (1) Growth-based methods, where a detectable signal is achieved by a period of subculture and growth, (2) Methods with direct measurement where individual cells are differentiated and visualized, and (3) Methods that measure the expression of specific cell components. Examples for growth-based methods are electrochemical methods, measurement of the consumption or production of gas, Bioluminescence, and Microcalorimetry. Examples for direct measurement are differentiation and visualization of individual cells, Solid Phase Cytometry, Flow Cytometry, and Direct Epifluorescent Filtration Technique (DEFT). Finally, examples for cell component analysis are immunological methods, Mass Spectrometry, Biochemical Assays based on physiological reactions, and NATs.

Apart from their basic principle of detection, different RMMs can be further divided in methods that are applied qualitatively (microorganisms present — yes/no), quantitatively (determination of the number of microorganisms present) and for identification purposes (for root cause analysis and for gathering information for patient treatment, in case the medicinal product has already been released and administered at the time of the positive test result). In order to replace one of the compendial methods for sterility testing or microbiological control, the RMM would have to be a qualitative method that detects the presence or absence of microorganisms. As for any analytical method that should be used instead of a compendial method, also RMMs need intensive validation in order to demonstrate that the alternative method yields equivalent or even better results. For validation of a qualitative RMM, Ph. Eur. Chapter 5.1.6 prescribes to address the validation parameters–accuracy, precision, specificity, limit of detection, and robustness and provides details for every required validation parameter.

When implementing RMM, the first and most crucial question is of course which method is the most suitable one for the specific CTP to be tested? Additionally, it is important to decide whether growth-based methods are used, that normally are more time-consuming, whether a method with direct measurement is used, that needs to be very sensitive with a low detection limit, or whether direct measurements are combined with short periods of pre-cultivation (e.g., in or on a pharmacopoeial liquid or solid culture medium).

The German PEI, Federal Institute for Vaccines and Biomedicines, and the US FDA both published their experiences with different RMMs (most of them developed for the transfusion setting and therefore not directly applicable to CBMPs) presenting advantages, disadvantages, and problems that have to be resolved in the future.[48, 55–57]

Störmer *et al.*[49] provide (among other approaches) a good summary of methods that were evaluated by the PEI for blood products and have the potential for further development and use for CBMPs. Presented are:

- Universal bacterial real–time PCR: This method uses the detection of highly conserved sequences of ribosomal nucleic acids by real–time PCR, offering a universal, rapid, and sensitive tool for detection. The method was evaluated in combination with a short pre-cultivation step of several hours, leading to a detection limit of <1 CFU/ml.

- Flow Cytometry using the BactiFlow cytometer (bioMérieux AES Chemunex GmbH, France): The method is based on the passage of non–fluorescent fluorogenes through the cell membrane of viable cells, followed by cleavage of the fluorogenes by intracellular esterases to produce fluorescence. Mammalian cells have to be enzymatically digested before application of the fluorogenes. Both bacteria and fungi can be detected with this system and the method can be used with or without pre-cultivation step. The sensitivity of the method without pre-cultivation of the test sample is 150 CFU/ml, with pre-cultivation it can be reduced to a sensitivity of theoretically 1 CFU/ml.

- Detection of microcolonies using the Milliflex Rapid (MR) and the Milliflex Quantum (MQ) (both Millipore S.A.S., France): These methods are based on membrane filtration, visualization and enumeration of microcolonies after a short incubation period with a theoretical sensitivity of 1 CFU/ml (practically 2–3 CFU/ml). Microcolonies are either visualized *via* ATP bioluminescence (using MR) or fluorescence technology (using MQ). The time for first detection of microcolonies in the PEI study was between four and 13 hours, depending on the system and the bacterial strain. The fluorescence technology (using MQ) allows repeated incubation up to the appearance of macroscopic visible colonies. Both methods also allow the identification of the contaminants using any differentiation method afterwards.

In addition to the presented methods, there are of course numerous other approaches that might be equally suitable and that can be adopted and validated for a variety of different cellular products.

To conclude about the future acceptance and significance of RMMs for CBMPs is difficult as they are hitherto not widely–used, despite their clear advantages for products with a short shelf life. Most of the obstacles for their implementation listed in Table 6.13 are associated with an initial increase in costs and labor, thus distracting manufacturers as long as the conventional methods are still accepted. Commercially available and pre-certified test kits might change this situation in the future. Apart from that the implication on product quality has not yet been shown and it remains to be demonstrated, if RMMs significantly improve biological safety of the CBMPs.

6.6.9.2 Pyrogens

Pyrogens (Greek: *Pyros* = fire) are substances that induce fever after parenteral administration. Lipopolysaccharide (LPS), a component of the cell membrane of Gram-negative bacteria, is one of the best-known pyrogens (belonging to the group of endotoxins, see 6.6.9.3) that elicit strong immune responses in animals and humans by activating the innate immune system, leading to the production of prostaglandins and pro-inflammatory cytokines and the generation of fever. Apart from Gram-positive and Gram-negative bacteria, pyrogens also originate from other biological sources as viruses and fungi as well as from chemical substances such as elastomers and rubber abrasion. The strength of the immune response is dependent on the individual pyrogen, its dose and the individual sensitivity of the challenged organism and can be as strong as septic shock and multi organ failure. Therefore, pyrogen testing is mandatory for all medicinal products that are administered parenterally or intrathecally.

The standard test procedure for analysis of pyrogens in both the European and the US Pharmacopoeia is fever reaction in mammal (rabbit) upon administration of the product that has to be tested (compare Ph. Eur. Chapter 2.6.8. "Pyrogens"[58] and USP Chapter <151> "Pyrogen Test")[59] The rabbit pyrogen test consists of measuring the rise in body temperature evoked by the intravenous injection of a sterile solution of the substance to be examined. This test method is widely used since many years in pharmaceutical industry and is thought to provide reliable and sensitive results, not only for endotoxins, that are known to be the strongest pyrogens, but also for various non-endotoxin pyrogens, thus providing significant advantages over the test for bacterial endotoxins (compare Section 6.6.9.3). But while the rabbit pyrogen test is widespread for conventional medicinal products, its application for CBMPs is limited as the human cells per se would stimulate the rabbits' immune system, leading to false positive results. On the other hand, some non-endotoxin pyrogens are species-specific causing false negative results as the rabbits' immune system would not react where administration of the product to humans would trigger an adverse reaction.[51] European authorities as well as the US FDA therefore accept the use of a LAL test for endotoxins *in lieu* of the rabbit pyrogens test in certain cases.[60]

Apart from the suitability or non-suitability of the rabbit pyrogen test for specific medicinal products, animal experiments are generally highly controversial since many years and there is a strong movement toward animal protection and replacement of those experiments with *in vitro* tests, wherever possible. This endeavor is not only subsidized by animal rights activists, but meanwhile also by the legislative bodies. The European Commission, to mention one example, published Directive 2010/63/EC on the protection of animals used for scientific purposes. The Directive designates the full replacement of procedures on live animals for scientific and educational purposes as the final goal that has to be achieved as soon as it is scientifically possible to do so. To achieve this goal, the European Commission created the European Centre for the Validation of Alternative Methods (ECVAM) to validate and support the acceptance of methods to replace, reduce or refine the use of laboratory animals, and to promote their scientific and regulatory acceptance.

To eventually replace the rabbit pyrogen test, efforts were made by ECVAM and other institutions such as the German PEI, Federal Institute for Vaccines and Biomedicines, to develop an equally suitable *in vitro* test system.[61–63] Finally, in 2010, the EDQM introduced the MAT to the European Pharmacopoeia (Ph. Eur. Chapter 2.6.30)[64] as suitable assay to replace the rabbit pyrogen test after product-specific validation. Although the MAT has not been introduced to the USP yet, the US FDA indicated in a guidance document concerning the use of pyrogen and endotoxins testing that alternative pyrogen tests such as the MAT may be substituted for the rabbit pyrogen test as long as equivalent pyrogen detection can be demonstrated.[60]

The MAT is based on the fact that monocytes are activated by pyrogens to produce a variety of pro-inflammatory cytokines such as interleukins IL-1β, IL-6 and tumor necrosis factor (TNF) that can be detected in an immunological assay (ELISA). As monocytes are able to react to a variety of different molecular structures, the MAT covers endotoxins as well as non-endotoxin pyrogens, although it has to be stated that the detection of non-endotoxin pyrogens remains a challenging issue for validation of the assay, as so far no standardized high-quality non-endotoxin pyrogens are available as internationally accepted reference standards.

The crucial components of the MAT are the monocytes that are used for incubation with the product to be tested. To achieve a reliable outcome, the monocytic cells must not be activated prior to use in the test system as this would lead to false positive results. A negative control is therefore important to exclude such cases. On the other hand, it is known that some cell donations are non-responding leading to false negative results. Use of a positive control such as LPS is therefore mandatory to demonstrate that the cells are potent to react in case a pyrogen is present in the sample to be tested. Source and qualification of the donors as well as the cells is therefore a key-issue of the compendial text. Possible cell sources are either whole blood or peripheral blood mononuclear cells (PBMCs) obtained from single or pooled blood donations. Alternatively, continuous monocytic human cell lines can be used. Donors must declare that they do not suffer from bacterial or viral infections and that they did not show any symptoms of such an infection seven days prior to donation. Furthermore, donors must not take non-steroidal anti-inflammatory drugs (NSAIDs) 48 hours prior to donation and steroidal anti-inflammatory drugs seven days prior to donation (for more details, see compendial text).[64] If cell pools are used they should consist of at least four independent donors, preferable are eight or even more. Cell pools have to be qualified prior to use with endotoxin standard.

As the availability of freshly prepared and qualified cells at the time of testing is highly elaborate, cryopreservation is an option offered by the European Pharmacopoeia as long as it can be demonstrated that the cryopreservation procedure and the cryoprotectant do not interfere with the test. If cryopreserved cells are used, the process of cryopreservation should be validated and the suitability of the thawed cells should be sufficiently demonstrated. Spreitzer et al.[61] and Koryakina et al.[65] present their validation work for the establishment of cryopreserved cells originating from whole blood and PBMCs, respectively. Meanwhile, commercially available test kits that use cryopreserved cells are offered by different providers.

Apart from qualification of donors and cells, it is essential to demonstrate that the product to be tested does not interfere with the monocytes (either through direct, pyrogen-independent stimulation of the cells leading to false positive results or by inhibition of the monocytic cell function leading to false negative results). Therefore, a matrix validation is obligatory for every product, even if the method itself is already validated. For CBMPs, it might not be unlikely that either the cells or raw materials and excipients such as cytokines that are (still) present in the product are potent stimulators of the monocytes. In these cases, the MAT is no option for pyrogen testing of the CBMP and it has to be discussed with the authorities, if a test on bacterial endotoxins is sufficient.

6.6.9.3 Bacterial endotoxins

Endotoxins are an integral part of the outer membrane of Gram-negative bacteria consisting of LPS. They are known to be toxic and elicit strong immune responses when administered to humans or animals. As endotoxins belong to the most common pyrogens and are biologically active already in low amounts, all medicinal products for parenteral applications have to be analyzed for their endotoxin content. Endotoxins are small enough to pass through a 0.2 μm filter and are resistant to common autoclaving and dry heat sterilization processes, therefore they are very difficult to remove from a product once it has been contaminated.

The general pharmacopoeial chapters for the bacterial endotoxins test are currently being harmonized between Europe (Ph. Eur. Chapter 2.6.14 "Bacterial Endotoxins"),[66] USA (USP <85> "Bacterial Endotoxins Test")[67] and Japan (JP 4.01 "Bacterial Endotoxins Test"). The ICH guideline Q4B "Annex 14 to note for evaluation and recommendation of pharmacopoeial texts for use in the ICH regions on bacterial endotoxins tests- general chapter" is in the final stage of implementation and considers the interchangeability of the three chapters, under conditions that: (1) All three described methods can be used for the test (in the case of doubt, the gel–clot test should be used), (2) The reference standards are interchangeable as they have been calibrated against the WHO International Standard for Endotoxin, and (3) the test approach described in Q4B section "Photometric quantitative techniques, Preparatory testing, Test for interfering factors" must be followed (for details, see ICH Q4B).

Since endotoxins represent the most frequent and hazardous pyrogens, and the sensitivity of the endotoxin test is higher than that of the rabbit pyrogen test, the endotoxin test is very often preferred for product release testing.

The assay utilizes the ancient ability of the horseshoe crab to respond to bacterial infection by hemolymph clotting. The clotting reaction is initiated by binding of LPS to Factor C present in amebocytes (white blood cells) of the horseshoe crab and has a protective function, as it leads to agglutination of pathogens making them available to antibacterial factors. In the endotoxin test, the amebocyte lysate from the horseshoe crab (*Limulus polyphemus* or *Tachypleus tridentatus*) is mixed with the substance to be tested and analyzed for the formation of clotting reaction visually or photometrically.

The pharmacopoeial chapters describe three different techniques for the LAL test. The gel–clot technique is based on the analysis of the gel formation and still serves as a gold standard when photometric techniques produce ambiguous results. The turbidimetric technique is based on the measurement of cloudiness as a result of cleavage of endogenous substrate. The chromogenic technique utilizes a synthetic peptide–chromogen complex for detection of color development after substrate cleavage.

The endotoxin amount is expressed in international units (IU). The endotoxin reference standards used in each test are calibrated against an International Standard stated by the WHO so that the equivalence in IU can be established. One IU of endotoxin is equal to one Endotoxin Unit (E.U.). The acceptable endotoxin limit depends on the route of administration, the overall volume and concentration of the medicinal product and the duration of administration. For intravenous and intrathecal administration routes, the endotoxin limits are defined in the respective pharmacopoeial chapters (5 IU per kg body weight per hour for intravenous administration, 2.5 IU per kg body weight per hour for intravenous radiopharma-ceuticals, and 0.2 IU per kg body weight per hour for intrathecal administration). In other cases, the acceptable limits have to be established during product development.

Since the test is aimed to detect minimal amounts of endotoxins, the use of depyrogenized glassware, pyrogen-free solutions and materials is strictly required. The product-specific validation has to be performed on each new product to verify the performance and reproducibility of the chosen test method. Special attention has to be paid to the endotoxin recovery and problematic endotoxin masking. The method is susceptible to a number of factors, such as presence of different salts, acids, and alcohols in the matrix; inhibition *via* citrate, Heparin, and EDTA; and false signal increase induced *via* Trypsin and β-glucans. Many further examples can be named. Training of personnel and verification of the training effectiveness have to be performed periodically to assure the method performance.

It might be advisable to authorize a specialized contract laboratory that routinely conducts Bacterial Endotoxins tests using the LAL technique, at least if not many batches have to be tested per year as this is in most cases time- and cost-saving. As for any other outsourced activity with potential influence on product quality or validity of analytical results, there should be a written contract between the manufacturer of the product to be tested (Contract Giver) and the contract lab (Contract Acceptor) which clearly establishes the duties of each party (compare EU GMP Guidelines, Chapter 7 "Outsourced Activities").[68]

6.6.9.4 *Mycoplasma*

Mycoplasma infection of cell cultures is a well-known problem in many cell culture labs with infection rates varying between 15% and 80 % depending on cell type, cell source, and culture methods.[69] Mycoplasma are originating either from the donor of the cells or from personnel responsible for the culture process. Unlike other bacteria or fungi, contamination with mycoplasma is not always easily detectable in the cell culture by turbidity of the cell culture medium or by change of medium color. Special culturing methods or analysis of mycoplasma DNA is often necessary for their detection.

Mycoplasma contamination of CBMPs is critical for two reasons: 1. Mycoplasma would be administered directly to the patient together with the contaminated cell product and thus exert negative reactions and adverse events directly, and 2. Mycoplasma can alter the characteristics of contaminated cells significantly and thus negatively influence both efficacy and safety of the CBMP indirectly. There-fore, mycoplasma testing of cultured cells used as CBMPs is required by almost all regulatory authorities worldwide.

Guidance for the analysis of mycoplasmas is provided, for instance, by the European Pharmacopoeia (Ph. Eur. Chapter 2.6.7 "Mycoplasma"),[70] by the US Pharmacopoeia (USP chapter <63> "Mycoplasma Test")[71] and by the US FDA ("Guidance for Industry: Characterization and Qualification of Cell Substrates and Other Biological Materials Used in the Production of Viral Vaccines for Infectious Disease Indications),"[72] and 21 CFR 610.30 "Test for Mycoplasma".[73]

The conventional assays for detection of mycoplasma recommended by the European, Japanese, and US pharmacopoeia are direct and indirect culture methods. With the direct method, mycoplasmas are cultured in broth with subsequent subculture on agar plates or on agar plates directly. Where the test for mycoplasmas is prescribed for a virus harvest, for a bulk vaccine or for the final batch, the direct culture method has to be used. With the indirect culture method, mycoplasmas are cultured in indicator cells with subsequent subculture on cover or chamber slides, fluorescence staining of mycoplasma DNA, and microscopic analysis of typical mycoplasma fluorescence patterns (extranuclear fluorescence spots or filaments). Where the test for mycoplasmas is prescribed for a MCB, for a WCB, for a virus seed lot or for control cells, both the direct culture method and the indirect indicator cell culture method can be used. The indicator cell culture method may also be used for screening of media.

Nimset, R.W., *et al.*[74] compared the culture methods defined by the European and the US Pharmacopoeia and explained the slight methodological differences between both approaches. Independent of these small differences, culture assays provided by diverse Pharmacopoeia are considered to be reliable and safe on one hand but time consuming on the other hand as culture and subculture is required for at least six days (culture in indicator cell lines) or even 28 days (culture in broth or on agar plates). Hence, these assays are not suitable as in-process controls, as they do not allow exerting influence on the culture process in due time and they are also not suitable as release tests for cellular products with short shelf life. The European Pharmacopoeia therefore introduced NAT-based method for detection of mycoplasma DNA to Chapter 2.6.7. With this method, test results are available within a few hours, thus NAT-based methods can be used as in-process controls that permit immediate decisions, and as release test for finished products with short shelf life. A prerequisite for the use of these NAT-based methods is validation of the analytical procedure following the specifications prescribed by the European Pharmacopoeia. Real-time PCR based test kits with certified conformance to the European Pharmacopoeia are meanwhile commercially available, significantly reducing validation efforts. One big disadvantage of NAT-based methods of course is that they cannot discriminate between viable and non-viable mycoplasma (deriving, for example, from inactivated raw materials as Fetal Bovine Serum) potentially leading to false positive results. In case mycoplasma detection of cellular products is NAT-based, it is therefore advisable to use critical raw materials with respect to a potential contamination with mycoplasma DNA, only if they are tested either by the supplier (confirmed in a CoA) or by in-house release testing prior to use. Volokhov *et al.* provided an overview of non-microbiological techniques for Mycoplasma testing and discussed the pros and cons of their application for the testing of mycoplasmas in biologics and cell substrates.[75]

As clean room personnel is a possible source of mycoplasma (e.g., through *Mycoplasma pneumoniae*), hence initial and periodic health checks on clean room personnel are mandatory together with commitment of personnel to report any health condition that could adversely affect the microbial quality of the products produced.

In addition to these health checks there should be written procedures in place that define actions to be taken after positive results of mycoplasma testing. This should include corrective action/preventive action (CAPA) for every positive microbiological result. Root cause analysis is mandatory in this respect. Furthermore, there should be a validated cleaning procedure established for decontamination of clean rooms and laminar air flow work-benches.

6.6.10 *Certificate of Analysis (CoA)*

For every batch of a finished medicinal product, the manufacturer has to provide a CoA that lists all test results of qualitative and quantitative analysis obtained for the finished product together with the corresponding acceptance criteria and reference to the test methods used. In addition, a clear statement is mandatory on whether the batch complies with the requirements defined in either the MA or the CTA [product specification file (PSF)].

The EU GMP Guidelines define CoAs as follows: *CoAs provide a summary of testing results on samples of products or materials together with the evaluation for compliance to a stated specification.*[45]

WHO provides a model CoA in its Technical Report Series No. 902 for use by manufacturers of pharmaceutical substances, excipients, and medicinal products.[76]

For a CTMP, a CoA can look like the example provided in Table 6.14.

6.7 Genetic Stability and Tumorigenicity

The analysis of genetic stability and potential tumorigenicity belongs to specific requirements for CBMPs (Commission Directive 2003/63/EC). It reflects the need to assure product's identity and integrity *via* analysis of its genome, which might

Table 6.14:   Template CoA for a CBMP.

Letter Head of Manufacturer
Certificate of Analysis

Name of product	Cell product XY
Marketing Authorization number/ Clinical Trial Authorization number	123456
Strength/potency	X, X x 10^X CDY^+/CDZ^+ cells per transfusion bag
Dosage form	Suspension for intravenous application
Package size and type	XXX mL per transfusion bag
Batch number	789XYZ
Date of manufacture	dd/mm/yyyy
Expiry date	dd/mm/yyyy (additionally hh: mm if applicable)
Results of analysis	

Type of Test	Test Procedure	Result	Acceptance Criterion	Compliance with Acceptance Criterion
Appearance				yes/no
Identity				yes/no
Purity				yes/no
Impurities				yes/no
Dosage content				yes/no
Concentration				yes/no
Overall cell content				yes/no
Cell dose				yes/no
Viability				yes/no
Potency				yes/no
Microbiological control				yes/no
Mycoplasma				yes/no
Bacterial endotoxin				yes/no
Name and title of authorized person	Head of QC			
Date of signature and signature of authorized person	dd/mm/yyyy*<signature>*			

Note: Listed types of tests are meant to be examples only. Not all of them might be relevant for all cellular products and additional types of tests might be required for specific cell types.

be unwillingly compromised by manipulation steps during manufacturing, such as *in vitro* cultivation or treatment with potentially mitogenic agents. Since genetic instability is often associated with and brings the danger of pro–cancerogenic changes, the elucidation of this phenomenon is an essential component in assuring the patient safety. As such, the genetic integrity of manufactured cells can be regarded as a constituent of biological stability, identity and purity of the cell-based therapeutic product. Whether the analysis of genetic stability should be introduced as release QC, in-process control or is sufficiently and satisfactorily elucidated during the product development, depends on the particular manufacturing process and characteristics of cells used, so that no universal recipe can be given to that. The following groups of products and cell-based intermediates have to be analyzed:

- *Somatic cells* that are cultivated *in vitro* or otherwise substantially manipulated *ex vivo*.
- All *MCBs/WCBs* used in manufacturing.
- *GM cells*: As the genome of the cells is modified by the introduced vector, genetic safety of the resulting product should be verified. In addition to general vector safety controls, such as control of vector copy number and RCR (where applicable), potential tumorigenicity of the GM cells should be examined.

6.7.1 *Overview and methodologies*

6.7.1.1 *Karyotyping/FISH*

The classical cytogenetic method often used is karyotyping. This technique allows for the chromosomal analysis of the whole metaphases by G-banding (Giemsa-staining) with resolution of about 5–10 Mb.[77] A modification of the method, spectral karyotyping (SKY) increases the resolution to about 1–2 Mb.[78] The molecular events below this threshold as well as loss of heterogenicity (LOH) rearrangements remain undetected. As a rule, 20 to maximum 50 metaphases are analyzed. The suggested acceptable limit for the test to pass is less than two identical rearrangements on 20 metaphases analyzed.[79] Since observed aberrations can be attributed to a single cell, the frequency of conspicuous cells in the sample can be quantified and the sensitivity of the sample analysis is rather high, which makes karyotyping an attractive method. However, the low quantity of analyzed cells in regard to the end product size (20–50 cells in the QC sample *vs.* millions of cells in the end product) does not provide a representative sample for the analysis of the cell population as whole, so that rare but meaningful aberrations may escape. Furthermore, for the visualization of chromosomal pattern by Giemsa-staining, metaphases have to be obtained, which requires an additional cultivation step prior to analysis, so that artefacts different from the original culture may arise. Alternatively, a parallel culture, equal to the original product in respect to cultivation conditions and the number of cell divisions can be used for karyotype analysis. Still, it has to be taken into account that the genetic status of the assay culture may eventually differ from that of the original cell population due to late mutational events. To exclude cultural artefacts and to confirm the persistence of the karyotype aberration in the analyzed cell population, fluorescent *in situ* hybridization (FISH) with probes specific for the altered area is often applied as a complementary method. Karyotyping is currently considered by many to be a method of choice for an initial chromosomal analysis.

6.7.1.2 *Molecular-based techniques*

An array-comparative genomic hybridization (aCGH) is a method based on hybridizing the control and sample DNA with different fluorophores and measuring the resulting fluorescent signals' intensity. This method dramatically increases the resolution of mutational analysis (down to 100 kb), but fails to recognize balanced translocations and inversions, LOH or loss and acquisition of an additional chromosomal set (polymorphy). The single nucleotide polymorphism (SNP) array based on the DNA labeling with allele-specific probes possesses a couple of advantages over the aCGH, keeping a high method resolution (down to 50 nucleotides) dependent on the number of probes used.[80] However, this method is also not able to detect balanced chromosomal aberrations. Moreover, since the analysis is performed on the DNA sample of pooled cells, the sensitivity of both methods is rather low and recognizes only chromosomal aberrations well established in the population (20%). Molecular based methods surely provide important supportive information for genetic characterization of the cell product. Yet, if we strive for making cellular products financially available for all patient groups, wide genomic analysis is not applicable as a routine release test nowadays, because of its high costs.

The common hurdle in the analysis of genetic integrity by both karyotyping and DNA-based techniques is, however, the data interpretation. While some chromosomal aberrations are well known in medical genetics and described in the scientific literature, the majority of collected data still cannot be linked to functional effects. The significance of detected aberrations often cannot be properly estimated. Furthermore, transient artefacts without selective advantage cannot be distinguished from mutations that will prevail in the genome. Our knowledge about the cancer mutations and pathway activation is rapidly growing but the analysis of the bulk data still remains challenging. One of the attempts to systematically couple the observed DNA aberrations with functional changes is the profiling of genetic instability *via* the analysis of the RNA expression proposed by Ben-David and Benvenisty.[81] This method is based on bioinformatical analyses of correlation between copy number and gene expression levels. Beside the prospective sample analysis, the methodology allows for retrospective evaluation of cell lines from available gene expression databases. However, low sensitivity (1/3–1/2 of cells should carry aberrations to be detected) and strong dependency on the number of expressed genes in particular cell type under particular conditions make the methodology barely acceptable as a routine QC.

6.7.1.3 *Telomere length and telomerase activity*

More straightforward in respect to data evaluation is the analysis of cell properties associated with the escape from senescence and tumor formation. The control of telomere length and telomerase activity is often applied to ensure that cell population does not exhibit uncontrolled growth. In contrast to pluripotent stem cells (PSCs) that remain immortal, normal somatic cells as well as adult stem cells undergo telomere shortening during their lifespan, which eventually leads to senescence.[82–85] The restoration of the telomere length after each division in embryonic and many tumor cells is due to the activity of the enzyme human telomerase reverse transcriptase (hTERT), which is detected in these cells at high levels. Multipotent stem cells, except MSCs, also exert a certain hTERT activity, which is just enough to keep their high proliferative potential, but not to prevent the gradual telomere erosion. MSCs of different origin appear to lack detectable telomerase complex. However, some authors argue that its absence in MSC has to be explained by the heterogeneity of analyzed populations, and a minor fraction of truly multipotent and highly proliferative MSC normally possess an active hTERT, which cannot be detected at the current state of technology.[82] In agreement, the telomerase activity of the MultiStem® (Athersys, Inc.) product based on propagated multipotent adult progenitor cells (MAPS) is considerably higher than that of MSC preparations.[86]

The maintained telomerase activity and the arrest of telomere erosion are detected in about 90% of tumor cells and is a mechanism by which cells escape senescence and remain immortal.[87] This makes the analysis of telomerase activity a promising marker for the control of cell-based products. The market offers a variety of assays, which are mostly based on different modifications of the traditional PCR-based telomerase repeat amplification protocol (TRAP) that analyzes the amplification of the telomerase-specific TAGGG-repeat. It is advisable to support the control of the hTERT activity with the direct analysis of the telomere length, i.e., by labeling chromosomal DNA with TAGGG-specific probes.[88] The performance of both methods strongly depends on the cell type and cultivation conditions used. Moreover, the dynamics of telomere shortening differ between cell types. Therefore, this method requires very accurate establishment and careful choice of controls and cut-off levels. The control of telomere length/telomerase activity can be supported by the analysis of pro-oncogenes or senescence-associated genes expression. Like in the cases above, the assay sensitivity might not be sufficient to detect potentially tumorigenic events present in cell populations with low frequency.

6.7.1.4 *Soft agar colony formation assay*

Another method for discerning potentially malignant cells is the soft agar colony formation assay. This semi–quantitative method is based on analysis of anchorage-independence and loss of contact inhibition, which is a hallmark of tumor cells. The soft agar assay allows for detection of spheroids that can be formed only by non-adherent growing cells, and shows good prediction results for the *in vivo* cell behavior. The sensitivity and limit of detection may highly vary on the chosen protocol and have to be carefully evaluated during the method establishment. The uncomplicated analysis of results, the reasonably high sensitivity and low assay costs make this method attractive. The disadvantage is the long assay time (about two weeks) and that its result does not offer an insight into the molecular basis of the findings. Therefore, the combination of the soft agar assay with supportive karyotyping and FISH is advisable to correlate the genomic and functional status of cells.

6.7.2 *Status quo of the scientific and regulatory opinion*

The major objective of assuring the DNA integrity of cell-based therapeutics is to exclude potential tumorigenic changes of the genetic material. Under the altered selection pressure *ex vivo*, cells with chromosomal aberrations that are rare or not viable *in vivo* might obtain selective advantage and spread over the cell population within just a few passages. Furthermore, epigenetic changes *in vitro* may contribute to cell dedifferentiation, faster genome disintegration and escape from senescence similar to that observed for tumor cells.

A special attention is paid to the safety of GM therapeutic products. Several cases of changed gene expression and clonal dominance with the risk of neoplastic transformation and leukemia occurrence have been described.[89–91] As the genome integrity of such cells is originally modified by introduction of the therapeutic gene, descriptive cytogenetic or molecular methods would not provide sufficient information to conclude about the product safety. The functional analysis such as telomerase activity, soft agar assay or analysis of pro-oncogenic proteins gets therefore a special importance and should be performed along with other safety analyses (for details, see "Note for Guidance on the quality, preclinical and clinical aspects of GTMPs").[15]

The issue of genetic integrity is by far best studied on cell lines and primary stem cells due to their propagating capacities *in vitro*. The phenomenon of acquiring genetic rearrangements in the course of adaptation to culture conditions is well known for human embryonic stem cells (hESCs) and their neural derivatives, and, besides ethical considerations, is one of the factors severely limiting their therapeutic use at present.[80,92,93] Several reports demonstrated genomic abnormalities in iPS (induced pluripotent stem cells).[94–97] Since the propagation of human HSCs in culture is technically limited, only little information exists about their genomic status *ex vivo*. The work of Ge *et al.*[98] described transient chromosomal abnormalities of expanded CD34+ cells from human umbilical cord that cleared away without signs of malignant transformation. There is no scientific consensus concerning the potential of MSC to undergo tumorigenic changes. The presence of malignant cells in MSC cultures was described in several publications.[99–101] The results of two of them were later revised since it appeared that the original cultures were contaminated with tumor cells of other origin.[100,101] Yet, many publications point out to a generally high stability of MSC's genome as well as their methylation pattern and RNA expression profile *in vitro*.[102–104] No adverse events have been reported in clinical studies with MSCs so far, supporting the supposition that their use is safe. However, the disposition of the cell culture to genomic variations may depend on features of a particular cultivation process as well as donor characteristics and has to be regarded every time anew. Furthermore, restricted sensitivity of the genome analysis does not allow excluding a single event of neoplastic transformation with certainty.

To build up consensus regarding the key aspects of tumorigenicity analysis in the MSC field, the members of CPWP (Cell Products Working Party) and CAT (Committee for Advanced Therapies) issued a publication representing their non-binding scientific and regulatory opinion.[79] They point out toward necessity of evaluating all MSC processes for genomic instability, i.e., by pushing samples of cells into senescence to prove their safety and by analyzing their karyotype by conventional cytogenetic analysis supported by FISH in case of detected abnormalities. According to the opinion of the authors, karyotyping or FISH analysis of each batch have to be introduced as a release assay, only if recurrent aberrations are identified in cell preparations (identical aberrations found in at least two independent cultures of the same origin). In all cases, a reference sample of each manufactured batch has to be available for possible genetic analysis. Special attention should be paid to the validity of the methods applied and to the accreditation state of the laboratory performing the analysis. Moreover, authors agreed that parameters such as population doubling level and growth rate have to be justified and controlled.

These general principles also well apply for other cell-based products. Factors such as proliferating potential of cells (initial or induced during manufacturing), duration of cultivation, and number of cell divisions performed *in vitro*, have to be taken into account. Furthermore, age and health of the donor may play a role in the initial cell quality, as genetic mutations accumulate with age in the body and can be disease-related. It especially concerns autologous manufacturing. Besides the matter of genomic stability, it may affect the therapeutic efficacy. Therefore, the control of cumulative population doublings is a useful and auxiliary practice to complement the deficiency of current methods of genome analysis. Furthermore, the best tool to mitigate the risks is to support the release methods by extensive studying of underlying biological properties of cellular product preparations throughout the whole pharmaceutical development.

6.8 Environmental Control of Microbial Contamination

As cell products cannot be sterilized [neither by heat or gas (ethylene oxide) nor by filtration], environmental control of microbial contamination is an important part of the control strategy of these products. In Europe, there is an ongoing debate on whether the principles for manufacturing of sterile medicinal products as defined in Annex 1 to the EU GMP Guidelines "Manufacture of Sterile Medicinal Products" are fully applicable to manufacture of CTPs, as these products by definition are not sterile. At least, these principles have to be taken into account for selection of environmental classification of the clean rooms and the associated environmental routine controls. Any exception of these rules should be justified by using QRM principles. However, many European authorities are not willing to accept lower standards than those laid down for the manufacture of sterile products (neither for the aseptic manufacture itself nor for environmental control) not even for cultured cells, where microbial contamination of the product would become evident easily and quickly.

6.8.1 *Routine microbial monitoring*

Every pharmaceutical manufacturer performing aseptic processing has to have a written procedure in place that defines where monitoring samples have to be taken (sampling plan), with which frequency, when samples have to be taken (during the manufacturing process or at the end), sample size or sample volume, which equipment has to be used or which techniques have to be applied and how they are executed and which alert and action limits have to be met.

Annex 1 to the EU GMP Guidelines does not specify which test methods have to be used where, as this is dependent on the process and the equipment

Table 6.15: Recommended limits for microbiological contamination in Europe.

Recommended Limits for Microbial Contamination (Average Values) According to
EU GMP Guidelines, Annex 1.

Clean Room Grade According to EU GMP Guidelines, Annex 1 (in operation)	ISO 14644 equivalent	Air Sample [cfu/m³]	Settle Plates (Diameter 90 mm) [cfu/4 hours][*]	Contact Plates (Diameter 55 mm) [cfu/plate]	Glove Print Five Fingers [cfu/glove]
A	ISO 4.8	<1	<1	<1	<1
B	ISO 7	10	5	5	5
C	ISO 7	100	50	25	—
D	ISO 8	200	100	50	—

Note: [*] Individual settle plates may be exposed for less than four hours.

used for production. Important is, that sampling methods do not interfere with zone protection (e.g., disturbing laminar air flow). The annex recommends the use of settle plates, volumetric air sampling and contact plates and defines limits for microbiological monitoring of clean areas and personnel, as summarized in Table 6.15.

In the United States US Pharmacopoeia chapter <1116> "Microbiological control and monitoring of aseptic processing environments" is the relevant compendial text. Further guidance is provided by the FDA Aseptic Guidance.[105]

The selection of sampling sites for routine microbial monitoring should be based on the results obtained from process qualification of the respective clean room.

For the sampling of gloves, it is important that the prints are taken directly after a manufacturing process with no disinfection steps in between. This should be clearly stated in the corresponding SOP. When glove prints are taken during manufacture and not at the end (e.g., to monitor especially critical production steps), gloves have to be changed after sampling to avoid contamination of the clean room environment and subsequently of the product.

6.8.2 *Alert and action levels*

In addition to the critical values for each method in each clean room grade as defined by official regulations and guidelines, appropriate alert and action levels have to be set. Exceeding these limits must lead to an investigation and if applicable, defined CAPA should be triggered.

The FDA Aseptic Guidance[105] offers definitions for alert and action level:

Alert Level is defined "*as an established microbial or airborne particle level giving early warning of potential drift from normal operating conditions and triggers appropriate scrutiny and follow-up to address the potential problem. Alert levels are always lower than action levels.*"

Action Level is defined as "*an established microbial or airborne particle level that, when exceeded, should trigger appropriate investigation and corrective action based on the investigation.*"

Specification of alert and action levels has to be based on monitoring data obtained within a certain time period, as otherwise they would not be significant. The longer the considered time period is and the more monitoring data are included, the more reliable are the obtained results.

Alert and action levels can be calculated using the following equations:

- Alert level $= M + 3\sqrt{M}$;
- Action level $=$ Alert level $+ 3\sqrt{M}$,

with M being the mean value of all considered results.

6.8.3 *Media growth promotion*

Almost any microbial monitoring method is based on agar plates (settle plates for passive air sampling, agar plates placed in active air samplers, and contact plates used for monitoring of surfaces, equipment, and personnel). Generally a microbiological solid growth medium has to be used that supports the growth of a wide range of bacteria, yeast, and molds. This medium should be supplemented with additives to overcome or to minimize the effects of sanitizing agents, at least for contact plates that are used for surface monitoring. As the quality of the plates is essential, apart from vendor qualification, control and release of every new batch of agar plates is mandatory. Many authorities ask for batch control before use by proving both sterility (no growth/CFUs after culture of unopened plates) and growth promotion by administering a certain number of CFUs of one or more defined microbial strains. Environmental isolates, that have been isolated from the environmental monitoring program, should be included in growth promotion testing.

Growth promotion of an agar plate is dependent on the quality of the agar that is altered by age (therefore the shelf life has to be defined and considered for each batch) and by drying-out when opened for longer time periods. This is often the case for settle plates that in many cases are opened for one or more hours to monitor complete production steps. It is important to demonstrate that micro-organisms are still able to grow after this opening time; therefore the maximum life time of the plate in opened condition has to be determined to prevent false negative results. Even if the supplier guarantees a certain opening time, it can be important to prove this in-house, as clean room conditions due to laminar air flow and high air change rates can influence this time span significantly.

6.9 Reference and Retention Samples

6.9.1 *Principles*

In Europe, Annex 19 to the EU GMP Guidelines "Reference and Retention Samples"[106] gives special guidance on the taking and holding of reference samples of starting materials, packaging materials and finished products and retention samples of finished products. Specific requirements for IMPs are given in Annex 13.[107]

The retention of samples is an integral part of GMP to fulfil two purposes: To provide a sample for analytical testing after product release and to provide a specimen of the fully finished product. Therefore two sample categories have to be differentiated according to Annexes 19 and 13:

- **Reference samples** are defined as samples of a batch of starting material, packaging material or finished product that are stored for the purpose of being analyzed, should the need arise during the shelf life of the batch concerned. Where stability permits, also reference samples from critical intermediates should be kept.
- **Retention samples** are defined as samples of a fully packaged unit from a batch of finished product or for each packaging run or trial period of IMPs. They are stored for identification purposes. For example, presentation, packaging, labeling, patient information leaflet, batch number, and expiry date; should the need arise during the shelf life of the batch concerned.

For finished products of conventional medicinal products, in many instances, the reference and retention samples will be presented identically, i.e., as fully packaged units. In such circumstances, reference and retention samples may be regarded as interchangeable.

6.9.2 *Duration of storage*

The duration of sample storage is prescribed by the European GMP Guidelines. Additional requirements may be defined in national laws or guidance documents.

According to EU GMP Guidelines Annex 19, reference and retention samples from each batch of finished product have to be retained for at least one year after the expiry date. The reference sample has to be contained in its finished primary packaging or in packaging composed of the same material as the primary container in which the product is marketed. Samples of starting materials have to be retained for at least two years after the release of product. That period may be shortened if the period of stability of the material, as indicated in the relevant specification, is shorter. As part of the starting materials of CBMPs are of human origin (blood, tissues or cells), special regulations have to be considered for these materials as samples are important for traceability and look back procedures (compare Sections 6.2.2. Starting Material, and 6.2.3. Donor Testing and Traceability). Packaging materials should be retained for the duration of the shelf life of the finished product concerned.

Reference and retention samples of IMPs (including blinded products) have to be kept for at least two years after completion or formal discontinuation of the last clinical trial in which the batch was used, whichever period is the longer. Consideration should be given to keeping retention samples of IMPs until the clinical report has been prepared to enable confirmation of product identity in the event of, and as part of an investigation into inconsistent trial results (Annex 13).[107]

6.9.3 *Location of storage*

Availability of retained samples is important in case investigations become necessary. Therefore location of storage is an issue covered by the EU GMP Guidelines, Annex 19.

As reference samples are for the purpose of analysis, they should be conveniently available to a laboratory with validated methodology. Samples of starting materials used for medicinal products should therefore be stored at the original site of manufacture of the finished product. Finished products should be stored at the original site of manufacture.

Retention samples represent a batch of finished product as distributed and may need to be examined in order to confirm non-technical attributes for compliance with the MA or EU legislation. Therefore in Europe, retention samples should in all cases be located within the European Economic Area (EEA). They should preferably be stored at the site where the QP certifying the finished product batch is located. Retention samples should be stored at the premises of an authorized manufacturer in order to permit ready access by the Competent Authority.

Sample storage outside the EEA is associated with additional requirements and accepted only if certain prerequisites are fulfilled, at least as far as medicinal products licensed in Europe or IMPs used in European clinical trials are concerned. Written agreements are mandatory in these cases.

6.9.4 *Sample size*

The size of reference and retention samples is an important issue as enough material has to be stored in order to enable a thorough investigation, in case this is necessary.

Annex 19 of the EU GMP Guidelines prescribes the following for licensed medicinal products:

The reference sample should be of sufficient size to permit the carrying out, on, at least, two occasions, of the full analytical controls on the batch in accordance with the MA File which has been assessed and approved by the relevant Competent Authority/Authorities. Where it is necessary to do so, unopened packs should be used when carrying out each set of analytical controls. Any proposed exception to this should be justified to, and agreed with, the relevant competent authority. Where applicable, national requirements relating to the size of reference samples and, if necessary, retention samples should be followed.

The same holds true for IMPs where sample size should be sufficient to permit the carrying out, on, at least, two occasions, of the full analytical controls on the batch in accordance with the IMPD submitted for authorization to conduct the clinical trial.

Of course these regulations can hardly be followed for many CBMPs and it is therefore important to discuss this issue with the competent authority (compare Section 6.9.6. Reference and Retention Samples for CBMPs).

6.9.5 *Written agreements*

Samples should be kept by the manufacturer and at the site of manufacturing of the medicinal product, whenever feasible. If different parties are involved (e.g., more than one manufacturer), retention of samples has to be defined in written agreements in order to control the taking and location of reference and retention samples. In any case, the QP who certifies a batch for sale has to ensure that all relevant reference and retention samples are accessible at all reasonable times.

For IMPs, it is important that the sponsor of the clinical trial and manufacturer(s) of the IMP define in a Technical Agreement who is responsible for the retention of samples, what kind of samples have to be stored and where, and that timely access by the competent authorities is guaranteed.

Written agreements are also required, if sample storage for European medicinal products (either licensed in Europe or used in a European clinical trial) should be located in third countries. Special rules have to be followed then.

6.9.6 *Reference and retention samples for CBMPs*

As clear and reasonable as the defined requirements for retaining of samples might be for conventional medicinal products, they are difficult or even impossible to fulfill for some CBMPs, as certain types of cells (e.g., autologous or allogeneic cells that are used in a directed way) are available in absolutely limited quantities, that do not allow for the storage of any reference material or at least not in quantities that enable full analytical control as defined in the MA or CTA.

The issue of retention samples, where a fully packaged unit from a batch of finished product would have to be stored is also not feasible for cell products that often are used in an autologous or directed allogeneic way as batch size in these cases often is only one packaging unit.

Apart from insufficient quantity of material, the short shelf life of non-cryopreserved cellular products is problematic as reference samples certainly would have to be cryopreserved to enable the prescribed storage times, but this procedure at the same time would significantly alter the cells and comparability to the original product would no longer exist, especially for parameters like viability.

Annex 2 to the EU GMP Guidelines therefore offers the possibility that a modified sample retention strategy may be developed and documented. This has to be discussed with the competent authorities. In any case, samples of starting material of human origin have to be retained for follow-up purposes and look back procedures. Details might be prescribed by national regulations. In Germany, for example, the Blood Working Party of the Federal Ministry of Health prescribes the storage of 1–2 mL of serum or plasma on the occasion of every donation of blood or blood components, divided in at least two aliquots and stored in separate lockable cups or containers at temperatures $\leq -30°C$.[108]

6.10 Stability

6.10.1 *General requirements for stability testing and relevant guidelines*

Stability elucidation is the keystone in ensuring integrity and biological activity of the pharmaceutical at the moment of its application. The requirements for stability data increase with the progress of the product development and the improved knowledge about its quality.

First, stability has to be assessed prior to the product testing in early clinical phases, and the provided data have to be sufficient to justify the indicated storage period before administration. It is possible that the set of data accumulated at this stage is rather incomplete. Also the MoA of the biological product might still be insufficiently studied, so that not all analytical methods are in place yet, or their status does not fulfill the regulatory requirements. Therefore, it is eligible to use development data as support for justification of the product shelf life. Nevertheless, the written stability protocol has to be provided. At late stages of development, identification of parameters critical to the product stability becomes essential, and stability indicative assays, such as quantitative potency assays, have to be established. For the manufacturing authorization, a completed real-time and real-condition stability study covering the target shelf life should be submitted, together with the information about applied analytical procedures and their validation status. Furthermore, the post-approval stability protocol and stability commitment should be provided.

In the European legislation, stability testing of medicinal products as a requirement for product authorization is described in the Commission Directive 2003/63/EC.[109] The FDA recommendations are included in the "Guidance for human somatic cell therapy and gene therapy".[110]

Recommendations on the design, performance, and evaluation of stability studies are presented in series of ICH Guidelines. The ICH Q1A (R2), Harmonised Tripartite Guideline on Stability Testing for New Drug Substances and Products,[111] is generally applicable for planning a stability assessment of different kinds of pharmaceutical products. However, it mostly provides examples best suited for chemical pharmaceutics. The ICH Q5C[112] takes into account specific features of biologics, such as necessity of temperature-controlled storage conditions and complex tests for analysis of biological activity. Whereas ICH Q5C[112] covers a broad range of products of biological origin such as cytokines, antibodies, growth factors, and vaccines, cell-based therapeutics and whole blood products are not included in the scope of this guidance. Nevertheless, both ICH Q1A (R2)[111] and ICH Q5C[112] provide general considerations and directions that constitute a useful base for setting up a faithful stability protocol for a cell-based product. The annexes Q1B–Q1E[113–116] complement ICH Q1A (R2)[111] and contain further recommendations on special aspects of the parenteral guideline.

In addition to documents directly dedicated to product stability, several further ICH and EMA guidelines can be consulted for specific questions. The overview of relevant documents is presented in Table 6.16.

None of these guidelines directly address ATMPs. The novelty and great divergence of ATMPs make it difficult to tailor a specific guidance for their analysis yet. Nevertheless, a number of general requirements exist that should be followed, if possible, for setting up a stability protocol.

Table 6.16: List of guidelines relevant for stability study design and data evaluation of biological products.

Harmonized Stability Guidelines		
Document Reference Number	Document Title	Remarks
ICH Q1A (R2).	Stability Testing of New Drug Substances and Products.	Describes stability data required for product registration "within the three regions of the European Union, Japan, and the United States"; mostly contains examples of chemical products.
ICH Q1B.	Stability Testing: Photostability Testing of New Drug Substances and Products.	Describes assessment of light sensitivity.
ICH Q1C.	Stability Testing for New Dosage Forms.	Stability requirements for submission of new dosage forms of existing active substances.
ICH Q1D.	Bracketing and Matrixing Designs for Stability Testing of New Drug Substances and Products.	Describes principles and examples for reduced study designs.
ICH Q1E.	Evaluation of Stability Data.	Describes principles of data evaluation and establishment of shelf life.
ICH Q5C.	Stability Testing of Biotechnological/Biological Products.	Specifically applies for biologics; blood products as well as cell-based products are not included.
Guidelines providing supportive information		
ICH Q3A (R).	Impurities in New Drug Substances.	Considerations for setting up specifications for chemical degradation products in drug substances.
ICH Q3B (R2).	Impurities in New Drug Products.	Considerations for setting up specifications for chemical degradation products in drug products.
ICH Q6B.	Specifications: Test Procedures and Acceptance Criteria for Biotechnological/Biological Products.	Contains considerations for setting up stability indicating pattern and stability specifications.

(Continued)

Table 6.16: (*Continued*)

Document Reference Number	Document Title	Remarks
EMA Guidelines		
CPMP/ QWP/ 556/96.	Note for Guidance on Stability Testing of Existing Active Substances and Related Finished Products.	Extention of ICH guidelines that sets up stability requirements for existing active substances and finished products.
CPMP/ QWP/ 609/96/ Rev 2.	Guideline on Declaration of Storage Conditions: A: In the Product Information of Medicinal Products. B: For Active Substances.	Instructions on labeling of active substances and finished medicinal products.
CPMP/ QWP/ 155/96.	Note for Guidance on Development Pharmaceutics.	Considerations for formulation development and establishment of parameters crucial for quality of finished product.
CPMP/ QWP/ 2934/99.	Note for Guidance on In-Use Stability Testing of Human Medicinal Products.	Describes design of study to assess the stability after container opening for multidose products.
CPMP/ QWP/ 159/96.	Maximum shelf life for sterile products after first opening or following reconstitution.	Contains recommendations on storage time of sterile products after container opening.

Drug substance/drug product. The stability of both, drug substance and drug product should be elucidated. If processing of the drug substance occurs not immediately, the time before further processing steps should be defined and analyzed for its influence on the product stability. Furthermore, critical product intermediates have to be identified and their stability analyzed. If the declared storage period of a drug substance or drug product exceeds six months, the real-time and real-conditions stability data covering at least six months should be provided at the moment of submission. For products with a shorter shelf life, a case-to-case decision can be made.

Origin and size of batches. The size of batches should be representable of the manufacturing scale or be at minimum of the pilot scale. If the pilot-scale batches are used, a commitment to elucidate the stability of the first three manufacturing batches post-approval has to be made, and the post-approval stability program has to be presented. In all cases, the manufacturing protocol and product quality should be representative of the product.

Defined container and container closure system. The container closure system used in stability studies should be identical to that of the product. If several primary containers are intended to be used for the product packaging, each of them should be included in the stability program.

Defined storage conditions. Biological products normally require storage under strictly defined and controlled conditions. Exemplarily, for cryopreserved cellular products exact storage conditions might be declared as "in the vapor phase of liquid nitrogen at $\leq -145°C$" or "in the liquid nitrogen at $\leq -145°C$", and a refrigerated storage can be defined as $5 \pm 3°C$ or $2 - 6°C$ depending on existing data. Definitions such as "room temperature" are not acceptable. If additional special conditions are required for regular storage (i.e., upright storage, light-protective storage), they should be included in the test program and their impact on the product quality should be assessed.

Testing periods. Testing periods are normally defined depending on the expected shelf life. The strategy for definition of testing periods is precisely described in ICH Q5C for drug products with an expected shelf life between 0.5 and five years. Please note that data extrapolation is not acceptable for biologics, since no precise prediction on the dynamics of product degradation can be made. Therefore, the shelf life is always set up based on real-time data.

Accelerated and stress testing. Should be included in the stability program, if applicable. During accelerated testing, the product is subjected to temperature conditions one step higher than regular (i.e., $25 \pm 5°C$ for regular storage conditions of $5 \pm 3°C$). This testing generally serves for preliminary assessment of the shelf life and degradation pattern. The applicability of the accelerated testing for cell-based products is a case-by-case decision. Stress testing includes various extreme conditions that the product can be accidentally exposed to, such as temperature change during transportation, temperature conditions, and handling at the clinical side.

Defined stability acceptance criteria including their justification. The principle of setting up stability specifications is described in ICH Q5C[112] and ICH Q6B.[44] In addition, ICH Q3A (R2)[117] regards specifications for chemical degradation products. For setting up suitable stability specifications, determination of the product-specific and stability-indicating profile is required. It is generally accepted that the product analysis after storage should go beyond its physico–chemical characterization and include tests for defining its biological activity (potency testing). The methods should be validated.

Stability in use. Elucidation of *stability in use* usually covers the time between container opening and begin of product administration. CPMP/QWP/2934/99[118] describes design of in-use stability studies for multidose products. CPMP/QWP/159/96[119] makes the emphasis on the control of sterility of aseptic products after opening. If reconstitution is required prior to administration, its duration and conditions also have to be studied; the duration of administration itself is not included.

The stability in use should also be proven for cell therapeutics. In case of cryopreserved therapeutics, it has to be taken into consideration that the stability issue becomes crucial from the moment they are taken out of the cryotank, already before container opening, as cells might rapidly degrade. Therefore, the protocol for in-use stability of cryopreserved products should include thawing of cells as an initial point. The quality of the product including its potency as well as absence of microbiological contamination by the time of administration has to be shown.

6.10.2 *Specifics of cell-based products*

The presence of living cells in the active substance defines several pivotal characteristics of ATMPs and has a great impact on the design of the stability protocol. Cellular drug substance represents a homogenous or heterogeneous population of living cells possessing defined therapeutic characteristics and prepared in an aseptic way. In accordance with it, viability, integrity, potency as well as microbiological safety are crucial for the quality of the product and have to be maintained at the moment of its application. In contrast to microbiological requirements for aseptic products, which usually do not allow much variation, the specifications for other parameters are very individual for each product. To reliably establish product shelf life, following questions have to be answered:

- What is the desired quality after storage?
- Which assays and specifications are indicative of this quality?
- How the process and product variations impact the stability after storage?
- To which conditions the product is realistically subjected during the storage and before application?

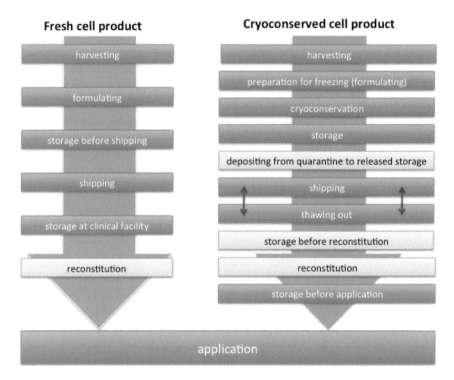

Figure 6.1: Illustrative lifecycle of a CBMP from harvesting to application. From the last preparation steps till application, a cell product is subjected to complex factors and conditions that may impact its stability. Examples of storage conditions for fresh and cryoconserved cell products are shown. Optional steps are shown in light gray; the order of events such as shipping and thawing out might be reversed (indicated by arrows).

The latter is often underestimated and presented in a stability protocol in a simplified way. Figure 6.1 illustrates the complexity of factors a cell product can be exposed to before its application. Understanding of real specification limits, such as variation of temperature conditions during transport and at the clinical side, duration of intermediate storage steps and of reconstitution is needed to discern their influence on the product stability and to develop a protocol that truly reflects and predicts shelf life of the analyzed product.

Furthermore, factors, such as heterogeneity of starting material, biological nature of manufacturing process and general fragility of the cell product have to be taken into consideration, as they may substantially contribute to the product variability which, in turn, influences the stability protocol. Therefore, the conceptual design of formal stability studies as well as the reliability of obtained results depends, in many ways, on the preceding developmental work.

6.10.2.1 *Fresh versus cryopreserved cell products*

Usually cells become easily susceptible to damage already during harvesting, when taken out of their optimal *in vitro* cultivation conditions. There are no options other than cryopreservation known that allow for greatly extending the stability period of cells after the final formulating of products. Therefore, relatively early in the product development the decision has to be made if cryoconservation should be applied to the product. If cells have to be administered freshly, their stability period is usually rather short. Many cellular products that are currently in clinical studies have declared shelf life of 48–72 hours. This requires tight coordination between the product manufacturing and its application. If the transportation of the product to the clinical side has to be performed, the required time may become predominant in the whole shelf life. Furthermore, the conditions and duration of handling steps before product administration have to be taken into consideration.

Cryopreservation of cells, when feasible, may extend the storage time of cell products to years. If the product or its intermediates can be cryopreserved without significant loss of viability or activity, generating off-the-shelf products becomes possible, which is an attractive marketing strategy. Furthermore, cryopreservation facilitates clinical planning and allows for choosing optimal administration time depending on the health state of the patient. However, the process of cryopreservation introduces several critical factors that have to be carefully analyzed with respect to their influence on the quality of the final product. Establishment and validation of freezing and thawing protocols as well as elucidation of cell quality after thawing are actions that have to be undertaken before designing a long-term stability study. The suitability of the protocol depends not only on the type of cells and excipients but also on the primary container used, since the nature of packaging material and its permeability play great role in the process of cryopreservation. Moreover, the performance of the protocol highly depends on the kind of freezing device used. The freezing device has to be qualified, in order to confirm the process consistency and to discern factors that may affect characteristics of the cryopreservation, such as the position of the product in the freezing device. Furthermore, the quality of the cryoconservation may depend on the fitness of cells that are subjected to it, so that variability of the cell product as well as the duration and conditions of preparation steps for cryoconservation have to be taken into account. As only very restricted molecular activity takes place at temperatures of liquid nitrogen, which allows the product to be kept well preserved for years, the active nature of the cryopreservation process puts a new accent in the elucidation of the product stability.

6.10.2.2 *Potency assays*

To control the product functionality, a performance of a quantitative potency assay for shelf life elucidation is requested by regulators. Potency assays for cell products often require complex biological analysis since the MoA cannot be reduced to a single parameter (compare also Section 6.6.8. Potency). If no surrogate markers are established or can be reliably analyzed in a quick assay, the duration of such a complex potency assay may take considerable time. Furthermore, if the analysis is performed on living cells, it often requires their maintenance under conditions different from the drug product composition. Exemplarily, for cryopreserved products, the excipients such as DMSO may interfere with the analysis and often have to be removed or diluted. Similarly, it might be necessary to take cells into culture or even adapt them to culture conditions over a certain period of time before their activity can be analyzed in an *in vitro* assay. In these cases, the potency assay is performed on the active substance and not on the finished drug product. This belongs to specifics of cell manufacturing and is often unavoidable at the current stage of knowledge. Nevertheless, it has to be regarded and justified whether the performed assay truly reflects the potency of the product in its final formulation.

Although cellular degradation products usually do not directly interfere with the performance of the potency assay, their influence has to be elucidated in order to discern effects of diminished viability (reduced dose) from the potency loss of living cells. Furthermore, decrease in potency can be a factor indicative of on-going product degradation (e.g., pro-apoptotic events). For the proper evaluation of potency results, international, national or in-house reference standards are recommended. The use of reference materials is discussed in detail in Section 6.11.5 (Reference Material and Reference Standards).

6.10.2.3 *Small batch size-reduced design*

Many cell-based products are characterized by a small batch size. A common pharmaceutical stability protocol, according to which only a relatively small part of a batch is dedicated to stability study and the whole stability program is covered by just a few batches is hardly applicable in this case. A characteristic case is autologous manufacturing, where only one product batch is normally produced from one starting material (i.e., from one apheresis product or bone marrow aspiration).

Aseptic way of cell product preparation and storage excludes taking multiple aliquots from the same primary container in the course of a long-term stability study. Furthermore, ethical considerations and scarceness of material often make "manufacturing just for testing" impossible or not desired. Therefore, reduced design is often applied for cell-based therapeutics. The principles of reduced design are described in ICH Q1D. In contrast to the full design, where each sample is analyzed for all stability-relevant parameters at each time point, reduced design allows to diminish the amount of the required material due to application of bracketing or matrixing. Bracketing means leaving intermediate conditions out of the protocol and including only test points of extremes. This can be applicable for parameters such as different fill size in the same container, different container sizes or different strengths of the drug product under condition that the product formulation remains unchanged. Bracketing implicates that the stability behavior characteristic for the intermediates lays within the range identified for the extremes. It has to be noticed that bracketing is not applicable to drug substances.

In the matrixing approach, only a subset of samples is elucidated for all stability factors at each time point so that the total set of samples covers all variations (i.e., variations of batch quality, batch size, and storage conditions). It implicates that the stability pattern detected for the subset of samples is fully representative of the stability of the drug product. It is recommended to include the analysis of initial and final points for all batches. It surely becomes impossible if the maximum of two aliquots can be made from the same batch. In this case, an alternative strategy such as increasing the total number of analyzed batches or the data pooling approach for low variable parameters should be considered and justified. It is preferable to elucidate all test parameters with the same frequency, i.e., to include equal amount of samples for each test point in relation to the total.

In order to design an adequate reduced stability protocol, knowledge about the product variability and the expected shelf life is essential. Whereas the full stability design allows for learning more about the product step-by-step, as every stability point is thoroughly analyzed for all factors, the frequency of analysis in the reduced design is dependent on the precision of prediction and requires a preparatory developmental work. Thus, highly variable factors should be discerned and studied before applying matrixing in order to define a minimal number of samples that brings statistically evaluable results and to reliably estimate their influence on the product shelf life. It is also advisable to perform the analysis of trends before designing a stability program. It has to be taken into account that due to diminishing the number of batches per time point, the matrixing design is less sensitive to stability trends. It is generally not advisable to combine bracketing and matrixing in the same protocol, as it can lead to difficulties in the data analysis and shelf life justification. The principles and approaches of stability data evaluation are discussed in ICH Q1E.

6.11 Validation of Analytical Procedures

6.11.1 *Validation principles*

In the Glossary of the EU GMP Guidelines validation is defined as '*action of proving, in accordance with the principles of GMP, that any procedure, process, equipment, material, activity or system actually leads to the expected results.*'

Chapter 6 of the EU GMP Guidelines further points out that '*The QC Department as a whole has to validate and implement all QC procedures. Not only test methods that are used for QC of the final product but also methods for in-process controls (even if they are performed in production) and test methods that are performed during process validation only, have to be validated*'.

Validation of analytical procedures is necessary in order to ensure that they deliver reliable results and to demonstrate that they are suitable for their intended purpose. This is especially important in early phases of clinical trials where the production process is in many cases not yet fully validated and often still variable. Prerequisite for the validation of an analytical procedure is qualified and where necessary calibrated equipment as well as trained personnel.

There are two different validation approaches for analytical procedures: (1) Newly developed procedures that are not described in a relevant pharmacopoeia and are not certified or pre-validated by a supplier (e.g., CE-certified test kits) have to be fully validated according to the relevant guidelines; (2) Analytical procedures that are based on a compendial method described in a relevant pharmacopoeia or are otherwise pre-validated do not require full validation. In these cases, it is sufficient to verify their suitability under the conditions of use (personnel, instruments, and laboratory, etc.). Most importantly it has to be demonstrated that the sample matrix does not negatively interfere with the test procedure; thus, this approach is termed matrix validation. The US Pharmacopoeia defines the necessary validation work for procedures that are based on the pharmacopoeia in general chapter <1225> "Validation of Compendial Procedures". Generally, it is important to point out that the validation of analytical procedures has to be completed before process validation can commence.

Apart from the requirement of initial validation of an analytical procedure prior to use, it has to be defined under which circumstances the method has to be revalidated. According to ICH Q2 (R1), this is typically the case when the synthesis (production) of the drug substance is changed, when the composition of the finished product is changed, or when the analytical procedure itself is changed. But of course also other types of changes might require revalidation of an analytical procedure. This has to be decided on a case-by-case basis usually by use of change control management principles. The degree of revalidation required depends on the nature and the significance of the change.

6.11.2 *Validation characteristics*

The main guidance document for validation of analytical procedures is ICH Q2 (R1) "Validation of Analytical Procedures: Text and Methodology".[120] The guideline defines the following validation characteristics: Accuracy, Precision (Repeatability, Intermediate Precision, and Reproducibility), Specificity, Detection Limit, Quantitation Limit, Linearity, and Range. Which or how many of these characteristics have to be addressed in a validation approach is dependent on the type of the analytical procedure. ICH Q2 (R1) defines the extent of required analytical tests for different types of analytical procedures as summarized in "Table 6.17: Required Analytical Tests for Validation of Analytical Procedures". Following these

Table 6.17:   Required analytical tests for validation of analytical procedures.

Characteristics / Type of Analytical Procedure	Identification	Testing for Impurities Quantitative	Testing for Impurities Limit	Assay Content and Potency
Accuracy	−	+	−	+
Precision				
Repeatability	−		⁻	⊦
Intermediate Precision	−|(1)		−	+(1)
Specificity(2)	+	+	+	+
Detection limit	−	−(3)	+	−
Quantitation limit	−	+	−	−
Linearity	−	+	−	+
Range	−	+	−	+

Notes:−Signifies that this characteristic is not normally evaluated.
⊦ Signifies that this characteristic is normally evaluated.
(1)In cases where reproducibility has been performed, intermediate precision is not needed.
(2)Lack of specificity of one analytical procedure could be compensated by other supporting analytical procedure(s).
(3)May be needed in some cases.
Source: Table modified from ICH Guideline Q2 (R1).[120]

principles, an analytical method used for determination of identity has to be only specific. If a method is used for quantification of the target cell fraction (content assay); accuracy, precision, linearity, and range would have to be validated additionally.

Generally, the different validation parameters do not have to be addressed individually. To save time, work, and sample volume, it is advisable to combine certain parameters in one approach. Reasonable is the combination of parameters where spiking experiments on different levels of concentration are performed (e.g., accuracy and precision). If linearity is included, it might be necessary to exclude the results of samples with very low concentrations (e.g., those analyzed for the assessment of the detection limit) as demonstration of linearity tends to be challenging, the closer the detection limit is approached.

Viability is not mentioned as type of analytical procedures in ICH Q2 (R1). Analysis of viability is a compendial method in Europe (Chapter 2.7.29)[27] and full validation might therefore not be necessary anyway. If this is not the case, viability can be regarded as a content assay since a certain type of cells (viable cells) has to be analyzed quantitatively.

ICH Q2 (R1) is a helpful guidance document for validation of analytical procedures that offers straight-forward advice on how to conduct validation work, but its scope is actually limited to conventional pharmaceutical methods such as chromatography (e.g., HPLC, GC) used for chemically-based small molecule drug products. Of course several validation principles are assignable also to methods used for analysis of cellular products, but these methods pose special challenges that are not addressed by ICH Q2 (R1). Traditional validation parameters are not applicable in these cases. Altogether there is currently few specific literature available for validation of methods such as flow cytometry, neither on the basis of scientific literature nor as regulatory guidance documents. One exception, at least for validation of bioassays in general- is USP general chapter<1033> "Biological Assay Validation" that was included in the US Pharmacopoeia in 2012. It introduces bioassay validation by the use of Design of Experiments (DoE), a statistical approach that allows analysis of interactions between different variation factors of the assay to be validated. Chapter <1033> contains a bioassay validation example based on the principles of DoE.

6.11.2.1 *Accuracy and precision*

'*The accuracy of an analytical procedure expresses the closeness of agreement between the value which is accepted either as a conventional true value or an accepted reference value and the value found. This is sometimes termed trueness.*' ICH Q2 (R1).[120]

'*The precision of an analytical procedure expresses the closeness of agreement (degree of scatter) between a series of measurements obtained from multiple sampling of the same homogeneous sample under the prescribed conditions. Precision may be considered at three levels: Repeatability, intermediate precision and reproducibility.*' ICH Q2 (R1).[120]

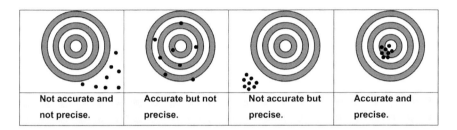

| Not accurate and not precise. | Accurate but not precise. | Not accurate but precise. | Accurate and precise. |

Figure 6.2: Validation characteristics: accuracy *versus* precision.

The "bull's eye" of the target is thought to be the true value. A shooter with low accuracy and low precision produces a pattern that is random; the target is only hit by chance. A shooter with accuracy but low precision hits the target, but the pattern still is rather random than tight. A shooter with high precision but low accuracy produces a tightly clustered pattern outside the bull's eye and the target. The optimal shooter is one who shoots accurately and precisely. In this case, a tight cluster is found in the bull's eye area.[121]

As there is sometimes confusion between the meanings of 'accuracy' compared to 'precision', it is worth to oppose both terms before dwelling on them individually and in more detail. As defined by ICH Q2 (R1), accuracy describes the difference between the measured value and the true value. Whenever a measured value is near the true value it is highly accurate. Precision on the other hand describes the differences in results for a set of measurements, regardless of their accuracy. A highly precise method is one in which repeated application of the method on a sample gives results which agree closely with one another. Precision is related with uncertainty: Measurements with high precision have low uncertainty and *vice versa*. To express accuracy and precision mathematically, the terms error and deviation are used. Figure 6.2 illustrates the terms accuracy and precision with the help of a target and a shooter.[121]

It is important to point out that accuracy and precision both not only depend on the weapon that is used for shooting but also on the shooter. Assigned to an analytical method this means that the reliability of a result depends on the instrument used as well as on the analyst who performs the method. Therefore, it is essential to have well trained personnel who works carefully and uses qualified and where necessary, calibrated instruments in order to obtain valid results.[121]

6.11.2.2 *Accuracy*

The validation of accuracy is necessary for all analytical procedures that are used for determination of potency and content. If impurities are analyzed, validation of accuracy is required whenever the method is used quantitatively (in contrast to a limit test, where accuracy would not necessarily have to be validated).

ICH Q2 (R1) offers three different methods to address accuracy:

1. **Analysis of an analyte with known purity** (either pure or spiked to drug substance/drug product):

   a. Analysis of the drug substance (API): Application of the analytical procedure to be validated to an analyte of known purity (e.g., reference material).
   b. Analysis of the drug product: Application of the analytical procedure to be validated to a synthetic mixture of the drug product components to which known quantities of the drug substance to be analyzed have been added. In cases where it is impossible to obtain samples of all drug product components to produce a synthetic mixture, it may be acceptable to add known quantities of the analyte to the drug product.
   c. Analysis of impurities: Application of the analytical method to be validated to drug substance/drug product spiked with known amount of impurities.

2. **Comparison of the results** of the analytical procedure to be validated with the results of a second well-characterized procedure, the accuracy of which is stated and/or defined.
3. **Accuracy may be inferred** once precision, linearity, and specificity have been established.

For CBMPs, method 1 might be challenging as reference material with known purity is often not available (compared to chemical substances where pharmacopoeial or WHO reference standards can be used in many cases and where purity of a drug substance can be addressed by numerous different analytical methods).

For flow cytometric analysis, it might be possible to use commercially available control cells as reference material for spiking experiments (e.g., to serve as cellular impurities typically originating from the starting material or as non-target cells) as they are delivered with specified amounts of the different cell populations that are contained. But of course these control cells are not offered for all types of potential impurities or non-target cells that are required for spiking and the cells are usually fixed leading to different characteristics in the flow cytometer (e.g., scatter and/or auto-fluorescence). This can either negatively influence their recovery rate or the instrument settings have to be changed for their analysis, leading to an alteration of the method to be validated. Alternatively blood samples which contain predefined amounts of different cells as analyzed, for example, with an hematology analyzer can be used. Cell lines that are known to express or not to express certain markers might be another option, but again their different properties in flow cytometry (e.g., the size of immortalized cell lines is often significantly altered compared to primary cells) might oppose their use in flow cytometry. Finally, if the drug product consists of cells that are induced or differentiated in cell culture, it might be possible to use cells that do not undergo this induction or differentiation process to mimic non-target cells, but very often cell culture leads to significant up- or down-regulation of certain markers, which causes different isotype binding or changes the size, shape or granularity of the cells, making the two cell populations (matrix and spiked cell population) again not really comparable.

However, even if cells that are used as non-target cells or cellular impurities in spiking experiments are not characterized as profoundly as is the case for chemical reference material, these experiments nevertheless provide valuable information on the assay and are therefore commonly accepted by the authorities. But of course an optimal strategy has to be developed anew for each new cellular product and intensive analysis in various qualification experiments is required before validation can commence.

For validation of the viability assay, it is possible to kill cells deliberately by freezing without cryoprotectant or chemical treatment (e.g., fixation) and spike them to the vital product. Of course it is important to address the overall viability of the vital product before non-viable cells are added. As already mentioned above, determination of viability (either by manual count in a hemocytometer or by flow cytometry) is a compendial method in the European Pharmacopoeia and full validation might therefore not be necessary.

6.11.2.3 *Precision*

The validation of precision (repeatability and intermediate precision) is necessary for all analytical procedures that are used for determination of potency and content. If impurities are analyzed, validation of precision is required, whenever the method is used quantitatively (in contrast to a limit test, where precision would not necessarily have to be validated).

According to ICH Q2 (R1), precision should be investigated using homogeneous, authentic samples. However, if it is not possible to obtain a homogeneous sample, it may be investigated using artificially prepared samples. The precision of an analytical procedure is usually expressed as the variance, standard deviation or coefficient of variation of a series of measurements.

There are three different types of precision as defined by ICH Q2 (R1):

1. **Repeatability** is defined as the precision under the same operating conditions over a short interval of time, also termed **intra-assay precision**. Repeatability is demonstrated with a minimum of nine determinations covering the specified range for the procedure or with a minimum of six determinations at 100% of the test concentration.

2. **Intermediate Precision (inter-assay precision)** is defined as precision under variations within a laboratory (different days, different analysts, and different equipment, etc.). Intermediate precision may not be confused with robustness (compare Section 6.11.2.9. Robustness) where different variations with suspected influence on the results are applied on purpose.

3. **Reproducibility** is defined as precision between laboratories (inter-laboratory trials; collaborative studies, usually applied to standardization of methodology). Reproducibility is not essential (and these data are not part of the MA dossier) but if it is analyzed, intermediate precision can be omitted.

Precision, particularly repeatability, is a validation parameter that can be easily addressed also with CBMPs. For analysis of intermediate precision it might be difficult to include the variation factor of analysis on different days as normally the same sample should be analyzed on various days and the results should be compared with one another. For CBMPs that are not cryopreserved, this is difficult as due to the short shelf life, samples will change within some hours or at least some days leading to significantly altered characteristics. It might therefore be necessary to skip the variation of analysis on different days or to validate reproducibility rather than intermediate precision.

Generally, it might be necessary to set the acceptable limits for variance, standard deviation or coefficient of variation broader than they are usually defined for chemical substances and physico–chemical analytical procedures (where CVs of 2–3% are common) as biotechnological and immunological methods tend to be more variable. Acceptance criteria should be based on the experience that is gained during assay development.

6.11.2.4 *Specificity*

'*Specificity is the ability to assess unequivocally the analyte in the presence of components which may be expected to be present. Typically these might include impurities, degradants, and matrix, etc. Lack of specificity of an individual analytical procedure may be compensated by other supporting analytical procedure(s).*

This definition has the following implications:

- *Identification: To ensure the identity of an analyte.*
- *Purity Tests: To ensure that all the analytical procedures performed allow an accurate statement of the content of impurities of an analyte, i.e., related substances test, heavy metals, and residual solvents content, etc.*
- *Assay (content or potency): To provide an exact result which allows an accurate statement on the content or potency of the analyte in a sample.'* ICH Q2(R1).[120]

The validation of specificity is required for all analytical procedures independent of their purpose. The procedures used for validation of specificity are dependent on the objective of the analytical procedure and vary between methods used for identification and those used for potency, content, and assessment of impurities.

1. **Identity**: The specificity of an analytical procedure used for assessment of identity can be validated by demonstrating its potential to discriminate between compounds of closely related structures. This means that the analytical procedure must obtain positive results from samples containing the analyte, and negative results from samples not containing the analyte. In addition, the identification test may be applied to materials structurally similar or closely related to the analyte to confirm that a positive response is not obtained.

2. **Potency, Content, and Impurities**: Generally it has to be demonstrated that the analytical procedure is able to discriminate the analyte in the presence of impurities, degradation products, and/or excipients.

   a. If impurities are available: Pure substances (drug substance or drug product) are spiked with appropriate levels of impurities and/or excipients. Additionally, unspiked samples are analyzed and the results of all assays are compared. It must be demonstrated that the analytical procedure is unaffected by the presence of the spiked substances by obtaining equal results for spiked compared to unspiked samples.

   b. If impurities are not available: If standards of impurities or degradation products are not available, specificity may be demonstrated by comparing the test results of samples containing impurities or degradation products to a second well-characterized procedure. This could include samples stored under relevant stress conditions.

Specificity is difficult to address for most analytical procedures used for CBMPs as again reference standards are not available; neither for drug substance and drug product nor for non-target cells, impurities or degradation products.

For all analytical methods that are based on the binding of an antibody to a specific antigen, it is important to know that specificity of an antibody is not only a matter of its clone (that determines the detection of a certain epitope) but also of the amount of antibody in relation to the target. If not enough antibody is used, results can be false negative and the antigen is not detected even though it is recognized by the antibody. If on the other hand too much antibody is used unspecific staining increases. This has to be considered especially whenever an antibody-dependent method should be validated over a great range, as the antibody–antigen-ratio changes significantly from the sample with the lowest concentration of target to the one with the highest concentration. For methods such as flow cytometry, it is mandatory to titrate each antibody during assay development and to evaluate which amount and/or which concentration is the most suitable one. Commonly, mean fluorescent intensities (MFI) of the negative (e.g., isotype control) as well as the positive population are analyzed and compared to determine the amount of antibody that best discriminates positive from negative populations. This is particularly challenging if not only positive and negative but low, intermediate, and high populations have to be distinguished. Non-viable cells are another problem as they are known to unspecifically bind antibodies.

Whenever possible certified antibodies (e.g., in Europe CE-certified) should be used as these are well characterized (commonly also in terms of their specificity and cross-reactivity to unrelated targets) and potentially data from the supplier can be used for demonstration of specificity.

6.11.2.5 *Detection limit*

'*The detection limit of an individual analytical procedure is the lowest amount of analyte in a sample which can be detected but not necessarily quantitated as an exact value.*' ICH Q2 (R1).[120]

The validation of the detection limit is required for analytical procedures that are used for detection of impurities on the basis of a limit test. Whenever impurities should be analyzed quantitatively, instead of the detection limit, the quantitation limit has to be validated (see Section 6.11.2.6).

ICH Q2 (R1) defines three different approaches for determination of the detection limit, depending on whether the procedure is instrumental or non-instrumental. The three approaches are either based on visual evaluation, on the signal-to-noise ratio or on the standard deviation of the response and the slope.

1. **Visual Evaluation**: The detection limit is determined by analysis of samples with known concentration of the analyte. The detection limit is the minimum level at which the analyte can be reliably detected.
2. **Signal-to-noise ratio**: This approach can only be used for methods that exhibit baseline noise (e.g., ELISA). Samples with known low concentration and blank samples are required for this approach. The measured signals of all samples are compared and the signal-to-noise ratios are calculated. The minimum concentration at which the analyte can be reliably detected shows a signal-to-noise ratio of at least 2:1, better 3:1.
3. **Standard deviation of the response and the slope**: Using this approach, the detection limit (DL) is calculated with the following formula:

$$DL = \frac{3.3\sigma}{S}$$

Where σ = the standard deviation of the response
S = the slope of the calibration curve
The slope S may be estimated from the calibration curve of the analyte. The estimate of σ may be carried out in a variety of ways, for example:

a. Based on the standard deviation of the blank: An appropriate number of blank samples have to be analyzed and the standard deviation σ of these responses has to be calculated.
b. Based on the calibration curve: Several samples containing an analyte in the range of the detection limit have to be analyzed in order to generate a specific calibration curve. The residual standard deviation σ of a regression line or the standard deviation of y-intercepts of regression lines may be used as standard deviation.

Determination of the detection limit is particularly important for those assays that analyze critical safety parameters and where demonstration of the complete absence of a certain impurity in the sample is desired. This applies i.e., to soft agar colony assay (demonstration of absence of tumorigenic cells) or RCV assay (demonstration of absence of retroviral particles in the sample). The sensitivity of the method is very important in these cases. To reduce the sampling error, the sample size should be as big as possible.

Whenever an impurity does not implicate safety concerns and is allowed to be present in low amounts, the quantitation limit is more important to be determined than the detection limit.

Amounts of impurities that are detected but are below the quantitation limit are often declared as "defined".

6.11.2.6 *Quantitation limit*

'*The quantitation limit of an individual analytical procedure is the lowest amount of analyte in a sample which can be quantitatively determined with suitable precision and accuracy. The quantitation limit is a parameter of quantitative assays for low levels of compounds in sample matrices, and is used particularly for the determination of impurities and/or degradation products.*' ICH Q2 (R1).[120]

The validation of the quantitation limit is required for analytical procedures that are used for quantitative detection of impurities. Whenever impurities should be addressed by only a limit test, instead of the quantitation limit, the detection limit has to be validated (see Section 6.11.2.5).

Same as for the detection limit, ICH Q2 (R1) defines three different approaches for determination of the quantitation limit, depending on whether the procedure is instrumental or non-instrumental. The three approaches are either based on visual evaluation, on the signal-to-noise ratio or on the standard deviation of the response and the slope.

1. **Visual Evaluation:** The quantitation limit is determined by analysis of samples with known concentration of the analyte. The quantitation limit is the minimum level at which the analyte can be quantified with acceptable accuracy and precision.

2. **Signal-to-noise ratio:** This approach can only be used for methods that exhibit baseline noise (e.g. ELISA). Samples with known low concentration and blank samples are required for this approach. The measured signals of all samples are compared and the signal-to-noise ratios are calculated. The minimum concentration at which the analyte can be reliably quantified shows a signal-to-noise ratio of 10:1.

3. **Standard deviation of the response and the slope:** Using this approach, the quantitation limit (QL) is calculated with the following formula:

$$QL = \frac{10\sigma}{S}$$

Where σ = the standard deviation of the response
S = the slope of the calibration curve
The slope S may be estimated from the calibration curve of the analyte. The estimate of σ may be carried out in a variety of ways, for example:

a. Based on the standard deviation of the blank: An appropriate number of blank samples have to be analyzed and the standard deviation σ of these responses has to be calculated.

b. Based on the calibration curve: Several samples containing an analyte in the range of the quantitation limit have to be analyzed in order to generate a specific calibration curve. The residual standard deviation σ of a regression line or the standard deviation of y-intercepts of regression lines may be used as standard deviation.

6.11.2.7 *Linearity*

'*The linearity of an analytical procedure is its ability (within a given range) to obtain test results which are directly proportional to the concentration (amount) of analyte in the sample.*' ICH Q2 (R1).[120]

Conventional methods usually show a linear relationship between concentration and test result that should be evaluated across the defined range (see Section 6.11.2.8). Linearity may be demonstrated using the analytical procedure to be validated directly on the drug substance and/or on synthetic mixtures of the drug product components. ICH Q2 (R1) recommends using at least five different concentrations for establishment of linearity. Once the results of the measurements are available, the linear relationship should be evaluated by appropriate statistical methods, for example, by calculation of a regression line by the method of least squares. In some cases, mathematical transformation of the test results may be necessary in order to obtain linearity. Usually the data are evaluated using the correlation coefficient, the y-intercept and the slope of the regression line as well as the residual sum of squares.

Some analytical methods such as immunoassays do not demonstrate linearity after any mathematical transformation. In these cases, the analytical response should be described by an appropriate function of the concentration of an analyte in a sample.

Demonstration of linearity across the defined range is usually feasible also for analysis of CBMPs. If for example, target cells are spiked in five different amounts to non-target cells, a flow cytometric analysis should demonstrate linear relationship. The same holds true for ELISA where different concentrations are used for calibration purposes and the equation of the regression line is used for the calculation of the sample's test result.

In many cases, not the whole linear range of a method has to be covered to study the different validation parameters, i.e., a method with a specification of $> 95\%$ does not necessarily have to be evaluated down the lowest linear concentration (compare Section 6.11.2.8. Range).

6.11.2.8 *Range*

'*The range of an analytical procedure is the interval between the upper and lower concentration (amounts) of analyte in the sample (including these concentrations) for which it has been demonstrated that the analytical procedure has a suitable level of precision, accuracy, and linearity.'* ICH Q2 (R1).[120]

Unlike all other validation parameters, the range of an analytical method is defined rather than analyzed or measured. According to ICH Q2 (R1), it is normally derived from linearity studies and depends on the intended application of the procedure, leading to completely different ranges for methods that analyze, for example, the content of a drug product compared to one analyzing impurities. The defined range should at least cover the product specification range. Thus, the range of a method used to analyze the content of the finished drug product will have to be set minimally at 80–120% of the test concentration (*Note*: these limits are defined by ICH Q2 (R1) for conventional medicinal products; they can of course vary for CBMPs) whereas the range of a method used for quantitative detection of an impurity will be defined around the limit of quantitation.

Definition of the range is necessary for all analytical procedures that are used for determination of potency and content. If impurities are analyzed, definition of the range is required whenever the method is used quantitatively (in contrast to a limit test, where the range would not necessarily have to be defined).

6.11.2.9 *Robustness*

'The robustness of an analytical procedure is a measure of its capacity to remain unaffected by small, but deliberate variations in method parameters and provides an indication of its reliability during normal usage.

The evaluation of robustness should be considered during the development phase and depends on the type of procedure under study. It should show the reliability of an analysis with respect to deliberate variations in method parameters.' ICH Q2 (R1).[120]

Robustness in contrast to the above mentioned parameters is not required for validation (and is therefore not listed in Table 6.17) but should be addressed whenever it is known that variations of analytical conditions could have a potential influence on the result. Robustness should already be considered prior to validation in the development phase of an analytical procedure. ICH Q2 (R1) lists examples of typical variations for chromatography-based methods that are mostly not suitable for analysis of CBMPs where immunological methods are predominantly used. Nevertheless, stability of analytical solutions (e.g., stability of an antibody master mix) or flow rate (e.g., for flow cytometric analysis) are examples that are also applicable to the analysis of cell preparations. Further possible variations for flow cytometry could, for example, be the cell concentration of the sample to be analyzed (involving a variation in cell-to-antibody ratio), the total amount of analyzed events (this could be especially important when rare populations are analyzed, e.g., as impurities), a variation in incubation times and the time between antibody-staining of the cells and their analysis with the flow cytometer (either to validate a potential delay for the beginning of the measurement or because a huge number of samples has to be analyzed and/or measurement of one single tube takes a long time leading to a significant difference in holding times of individual samples). Also longer waiting times between cell harvest (e.g., by trypsinization) and analysis can potentially influence the result of an analytical procedure. It might also be advantageous to validate potential instrument break downs that either lead to a delayed processing and/or analysis or generate worst case scenarios for certain assay parameters (e.g., incubation temperature).

6.11.3 *System suitability test (SST)*

'*System suitability testing is an integral part of many analytical procedures. The tests are based on the concept that the equipment, electronics, analytical operations and samples to be analyzed constitute an integral system that can be evaluated as such. System suitability test parameters to be established for a particular procedure depend on the type of procedure being validated. See Pharmacopoeias for additional information.*' ICH Q2 (R1).[120]

The fundamentals for obtaining reliable and valid analytical results over the entire life cycle of an analytical procedure are instrument qualification and method validation (both conducted initially and repeated at least after significant changes following a change control procedure). But these basic GMP operations might not be sufficient for instruments with complex functionality that exhibit a higher relative standard deviation anyway and are susceptible even to small variations. In these cases, it might be necessary to assure that the instrument's performance is acceptable (according to the analyst's expectations and according to the criteria that are defined for a certain analytical procedure) at the time of the analysis.[122] Pharmacopoeias therefore request system suitability tests for some methods (e.g., chromatography-based methods and flow cytometry).

6.11.4 *Method transfer*

The transfer of analytical methods may appear in many forms during the product life span. It can include the transfer from the developing laboratory to the testing laboratory within the same company, expansion of manufacturing sites (intercompany transfers), transfer of developed process and methodology to a contract manufacturer or outsourcing of testing (intra-company transfers).

WHO guidelines on transfer of technology in pharmaceutical manufacturing (Annex 7)[123] define transfer of technology as '*a logical procedure that controls the transfer of any process together with its documentation and professional expertise between development and manufacture or between manufacture sites'.*

At the outset of any transfer activity, a written agreement between the transferring and receiving sites has to be put in place that defines the objective, scope, and responsibilities of the involved parties. An example on how responsibilities can be divided between the transferring and receiving units is given in the WHO guidelines and covers in detail, all essential steps of the method transfer. In some cases, a third managing site is involved in the transfer activities.

6.11.4.1 *Transfer of documentation/knowledge transfer*

The sending laboratory should provide the receiving laboratory with all documentation necessary to establish the method at the receiving site for the intended purpose: Test instructions, validation documentation, development documentation, and product-specific acceptance criteria. For the receiving site, it is very important to obtain an understanding, as thorough as possible, of the current state of the method and of its critical (or most variable) steps, as both have direct influence on the complexity of the transferring activities. For this, the support of the transferring laboratory is invaluable. WHO guidelines on transfer of technology in pharmaceutical manufacturing[123] point out that *'any lack of transparency may lead to ineffective transfer of technology'.*

6.11.4.2 *Criteria for the successful transfer*

Criteria for the successful transfer have to be defined and agreed on between both sites. The acceptance criteria for the method transfer are not necessarily identical to the criteria resulting from the method validation at the transferring site, and have to be assessed and defined in a risk-based approach. It has to be proved that the method as it is going to be transferred is in agreement with the MA or, for IMPs with the relevant IMPD. The original validation should be reviewed in the context of its compliance with current ICH requirements (compare EU GMP Guidelines, Chapter 6).[1] For pharmacopoeial methods, it is advisable to prove the compliance with the current Pharmacopeia edition. Furthermore, when the method transfer takes place between countries belonging to different regulatory zones, the Pharmacopeia requirements of the participants have to be compared and possible gaps identified. This analysis has to be made very early in the method transfer, since it can have great influence on the extent of the validation activities in the receiving laboratory. Ideally, this analysis is performed before the timelines and responsibilities of the receiving site are determined contractually.

6.11.4.3 *Gap analysis*

A gap analysis regarding the necessary personnel, equipment, and materials should be performed. All new equipment and materials have to be qualified before the formal method transfer begins.

6.11.4.4 *Staff training*

Participation of the transferring site in the personnel training of the method is very much advisable. It helps to establish an equivalent method performance at the receiving site and to introduce the personnel into the critical steps of the methods and little practical tricks that assure best performance.

6.11.4.5 *Written transfer plan*

A Written transfer plan should exist that specifies timelines, design, and extent of experiments as well as acceptance criteria for the method transfer. Usually both, transferring and receiving unit participate in the preparation of the transfer plan. At the least, both sides have to formally agree with the plan. After the execution of experiments, the results have to be summarized in the transfer report, which includes the description and (statistical) evaluation of the performed experiments, raw data, description and evaluation of the deviations occurred in the course of the method transfer. The deviations have to be elucidated and closed for the method release. The validation report has to be reviewed and approved by all involved sites.

6.11.4.6 *Execution*

Since most method transfers are unique, there is no common recipe for their execution. USP chapter <1224> "Transfer of analytical procedures"[124] describes different types of method transfers. We do not intend to repeat the pharmacopoeial text here, but briefly discuss the outlined methods with regard to their applicability for cell-based products.

- **Comparative testing** is the most commonly used strategy. In comparative testing, the same lot (or lots) of product is tested by both laboratories. When testing of the same lot is not feasible, for example due to short shelf life of the product or instability/limited availability of tested intermediate, different lots can be used and compared for their compliance with pre-determined acceptance criteria.

Although USP Chapter <1224> explicitly states that the analysis of one lot can be sufficient since not the manufacturing but the method is being evaluated, this has to be critically accessed in the case of cellular products, especially when alternative, non-pharmacopoeial techniques are transferred. Particularly for autologous products, the possible influence of the donor material on the end product should not be underestimated, and the variability of the tested material has to be sufficiently covered during the method transfer. It is not advisable to elucidate only "good" batches, since it can mask deficiencies of the method transfer and lead to OOS results due to analytical errors later on. Furthermore, in many cases one batch of the product might simply not be large enough to perform the whole set of planned experiments.

The test results have to be critically evaluated by the transferring unit. Formal compliance to acceptance criteria as well as all deviations and trends have to be carefully accessed. Where applicable, round robin tests can be used as supportive element to ensure the correct method performance.

- **Co-validation between two or more laboratories**. In this case, the transferring unit involves the receiving unit in the method validation activities, thus collecting the data for the reproducibility between the two (or more) sites.
- As indicated above, **revalidation or partial revalidation** of the method might be required. Most often, critical issues are the overall performance of the method, inter- and intra-laboratory precision, variability as well as specific points that may influence robustness. Furthermore, if trends are observed during the method transfer, their nature should be thoroughly elucidated since they may point out to systematic errors in the method performance, which are not obvious due to broad acceptance criteria or sub-optimal transfer design. For further details on method validation, see Section 6.11 (Validation of Analytical Procedures).
- **Transfer waiver**. Sometimes, the risk assessment might show that the generation of inter-laboratory experimental data can be omitted, for instance if the receiving laboratory already performs the validated method with a product of comparable composition or the pharmacopoeial analytical procedure is being transferred without modification. In this case, it is sufficient to show the successful method performance in the receiving laboratory. Also for some purely qualitative methods, the comparison between laboratories might not be necessary, since it does not provide any additional information. The protocols and training *via* the sending laboratory might thus be sufficient to implement the method. In any case, the justification of the transfer waiver and the formal release of the method by all involved sides must be existent in written form.

6.11.4.7 *Method transfer for CBMPs*

Method transfer in the field of cell therapies is often represented by extremes. Thus, the transfer of a complex, highly product-specific and unique protocol for the flow cytometric analysis might require a strategy that unites comparative testing with at least partial revalidation at the receiving site. Since flow cytometric analysis is subjective by nature and minimal differences in evaluation strategies may have great impact on the results, it is very important to perform extensive training of personnel and to clearly communicate the rationales and philosophy that lay behind the chosen evaluation strategy. If the transfer occurs between the developing laboratory and the GMP facility, a re-evaluation of the established protocol with regard to its compliance with GMP standards might be needed. Furthermore, technical characteristics of flow cytometers from different manufacturers may have more influence on the numerical parameters as expected; therefore it is almost unavoidable to perform at least partial revalidation, if identical instruments are not used in both laboratories. Obtained results must be subjected to a critical assessment by the transferring site.

On the other hand, for the analysis of stem and progenitor cells from peripheral blood, a complex flow cytometric method, which however is commonly used for medical applications and often established in experienced flow cytometric laboratories, the regular successful participation in the round robin tests deem sufficient to qualify the method if all other conditions are met (i.e., training is performed by trained personnel with a qualified equipment). Furthermore, product-specific cell-based semi-quantitative or qualitative tests are often applied for the analysis of cellular products which requires specific approaches for successful method transfer.

6.11.5 *Reference material and reference standards*

Reference standards are highly characterized physical specimens of drug substances, excipients, impurities, degradation products, and other substances that serve as a calibrated basis of comparison for substances of the same kind. Many pharmacopoeial assays require the use of a reference standard to prove identity, strength, quality, or purity of a test sample. Therefore, official reference standards are offered, for example, by the European and the US pharmacopoeial committees (EDQM Reference Standards in Europe and USP Reference Standards in the US). Also the WHO offers official reference standards.

Reference standards can be differentiated into primary and secondary. ICH guideline Q7[125] offers a definition for both types.

Primary Reference Standard: A substance that has been shown by an extensive set of analytical tests to be authentic material and should be of high purity. This standard can be: (1) Obtained from an officially recognized source, or (2) Prepared by independent synthesis, or (3) Obtained from existing production material of high purity, or (4) Prepared by further purification of existing production material.

Primary reference standards obtained from an officially recognized source are normally used without testing, if stored under conditions consistent with the supplier's recommendations.

Secondary Reference Standard: *A substance of established quality and purity, as shown by comparison to a primary reference standard, used as a reference standard for routine laboratory analysis.*

Secondary reference standards should be appropriately prepared, identified, tested, approved, and stored. The suitability of each batch of secondary reference standard should be determined prior to first use by comparing against a primary reference standard. Each batch of secondary reference standard should be periodically re-qualified in accordance with a written protocol.

Definitely reference standards are valuable measures to prove the quality of a certain type of analysis, to demonstrate that assays do not significantly change over time and to verify that a given sample meets the required specifications. But reference standards for CBMPs are of course not readily available from officially recognized sources. Nevertheless, many authorities and guidance documents (e.g., European Directive 2009/120/EC)[14] request a reference standard, relevant and specific for at least the finished product. In these cases, in-house primary reference standards have to be generated and appropriately tested for identity and purity.

But even preparation of in-house standards for cellular material can be challenging, as primary cells or tissues are quite variable with respect to their quality and not at all standardized, especially when autologous material is used. Reference standards might be processed from material of voluntary healthy donors in these cases. Also banking of cells from a healthy donor could be a possibility, although full comparability cannot be achieved with this approach. At least banked material can be used to demonstrate that test systems and analytical methods are working within the required ranges. When a reference standard for a finished cell-product is produced, the material has to be processed under absolutely controlled conditions and must pass all in-process controls and final release tests. Additional testing is required including tests that are usually not performed with the finished product to fully characterize the reference material. Stability is an additional issue that has to be addressed since reference standards are supposed to be used over longer periods of time and should not significantly change.

Stability and storage of reference material is a special issue whenever a CBMP is not cryopreserved. Reference standards that have to be cryopreserved for storage cannot be fully comparable to the medicinal product then, at least not with respect to characteristics like viability. Even identity might be compromised as some cell surface markers are up- or down-regulated due to freezing processes.

6.11.6 *Standards and controls*

6.11.6.1 *Principles*

Without appropriate controls — negative as well as positive controls — significance and validity of many analytical methods is poor. Apart from reference standards, different kinds of controls are needed for the performance and control of different test methods.

Reference standards are commonly used as positive controls to verify whether a test produces acceptable results. Whenever the specified result for a defined test method is negative (e.g., mycoplasma testing, endotoxin testing or testing for product and process related impurities), reference material cannot serve as positive control, thus artificial positive controls have to be used such as defined nucleic acid sequences for NAT-based technologies (e.g., DNA sequences specific for certain mycoplasma ssp. or vector/plasmid DNA sequences used for genetic modification), LPS for endotoxin testing, or non-target cells that could be part of the drug product as impurity.

For quantitative analytical test methods calibration standards are required. Examples are calibration standards for ELISA-based techniques, where several dilutions of a defined reference material are measured in order to generate a calibration line. Counting reference beads for single platform quantitative flow cytometric analysis that are added to the specimen in a known concentration and measured simultaneously with the cells, is another example.

Negative controls are needed for some test methods to discriminate negative from positive results. For ELISA-based techniques a blank is, for example, used as negative control to determine the optical density obtained by mere sample buffer Negative controls are especially important in flow cytometry for setting the right negative–positive-boundary. Isotype controls are most commonly used for these purposes. For more detailed information on isotype controls and other controls used in flow cytometry, compare the subsequent section 6.11.6.2.

For NAT-based methods, negative controls are important to demonstrate that results are not positive due to contaminations with nucleic acid sequences as single copies can be sufficient to obtain false positive results and especially plasmid DNA (if for example, used as control) is known to be sticky. The PCR master mix without the test sample serves as negative control in most assays. A further negative control for analysis of RNA could be a sample prepared without reverse transcriptase.

Additionally to the above mentioned positive and negative controls, standards are required for instrument set-up and/or performance check, for system suitability testing or calibration of the instrument. For system suitability testing, some companies offer appropriate fixed control cells in defined quantities (low, medium, and high) together with acceptance criteria that have to be met when the control cells are measured (e.g., for automated hematology analyzers). These control cells are used on a daily basis and meeting the acceptance criteria is a prerequisite to use the system for QC purposes.

6.11.6.2 *Standards and controls in flow cytometry*

USP chapter <1027> Flow Cytometry[26] provides a valuable overview on different types of standards and controls used for flow cytometric analysis. Some of the main issues for standards and controls as presented by this USP chapter are summarized below.

Standards

As flow cytometers are highly engineered and precise instruments based on laser technology, the optical alignment is essential for the quality and validity of the obtained results. For instrument set-up and calibration, accurate standards are required to maintain this precision. Microsphere-based fluorescence standards are therefore used that can be categorized by their purpose in three different types:

- Type I standards are alignment standards that are used to make adjustments to the instrument's optical alignment. These are typically used by field service engineers and by users of operator-adjusted systems to check the optical signal alignment in order to improve instrument sensitivity. These particles are typically small (∼2 mm) and bright, and they provide the most uniform illumination.
- Type II standards are reference beads and are the most commonly used bead standards. These typically are used on a daily basis, have dim to moderate fluorescence intensity, and can be obtained with various attached fluorophores. These can be used to mimic cells and, with dedicated software, to determine relative instrument sensitivity.
- Type III standards are used for fluorescence calibration. These are used for specialized applications that require calibration of one or more fluorescence detectors for quantitation of molecules of fluorochrome. Determination of the ratio of fluorophores to antibody (F/P ratio) allows subsequent calculation of the number of antibodies bound per cell.

Controls

Unlike the above mentioned standards that are required for instrument set-up and calibration, controls are needed to discriminate negative from positive signals. This is especially important in flow cytometry as false positive signals can originate from the use of too much antibody, from insufficient cell washing, from unspecific binding of antibody (e.g., due to inadequate blocking of Fc-receptors), from improper compensation or from improperly high instrument photomultiplier tubes (PMT) gain. Negative controls such as isotype or Fluorescence minus one (FMO) controls are necessary to demonstrate the characteristics of cells that are definitely negative for a certain marker.

In contrast false negative results can be generated from wrong or improper instrument parameters (poor laser alignment, improper compensation, improper setup, inconsistent gain settings, or weak laser output), from insufficient staining procedures or reagents (insufficient antibody concentration, poor reagent quality such as fluorochrome fading or degradation of tandem dyes) or from cell physiology (labile or secreted target antigen, or inaccessible target antigen). Positive controls can demonstrate that the assay (sample preparation in combination with instrument parameters) is able to produce reliable results.

Another reason for the importance of controls in flow cytometry is the way of data analysis. For most applications, gating is performed manually and the operator decides where to draw the boundary between positive and negative signals. Negative controls are therefore relevant independent reference points for gating.

Relevant controls in flow cytometry are (compare USP chapter <1027>):

- **Isotype controls**: An isotype control is a negative-control antibody that should not react with the antigen of interest and is the same isotype as the test antibody. Myeloma protein or immunoglobulin that has no specificity to the species being tested and has the same Ig chain class and sub-class as the test antibody is conjugated to a fluorochrome identical to that on the test antibody. Ideally, very little or no binding occurs when the isotype control is used in parallel with the test. Idiotypic non-specific binding frequently occurs, however, and is independent of the isotype of the antibody. This is most likely related to other differences in antibody chemistry and can be especially problematic with rare-event detection assays, such as those for HSC assays in peripheral blood.
- In addition to isotype controls, the European Pharmacopeia offers the possibility of using **isoclonic controls** (e.g., for numeration of HSCs).[28] In these cases, the unconjugated detection antibody is incubated with the test sample before staining with the fluorochrome-conjugated antibody. All epitopes should then be blocked with the unstained antibody (use of sufficient amount of antibody assumed) resulting in a negative population.
- **FMO controls** are used to control non-specific staining during a multicolor assay. After compensation has been set, a tube containing all of the fluorochrome-labeled antibodies, except one, is run. If the compensation has been properly

set, any positive fluorescence in the parameter corresponding to the missing fluorochrome-labeled antibody is caused by non-specific staining and can be an indication of excess antibody or degradation of related tandem dyes. Although FMO controls are very useful for estimating the sensitivity of a particular detector in the context of other reagents, the controls do not take into account non-specific binding that can occur with the addition of the test antibody. FMO control tubes are most appropriately used for troubleshooting or when establishing a new multicolor reagent cocktail.

- **Process controls**: Also known as system suitability standards, account for sample preparation and data acquisition. They can include commercially available preserved control cells, cell lines, or primary cells such as normal peripheral blood cells. Process controls can also be used to test new lots of antibody reagent against old lots.

- **Biological controls**: When treated or stimulated cells are compared to untreated or unstimulated cells, the untreated or unstimulated cells may in some cases be the most useful control for setting a positive/negative boundary. However, use of isotype controls may also apply to these situations, because stimulation may lead to Fc receptor up-regulation, leading in turn to increased background staining, the presence of which can be elucidated by an isotype control.

Calibration of the instrument with internal controls as well as the use of positive controls is also requested by the European Pharmacopoeia (Ph. Eur. 2.7.24. Flow Cytometry):[25] '*The system's optical alignment must be validated before analysis using adapted fluorospheres and the optimum fluidic stability is checked. The data obtained are reported and allow the periodical review of control values against the mean performance value. A positive control is highly desirable to prove that the test antibody is functional and to allow the proper setting of the flow cytometer. The positive control must include samples known to be positive for the marker of interest.*'

6.12 Deviation Management and OOS Results

The QC Department has different responsibilities in conjunction with deviation management:

- QC has to document and investigate all deviations occurring in its own department.

- QC might be involved in deviation management of other departments (particularly production) to evaluate the impact of a deviation on the quality of the product.

- QC has to participate in the investigation of any complaint that is related to the quality of the product. This can require QC of reference or retention samples or returned product.

Deviations within the QC department not necessarily have to but might lead to the generation of OOS results that have to be handled carefully. Every QC department therefore has to have a written procedure in place to handle results that do not comply with the defined specifications. The most important question to answer in this respect is the reason for the OOS result, as it is fundamental to know if the result is caused by analytical error or whether the result reflects the actual condition of the tested material or product. To clarify this, a root cause analysis has to be performed by the Head of QC or an authorized person with sufficient competence. The investigation must consider the original test reports as well as the information provided by the operator(s) who obtained the suspected result. Investigation of OOS results and a research regarding the cause of the OOS result is necessary even if a batch is rejected because of the result, as it has to be determined if the result is associated with other batches of the same product or even with other products.

Investigation of OOS results is requested by the EU GMP guidelines in the chapter Quality Control[1] as well as by the FDA regulations in §211.192 on production record review.[126]

FDA Guidance for Industry on "Investigating OOS Test Results for Pharmaceutical Production"[127] contains non-binding recommendations for handling OOS results. Specifically the guidance document discusses how to investigate OOS test results, including the responsibilities of laboratory personnel, the laboratory phase of investigation, additional testing that may be necessary, when to expand the investigation outside the laboratory, and the final evaluation of all test results.

The Official Medicines Control Laboratory (OMCL) guideline on the Evaluation and reporting of results[128] provides a model template for investigation of OOS results that is partially suitable for CTPs as well.

Phase I of the investigation should start with identifying and assessing the obtained OOS test result to determine whether the source of the result is an aberration of the measurement process or the manufacturing process. To address this question, it is essential to find out if one or more analytical errors occurred. Possible analytical errors are listed in Table 6.18. An assessment of QC data and reports including raw data and calculations should be included in the investigation, as well as information from QC personnel, especially the analyst who performed the suspected assay.

Table 6.18: Investigation of OOS results: List of possible analytical errors.

Investigation of OOS Results: Possible Analytical Errors

- System suitability test missing or failed.
- Instrument calibration missing.
- Wrong instrument parameters.
- Wrong instrument used.
- Deviation from the specified method.
- Wrong method used.

• Mistakes of general character.	✓ Solutions or reagents expired.
✓ Weighting error.	✓ Reagents not dissolved completely.
✓ Use of wrong reagents.	✓ Error during filtration.
✓ Improper storage of reagents.	✓ Carry-over of reagents.
✓ Improper storage of solutions.	
• Mistakes in result calculation.	✓ Wrong factor used.
✓ Calculation error.	✓ Data transfer error.
✓ Formula wrong.	
• Mistakes in pipetting or dilution.	✓ Dilution error.
✓ Pipetting device with wrong volume.	✓ Carry-over.
✓ Pipettes with wrong tips.	

- Environmental conditions (inadequate temperature, etc.).

If the investigation uncovers an obvious technical reason for the OOS result, it is permitted to invalidate the suspected result and repeat the analysis. In this case only the result obtained by the repeated assay is considered.

If phase I of the investigation does not reveal analytical errors and no reason for the OOS result is found, a full scale investigation is necessary. A review of the production and sampling procedure should be performed. If the investigation successfully identifies the root cause of the OOS result in the production process, the OOS investigation may be terminated and the product has to be rejected. If no reason is found in production and sampling, a repetition of the initial test and/or additional laboratory tests are necessary to either confirm the OOS test result or disprove it. In this case, the aspects listed in Table 6.19 have to be considered and predefined before laboratory tests are performed.

Unless invalidated, the initial OOS result is not rejected and it is included in the evaluation of the product. It is important that the number of replicates for retesting is defined in advance to avoid "testing into compliance". The number of retests must not be adjusted depending on the test results obtained.

Table 6.19: Points to consider for retesting and re-sampling in connection with investigations of OOS results.

Repetition of Analytical Test Procedures after an OOS Result: Points to Consider

- Is resampling necessary?
- If resampling is necessary: Does a different sampling procedure have to be applied?
- Definition of number of replicates (n) for retest (with $n = x$).[1]
- Must a different operator than the one that obtained the OOS result perform the test?
- Must different batches of reagents than those with which the OOS result was obtained be used?
- Must a different instrument of the same type than the one with which the OOS result was obtained be used (if more than one adequate instrument is available)?
- Must another lab with the same validated test method be included to analyze an aliquot of the same or a new sample?

Note: [1]None of the guidance documents prescribes a defined number of replicates but it is important that the number of replicates is based on scientifically sound principles. For conventional medicinal products the number of replicates is often defined as $n \geq 6$. For CBMPs even two or three replicates can be difficult or even impossible to realise as sample volume is often reduced to the absolute minimum quantity due to scarce overall amount of in-process control samples and finished product.

Retesting and/or re-sampling procedures can either confirm the OOS test result or disprove it. If the OOS result is confirmed the batch has to be rejected, if it is disproven that batch can be released.

If the initial test result cannot be invalidated because of an analytical error, it has to be defined which results are reported and whether an average value is calculated or whether all individual results, including the initial OOS test result are reported and considered in batch release decisions.

6.13 Round Robin and Proficiency Tests

Round robin tests are inter-laboratory analyses of aliquots of one and the same test sample performed by several independent operators in independent facilities. As every participating lab is using its own equipment and method (that might slightly differ from each other) round robin tests help to show reproducibility of a test method. For the individual lab, round robin tests are important to demonstrate that the combination of equipment, test method and personnel leads to reliable and correct results within acceptable limits. This kind of approach is particularly important for analytical procedures that lack adequate standard controls (what is the case for most cellular products), that are susceptible to bias of the operator (what holds true especially for flow cytometry) and with no commercially available certified reagents or test kits (what is especially true for new types of cell products).

However, round robin tests in cell therapy are problematic for three reasons:

- The types of material offered by different institutions (whole blood, leukapheresis, and fixed cells, etc.) often do not reflect the type of material that is processed for the CTMP, especially when GM or cultured cells would have to be examined.
- The types of cells that have to be analyzed for the round robin test are either not the cells that are analyzed for the cell product or represent only a small part of the analyzed cells (and in most cases these are not the critical populations).
- Cellular materials, at least if they are not fixed, are sensitive to temperature conditions and time of transport, occasionally leading to bad quality of the cells when arriving at the test sites. As the material is transported individually to every participating centre, these effects often occur at just one single site and as transport conditions are often uncontrolled, it is difficult to prove what happened. Hence it is advisable to include the analysis of control cells to demonstrate that the method itself in combination with equipment, reagents and personnel was able to achieve correct results on the day of round robin test analysis. Some of the institutions that offer round robin tests exclusively use fixed cells to circumvent problems with material of insufficient quality, but this changes the characteristics of the cells significantly (e.g., scatter characteristics in flow cytometry) and makes comparability to the test methods used routinely even harder. Furthermore, these samples cannot be used to test methods for the determination of vitality/viability.

Despite of all these disadvantages and problems many authorities attach importance to the participation in round robin tests and check the availability of the corresponding certificates during inspections regularly. The European Pharmacopoeia in Chapter 2.7.24 "Flow Cytometry"[25] also asks for external controls to ensure reliability in the data obtained or to check inter-laboratory reproducibility and recommends the participation in proficiency testing studies. USP <1027> Flow Cytometry[26] similarly recommends participation in a proficiency testing program that reflects the test menu. According to USP, this could range from a formal program such as the one administered by the College of American Pathologists (CAP) to simple sharing of specimens and analysis with another laboratory.

In summary, it is highly advisable to take part in this kind of control measures, at least for every type of analytical procedure that is performed, even if analyzed materials or cells do not fully correspond to the routine tests. Certificates are often valid for six months or even a year, whereas the tests are offered in more frequent intervals. Therefore, failing in one of the tests (e.g., because of bad quality of the test material) is not too severe. For new methods, it might be advisable to check different providers at the time of assay development or validation to be able to choose the best performing one for routine. Vendor qualification of the institutions that offer round robin tests is an important tool to avoid problems in advance.

References

1. EudraLex — The Rules Governing Medicinal Products in the European Union, Volume 4: Good manufacturing practice (GMP) Guidelines, Part I, Chapter 6: QC.
2. Liumbruno, G.M., *et al.* Reduction of the risk of bacterial contamination of blood components through diversion of the first part of the donation of blood and blood components. *Blood Transfus.* 7, 86–93 (2009).
3. Pietersz, R.N.I. Bacterial contamination in platelet concentrates. *Vox Sang.* 106(3), 256–283 (2014).
4. Haemovigilance Report of the Paul-Ehrlich-Institute 2010 - Assessment of the Reports of Serious Adverse Transfusion Reactions pursuant to Section 63 c AMG. Paul-Ehrlich-Institute, Federal Institute for Vaccines and Biomedicines.
5. de Korte, D., *et al.* Effects of skin disinfection method, deviation bag, and bacterial screening on clinical safety of platelet transfusions in the Netherlands. *Transfusion* 46(3), 476–485 (Mar 2006).
6. V27: Implementation of Predonation Sampling (Votum 27 des Arbeitskreises Blut: Einführung des Predonation Sampling). Federal Ministry of Health, Germany, Blood Working Party (2002).
7. Jacobs, M.R. Microbial contamination of hematopoietic progenitor and other regenerative cells used in transplantation and regenerative medicine. *Transfusion* 53, 2690–2696 (2013).
8. Clark, P., Trickett, A., Stark, D., *et al.* Factors affecting microbial contamination rate of cord blood collected for transplantation. *Transfusion* 52, 1770–1777 (2012).
9. Vanneaux, V., *et al.* Microbial contamination of BM products before and after processing: A report of incidence and immediate adverse events in 257 grafts. *Cytotherapy* 9(5), 508–513 (2007).
10. Jacobs, M.R., *et al.* Microbial contamination of hematopoietic progenitor and other regenerative cells used in transplantation and regenerative medicine. *Transfusion* 53(11), 2690–2696 (Nov 2013).
11. EudraLex- The Rules Governing Medicinal Products in the European Union, Volume 4: Good manufacturing practice (GMP) Guidelines, Part I, Annex 2: Manufacture of Biological Active Substances and Medicinal Products for Human Use.
12. ICH Q5D: Derivation and Characterisation of Cell Substrates used for Production of Biotechnological/Biological Products, ICH Harmonised Tripartite Guideline. International Conference on Harmonisation of Technical Requirements for Registration of Pharmaceuticals for Human Use.
13. USP General Chapter <1046> Cell and Gene Therapy Products, United States Pharmacopoeia. U.S. Pharmacopeial Convention.

14. Directive 2009/120/EC amending Directive 2001/83/EC on the Community code relating to medicinal products for human use as regards advanced therapy medicinal products. European Parliament and Council; September 14, 2009.

15. Note for Guidance on the quality, preclinical and clinical aspects of gene transfer medicinal products (CPMP/BWP/3088/99). The European Agency for the Evaluation of Medicinal Products, April 24, 2001.

16. Guideline on quality, non-clinical and clinical aspects of medicinal products containing GM cells (EMA/CAT/GTWP/671639/2008). European Medicines Agency, April 13, 2012.

17. Ph. Eur. Chapter 5.14. Gene transfer medicinal products for human use, European Pharmacopoeia. The European Directorate for the Quality of Medicines & Healthcare (EDQM).

18. Circular of Information for the Use of Cellular Therapy Products. Circular of Information for Cellular Therapy Products Task Force (September 2013). (Available at: http://www.aabb.org/aabbcct/coi/Pages/default.aspx).

19. Richtlinien zur Gewinnung von Blut und Blutbestandteilen und zur Anwendung von Blutpordukten (Haemotherapie). Bundesärztekammer im Einvernehmen mit dem Paul-Ehrlich-Institute.

20. Directive 2006/17/EC implementing Directive 2004/23/EC as regards certain technical requirements for the donation, procurement and testing of human tissues and cells. European Parliament and Council; 8.2.2006.

21. Qualification of Excipients for Use in Pharmaceuticals. International Pharmaceutical Excipients Council (IPEC), 2008.

22. USP General Chapter <1032> Design and development of biological assays, United States Pharmacopoeia. U.S. Pharmacopeial Convention.

23. Kingsley, M. Statistical practices in assay development and validation implementing proper statistical methods ensures the development of safe and effective assays. *IVD Technol.* (2005).

24. Little, T.A. Assay Development and Method Validation Essentials. *Biopharm International* 25(11), Nov 01 (2012).

25. Ph. Eur. Chapter 2.7.24. Flow Cytometry, European Pharmacopoeia. The European Directorate for the Quality of Medicines & Healthcare (EDQM).

26. USP General Chapter <1027> Flow Cytometry, United States Pharmacopoeia. U.S. Pharmacopeial Convention.

27. Ph. Eur. Chapter 2.7.29. Nucleated cell count and viability, European Pharmacopoeia. The European Directorate for the Quality of Medicines & Healthcare (EDQM).

28. Ph. Eur. Chapter 2.7.23. Numeration of CD34/CD45+ cells in haematopoietic products, European Pharmacopoeia. The European Directorate for the Quality of Medicines & Healthcare (EDQM).

29. Ph. Eur. Chapter 2.7.28. Colony-forming cell assay for human haematopoietic progenitor cells, European Pharmacopoeia. The European Directorate for the Quality of Medicines & Healthcare (EDQM).

30. Ph. Eur. Chapter 2.2.31. Electrophoresis, European Pharmacopoeia. The European Directorate for the Quality of Medicines & Healthcare (EDQM).

31. USP General Chapter <1056> Biotechnology-derived Articles- Polyacrylamide Gel Electrophoresis, United States Pharmacopoeia. U.S. Pharmacopeial Convention.

32. Ph. Eur. Chapter 2.2.54. Isoelectric focusing, European Pharmacopoeia. The European Directorate for the Quality of Medicines & Healthcare (EDQM).

33. USP General Chapter <1053> Biotechnology-derived Articles- Isoelectric focusing, United States Pharmacopoeia. U.S. Pharmacopeial Convention.

34. Ph. Eur. Chapter 2.6.21. Nucleic acid amplification techniques, European Pharmacopoeia. The European Directorate for the Quality of Medicines & Healthcare (EDQM).

35. USP General Chapter <1125> Nucleic Acid-Based Techniques- General, United States Pharmacopoeia. U.S. Pharmacopeial Convention.

36. USP General Chapter <1126> Nucleic Acid-Based Techniques- Extraction, Detection, and Sequencing, United States Pharmacopoeia. U.S. Pharmacopeial Convention.

37. USP General Chapter <1127> Nucleic Acid-Based Techniques- Amplification, United States Pharmacopoeia. U.S. Pharmacopeial Convention.

38. USP General Chapter <1128> Nucleic Acid-Based Techniques- Microarray, United States Pharmacopoeia. U.S. Pharmacopeial Convention.

39. USP General Chapter <1129> Nucleic Acid-Based Techniques- Genotyping, United States Pharmacopoeia. U.S. Pharmacopeial Convention.

40. USP General Chapter <1130> Nucleic Acid-Based Techniques- Approaches for Detecting Trace Nucleic Acids (Residual DNA Testing), United States Pharmacopoeia. U.S. Pharmacopeial Convention.

41. USP General Chapter <766> Optical Microscopy, United States Pharmacopoeia. U.S. Pharmacopeial Convention.

42. Ph. Eur. Chapter 2.9.37. Optical Microscopy, European Pharmacopoeia. The European Directorate for the Quality of Medicines & Healthcare (EDQM).

43. Guideline on Human CBMPs, EMEA/CHMP/410869/2006. European Medicines Agency, May 21, 2008.

44. ICH Q6B: Specifications: Test Procedures and Acceptance Criteria for Biotechnological/Biological Products, ICH Harmonised Tripartite Guideline. International Conference on Harmonisation of Technical Requirements for Registration of Pharmaceuticals for Human Use.

45. EudraLex- The Rules Governing Medicinal Products in the European Union, Volume 4: Good manufacturing practice (GMP) Guidelines, Part I, Chapter 4: Documentation.

46. Guideline on Potency Testing of Cell Based Immunotherapy Medicinal Products for the Treatment of Cancer (EMEA/CHMP/BWP/271475/2006). European Medicines Agency, October 10, 2007.

47. Bravery, C.A., et al. Potency assay development for cellular therapy products: An ISCT review of the requirements and experiences in the industry. *Cytotherapy* 15(1), 9–19 (Jan 2013).

48. Montag, T., et al. Microbial safety of cell based medicinal products — What can we learn from cellular blood components? *Clin. Chem. Lab. Med.* 46(7), 963–965 (2008).

49. Störmer, M., et al. Bacterial safety of cell-based therapeutic preparations, focusing on haematopoietic progenitor cells. *Vox Sang.* 106, 285–296 (2014).

50. Akan, O.A., and Yildiz, E. Comparison of the effect of delayed entry into 2 different blood culture systems (BACTEC 9240 and BacT/ALERT 3D) on culture positivity. *Diagn. Microbiol. Infect. Dis.* 54(3), 193–196 (Mar 2006).

51. Montag, T., Störmer, M., and Schurig, U. Probleme der mikrobiellen Sicherheit bei neuartigen Therapien - Die Quadratur des Kreises. *Bundesgesundheitsbl* 53, 45–51 (2010).

52. Draft Guidance for Industry: Validation of Growth-Based Rapid Microbiological Methods for Sterility Testing of Cellular and Gene Therapy Products. U.S. Department of Health and Human Services, Food and Drug Administration, Center for Biologics Evaluation and Research, February 2008.

53. Parenteral Drug Association (PDA), [Hrsg]. PDA Technical Report No. 33: Evaluation, Validation and Implementation of Alternative and Rapid Microbiological Methods. October 2013. ISBN: 9780939459636.

54. Duguid, J., Balkovic, E., and du Moulin, G.C. Rapid Microbiological Methods: Where Are They Now? *Am. Pharm. Rev.* 14(7) (Nov/Dec 2011).

55. Caro, O., *et al.* Bacteria detection by flow cytometry. *Clin. Chem. Lab. Med.* 46(7), 947–953 (2008).

56. Montag, T. Strategies of bacteria screening in cellular blood components. *Clin. Chem. Lab. Med.* 46(7), 926–932 (2008).

57. Parveen, S., *et al.* Evaluation of growth based rapid microbiological methods for sterility testing of vaccines and other biological products. *Vaccine* 29(45), 8012–8023 (Oct 19, 2011).

58. Ph. Eur. Chapter 2.6.8. Pyrogens, European Pharmacopoeia. The European Directorate for the Quality of Medicines & Healthcare (EDQM).

59. USP General Chapter <151> Pyrogen Test, United States Pharmacopoeia. U.S. Pharmacopeial Convention.

60. Guidance for Industry: Pyrogen and Endotoxins Testing: Questions and Answers. U.S. Department of Health and Human Services, Food and Drug Administration (FDA), June 2012.

61. Spreitzer, I., *et al.* 10 years of experience with alternative pyrogen tests (monocyte activation tests). *AATEX 14, Special Issue; Proc. 6th World Congress on Alternatives & Animal Use in the Life Sciences, Tokyo, Japan.* August 21–25, 2007, 587–589.

62. Montag, T, *et al.* Safety testing of CBMPs: Opportunities for the monocyte activation test for pyrogens. *ALTEX* 24(2), 81–89 (2007).

63. Schindler, S., *et al.* Development, validation and applications of the monocyte activation test for pyrogens based on human whole blood. *ALTEX* 26(4), 265–277 (2009).

64. Ph. Eur. Chapter 2.6.30. Monocyte-activation test, European Pharmacopoeia. The European Directorate for the Quality of Medicines & Healthcare (EDQM).

65. Koryakina, A., Frey, E., and Bruegger, P. Cryopreservation of human monocytes for pharmacopeial monocyte activation test. *J. Immunol. Methods* 405, 181–191 (2014).

66. Ph. Eur. Chapter 2.6.14. Bacterial Endotoxins, European Pharmacopoeia. The European Directorate for the Quality of Medicines & Healthcare (EDQM).

67. USP General Chapter <85> Bacterial Endotoxins Test, United States Pharmacopoeia. U.S. Pharmacopeial Convention.

68. EudraLex- The Rules Governing Medicinal Products in the European Union, Volume 4: Good manufacturing practice (GMP) Guidelines, Part I, Chapter 7: Outsourced Activities.

69. Janetzko, K., *et al.* A single-tube real-time PCR assay for mycoplasma detection as a routine QC of cell therapeutics. *Transfus. Med. Hemother.* 41, 83–89 (2014).

70. Ph. Eur. Chapter 2.6.7. Mycoplasma, European Pharmacopoeia. The European Direc-
    torate for the Quality of Medicines & Healthcare (EDQM).
71. USP General Chapter <63> Mycoplasma Test, United States Pharmacopoeia. U.S.
    Pharmacopeial Convention.
72. Guidance for Industry: Characterization and Qualification of Cell Substrates and Other
    Biological Materials Used in the Production of Viral Vaccines for Infectious Disease
    Indications. U.S. Department of Health and Human Services, Food and Drug Admin-
    istration, Center for Biologics Evaluation and Research, February 2010.
73. 21 CFR 610.30: Test for Mycoplasma . U.S. Food and Drug Administration, Depart-
    ment of Health and Human Services Bde. Code of Federal Regulations, Title 21,
    Volume 7 (April 2014).
74. Nims, R.W., and Meyers, E. USP <63> mycoplasma tests: A new regulation for
    mycoplasma testing, what you need to know about USP chapter <63>. *BioPharm.
    Int.* 23(8) (Aug 1, 2010).
75. Volokhov, D.V., *et al.* Mycoplasma testing of cell substrates and biologics: Review of
    alternative non-microbiological techniques. *Mol. Cell. Probes.* 25(2–3), 69–77 (Apr–Jun
    2011).
76. WHO Technical Report Series, No. 902. World Health Organisation, WHO Expert
    Committee on Specifications for Pharmaceutical Preparations (2002).
77. Riegel, M. Human molecular cytogenetics: From cells to nucleotides. *Genet. Mol. Biol.*
    37(Suppl 1), 194–209 (Mar 2014).
78. Schrock, E., *et al.* Multicolor spectral karyotyping of human chromosomes. *Science*
    273(5274), 494–497 (Jul 26, 1996).
79. Barkholt, L., *et al.* Risk of tumorigenicity in mesenchymal stromal cell-based therapies-
    bridging scientific observations and regulatory viewpoints. *Cytotherapy* 15(7), 753–759
    (Jul 2013).
80. Lefort, N., *et al.* Human embryonic cells and genomic instability. *Regen. Med.* 4(6),
    899–909 (2009).
81. Ben-David, U., and Benvenisty, N. Analyzing the genomic integrity of stem cells.
    StemBook [Internet]. Cambridge, MA· Harvard Stem Cell Institute (Jun 10, 2008–
    2012).
82. Zimmermann, S., *et al.* Lack of telomerase activity in human mesenchymal stem cells.
    Leukemia 17, 1146–1149 (2003).
83. Bieback, K., *et al.* Replicative aging and differentiation potential of human adipose
    tissue-derived mesenchymal stromal cells expanded in pooled human or fetal bovine
    serum. *Cytotherapy* 14(5), 570–583 (May 2012).
84. Karimi, T., *et al.* Study of telomerase activity, proliferation and differentiation charac-
    teristics in umbilical cord blood mesenchymal stem cells. *Iranian J. Vet. Res., Shiraz
    Univ.* 13(3), 176–185 (2012).
85. Shibata, *et al.* Expression of the p16INK4A gene is associated closely with senescence
    of human mesenchymal stem cells and is potentially silenced by DNA methylation
    during *in vitro* expansion. *Stem Cells* 25(9), 2371–2382 (Sep 2007).
86. Boozer, S., *et al.* Global Characterization and Genomic Stability of Human MultiStem,
    a Multipotent Adult Progenitor Cell. *J. Stem Cells* 4, 17–28 (2009).
87. Kim, J., *et al.* Biological characterization of long-term cultured human mesenchymal
    stem cells. *Arch. Pharm. Res.* 32(1), 117–126 (Jan 2009).

88. Wieser, M., *et al.* Nuclear flow FISH: Isolation of cell nuclei improves the determination of telomere lengths. *Exp. Gerontol.* 41(2), 230–235 (Feb 2006).

89. Hacein-Bey-Abina, S., *et al.* LMO2-associated clonal T-cell proliferation in two patients after gene therapy for SCID-X1. *Science* 302, 415–419 (2003).

90. Boztug, K., *et al.* Stem-cell gene therapy for the Wiskott–Aldrich syndrome. *N. Engl. J. Med.* 363, 1918–1927 (2010).

91. Cavazzana-Calvo, M., *et al.* Transfusion independence and HMGA2 activation after gene therapy of human β-thalassaemia. *Nature* 467(7313), 318–322 (Sep 16, 2010).

92. Baker, *et al.* Adaptation to culture of human embryonic stem cells and oncogenesis *in vivo. Nat. Biotechnol.* 25(2) (February 2007).

93. Varela, *et al.* Recurrent genomic instability of chromosome 1q in neural derivatives of human embryonic stem cells. *J. Clin. Investig.* 122(2), 569–574 (2012).

94. Mayshar, Y., *et al.* Identification and classification of chromosomal aberrations in human induced pluripotent stem cells. *Cell Stem Cell* 7(4), 521–531 (Oct 8, 2010).

95. Pasi, *et al.* Genomic instability in induced stem cells. *Cell Death Differ.* 18, 745–753 (2011).

96. Hussein, S.M., *et al.* Copy number variation and selection during reprogramming to pluripotency. *Nature* 471(7336), 58–62 (Mar 3, 2011).

97. Laurent, *et al.* Dynamic changes in the copy number of pluripotency and cell proliferation genes in human ESCs and iPSCs during reprogramming and time in culture. *Cell Stem Cell* 8, 106–118 (2011).

98. Ge, J., Cai, H., and Tan, W.S. Chromosomal stability during *ex vivo* expansion of UCB CD34+ cells. *Cell Prolif.* 44(6), 550–557 (2011).

99. Wang, *et al.* Outgrowth of a transformed cell population derived from normal human BM mesenchymal stem cell culture. *Cytotherapy* 7(6), 509–519 (2005).

100. Torsvik, A., *et al.* Spontaneous malignant transformation of human mesenchymal stem cells reflects cross-contamination: Putting the research field on track-letter. *Cancer Res.* 70(15), 6393–6396 (Aug 1, 2010).

101. Garcia, S., *et al.* Pitfalls in spontaneous *in vitro* transformation of human mesenchymal stem cells. *Exp. Cell Res.* 316, 1648–1650 (2010).

102. Bernardo, *et al.* Human bone-marrow derived mesenchymal stem cells do not undergo transformation after long-term *in vitro* culture and do not exhibit telomere maintenance. *Cancer Res.* 67, 9142–9149 (2007).

103. Meza-Zepeda, L.A., *et al.* High-resolution analysis of genetic stability of human adipose tissue stem cells cultured to senescence. *J. Cell. Mol. Med.* 12(2), 553–563 (Apr 2008).

104. Villa, A., *et al.* Long-term molecular and cellular stability of human neural stem cell lines. *Exp. Cell Res.* 294(2), 559–570 (Apr 1, 2004).

105. Guidance for Industry: Sterile Drug Products Produced by Aseptic Processing- Current Good Manufacturing Practice. U.S. Department of Health and Human Services, Food and Drug Administration, 2004.

106. EudraLex- The Rules Governing Medicinal Products in the European Union, Volume 4: Good manufacturing practice (GMP) Guidelines, Part I, Annex 19: Reference and Retention Samples.

107. EudraLex- The Rules Governing Medicinal Products in the European Union, Volume 4: Good manufacturing practice (GMP) Guidelines, Part I, Annex 13: Investigational Medicinal Products.

108. V34: Look Back procedures (Votum 34 des Arbeitskreises Blut: Verfahren zur Rück-verfolgung [Look Back]). Federal Ministry of Health, Germany, Blood Working Party, 2006.

109. Directive 2003/63/EC amending Directive 2001/83/EC on the Community code relating to medicinal products for human use. European Parliament and Council, June 25, 2003.

110. Guidance for Industry: Guidance for Human Somatic Cell Therapy and Gene Therapy. U.S. Department of Health and Human Services, Food and Drug Administration.

111. ICH Q1A (R2): Stability Testing of New Drug Substances and Products, ICH Harmonised Tripartite Guideline. International Conference on Harmonisation of Technical Requirements for Registration of Pharmaceuticals for Human Use.

112. ICH Q5C: Stability Testing of Biotechnological/Biological Products, ICH Harmonised Tripartite Guideline. International Conference on Harmonisation of Technical Requirements for Registration of Pharmaceuticals for Human Use.

113. ICH Q1B: Stability Testing: Photostability Testing of New Drug Substances and Products, ICH Harmonised Tripartite Guideline. International Conference on Harmonisation of Technical Requirements for Registration of Pharmaceuticals for Human Use.

114. ICH Q1C: Stability Testing of New Dosage Forms, ICH Harmonised Tripartite Guideline. International Conference on Harmonisation of Technical Requirements for Registration of Pharmaceuticals for Human Use.

115. ICH Q1D: Bracketing and Matrixing Designs for Stability Testing of New Drug Substances and Products, ICH Harmonised Tripartite Guideline. International Conference on Harmonisation of Technical Requirements for Registration of Pharmaceuticals for Human Use.

116. ICH Q1E: Evaluation of Stability Data, ICH Harmonised Tripartite Guideline. International Conference on Harmonisation of Technical Requirements for Registration of Pharmaceuticals for Human Use.

117. ICH Q3A (R2): Impurities in New Drug Substances, ICH Harmonised Tripartite Guideline. International Conference on Harmonisation of Technical Requirements for Registration of Pharmaceuticals for Human Use.

118. Note for Guidance on In-use stability testing of human medicinal products (CPMP/QWP/2934/99). The European Agency for the Evaluation of Medicinal Products, March 1, 2001.

119. Note for Guidance on maximum shelf-life for sterile products for human use after first opening or following reconstitution (CPMP/QWP/159/96corr). The European Agency for the Evaluation of Medicinal Products, January 28, 1998.

120. ICH Q2 (R1): Validation of Analytical Procedures: Text and Methodology, ICH Harmonised Tripartite Guideline. International Conference on Harmonisation of Technical Requirements for Registration of Pharmaceuticals for Human Use.

121. ORA Laboratory Manual, Volume III, Other Lab Operations, Section 4- Laboratory Applications of Statistical Concepts. U.S. Department of Health and Human Services, Food and Drug Administration, FDA Office of Regulatory Affairs, Office of Regulatory Science, 2013.

122. USP General Chapter <1058> Analytical Instrument Qualification, United States Pharmacopoeia. U.S. Pharmacopeial Convention.

123. WHO guidelines on transfer of technology in pharmaceutical manufacturing, Annex 7, WHO Technical Report Series, No. 961. 2011.

124. USP General Chapter <1224> Transfer of the analytical procedures, United States Pharmacopoeia. U.S. Pharmacopeial Convention.

125. ICH Q7: Good Manufacturing Practice Guide for Active Pharmaceutical Ingredients, ICH Harmonised Tripartite Guideline. International Conference on Harmonisation of Technical Requirements for Registration of Pharmaceuticals for Human Use.

126. Records and Reports, Section 211.192: Production record review. *Part 211- Current Good Manufacturing Practice for Finished Pharmaceuticals*. U.S. Department of Health and Human Services, Food and Drug Administration. Bde. Code of Federal Regulations, Title 21, Volume 4.

127. Guidance for Industry: Investigation Out-of-Specification (OOS) Test Results for Pharmaceutical Production. U.S. Department of Health and Human Services, Food and Drug Asministration, 2006.

128. OMCL Guideline on the evaluation and reporting of results. EDQM- The European Directorate for the Quality of Medicines & Healthcare. PA/PH/OMCL (7) 28 DEF CORR.

Cell Banking 7

Elena Meurer

7.1 Introduction and Overview

Development of appropriate banking strategies is highly relevant for cell-based products, mainly because it secures the availability of the product independent of the patients' status, and in amounts mandatory and sufficient to serve the market after marketing authorization (MA).

In contrast to chemically synthesized pharmaceutical products and biologics that are not dependent on the primary cell material, the batch size of cellular products often represents just one or a few individual therapeutic doses. The reasons for the small batch size are the absolutely restricted availability of blood and tissue used as a starting material, the limited capacity of adult primary cells to propagate, and sometimes the low abundance of the target cell type in the starting material. Frequent changeover of the primary starting material taken together with its high batch-to-batch variability affect the homogeneity and may influence the quality of the final product, especially because the manufacturing process is often complex, elaborate, and manual. The appropriate upscale solutions have not yet been developed for all cell types of interest. While suspension cells generally appear less problematic for up-scaling, large-scale production of adherent cells with specific requirements for an attachment surface might represent a challenge. A well-known example is human mesenchymal stem cells (MSCs), which are large in comparison to most of other cells *in vitro* and thus require large cultivation surface. Different solutions have been employed to increase the cultivation space, starting from the simple increase in quantity of cultivation flasks and development of compact multi-layer 2D systems to the utilization of bioreactors on the basis of micro–carriers or complex 3D-matrices (for more information on up-scaling, see chapter 'Process

Development and Manufacturing'). These diverse strategies are associated with different biological restrictions, and there seems to be no universal, well-accepted technological solution at the moment. Thus, in addition to the problem of small batches, the production of large uniform cell quantities, which is the basis of any classical cell banking, can be technologically tricky and tedious.

So far, the most extensive clinical experience comes from the banking of blood preparations, where different approaches have been established and proven successful. The banking can be performed for an individual patient or for the public use with the entry in the national and international registries. The examples of the individual banking are autologous banking of hematopoietic stem cells (HSCs), directed cord blood banking, and genetically modified HSCs. The public banks store cell material, (blood components, HSCs from cord blood and other sources) for the allogeneic use. Bone marrow or mobilized peripheral blood stem cells (PBSCs) for allogeneic transplantation are usually not banked, but the donors are registered, pertaining to certain selection criteria. Typically, only one batch of the final product is prepared for one patient. Moreover, the cell dose obtained from one batch of the stored material (such as cord blood unit for the HSC transplantation) does not always appear sufficient for an adult patient, so that transplants combined from two units might be required.[1] The quality criteria for the release of the blood preparations are minimally cell enumeration and infectious diseases markers. The analysis of ABO blood group, the human leukocyte antigen (HLA) markers and sometimes other genetic markers before storage, constitute the basis for the allogeneic use of the banked product. Even though these parameters are not required for the autologous application, they are usually analyzed and used for the identity control. This also allows for eventual redirecting of the stored material from the originally defined recipient to the public use, the hybrid strategy utilized by some banks. Further quality parameters might be required to secure comparable quality between the banks, and to improve the selection of units with high engraftment rate after transplantation.[2,3]

In contrast to HSCs, the proliferation potential of MSCs can be relatively easily exploited *in vitro*. A number of clinical studies have been performed with MSCs or its sub-populations isolated from different sources. It is absolutely essential to introduce the banking system at the latest by the time of clinical approbation of the cellular product in the Phase III, whereas the cell number required for clinical phases I and II can be achievable even otherwise. Exemplarily, in the Phase II studies with the allogeneic MSC-based product Remestemcel-L (Prochymal®, Osiris Therapeutics, Inc., Columbia, MD, US) used in acute graft-versus-host disease (aGvHD), four and six bone marrow aspirates were expanded to treat 12 and 32 patients, respectively. The proliferation potential of MSCs was substantially stretched for the recently completed Phase III (up to 10,000 doses from one bone marrow donor).[4] It has been widely discussed, whether this could be one of the factors that negatively influenced the clinical efficacy of the Phase III in comparison to earlier clinical studies,[5] especially since the correlation of the MSC expansion with the survival rate has earlier been shown.[6]

Another example is MultiStem®, an allogeneic off-the-shelf product consisting of multipotent adult progenitor cells (MAPCs), a primitive population with high proliferating capacities within a stromal cell compartment. This product has been tried in clinical studies for multiple therapeutic applications.[7] The cells obtained from a single donor are characterized and banked. A master cell bank (MCB) and working cell bank (WCB) system is used to produce more than hundreds of thousands of doses from each banked starting material.[7] Clear advantages of this approach are the great quantity and homogeneity of the obtained product. However, this is a rather rare example in the field of cell therapy, as most of today's manufacturing protocols for different cell types allow for just one or a few doses being made from a single starting material.

7.2 Definitions and Guidelines

The features of the starting material greatly influence the features of banking of cell therapeutics, be it the banking of processed blood and tissue or of *in vitro* cultured primary cells. In fact, the typical cell bank system, as we know it for virus or antibody production, can be applied only when the starting material possesses a substantial proliferation potential or this potential is increased *via* chemical or genetic modifications of cells. As already mentioned above, the examples of such cell therapeutics are scarce. The International Conference on Harmonization (ICH) Q5D even states that "primary cells are not banked".[8]

USP chapter ⟨1046⟩ "Cellular and tissue-based products" defines a cell bank as follows:

> "A cell bank is a collection of cells obtained from pooled cells or derived from a single cell clone or donor tissue that is stored in bags or vials, under defined conditions, which maintain genotypic and phenotypic stability. The cell bank system usually consists of a MCB and a WCB, although alternative approaches are possible".[9]

The recommendations for banking of cell material as given in "Guideline on human cell-based medicinal products" (EU):

> "Where cell lines are used, an appropriately characterized MCB and WCB should be established, whenever possible. Cell banking and characteri-

zation and testing of the established cell banks should comply with the ICH guideline Q5D".[10]

ICH Q5D "Quality of Biotechnological Products: Derivation and Characterization of Cell Substrates used for Production of Biotechnological/Biological Products" gives definition of a cell bank as "a collection of appropriate containers, whose contents are of uniform composition, stored under defined conditions. Each container represents an aliquot of a single pool of cells".[8]

Thus, the establishment of a typical cell bank presumes the homogeneity or even the clonal origin of cell material, known for continuous cell lines and hardly applicable for cell lines with a finite *in vitro* life span. Therefore, as an alternative to the classical two-tiered banking approach, other storage strategies can be developed and utilized for cellular products. Even though primary cells are not addressed in ICH Q5D, the general considerations described in its Annex I "Primary Cell Substrates" can be applied to establish an appropriate protocol for storage of primary cell material.

7.3 MCB and WCB

The typical cell bank is two-tiered (consisting of MCB and WCB) or one-tiered (MCB only). The MCB represents aliquots of homogenous cell material obtained from a qualified primary source or from a preliminary cell bank. These aliquots may serve to derive a WCB by means of cell propagation. The WCB is then used to obtain a final product. Sometimes, in early clinical phases, the cells of the MCB are also used to manufacture the final product, and only later to create a WCB. In the one-tiered system, the MCB is directly used to make the product.

The ICH Q5D and USP ⟨1046⟩ give detailed recommendations on qualification, manufacturing and testing of cell banks. Comprehensive and as complete as possible documentation of the bank history, such as origin and qualification of the starting material and description of all manipulations performed with cells before the creation of the MCB, is central for the bank qualification. The use of cell lines with the laboratory history as a basis of a cell bank dramatically complicates the bank characterization in terms of both safety and traceability. As requirements for product characterization increase with advance of its clinical approbation, it is advisable to address the characterization of the MCB as early as possible to assure its full compliance and to avoid the unfavorable situation, where a new MCB has to be created in order to enter later clinical phases.

The requirements on procurement and characterization of blood and tissue as starting material for cell-based therapeutics are extensively described in the chapter 'Quality Control', and will not be repeated in this chapter.

Safety testing is one of the central aspects of cell bank characterization. Usually, the full assessment of adventitious agents and endogenous viruses is performed on the MCB. The safety testing of WCB mostly includes analysis of microbial and viral contaminations that could be introduced during the WCB manufacturing, and end-of-production safety testing. The recommendations for testing of viral safety are described in ICH Q5A "Viral Safety Evaluation of Biotechnology Products Derived from Cell Lines of Human or Animal Origin" and can be applied to cell therapeutics as well.[11]

The testing of MCB/WCB may also pose significant costs and time constraints. According to USP chapter ⟨1046⟩, tests for identity, sterility, purity, viability, and the presence of viruses and mycoplasma represent minimal requirements for MCB and WCB testing. However, the qualification of cell banks usually goes beyond these characteristics. The pivotal consideration is which of the parameters are necessary and sufficient to ensure that the MCB or WCB will serve as a safe and reliable source of a cellular product of required quality. These criteria should be reflected in an MCB/WCB specification. Beside the parameters mentioned above, usual subjects of characterization are cellular age (minimally expressed as population doublings or number of sub-cultivations), growth kinetics, genetic stability (on molecular or chromosomal level), morphologic or phenotypic assessment, specific biochemical, functional, and immunological markers.

7.4 Alternative Banking Strategies. Banking of Blood and Tissue as a Source of Therapeutic Cells

If only a few therapeutic doses can be made from one batch of starting material, there is often no possibility or strict need to bank the starting material or product intermediates. However, since banking may facilitate manufacturing and commercialization of cellular products in many respects, it is an attractive alternative to the manufacturing from "fresh" material followed by immediate product application.

It, however, requires a principally different approach toward the storage of material. The most common example of such an approach is the banking of HSC preparations from blood and tissue, i.e., collection and storage of material from different donations with shared quality specifications. Instead of uniformity or clonality, the diversity of the stored material is utilized here to the great advantage, as it allows for selecting the best available HLA-match from a large amount of units.

This banking strategy that became widely accepted in the transplantation field also appears attractive for a broad range of novel cell-based therapeutic applications. Due to the donor-specific variability of blood and tissue, the characterization of the starting material as well as of resulting cell preparations gets special significance. The banking implies that either any of the banked units or that suitable for the particular application material which is selected on the basis of material specifications can be equally used. Thus, specifications have to be set, such as, to enable the manufacturing of samples of equal quality, despite the original diversity, and/or to recognize the diversity of samples. This requires an extensive analysis of comparability of starting materials and deep scientific understanding of quality requirements. Ideally, the product requirements have to be understood so well as to allow for a successful pre-selection of the starting material in form of a product-specific material specification.

This is one of the factors that impede the universal use of existing blood and tissue banks at the moment. Due to complicated ethical and regulatory access to blood and tissue as a source of cell therapeutics, the world-wide existing HSC banks appear to be an attractive platform, also for other cell-based products. This approach may be feasible for MSC that can be cryopreserved as a part of the same fraction of starting material. However, it has to be kept in mind that cellular preparations from these banks are manufactured and tested with the primary goal to serve as the source of HSC. Although the extent of manipulations that lead to cryo-conservation of samples might be very diverse (i.e., supplementation with cryopreservation solution, erythrocyte depletion, and cell fractionation), they are all optimized for preservation of functional HSC. Consequently, the specifications of the HSC preparations are fitted to the requirements of stem cell transplantation and might not be sufficient or optimal for ATMP applications. Furthermore, the quality of the stored material offered by existing private banks may significantly differ and the best-practice standards are not necessarily followed. Therefore, it might be worth investing in the development of optimal purification and storage procedures for specific cell fractions with specifications and functional tests best suitable for a particular product.

Also other banking strategies such as storage of pooled material (analog to pooled platelet units) or processing of starting material to a cellular intermediate prior aliquoting and banking may be considered for large-scale cell storage. The specifics of these strategies have to be reflected in the bank characterization. The use of pooled material might require special safety considerations due to potential risk of distribution of adventitious agents. For example, the parameters such as maximal pool size must be connected to the sensitivity of methods used for viral and microbial control. Since the pooling of cell products is still not established and generally accepted, this approach, if chosen, should be extensively discussed with the regulatory agencies.

In all cases, following general requirements are valid:

- All aspects of donation and testing of blood and tissue as starting material for manufacturing of cell-based therapeutic products have to comply with regulations (see chapter 'Quality Control').
- Specifications of the starting material might be necessary to include product-specific parameters.
- All manipulations performed prior banking have to take place under manufacturing license according to cGMP requirements.
- The assessment of all critical materials should be made and the materials appropriately qualified and tested.
- The banking system has to be defined and described, including the listing and qualification of all ancillary materials, size of the bank, primary containers, and closure systems. The configuration and size of a bank must be suitable for planned clinical studies or to serve the market after MA, as legally required.
- Manufacturing process of the banked material must be validated.
- The extensive testing according to defined quality specifications must be performed (following the recommendations of ICH Q5D or its Annex I "Primary Cell Substrates").
- The storage period must be defined and the applicability of the bank material at the end of the storage period has to be shown (stability study).
- All aspects of the cryo-conservation process, in-use stability, shelf-life and logistics must be carefully evaluated and defined.

7.5   Summary

The definition of a specific banking strategy as part of the up-scaling is of pivotal importance for bringing cell-based therapeutics into the market and to provide robust and stable products to the patient. Since qualitatively comparable, off-the-shelf cellular products is one of the most credible means to make cell therapies available to all social classes of patients enforcing the need for development of appropriate banking strategies.

The off-the-shelf availability may be achieved through individual manufacturing of patient-specific products, allogeneic banking of the final product or *via* establishment of a MCB and WCB with further cell expansion to the final product. The access to human starting material, the traceability and testing of starting material, intermediates and end product and the up-scaling technology in the field of cell and gene therapy are often defined on a case-by-case basis. Therefore, the advice from competent authorities is recommended.

References

1. Petrini, C. Umbilical cord blood banking: From personal donation to international public registries to global bioeconomy. *J. Blood Med.* 5, 87–97 (2014).
2. Querol, S., Gomez, S.G., Pagliuca, A., Torrabadella, M, and Madrigal, J.A. Quality rather than quantity: The cord blood bank dilemma. *Bone Marrow Transplant.* 45, 970–978 (2010).
3. Allan, D., Petraszko, T., Elmoazzen, H., and Smith, S. A review of factors influencing the banking of collected umbilical cord blood units. *Stem Cells Int.* 2013, Article ID 463031, 7 pages (2013).
4. Chen, GL, Paplham, P., and McCarthy, P.L. Remestemcel-L for acute graft-versus-host disease therapy. *Expert Opin. Biol. Ther.* 14(2), 261–269 (2014).
5. Galipeau, J. The mesenchymal stromal cells dilemma — does a negative phase III trial of random donor mesenchymal stromal cells in steroid resistant graft-versus-host disease represent a death knell or a bump in the road? *Cytotherapy* 15(1), 2–8 (2013).
6. von Bahr, L., Sundberg, B., Lönnies, L., Sander, B., Karbach, H., Hägglund, H., Ljungman, P., Gustafsson, B., Karlsson, H., Le Blanc, K., and Ringdén, O. Long-term complications, immunologic effects, and role of passage for outcome in mesenchymal stromal cell therapy. *Biol. Blood Marrow Transplant.* 18, 557–564 (2012).
7. Vaes, B., Hof, V.W., Deans, R., and Pinxteren, J. Application of MultiStem allogeneic cells for immunomodulatory therapy: Clinical progress and pre-clinical challenges in prophylaxis for graft-versus-host disease. *Front. Immunol.* 27(3), 345 (November, 2012).
8. ICH Q5D: Derivation and Characterization of Cell Substrates used for Production of Biotechnological/Biological Products, ICH Harmonised Tripartite Guideline. S.l.: International Conference on Harmonization of Technical Requirements for Registration of Pharmaceuticals for Human Use.
9. USP General Chapter ⟨1046⟩ Cellular and tissue-based products. S.l.: US Pharmacopeial Convention.
10. Guideline on Human Cell-based Medicinal Products, EMEA/CHMP/410869/2006. S.l.: European Medicines Agency, May 21, 2008.
11. ICH Q5A: Viral Safety Evaluation of Biotechnology Products Derived from Cell Lines of Human or Animal Origin, ICH Harmonized Tripartite Guideline. S.l. : International Conference on Harmonization of Technical Requirements for Registration of Pharmaceuticals for Human Use.

Product Release   8

Andrea Hauser and Christine Günther

8.1 Introduction

The formal release of a finished product batch is the last step of manufacturing a medicinal product and allows its subsequent sale or supply. Companies or institutions performing finished product batch release need a manufacturing license even if this is the only manufacturing step they are executing. Release of a finished product batch in most countries is also required upon importation of that batch from another country [in Europe this applies to all medicinal products that are imported from outside the European Union (EU) or European Economic Area (EEA)].

The principles and responsibilities for product release slightly differ, depending on the country or region. A specific feature of product release in Europe is the responsibility of the so called Qualified Person (QP) who is personally liable. For this reason, there is no drug master file system established in Europe, as the QP needs to be informed in detail of the manufacturing and quality control (QC) processes and this would not be the case if suppliers are able to hand in documents concerning raw materials or active substances under disclosure. In the US, no equivalent to the European QP exists, at least not in terms of the above mentioned personal responsibility and liability. There, batch release is executed by a responsible person within the Quality Unit (QU).

The term "release" can be used for different processes within the life cycle of a medicinal product as release procedures can occur on different stages of manufacturing. There might be release of the starting material or active pharmaceutical ingredient (API) for use in the manufacturing process, release of intermediates for further processing, release of bulk products for final formulation, filling or packaging or release of a finished product batch for sale or supply. This chapter focuses on release of the finished product batch for sale or supply. It, furthermore, does not cover batch release performed by official control authorities (as for example, required for blood or certain immunological products).

For cell-based medicinal products (CBMPs), specific questions and challenges may pose difficulties to the QP in releasing a product. The interface between human blood-derived products, tissue-derived products, and Advanced Therapy Medicinal Products (ATMPs) on the one hand and the interface between Good Manufacturing Practice (GMP) and Good Clinical Practice (GCP) for investigational medicinal products (IMPs) on the other hand is challenging. The GMP principles fully apply but in many cases a risk-based approach is required in order to be able to release a finished product batch.

In this chapter, we provide an overview of the requirements for product release in general and address specific issues for product release of CBMPs. As the requirements for certification and batch release are generally similar in all countries and regions that have implemented the GMP rules, here we focus on the European system with the special role of the QP. In the USA, information is provided by the US Food and Drug Administration (FDA) in the Code of Federal Regulations (CFR) Section 211.192 "Production record review".[1]

8.2 General Principles

Every finished product batch of an MP or IMP must be certified and released by a QP residing within Europe (either a member state of the EU or the EEA), before sale or supply of this batch is permitted. This holds true for products that are manufactured in parts or completely within the EU/EEA, even if they are produced for export reasons only; as well as for products that are produced in a non-European country and are imported to the EU/EEA for sale or supply. In the latter case, an authorization for importation is required. Differences have to be considered depending on the country of origin from which the batch is imported as there are relieved requirements for countries that share a Mutual Recognition Agreement (MRA) with the EU (MRA partners are Australia, Canada, Japan, New Zealand, and Switzerland), compared to all other so called third countries. Details are provided in Annex 16 to the EU GMP Guidelines.[2]

Although release of a finished product batch in Europe is intimately connected with the QP, it is important to differentiate between responsibilities that lie within the competence of the pharmaceutical manufacturer of a medicinal product and thus have to be accounted for by the QP and those of the marketing authorization holder (MAH) (for licensed medicinal products) or the Sponsor of a clinical trial (for IMPs). While it is the QP's responsibility to assure that a particular product batch has been manufactured in accordance with all applicable rules and regulations, it is the responsibility of the MAH or the Sponsor to define basic requirements for product release in the marketing authorization (MA) or clinical trial authorization (CTA). In other words, the MAH or the Sponsor are ultimately responsible for an IMP's general features such as safety, quality, and efficacy, whereas the QP is responsible to verify that a defined product batch meets the release criteria as laid down in the MA or CTA. This split of responsibilities can be challenging whenever a medicinal product is produced by a contract manufacturer that has no direct access to the MA or CTA. In these cases, a written contract between both parties following the principles of the EU GMP guidelines chapter 7 "Outsourced Activities" is mandatory. It has to be determined that the contract manufacturer always has the updated information on all essential quality attributes and the available release criteria. On the other hand, whenever a medicinal product is produced by a contract manufacturer who is not responsible for the release of the finished product batch, the QP who certifies and releases the finished batch needs to have all documents available that are required to evaluate the quality of the batch. For this reason, the written contract should determine which documents have to be provided by the contract manufacturer to the QP for product release.

Apart from the defined release criteria laid down in the MA or CTA, the QP additionally has to certify that a specific product batch was manufactured in accordance with the EU GMP guidelines (or at least equivalent, when the product was manufactured outside the EU/EEA) and in compliance with national laws in force in the member state where the medicinal product is released. If a medicinal product is exported to another country, the QP also has to certify that the product was manufactured in accordance with applicable national laws of the destination country. It is important to know that even products that are produced for export reasons only, have to be released by a QP in Europe before sale or supply and that the European GMP rules have to be followed even if the destination country is non-European.

In summary, the general principles for certification and batch release of an IMP in Europe mean for the QP to certify that the batch has been manufactured:

1. In accordance with the MA or CTA including the product release specifications;
2. In accordance with the EU guidelines for GMP for medicinal products (or those of another country, if considered to be at least equivalent);
3. In compliance with national laws in force in the member state where the batch is certified (if applicable, and if different in the destination country).

In addition to the above mentioned requirement that a QP has to certify a finished product batch and thus guarantees that — to the QP's best knowledge — the batch has been produced in accordance with all applicable rules and regulations, there is one further reason for the requirements of such a formal and strict release procedure i.e., in the event that a defect needs to be investigated or a batch needs to be recalled, it has to be ensured that the QP who certified that batch as well as the relevant records (manufacturing records, QC records, investigations, reports, and QA documents, etc.) is readily identifiable.[2] It is laid down in Chapter 8 of the EU GMP Guidelines on complaints, quality defects, and product recalls[3] that the QP has to be made formally aware of any investigations, any risk-reducing actions and any recall operations, in a timely manner.

Essential information on batch certification and product release is provided by the EU GMP Guidelines Part 1 Annex 16 "Certification by a Qualified Person and Batch Release"[2] with special requirements for IMPs being provided in Annex 13 Manufacture of Investigational Medicinal Products.[4]

8.3 Required Qualification to Act as QP

To act as QP, specific expertise defined by the European Commission (EC) and additional national laws in each European member state is necessary. Directive 2001/83/EC,[5] Articles 48 and 49, lay down the required qualification for acting as QP for conventional medicinal products for human use. For this type of medicinal products (small molecules, chemical substances, etc.), the QP is basically required to be in possession of a diploma, certificate or other evidence of formal qualifications awarded on completion of a university course of study in pharmacy. Other types of university courses and degrees such as medicine, chemistry and biology are acceptable, but in these cases several additional theoretical and practical university courses covering a range of different pharmaceutical subjects are required. Apart from the formal academic qualification, additional practical experiences over at least two years in the field of qualitative analysis of medicinal products, quantitative analysis of active substances, and the testing and checking necessary to ensure the quality of medicinal products in a facility or company that is authorized to manufacture medicinal products are required.

As uniform as the qualification requirements might be for conventional medicinal products, as heterogeneous they are for special types of products such as blood, blood products, tissues, cells, and ATMPs. In most European member states, products of human origin that are not substantially manipulated, and that are therefore not considered to be an ATMP, do not have to be released by a QP according to Article 48 of Directive 2001/83/EC,[5] and production and product release do not have to follow the requirements of the EU GMP Guidelines. For human tissues and cells, Directive 2004/23/EC[6] defines in Article 17, the requirements for a "Responsible Person" who has to ensure that human tissues and cells intended for human applications are procured, tested, processed, stored, and distributed in accordance with the Directive and the laws in force in the Member State. Qualification requirements are the possession of a diploma, certificate or other evidence of formal qualifications in the field of medical or biological sciences, awarded on completion of a university course of study or a course recognized as equivalent by the Member State concerned and at least two years practical experience in the relevant fields. Equivalent to Directive 2004/23/EC for human tissues and cells, Directive 2002/98/EC[7] on human blood and blood components defines in Article 9, the requirement for a "Responsible Person" who ensures that every unit of blood or blood components (when intended for transfusion) has been collected and tested, processed, stored, and distributed in compliance with the laws in force in the Member State. The formal and practical qualification requirements are comparable to those mentioned above for tissues and cells. Germany established an important exception to the above mentioned requirements for blood and blood components (including peripheral blood stem cells) as these products have to be produced and released following the EU GMP Guidelines. Qualification requirements for these QPs are nevertheless different from those mentioned above for conventional medicinal products, in so far as a university degree or diploma in pharmacy is not mandatory, but rather practical experience in transfusion medicine. For human tissues and cells (including bone marrow), Germany has established the facilitated rules of a Responsible instead of a QP, and manufacturing as well as product release do not have to follow the GMP rules.

For ATMPs (tissue-engineered products, somatic cell therapy medicinal products, and gene therapy medicinal products), strict compliance with the GMP rules is mandatory since Regulation (EC) No 1394/2007[8] came into force. Qualification requirements for QPs basically have to follow the principles laid down in Directive 2001/83/EC.[5] The requirements for the necessary practical experiences are regulated nationally and are highly diverse within Europe. In Great Britain, for example, the Medicines and Healthcare Products Regulatory Agency (MHRA) was able, for a brief time after Regulation (EC) No 1394/2007[8] came into force, to grant "transitional QP" status to non-pharmacists for ATMP release. These QPs with transitional status, however, are only allowed to release ATMPs that are classified as IMPs; they would not be allowed to release licensed ATMPs. In Germany, different kinds of university degrees (e.g., pharmacy, biology, and medicine) are possible together with practical experience of two years, particularly in a field with medical relevance such as genetic engineering, microbiology, cell biology, virology, or molecular biology that is not restricted to facilities with a manufacturing license. Generally in a number of European member states, it is quite challenging to find QPs with sufficient qualification for ATMPs as laid down by national laws and regulations and it is intensively discussed whether a harmonization within Europe is necessary and how training courses or even university courses can be established to educate and qualify a sufficient number of QPs for ATMPs. It is further under discussion whether training or university courses can, at least in part, substitute for the required practical experiences in companies or facilities that are manufacturing the relevant products, as it is utterly impossible to standardize the quality of this two-year period. But so far, e.g., in Germany, no course, degree or diploma is accepted as QP qualification to replace the two-year period of practical experience.

Apart from all the above mentioned formal and practical requirements for QPs, Annex 16 of the EU GMP Guidelines[2] points out one additional expertise: Detailed knowledge and experience [e.g., of the manufacturing steps or the quality management system (QMS)] to fulfill her/his duties as otherwise it is hardly feasible to evaluate correctly, the deviations and Out-of Specification (OOS) results that might occur in production and/or QC.

The fact that the qualification of a QP always is connected to a certain type of product is the reason why, e.g., German regulatory agencies do not provide certificates for individual persons that confirm their qualification to act as QP. A formal confirmation can be solely achieved by an application for a specific (type of) product and subsequent entry in the manufacturing authorization. Whenever it is unclear whether the formal qualification is sufficient to act as QP, this should be discussed with the authorities.

Often QPs take the responsibility for medicinal products which might be applied to thousands of patients. Their position in a company or institution and their legal protection do not always reflect this. As mentioned above, education and professional requirements are not harmonized. Moreover, there are decisions which have to be discussed intensely and may also have significant impact on commercial aspects. Associations as the European QP association (EQPA, http://www.qp-association.eu), the German (GQPA, http://www.german-qp.de) or the Austrian (AQPA, http://www.austria-qp.at) may offer valuable support and further education.

8.4 Batch Record Review (BRR)

Before certification and formal release of a finished product batch, the QP has to verify that production and QC meet the defined specifications and acceptance criteria. This is done by reviewing the batch documentation and associated documents such as environmental monitoring reports- a process commonly referred to as BRR. The term is not legally defined and not mentioned in the EU GMP guidelines, but it is obvious that without reviewing the complete documentation belonging to a specific product batch, certification and batch release are not possible. On the other hand, it is evident that in many cases the responsible QP cannot review all documents personally, thus the BRR is rather a process with different personnel involved at different levels and stages and with the QP being responsible to review the completed batch documentation (at least selected documents) and to evaluate critical deviations and OOS results in full detail. As the QP remains personally responsible for a released product batch, it is important that she/he authorizes the procedure for the BRR and eventually trains involved personnel on the process and on important points.

To define the process of BRR, a detailed SOP is mandatory that defines whose responsibility it is to sign, check, double-check or authorize which kind of document and when and to whom the document has to be provided. As commonly numerous different types of documents have to be checked and reviewed and as it has to be assured that the batch documentation is complete, the use of a checklist is very useful in most cases. Relevant issues, topics and documents for the BRR are determined by the QP's routine duties as defined in Annex 16 to the EU GMP Guidelines. Following these routine duties, a QP should ensure that at least the following requirements are met before she/he certifies the batch:

- Manufacture (including relevant QCs) must be in compliance with the provisions of the MA or CTA;
- Manufacture (including relevant QCs) has to be in accordance with GMP;
- Manufacturing and testing processes must have been validated (including qualification of the relevant equipment, machines, and instruments);
- Actual production conditions and manufacturing records must be considered (e.g., environmental monitoring reports of the production area, cleaning of instruments and machines);
- Deviations, OOS results, Corrective Action/Preventive Action (CAPA) procedures or planned changes in production or QC must have been evaluated and authorized by the responsible persons and in accordance with a defined QMS;

- Any changes requiring variation to the MA or Manufacturing Authorization must have been notified to and authorized by the relevant authority;
- All necessary checks and tests must have been performed, including any additional sampling, inspection, test or checks initiated because of deviations or planned changes;
- All necessary production and QC documents have been completed and endorsed by the staff authorized to do so. This includes final review and authorization of the production records by the Head of production and subsequently by the Head of QC, as well as final review and authorization of the QC records by the Head of QC.
- All audits have been carried out as required by the quality assurance system (QAS).

To support the QP in the process of BRR, in most cases either Quality Assurance (QA) or QC personnel do assist and pre-evaluate to verify that the documentation is complete, plausible, readable, correct, signed by responsible persons, and double checked where necessary, reproducible, and traceable (especially comments). The principles of GMP compliant documentation as laid down in Part I, Chapter 4 of the EU GMP Guidelines have to be followed.[9]

The QP should at least review selected documents of the batch record and evaluate deviations and OOS results. Authorities increasingly demand that the curriculum of review is documented, for example, with a list of raw data or documents that have been reviewed. Furthermore, the justification for product release (or rejection) should be documented. This is mandatory whenever major deviations occur as the decision for product release must, in these cases, be risk based (for further details, compare Section 8.5).

Another valuable document for the QP, not directly related to an individual batch is the Product Quality Review (PQR), which has to be provided for authorized products annually including trending analysis (details are provided in Chapter 1 of the EU GMP Guidelines).[10] The document is a valuable and helpful basis for evaluating general GMP compliance and effectivity of the Quality Assurance System (QAS). It is strongly recommended to evaluate and analyze IMPs accordingly. The continuous optimization of the product and process during clinical development is based on the thorough analysis of manufactured batches (see also chapter "Quality Management").

Figure 8.1 provides a flow chart on the procedure of BRR and release of the finished product batch. Please note that this is a simplified overview without potential reprocessing or reworking steps (hardly feasible for ATMPs anyway). Also intermediate release steps by multiple QPs at different stages of manufacturing or performed

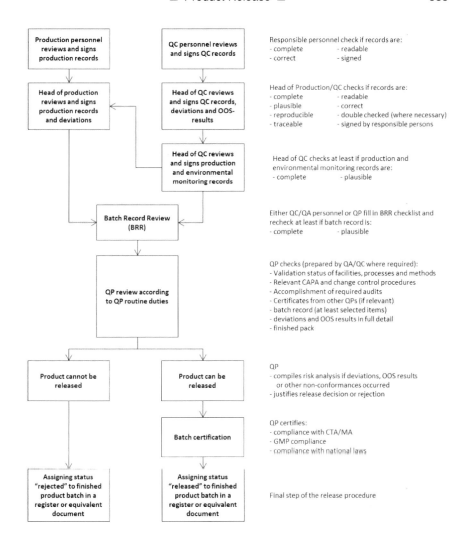

Figure 8.1: Schematic overview on BRR and finished product batch release.

Note: Please note that this is a simplified overview that does not contain any intermediate release procedures (such as, for example, release of the starting material, bulk release or release for packaging) and does not cover manufacturing at different sites or by different (contract) manufacturers. Also importation of a medicinal product from a country outside the EU/EEA is not reflected. BRR: Batch Record Review; CAPA: Corrective Action/Preventive Action; CTA: Clinical Trial Authorization; MA: Marketing Authorization; OOS: Out-of Specification; QA: Quality Assurance; QC: Quality Control; and QP: Qualified Person.

by various (contract) manufacturers are not considered. Furthermore, importation of medicinal products from countries outside the EU/EEA is also not reflected.

For conventional medicinal products, it is quite common that different manufacturing sites (either within one and the same company or at different contract manufacturers) participate in the production of a single product batch and therefore several QPs are involved at different production stages. In these cases, the overall responsibility nevertheless remains with the QP who certifies and releases the finished product batch. However, it is acknowledged that in an industrial situation usually one single QP simply cannot be closely involved with every stage of manufacture, and that the QP being responsible for final release may therefore need to rely in part on the advice and decision of other QPs. Before doing so, the QP being responsible for final release has to ensure that this reliance is well founded; either from personal knowledge or from the confirmation by other QPs within a quality system which she/he has accepted.[2] Whenever a QP wishes to rely on the decision of another QP, there should be a written agreement in place in order to clearly define the matters that are confirmed. It is important that the QP being responsible for certifying the finished product batch is notified of any deviations, OOS results, and non-compliances with GMP, investigations, complaints or other matters which should be taken into account for the certification procedure.[2]

Apart from QP confirmations on different stages within the manufacturing process there are increasing demands to include the active pharmaceutical ingredients (APIs) that serve as starting material for the production of a medicinal product and therefore also underlie the GMP principles as laid down in part II of the EU GMP Guidelines.[11] The European Medicines Agency (EMA) published in 2014, the "Guidance for the template for the QP's declaration concerning GMP compliance of active substance manufacture- The QP declaration template".[12] The guidance document emphasizes the importance of providing a valid QP declaration for active substances used as starting material for the production of medicinal products for human or veterinary use to facilitate the validation of regulatory submissions for MA. The aim of this QP declaration on active substances is to verify their GMP compliance, to define and fully understand their supply chain and to verify that they have been sourced through this supply chain. The QP declaration on APIs is not (yet) required for APIs used for the production of IMPs and it is not required for blood or blood components as these are not considered to be medicinal products and are subject to the requirements of Directive 2002/98/EC.[7]

For CBMPs, manufacturing sites in Europe are still rare due to the requirements for full GMP compliance and many products are produced in small companies or in academic institutions without possibilities of outsourcing or contract manufacturing.

Therefore, involvement of several QPs in the production of a single ATMP product batch is not common, yet.

8.5 Batch Certification and Product Release

After verifying by the process of BRR that all prerequisites for product release are fulfilled, the last steps of the release procedure are certification of the batch and formal release by documenting the batch in a register or equivalent document with status "released".

The EMA has defined the requirements for batch certification in a document called "Internationally Harmonised Requirements for Batch Certification in the context of Mutual Recognition Agreements, Agreements on Conformity Assessment and Acceptance of Industrial Products and other appropriate arrangements on GMP with the European Union".[13] The document defines the content of a batch certificate for medicinal products. It is actually not mandatory to use the template provided by the document, at least as long as the medicinal product is not transferred to other countries, even though the provided information is useful for setting up an appropriate certificate of compliance. Table 8.1 provides a model certificate based on the requirements defined by the EMA.

The certification of a finished product batch has to be recorded in a register or equivalent document provided for that purpose. The record must be kept up to date as operations are carried out. Recalls of released batches also have to be documented in the register or equivalent document.

After certification, the last step of the release procedure is assigning the release status to the product. This final step effectively releases the batch for sale, supply, or export.

8.6 Specifics of CBMPs

CBMP is a term that summarizes all different kinds of products ranging from non-substantially manipulated cellular products or tissues to ATMPs containing major manipulations and being produced by extensive processing steps. As not all of these products are regulated equally, for manufacture and product release it is important to know whether the GMP rules have to be followed or whether the facilitated rules for blood, blood components, cells, and tissues apply. In Europe, the borderline for GMP-compliance is drawn whenever a product is classified as ATMP.

Table 8.1: Template for batch certification of a finished product batch.

Letter Head of Manufacturer	
Certificate of Compliance	
1. Name of Product	Proprietary, brand or trade or proper name in the importing country, as applicable. For IMPs, the code number as referred to in the CTA.
2. Importing Country	Name of importing country.
3. MA Number or CTA Number	The MA number of the product in the importing country. For IMPs, the CTA number or trial reference to be provided when available.
4. Strength/Potency	Identity (name) and amount per unit dose required for all active ingredients/constituents. IMPs include placebos and the manner in which this information is provided should not unblind the study.
5. Dosage Form	For example, tablets, capsules, and ointments, etc.
6. Package Size and Type	This would be the contents of container and vials, bottles, and blisters, etc.
7. Batch Number or Lot Number Related to the Product	Unique combination of numbers, letters or symbols that identifies a batch and from which the production and distribution history can be determined.
8. Date of Manufacture	In accordance with national (local) requirements of the importing country.
9. Expiry Date	The date placed on the container/label of a product designating the time during which the product is expected to remain within the authorized shelf life specifications authorized by the importing country, if stored under defined conditions, and after which it should not be used.
10. Name, Address and Authorization Number of all Manufacturing and QC Sites	All sites involved in the manufacture including packaging/labeling and QC of the batch should be listed with name, address and authorization number. The name and address must correspond to the information provided on the manufacturing authorization.

(Continued)

Table 8.1: *(Continued)*

Letter Head of Manufacturer

---

11. Certificates of GMP Compliance of all Sites Listed under 10 or, if Available, EudraGMP Reference Numbers	Certificate numbers and/or EudraGMP reference numbers should be listed under this item.
12. Results of Analysis	Should include the authorized specifications, all results obtained and refer to the methods used (may refer to a separate certificate of analysis which must be dated, signed, and attached).
13. Comments/Remarks	Any additional information that can be of value to the importer and/or inspector verifying the compliance of the batch certificate (e.g., specific storage or transportation conditions).
14. Certification Statement	This statement should cover the fabrication/manufacturing, including packaging/labeling and QC. The following text should be used: "I hereby certify that the above information is authentic and accurate. This batch of product has been manufactured, including packaging/labeling and QC at the above mentioned site(s) in full compliance with the GMP requirements of the local Regulatory Authority and with the specifications in the MA of the importing country or product specification file (PSF) for IMPs. The batch processing, packaging and analysis records were reviewed and found to be in compliance with GMP".
15. Name and Position/Title of Person Authorizing the Batch Release	Including the name and address, if more than one site, is mentioned under item 10.
16. Signature of Person Authorizing the Batch Release	⟨signature⟩
17. Date of Signature	dd/mm/yyyy

Note: Table modified after EMA document on "Internationally Harmonised Requirements for Batch Certification".[13]

Almost all ATMPs are currently IMPs with only a minority of licensed products. Special requirements for IMPs are therefore relevant for product release of the majority of these products (for further details, compare Section 8.7). But not only their status as investigational causes specific challenges for the release of ATMPs, but also a whole range of particularities that are immanent for production and QC of this type of products (most of them are discussed in full detail in the chapters "Process Development and Manufacturing" and "Quality Control").

Specific challenges for product release of ATMPs are:

- **Starting material**: The cellular starting material for ATMPs (human blood, tissues, and cells) underlies high biological diversities dependent on the donor and/or the procurement procedure (e.g., apheresis products or cord blood units), thus standardization is difficult. Establishment of suitable specifications and acceptance criteria is challenging, leading to an increased number of deviations already at the first step of manufacture. Additionally, processing of the starting material in many cases has to be initiated before its analysis is completed as manufacturing processes tend to be time consuming and cellular viability is beginning to be affected already several hours after procurement.

- **Raw/Ancillary materials**: Many of these materials (e.g., cytokines, growth factors, culture media, human, or animal serum) are not available in pharmaceutical grade or otherwise appropriate quality, although they exert a significant impact on the cells and/or the manufacturing process. This might lead to less robust manufacturing processes, causing deviations and/or OOS results that have to be evaluated carefully with respect to their impact on product safety.

- **Process validation**: Manufacturing processes for ATMPs can hardly be validated as thoroughly and completely as is the case for conventional medicinal products containing small molecules. One reason for this is that material of human origin is not readily available, as it is unethical to put voluntary donors at risk for the mere purpose of data collection. Worst case scenarios, therefore, often cannot be studied in full detail leading to difficulties in evaluating deviations correctly.

- **Manufacturing process**: Manufacturing processes for ATMPs tend to be much more variable than those of conventional medicinal products. Particularly at early stages of clinical trials and for production of the first routine batches, it is difficult to define appropriate in-process controls and the corresponding acceptance criteria. If those acceptance criteria are not met, it might be unclear whether the safety of the product is actually affected. Apart from variability, manufacturing processes of CBMPs are often more complex than those of conventional medicinal products and technologies vary significantly when applied to different types of cells (e.g., culture processes). QPs thus have to be involved closely in or must have detailed knowledge of the process development and validation of the procedures they are responsible for. This is necessary for the correct evaluation of deviations or OOS results.

- **Diversity of products**: Due to a multitude of diverse products, comparability within one and the same company/facility or among different manufacturers is difficult leading to the fact that a certain routine in production and QC is achieved significantly later compared to conventional medicinal products.

- **Analytical methods**: Only for some methods and/or products, internationally accepted reference standards are available making it more difficult to evaluate potential OOS results. Furthermore methods for analysis of cells tend to be more variable than physico-chemical methods leading to OOS results.

- **Contract laboratories**: Only a very limited number of highly qualified and experienced external contract laboratories are available.

- **Finished product batch**: During clinical development high inter-batch variability is to be expected.

- **Release procedure**: In case of individual (autologous or allogeneic directed) batches, the release procedure is time-consuming. Release of short shelf-life products has to be conducted immediately after or in parallel to the final release testing (for details, compare Section 8.8). The QP therefore has to be available whenever a product batch is about to be finished. In some cases, the release has to be performed in two stages and products have to be shipped in quarantine status making it necessary to include the site of administration in the release process (quarantined product only to be administered or handed over after certification and final batch release by the responsible QP). Assignment of part-time QPs is hardly possible, even if only a small number of batches are produced.

- **Risk management**: Due to an expected higher level of deviations and OOS results in a significant number of cases, a thorough risk analysis is mandatory before a product can be released (also compare, Section 8.9). Despite the detailed knowledge of the QP that is required to compile such a risk analysis, it has to be considered that the procedure is time consuming; a fact that is especially important for short shelf-life products.

- **IMPs**: As most ATMPs are classified as IMPs that are used within clinical trials, a two–step release procedure (QP and Sponsor) is required (for details, see section 8.7).

- **Interface GMP and GCP**: For IMPs that have to be administered to the patient shortly after arrival at the clinical trial site (either because of their short shelf-life or because they cannot be stored there properly, e.g., in liquid nitrogen), it is important that the IMP manufacturer and the Sponsor (or investigator) communicate closely on possible dates and time. In addition, immune monitoring might be required continuously or for a short time-period after administration of the IMP requiring additional organization and timing. Also products which are shipped to the clinic prior to certification and final release need special consideration. Pharmacovigilance aspects, safety signal monitoring and recall procedures are some other points of intersection between GMP and GCP and should be carefully checked for relevance.
- **Administration of ATMPs**: Some ATMPs need a last manufacturing step immediately before administration to the patient, as often more than mere reconstitution is required for application (e.g., for cryopreserved products that have to be thawed). QPs therefore might have an extended responsibility.
- **Traceability**: Specific requirements for traceability apply for human-derived products that are processed to ATMPs (blood, stem cells, tissue, and plasma-products, etc.). Traceability is of special importance for infectious diseases and adventitious agents which might be transmitted. Special consideration has to be paid to adequate donor-testing, availability of samples for retesting and the identification of donors (despite anonymization/pseudonymization procedures required by GCP). The interface between GCP and GMP is crucial in this respect. Look-back procedures, product recalls, and reports of safety signals (adverse events) also require full traceability of the products.
- **Hospital Exemption**: Application of novel ATMPs is usually restricted to authorized clinical trials. An alternative approach in Europe may be the so called 'Hospital Exemption' (HE; see chapter "Clinical Development of Cell-Based Products"). The 'Hospital Exemption' clause is not established in every EU/EEA country and the responsibility for implementation is allocated to the individual Member States, leading to a highly diverse regulatory landscape. It is important to know whether ATMPs that should be applied following the 'HE' clause have to be manufactured under the requirements of a manufacturing license and therefore have to be released by a QP (as is the case, e.g., in Germany). The QP then has to certify that the medicinal product meets (apart from GMP and other requirements) the specifications as laid down in the 'HE' authorization.
- **Application in case of Necessity**: In some instances, individual patients require medication because of life-threatening disease condition which is not otherwise treatable. These special circumstances are usually legally implemented in every

country in one or another way, in Germany, for example, in Section 34 "Necessity" of the German Criminal Code: '*A person who, faced with an imminent danger to life, limb, freedom, honour, property or another legal interest which cannot otherwise be averted, commits an act to avert the danger from himself or another, does not act unlawfully, if, upon weighing the conflicting interests, in particular the affected legal interests and the degree of the danger facing them, the protected interest substantially outweighs the one interfered with. This shall apply only if and to the extent that the act committed is an adequate means to avert the danger*'.[14] In case of necessity, a medicinal product that was manufactured under a manufacturing license and released by a QP is administered to a patient without legal permission (no MA, CTA or HE authorization, although one of the authorizations would be required). The manufacturer may release the product for individual application and takes the whole responsibility. Information of the authority is advisable for ATMPs. In any case, thorough documentation is required and consultation of the legal department might be reasonable especially when deviations, OOS results or other non-conformances are involved.

8.7 Specific Guidance for IMPs

As only an absolute minority of ATMPs are authorized, in most cases the special requirements for IMPs as defined in Annex 13 to part I of the EU GMP Guidelines[4] have to be followed for product release. IMPs are to a high degree allocated to academic institutions where they are used within Investigator Initiated Trials.

Basically, it is important to differentiate between responsibilities of the Sponsor of a clinical trial in which a certain medicinal product is used and the pharmaceutical manufacturer of the IMP (comparable to the split of responsibilities between MAH and pharmaceutical manufacturer). The Sponsor lays down specifications and release criteria of an IMP in the IMP dossier (IMPD) that is part of the CTA. If the IMP manufacturer has no direct access to the IMPD (e.g., in case of contract manufacturing), he must at least have detailed knowledge of relevant information concerning manufacture and QC of the IMP. Establishment of a PSF that is shared by the Sponsor and the IMP manufacturer is helpful in these cases. Strict adherence to change control principles is required for both parties for fulfillment of the relevant duties (compare Figure 8.2a).

One particularity for IMPs is the required two-step process for finished batch release: The IMP has to be released by the QP first following a second release step by the Sponsor. While the QP releases the product batch according to the release

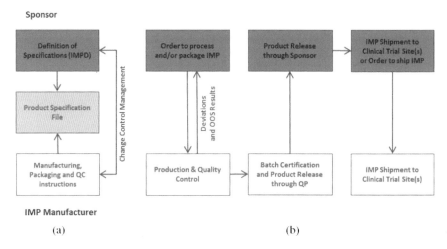

Figure 8.2: Schematic overview on split responsibilities between the sponsor of a clinical trial and the IMP manufacturer.

Notes: (a) The IMP manufacturer must have knowledge of the relevant product specifications and release criteria that have been defined by the Sponsor within the IMPD. This can be done by setting up a PSF that contains the relevant details and is shared by both parties. The minimal content of a PSF is described in Annex 13 to the EU GMP Guidelines.[4] It is important that the Sponsor as well as the IMP manufacturer strictly adhere to change control principels and that information on planned changes are provided to the other party before the change is implemented. (b) Manufacture of an IMP has to be initiated (ordered) by the Sponsor. The IMP manufacturer has to report at least every critical deviation or OOS result that occurs during production or QC to the Sponsor. This has to be defined in a written contract. IMPs have to be released for supply in a two-step procedure: After product release through the QP, the IMP must be released additionally by the Sponsor for use in the clinical trial before shipment to the clinical trial site(s), and administration to the patient is permitted. IMP: Investigational Medicinal Product: IMPD: Investigational Medicinal Product Dossier, QC: Quality Control; QP: Qualified Person; OOS: Out-of Specification.

criteria as laid down in the IMPD and according to GMP principles and national laws, the Sponsor has to release the IMP for application within the authorized clinical trial protocol (compare Figure 8.2b).

Supplementary to Annex 16 of part I to the EU GMP Guidelines[2] Annex 13[4] provides guidance for QPs in connection with the certification and batch release of IMPs. According to Annex 13, IMP batch release may not occur until after the QP has certified that the requirements of Article 13.3 of Directive 2001/20/EC[15] have been met (basically GMP compliance). It is important to differentiate between products that have been manufactured in the EU/EEA and those manufactured in an MRA partner state or third country with subsequent import into the EU/EEA.

Annex 13 summarizes the elements that need to be considered for the most common circumstances for manufacture and import of IMPs and the various duties a QP has to fulfill depending on the IMP's country of origin.

Equivalent to a QP's routine duties as defined in Annex 16 to the EU GMP Guidelines[2] (compare Section 8.4. 'Batch Record Review'). Annex 13[4] defines the elements a QP should take into account for assessment of each IMP batch for certification prior to release. These elements may include as appropriate:

- Batch records, including control reports, in-process test reports and release reports demonstrating compliance with the PSF, the order, protocol, and randomization code. These records should include all deviations or planned changes, and any consequent additional checks or tests, and should be completed and endorsed by the staff authorized to do so, according to the quality system.
- Production conditions (e.g., cleaning status of instruments, environmental monitoring reports, etc.).
- Validation status of facilities, processes, and methods.
- Examination of finished packs.
- Where relevant, results of any analyses or tests performed after importation.
- Stability reports.
- The source and verification of conditions of storage and shipment.
- Audit reports concerning the quality system of the manufacturer (in case of contract manufacturing),
- Documents certifying that the manufacturer is authorized to manufacture IMPs or comparators for export by the appropriate authorities in the country of export.
- Where relevant, regulatory requirements for MA, applicable GMP standards, and any official verification of GMP compliance.
- All other factors of which the QP is aware of that are relevant to the quality of the batch.

The Sponsor should ensure that the elements taken into account by the QP when certifying the batch are consistent with the information notified pursuant to Article 9(2) of Directive 2001/20/EC[13] (=information laid down in the CTA to the competent authority of the Member State in which the sponsor plans to conduct the clinical trial).

Because of the special requirements for clinical trials as well as for IMPs, persons who want to act as QPs for an IMP are required to have broad knowledge of pharmaceutical development and clinical trial processes in addition to the usual QP qualification and expertise. Special consideration should be paid to the interface of GMP and GCP in the field of CBMPs, as often considerably more interaction is required between both sides than is the case for conventional IMPs. This is particularly true for IMPs with a short shelf-life that have to be administered to the patient within a short time-period after shipment to the clinical trial site. Product release and shipment have to be coordinated with the sponsor or the investigator directly in order to enable the treatment of the patient.

Furthermore for some CBMPs, a last manufacturing step is required immediately before administration of the product to the patient. Usually manufacturing steps for IMPs carried out directly at the investigator site are packaging and labeling steps (e.g., for blinding procedures) or reconstitution prior to administration. These steps can be executed by, or performed under the supervision of a clinical trials pharmacist, or other health care professional, in most Member States and need not be covered by a manufacturing authorization. The QP is not required to certify these activities (but the sponsor is nevertheless responsible for ensuring that the activity is adequately documented and carried out in accordance with the principles of GMP and should seek the advice of the QP in this regard). For ATMPs however more than mere reconstitution might be required for administration (e.g., thawing of cryopreserved products) and it should be evaluated early whether a manufacturing authorization is required and whether the QP has to assume extended responsibility.

8.8 Batch Release of Short Shelf-Life Products

A finished product batch usually must not be released before the whole range of required analytical tests is completed and all test results (including those of contract laboratories) are available. This is utterly not possible for medicinal products with a short shelf-life of only some hours or days as tests such as microbiological control and sterility testing would exceed this time frame, at least if compendial methods are used that require seven days or more. In these cases, release criteria have to be defined thoroughly in order to allow product release shortly after final formulation, leaving enough time for shipment, while at the same time guaranteeing product safety. This is acknowledged by Annex 2 to the EU GMP Guidelines[16]:

'For biological medicinal products with a short shelf-life, which for the purposes of the annex is taken to mean a period of 14 days or less, and which need batch certification before completion of all end product quality control tests (e.g., sterility tests) a suitable control strategy must be in place. Such controls need to be built on enhanced understanding of product and process performance and take into account the controls and attributes of starting and raw materials. The exact and detailed description of the entire release procedure, including the responsibilities of the different personnel involved in assessment of production and analytical data is essential. A continuous assessment of the effectiveness

of the quality assurance system must be in place including records kept in a manner which permit trend evaluation. Where end product tests are not available due to their short shelf-life, alternative methods of obtaining equivalent data to permit initial batch certification should be considered (e.g., rapid microbiological methods). The procedure for batch certification and release may be carried out in two or more stages:

a) *Assessment by designated person(s) of batch processing records, results from environmental monitoring (where available) which should cover production conditions, all deviations from normal procedures and the available analytical results for review in preparation for the initial certification by the Qualified Person.*

b) *Assessment of the final analytical tests and other information available for final certification by the Qualified Person.*

Also European Directive 2009/120/EC[17] amending Directive 2001/83/EC[5] as regards ATMPs allows to use an amended characterization and control strategy for short shelf-life products in a way that test results of key intermediates and/or in-process controls can serve as release criteria, if certain release tests cannot be performed on the active substance or finished product in due time. These altered control strategies have to be justified and it is highly recommended to discuss with the competent authority which tests are essential. Typically the test on identity is required together with purity and potency (at least testing on surrogate parameters). If it is known that certain impurities (either product or process related) would pose the recipient at considerable risk, also testing on these impurities will be requested by the authorities. For sterility testing, it is widely accepted to use the so called negative-to-date concept, where test results from in-process controls (either cellular material or surrogates such as cell-culture medium) are used for product release. The use of rapid microbiological methods would be another alternative. For further details on microbiological control and sterility testing, compare chapter 'Quality Control'.

Whatever control strategy is chosen to enable product release, it is important to define whether certain analytical tests are required, even though their test results are not available at the time of product release. This is usually the case for microbiological testing of the finished product. The results of these tests have to be followed up closely and the Sponsor as well as the investigator have to be informed promptly in case of positive test results.

It should be mentioned here that the EMA published in 2012, the revised Guideline on Real Time Release Testing (RTRT)[18] (formerly Guideline on Parametric Release), aiming to provide better guidance for regulatory professionals to ensure their products consistently meet necessary specifications, and therefore to allow product release without the full range of end-product testing. Principles and requirements for Parametric Release are furthermore provided by Annex 17 to Part I of the EU GMP Guidelines.[19]

EMA explains in the guideline on RTRT that it *'is a system of release that gives assurance that the product is of intended quality, based on the information collected during the manufacturing process, through product knowledge and on process understanding and control'*. The guideline further points out that *'RTRT recognizes that under specific circumstances an appropriate combination of process controls (critical process parameters) together with pre-defined material attributes may provide greater assurance of product quality than end product testing and the context as such be an integral part of the control strategy'*.

The guideline provides amongst other things the requirements to implement RTRT, its use as part of a control strategy and its use with biological and biotechnological products. However, the guideline does not cover IMPs as critical process parameters that are required for RTRT are often not well enough defined (at least in early stages of clinical trials). For CBMPs, the use of RTRT will be challenging anyway, for some products maybe even impossible, as highly variable processes and materials (starting as well as raw materials) counteract the use of RTRT principles. A cultured product, for example, might meet all in-process specifications but might nevertheless show OOS results at the end-product level.

Again it should be discussed with the authorities what is possible and whether the use of RTRT for CBMPs might be accepted (at least in part and in combination with a reduced range of end-product testing).

8.9 Deviations, OOS Results and other Non-Conformances

Production and QC of a medicinal product is hardly possible without deviations. This is especially true for CBMPs that underlie high batch to batch variability of the starting material as well as the finished product batch and for which complex manufacturing processes are required, at least as far as ATMPs are concerned. Furthermore, analytical test methods are often more variable than conventional physico-chemical analytical procedures. Not all deviations have significant influence on product quality and of course not all of them prevent product release, but it is important to evaluate as thoroughly as possible their potential impact on product safety.

Basically deviations can occur in different ways and at different stages: There might be deviations to GMP principles, to the requirements and specifications laid down in the CTA or MA, to national laws or regulations or to internal quality standards or written operating procedures with no ranking that one type of deviation generally is more severe than another one. Another kind of non-conformance is OOS results. They might occur at the intermediate level as OOS results of in-process controls or at the level of the finished batch as OOS results of release testing. It is evident that OOS results that are proven to be product-related are more severe than most deviations, as they demonstrate divergency to defined quality attributes. And of course OOS results concerning the finished product are more severe than those affecting intermediate products. Apart from these general rules, every deviation, non-compliance or OOS result has to be evaluated individually and thoroughly to investigate its effects.

In general, it is the role and responsibility of the QP to make a decision whether to release or not to release a product batch. But whenever deviations and non-conformances occur, it is mandatory to follow the principles of quality risk management (QRM) and to thoroughly justify the release of the batch. As the QP is personally responsible, there should be written procedures in place that pre-define how to act in cases of non-conformance. If relevant, all non-conformances in production and QC have to be considered in total to evaluate potential inter-dependencies and they should of course not affect safety and efficacy of the concerned product batch. The QP may release products with deviations but should adhere strictly to written procedures and a risk-based approach. Specifically cell-based products with all their potential biologic variation may pose severe discussion on the appropriateness of a release. On the other hand, the risk analysis should include the condition of a patient and the availability of an alternative treatment.

EMA published in 2009, the "Reflection paper on a proposed solution for dealing with minor deviations from the detail, described in the MA for human and veterinary Medicinal Products" (also known as Reflection paper on QP discretion)[20] in order to define a harmonized approach for dealing with deviations and their influence on product release in the European Community.

According to the details set out in the reflection paper on QP discretion, it is proposed that a batch of finished product can be considered to continue to meet the defined requirements — and therefore being released — '*when*:

1. *The deviation is minor, one-off and unplanned in nature and relates only to the manufacturing process and/or the analytical control methods of either the starting materials or the medicinal product as described in the Marketing Authorisation or clinical trial application, and has no influence on the result of analytical testing.*
2. *The active substance and finished product specifications as described in the marketing authorisation or clinical trial application are complied with.*

3. *An assessment is performed by the manufacturer using an appropriate approach such as described in the International Conference on Harmonisation (ICH) Q9, Quality Risk Management, to establish and support a conclusion that the occurrence is a minor quality deviation that does not affect the safety and efficacy of the product.*
4. *The risk assessment should assess the need for inclusion of the affected batches in the ongoing stability program as required by Chapter 6 of the GMP Guide.*
5. *The risk assessment for biological medicinal products should consider in particular that even minor changes to the process can have an unexpected impact on safety or efficacy.*
6. *The Quality Risk Management Process is integrated into the manufacturer's Pharmaceutical Quality System, notably the documentation system established to comply with GMP, and records are available for inspection by the Competent Authorities.*
7. *Deviations must be properly recorded in the relevant batch documentation in accordance with GMP. All such deviations must be reviewed as part of the product quality review as required by Chapter 1 of the GMP Guide'.*

Although it is the QP's decision and responsibility whether to release or reject a batch, it is advisable to discuss the issue with the competent authorities.

References

1. Code of Federal Regulations (CFR), Chapter I, Subchapter C, Title 21- Food and Drugs, Part 211- Current Good Manufacturing Practice for finished Pharmaceuticals, Subpart J- Records and Reports, Section 211.192- Production record review. US Department of Health and Human Services, Food and Drug Administration, April 1, 2010.
2. EudraLex- The Rules Governing Medicinal Products in the European Union, Volume 4: Good manufacturing practice (GMP) Guidelines, Part I, Annex 16: Certification by a Qualified Person and Batch Release.
3. EudraLex- The Rules Governing Medicinal Products in the European Union, Volume 4: Good manufacturing practice (GMP) Guidelines, Part I, Chapter 8: Complaints, Quality Defects and Product Recalls.
4. EudraLex- The Rules Governing Medicinal Products in the European Union, Volume 4: Good manufacturing practice (GMP) Guidelines, Part I, Annex 13: Manufacture of Investigational Medicinal Products.
5. Directive 2001/83/EC on the Community code relating to medicinal products for human use. European Parliament and Council , November 6, 2001.
6. Directive 2004/23/EC on setting standards of quality and safety for the donation, procurement, testing, processing, preservation, storage and distribution of human tissues and cells. European Parliament and Council , March 31, 2004 .
7. Directive 2002/98/EC setting standards of quality and safety for the collection, testing, processing, storage and distribution of human blood and blood components and amending Directive 2001. European Parliament and Council, January 27, 2003 .

8. Regulation (EC) No 1394/2007 of the European Parliament and of the Council of November 13, 2007 on advanced therapy medicinal products and amending Directive 2001/83/EC and Regulation (EC) No 726/2004.

9. EudraLex- The Rules Governing Medicinal Products in the European Union, Volume 4: Good manufacturing practice (GMP) Guidelines, Part I, Chapter 4: Documentation.

10. EudraLex- The Rules Governing Medicinal Products in the European Union, Volume 4: Good manufacturing practice (GMP) Guidelines, Part I, Chapter 1: Pharmaceutical Quality System.

11. EudraLex- The Rules Governing Medicinal Products in the European Union, Volume 4: Good manufacturing practice (GMP) Guidelines, Part II: Basic Requirements for Active Substances used as Starting Materials.

12. Guidance for the template for the qualified person's declaration concerning GMP compliance of active substance manufacture "The QP declaration template". EMA/196292/2014. European Medicines Agency, May 21, 2014 .

13. Internationally Harmonised Requirements for Batch Certification in the context of Mutual Recognition Agreements, Agreements on Conformity Assessment and Acceptance of Industrial Products and other appropriate arrangements on GMP with the European Union. EMA/INS/MRA/387218/2011. European Medicines Agency, June 1, 2011.

14. German Criminal Code in the version promulgated on November 13, 1998, Federal Law Gazette I p. 3322, last amended by Article 3 of the Law of October 2, 2009, Federal Law Gazette I p. 3214. Translation provided by Prof. Dr. Michael Bohlander; ©2013 juris GmbH, Saarbrücken.

15. Directive 2001/20/EC on the approximation of the laws, regulations and administrative provisions of the Member States relating to the implementation of good clinical practice in the conduct of clinical trials on medicinal products for human use. European Parliament and Council, April 4, 2001.

16. EudraLex- The Rules Governing Medicinal Products in the European Union, Volume 4: Good manufacturing practice (GMP) Guidelines, Part I, Annex 2: Manufacture of Biological active substances and Medicinal Products for Human Use

17. Directive 2009/120/EC amending Directive 2001/83/EC on the Community code relating to medicinal products for human use as regards advanced therapy medicinal products. European Parliament and Council, September 14, 2009.

18. Guideline on Real Time Release Testing. EMA/CHMP/QWP/811210/2009-Rev1. European Medicines Agency, March 29, 2012.

19. EudraLex- The Rules Governing Medicinal Products in the European Union, Volume 4: Good manufacturing practice (GMP) Guidelines, Part I, Annex 17: Parametric Release.

20. Reflection paper on a proposed solution for dealing with minor deviations from the detail described in the Marketing Authorization for human and veterinary Medicinal Products. EMEA/INS/GMP/227075/2008. European Medicines Agency.

Clinical Development of Cell-Based Products   9

Volker Scherhammer, Sylvia Peter, and Christine Günther

9.1 Clinical Application of Mesenchymal Stem Cells (MSCs)

Emergence of biotechnology has brought along tremendous technological advancement in innovative therapies which are based on genes, cells, and engineered tissues. These new medicinal products, termed as Advanced Therapy Medicinal Products (ATMPs) are defined and categorized in the legislation (Part IV, Annex 1 to Directive 2001/83/EC)[1] as Gene Therapy (GT), Somatic cell therapy (SCT) and Tissue engineered products (TEPs).

These ATMPs have revolutionized the treatments for a number of diseases or injuries such as Alzheimer's, cancer, graft-*versus*-host disease (GvHD), to name a few.

The industry of ATMPs has historically faced some hurdles in entering the European markets due to the different regulatory procedures followed by the EU nations. The lack of understandable and consistent legal framework prompted the need for adopting a regulation for these Advanced Therapy products (ATPs) in EU.

The first clinical trial using culture-expanded MSCs was carried out in 1995 and 15 patients became the recipients of the autologous cells. Since then, a number of clinical trials have been conducted to test the feasibility and efficacy of MSCs therapy.[2,3] By 2013, the public clinical trials database (http://clinicaltrials.gov website) has shown 177 clinical trials using MSCs for a very wide range of therapeutic applications. In the European database (www.clinicaltrialsregister.eu as of January 16, 2014), 39 clinical trials with MSCs are registered. Most of these trials are in

Phase I (safety studies), Phase II (proof of concept for efficacy in human patients), or a mixture of Phase I/II studies. Only a small number of these trials are in Phase III (comparing a newer treatment to the standard or best known treatment) or Phase II/III. In general, MSCs appear to be well-tolerated, with most trials reporting lack of adverse effects in the medium term, although a few showed mild and transient peri-injection effects.[4] In addition, many completed clinical trials have demonstrated the efficacy of MSC infusion for diseases including stroke, liver cirrhosis, amyotrophic lateral sclerosis (ALS), and GvHD.[3,5-8]

9.2 Legislation and Guidance

Clinical trials conducted in the EU using ATMPs as investigational medicinal products (IMPs) are currently regulated under the Clinical Trials Directive and require national clinical trial applications (CTAs). For GT, SCT, TEPs, and all medicinal products containing genetically modified organisms (GMOs), the time limit for the Ethics Committee opinion and authorization by a national competent authority (NCA) is currently a maximum of 90 days (60 days for other IMPs) after receipt of a valid application, although with justification this can be extended to 180 days. In the case of cell therapies consisting of xenogeneic cells, there is no maximum time limit for the assessment of the CTA. A specific authorization is also required for the use of GMOs, but this requirement will not be covered further in this chapter.

The European Medicines Agency (EMA) guideline on First-in-Human (FIH) studies specifically excludes gene and cell therapy medicinal products; however, the general approach to first exposure of a human subject should be followed, with relevant precautions and risk assessments.

9.3 Legal Basis of ATMP Classification

According to Article 2(1)(a) of Regulation (EC) No.1394/2007,[9] an 'ATMP' means any of the following medicinal products for human use:

- A gene therapy medicinal product (GTMP) as defined in Part IV of Annex I to Directive 2001/83/EC.[1]
- A somatic cell therapy medicinal product (SCTMP) as defined in Part IV of Annex I to Directive 2001/83/EC.[1]
- A TEP as defined in Article 2(1)(b) of Regulation (EC) No. 1394/2007.[9]
  Source: Reflection paper on classification of ATMPs, EMA/CAT/600280/201.

9.4 Regulatory Definitions for ATMPs

9.4.1 *SCTMP*

SCTMP means a biological medicinal product which fulfills the following two characteristics:

(a) "Contains or consists of cells or tissues that have been subjected to substantial manipulation so that biological characteristics, physiological functions, or structural properties relevant for the intended clinical use have been altered, or of cells or tissues that are not intended to be used for the same essential function(s) in the recipient and the donor";

(b) "Is presented as having properties for, or is used in or administered to human beings with a view to treating, preventing, or diagnosing a disease through the pharmacological, immunological, or metabolic action of its cells or tissues."

For the purpose of point (a), the manipulations listed in Annex I to Regulation (EC) No 1394/2007,[9] in particular, shall not be considered as substantial manipulations: Cutting, grinding, shaping, centrifugation, soaking in antibiotic or antimicrobial solutions, sterilization, irradiation, cell separation, concentration or purification, filtering, lyophilization, freezing, and cryopreservation. It should be pointed out that this list is non-exhaustive.

9.4.2 *TEP*

Means a product that:

- Contains or consists of engineered cells or tissues.
- Is presented as having properties for, or is used in or administered to human beings with a view to regenerating, repairing, or replacing a human tissue.

9.4.3 *Combined ATMP*

Means an ATMP that fulfils the following conditions:

"It must incorporate, as an integral part of the product, one or more medical devices within the meaning of Article 1(2)(a) of Directive 93/42/EEC.[10] or one or more active implantable medical devices within the meaning of Article 1(2)(c) of Directive 90/385/EEC, and

— Its cellular or tissue part must contain viable cells or tissues, or
— Its cellular or tissue part containing non-viable cells or tissues must be liable to act upon the human body with action that can be considered as primary to that of the

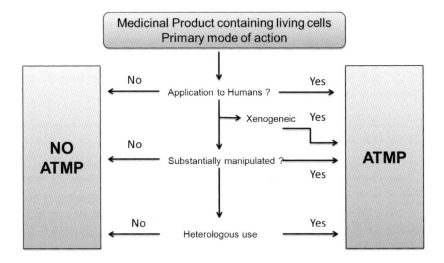

Figure 9.1: Decision tree: classification of ATMPs.

Source: (EMEA/CHMP/410869/2006).

devices referred to." (*Source*: Commission Directive 2009/120/EC of September 14, 2009 amending Directive 2001/83/EC of the European Parliament and of the Council on the Community code relating to medicinal products for human use as regards ATMPs).

9.5 Regulatory Framework in the EU

European countries may be classified into three groups based on their different positions regarding research with stem cells of human origin. Please note that this is a current statement and can change at any time:

(a) Countries with a restrictive political model (Germany, Iceland, Denmark, Lithuania, Slovenia, Austria, Norway, Ireland, and Poland), (b) Countries with a liberal political model (Sweden, United Kingdom, Belgium, and Spain. (c) Countries with an intermediate model (Latvia, Estonia, Greece, Finland, France, Switzerland, Hungary, the Netherlands, Bulgaria, Cyprus, Portugal, Turkey, Ukraine, Georgia, Moldavia, Romania, and Slovakia.

Guidelines on therapeutic products based on human cells are also established. Guidance is provided about the tests and criteria for the starting material, manufacturing process design, validation, characterization of cell-based products, and quality control (QC) aspects of the clinical development program.

The Directive recognizes that conventional non–clinical toxicology and pharmacology are different from cell-based products but should be strictly necessary for predicting side-effects (serious and non-serious adverse events) in humans. It also establishes the guidelines in terms of pharmacodynamics (PD) and pharmacokinetic (PK) studies which are required to define the safe dose(s) for application.

The guideline also describes the special consideration to Pharmacovigilance (PV) and risk management (RM) plan for these products.

As it can be seen, the guideline has therefore a multidisciplinary function and involves pre-clinical development, clinical development, manufacturing, QC of medicinal products based on human cells, and tissue engineering products. It also includes the development of autologous and allogeneic study protocols (not xenogeneic) based on cells; either isolated, combined with non–cell-components, or genetically modified.

However, the guideline does not address the development of non–viable cells or fragments from human cells.

The European Legislation is mainly based on three Directives:

- Directive 2003/63/EC- Annex 1 (amending Directive 2001/83/EC): Analytical, Pharmacotoxicological, and clinical standards and protocols in respect to the testing of medicinal products.
- Directive 2001/20/EC[11]- defining the regulations and administrative provisions of the Member States relating to the implementation of good clinical practice (GCP) in the conduct of clinical trials on medicinal products for human use.
- Directive 2004/23/EC,[12] which defines the quality, harvesting, processing, storage, distribution, and donation safety for tissues and human cells.

The EU regulation (1394/2007) on ATMPs became effective in December 2008 and is legally binding for all Member States of the European Union. ATMPs include cell therapy products (CTPs) and TEPs as per definition in the Directive 2001/83/EC. While in the United States and European Union, regulations are in place, in India, there is no well-defined regulatory framework for "stem cell-based products (SCBPs)". Till date, three Marketing Authorizations (MAs) have been granted for stem cell-based medicinal products (SCBMPs) by the EMA. The term "SCBP" is used to refer to products intended to be administered to a patient, that contain or are derived from stem cells.[13] There are several regulatory issues to be considered that relate to the safety, efficacy, and quality of SCBPs, while preparing a cell- and tissue-based therapy for clinical and commercial use.[14,15]

Initially, safety testing is critical, including assays for potential microbial, fungal, endotoxin, mycoplasma, and viral contamination; karyotype testing; and enrichment for the required cell population. Once safety has been established, the product must pass *in vitro* functional assays designed to act as surrogate measures for clinical effectiveness. EMA has released a "Reflection Paper" in 2011 [Reflection paper on SCBMPs which covers specific aspects related to SCBPs with an intention for MA application]. This reflection paper is relevant to all medicinal products using stem cells as starting material regardless of their differentiation status at the time of administration. SCBPs intended for clinical use should be produced *via* a robust manufacturing process, governed by QC, sufficient to ensure consistent and reproducible final product. EMA suggests a risk–based approach according to Annex I, part IV of Directive 2001/83/EC (Directive 2001/83/EC of the European Parliament and of the Council of November 6, 2001 on the Community code relating to medicinal products for human use) for SCBPs.

9.6 Application and Evaluation Procedure for ATMPs

The Committee for Advanced Therapies (CAT) provides a centralized procedure for ATMPs. The CAT members of the EMA formulate a draft opinion on the quality, safety, and efficacy aspect of the product for the final approval by the Committee for the Medicinal Products for Human Use (CHMP). The CHMP more or less follows the recommendation of the CAT.

The tasks of the CTA include the classification of the ATPs and the preclinical data given in the dossier. Applicants have to do the classification procedure in order to determine whether a given product based on cells, genes, or tissues meets the criteria for an ATMP. It is not a legal requirement for the applicant and an opinion is delivered within 60 days after the receipt of the request. The submitted and evaluated submission can be downloaded from the EMA homepage as non–confidential summaries. The ATMP classification procedure does not signify whether the product dossier will be evaluated by the centralized procedure or not and the CAT classification opinion is not legally binding for the NCAs.

Small and Medium-sized enterprises (SMEs) developing ATMPs can submit all the relevant quality data, and where available non-clinical data to the EMA for scientific evaluation by the CAT. It is a 90-day procedure and in the case of a favorable opinion by the CAT, the EMA will issue a corresponding certificate. Again the certification is not legally binding but it will facilitate the development and improve the CTA and marketing authorization applications (MAAs) based on the same data.

Table 9.1: Centralized and national components of the regulatory framework for ATMP development in the EU.

Type of Activity	Legislation	NCA	EMA/CAT
Cell and tissue donation, procurement, and processing	National	Inspection, authorization	N/A
Pre-clinical development	National	GLP inspection, consultation	Certification procedure (optional)
Clinical development	National	GCP, GMP inspections, authorization	N/A
ATMP classification	EU	Consultation	Procedure/opinion
ATMP certification	EU	N/A	Procedure/opinion/ certificate
ATMP evaluation	EU	N/A	Procedure/opinion
Transition period	EU	Consultation	ATMP evaluation
Hospital exemption	National	Consultation, GMP inspection, production license	N/A

Note: (GLP = good laboratory practice; GCP = good clinical practice; and GMP = good manufacturing practice).

9.7   EU Marketing Procedure

The final stage in the development of a gene therapy product (GTP) after conducting clinical trials is the marketing application. The EMA is a European agency for the evaluation of medicinal products, including GTMPs. The legislative framework for MA of human GTPs and other medicinal products is initially based on Regulation (EC) No 726/2004,[16] laying down Community procedures for the authorization and supervision of medicinal products for human and veterinary use, and establishing a European Medicines Agency. If the application concerns a product that contains a GMO, the MA dossier submitted directly to the EMA should also contain the environmental risk assessment in accordance with the principles set out in Annex II to Directive 2001/18/EC.[17] Regulation (EC) 726/2004[16] also describes that the competent authorities of 2001/18/EC[17] must be consulted. In addition, the regulation indicates that an application must be accompanied by a written consent to the deliberate release into the environment of GMOs for research and development purposes, provided for in part B of Directive 2001/18/EC.[17] Thus, there is a clear connection between MA of a GTP and the environmental risk assessment based on Directive 2001/18/EC[17] for clinical trials.

Regulation (EC) No 726/2004 and Directive 2001/83/EC[1] were amended by Regulation (EC) No 1394/2007 of the European Parliament and of the Council of November 13, 2007 on ATMPs.

9.8   CAT

In accordance with this ATMP regulation, the CAT has been established. The CAT is a multidisciplinary committee which gathers together the experts in Europe to assess the quality, safety, and efficacy of ATMPs and to follow scientific developments in the field. The main responsibility of the CAT is to prepare a draft opinion on each ATMP application submitted to the European Medicines Agency, before the CHMP adopts a final opinion on the granting, variation, suspension, or revocation of a MA for the medicine concerned. At the request of the EMA Executive Director or of the European Commission, an opinion is also drawn up on any scientific matter relating to ATMPs. The CAT is composed of different members, including five members or co-opted members of the CHMP. These members are appointed by the CHMP itself.

9.9   CHMP

The CHMP is the committee at the EMA that is responsible for preparing opinions on questions concerning medicines for human use. Assessments conducted by the CHMP are based on purely scientific criteria and determine whether the medicines concerned meet the necessary quality, safety, and efficacy requirements (in accordance with EU legislation, particularly Directive 2001/83/EC). These processes ensure that medicines have a positive risk-benefit balance in favor of patients/users of these products, once they reach the market place.

9.10   Gene Therapy Working Party (GTWP)

The CAT GTWP was a multidisciplinary group of European experts that provided recommendations to the CAT on all matters relating directly or indirectly to GT. It was established following the discontinuation of the GTWP of the CHMP. The GTWP was replaced by ad-hoc drafting groups in September 2012.

http://www.ema.europa.eu/ema/index.jsp?curl=pages/regulation/document_
listing/document_listing_000265.jsp&mid=WC0b01ac05800b378a&jsenabled=
true.

9.11 Specific Rules for Post-Authorization Surveillance of ATMPs

9.11.1 *Safety concerns*

ATMPs provide new possibilities for restoring, correcting or modifying physiological functions, or making a diagnosis. At the same time, because of their novelty, complexity, and technical specificity, they may bring along new unexplored risks to public health and to individual patients. The specific rules described in this guideline should facilitate early detection of such risks and provide a framework for effective mitigation of their consequences to public health or to individual patients.

When preparing a RM plan for a particular ATMP, comprehensive scientific consideration should be given to the important identified or potential risks, and to the important missing information.

The most relevant risks to ATMPs should be considered (listed in chronological order from manufacturing, handling, application, and clinical follow-up). Again this list is not exhaustive.

9.11.2 *Risks to living donors*

• Risks to living donors related to their conditioning prior to procurement (immuno-suppression, cytotoxic agents, and growth factors etc.).
• Risks to living donors related to surgical/medical procedures used during or following procurement, irrespective of whether the tissue was collected or not.
• Risks to patients related to quality characteristics of the product, in particular:

  — Species of origin and characteristics of cells (and related body fluids, biomaterials, and biomolecules) that are used during manufacturing and the performed safety testing.
  — Characteristics of vectors for GTMPs.
  — Biologically active substances used in manufacturing (e.g., enzymes, antibodies, cytokines, sera, growth factors, and antibiotics).
  — Quality assurance (QA) and characteristics of the finished product in terms of defined composition, stability, biological activity, and purity with reference to non-physiologic proteins, and fragments thereof.

— Risk related to transmissible diseases (viral, bacterial, parasitic infections and infestations, malignant disease, and others).

- Risks to patients related to the storage and distribution of the manufactured product:

  — Risks related to preservation, freezing, and thawing.
  — Risks of breaking the cold chain or other type of controlled temperature conditions.
  — Risks related to stability of the product.

- Risks to patients related to administration procedures, for instance:

  — Biologically active substances used in preparation of the product prior to administration (e.g., enzymes, antibodies, cytokines, sera, growth factors, and antibiotics).
  — Risks related to conditioning of the patient.
  — Risks of related medical or surgical procedures (such as anaesthesia, infusion, transfusion, implantation, transplantation or other application method, etc.).
  — Risks related to clinical follow-up (immunosuppression as co-medication or as necessary for treatment of complications, diagnostic procedures, and hospitalization, etc.).
  — Risks related to mistakes or violations of the standard procedures for administration of the product (e.g., different administration procedures used by different healthcare establishments/healthcare professionals resulting in different results).

- Risks related to interaction of the product and the patient, for instance:

  — Unwanted immunogenicity and its consequences (including anaphylaxis, GvHD, graft rejection, hypersensitivity reactions, immune deficiencies, etc.).
  — Risks related to both intended and unintended genetic modification of the patient's cells (apoptosis, change of function, alteration of growth and/or differentiation, and malignancy).
  — Early and late consequences of homing, grafting, differentiation, migration, and proliferation.

- Risks related to persistence of the product in the patient, for instance:

  — Availability of rescue procedures or antidotes and their risks.
  — Late complications, particularly malignancies, and autoimmunity.
  — Considerations on the potential impact of previous, concomitant, or future therapies (typical for the diagnosis or treatment of the respective disease), on the product, or *vice versa* impact of the product on those other therapies

(e.g., an immunoglobulin treatment later in life could impact on expression of the introduced gene by antibody interaction.).

- Risks related to re-administration, for instance:
  — Immune reactions- anaphylaxis, neutralizing antibodies.
  — Risks related to repeated surgical or administration procedures.
- Risks to close contacts, for instance:
  — Based on the environmental risk assessment, virus shedding, and its consequences.

9.12 Dynamics of the Disease and Effects of the Product

Detection of early complications (infectious diseases, complications linked to the related surgical procedures) and late complications (malignant diseases, emerging diseases, etc.) need different approaches. Moreover, they need to be considered in conjunction with the possible gradual increase or decrease of efficacy of the administered product over time. Design of the studies needs to take into account such dynamics, and good medical practice that may require specific timing of procedures, treatment adjustments, and laboratory investigations to be tailored for individual patients.

Source: EMEA/149995/2008.

9.13 Considerations on Safety Follow-Up of Living Donors

It is acknowledged that follow-up of living donors of tissues, cells, or blood is a legal responsibility of tissue establishments or blood establishments. Nevertheless, when the ATMP in question requires donation from living donors for its production, the Marketing Authorizations Holder (MAH) of such ATMP should take into account the risks identified for donors and design its PV plan in such a way that guarantee a data exchange with the establishment performing the procurement. The aim is to make sure that production of the product does not bring undue risk to living donors, and also to ensure that in the event that an infectious disease with a long latency emerges in the donor, the receivers may get appropriate screening and treatment (using the traceability system).

The particular design and length of such follow-up should be decided on a case-by-case basis, and needs to be proportionate to the nature of the procurement procedure, identified and potential risks to donors and health characteristics of donor.

9.14   Regulatory Framework in the US

In the US, use of CTPs is codified within the Code of Federal Regulations (CFRs) in the following sections: Investigational New Drug (IND) regulations (21 CFR 312),[18] biologics regulations (21 CFR 600),[19] and cGMP (21 CFR 211). In particular, US federal regulation on cellular therapy is divided into two sections of the Public Health Service Act (PHSA), referred as "361 products" and "351 products". Traditional blood and bone marrow progenitor cells as well as other tissues for transplantation fall into 361 products definition. The Food and Drug Administration (FDA) has established that cells or tissues used for therapeutic purposes and the regulation that pertains to processing of 361 products are codified under the Good Tissue Practice (GTP)[20] CFR, Part 1271, provides US regulations on Cells, Tissues, and Cellular and Tissue-Based Products (HCT/Ps).[21] This became effective in 2005 as rules for HCT/Ps. The FDA has also issued guidance documents about how the drug, biologic, and device regulations apply to cellular and genetic therapies.[22]

Classification of stem cell-based therapies (SCBTs) is based on indications to be treated. Restrictions are limited to research with federal funds. No limitations exist for research with human embryonic stem cells (hESCs), provided the funds come from private investors or specific states. The FDA has developed a regulatory framework that controls both cell- and tissue-based products, based on three general areas:

- Prevention of use of contaminated tissues or cells (e.g., AIDS or hepatitis);
- Prevention of inadequate handling or processing that may damage or contaminate those tissues or cells; and
- Clinical safety of all tissues or cells that may be processed, used for functions other than normal functions, combined with components other than tissues, or used for metabolic purposes.

The Center for Biologics Evaluation and Research (CBER), the division of US FDA that regulates SCBTs, has so far approved ApliGraf®, Carticel®, and Epicel®. Those cell-based therapeutics "that are, minimally manipulated, labeled or advertized for homologous use only, and not combined with a drug or device" do not require FDA approval.[23] In contrast, manipulated autologous cells for structural use, meet the definition of somatic cell therapy products (SCTPs) and require an "IND" exemption or the FDA license approval. In 2007, the "Guidance for Industry: Regulation of HCT/Ps- Small Entity Compliance Guide," and in 2009, the "Guidance for Industry on Current Good Tissue Practice (cGTP) and Additional Requirements for Manufacturers of HCT/Ps" (http://www.fda.gov) had been released.[24] Clinical studies employing MSCs underlie the IND mechanism. Accordingly, the investigators have to make an IND application, which necessitates detailed study protocols describing the clinical plan as well as the preparation and testing of the therapeutic cell product.[25]

Under the current FDA policies, there are at least two ways in which physicians may administer more than minimally manipulated stem cell products to patients. The first is under the FDA's program for expanded access to investigational drugs and biological products for use in treatment (what is sometimes referred to as "compassionate use") as long as these products are currently being tested elsewhere in a Clinical Trial and only if the expanded access does not interfere with the conduct of clinical investigations. FDA allows clinicians to charge for direct cost recovery and administrative costs associated with expanded access use.[26] The second is the off-label prescribing of FDA-approved stem cell products. Off-label prescribing is premised on the condition that the FDA does not have the authority to regulate medical practice and the assumption that physicians can be trusted to use their professional judgment in deciding how to treat their patients.

9.15 The Orphan Drug Act and the Development of SCBPs for Rare Diseases

About 30 million people living in the EU suffer from a rare disease. Rare diseases are defined as life-threatening or chronically debilitating conditions that affect no more than five in 10,000 people in EU. This is equivalent to around 250,000 people or less for each disease.

Sponsors of designated orphan medicines are eligible to benefit from the incentives offered which includes the following:

- Assistance with development of the medicine.
- Reduced fees for MAAs.
- Protection from market competition once the medicine is authorized.

9.15.1 *Rare diseases at a glance*

- Rare diseases are life-threatening or chronically debilitating conditions affecting no more than five in 10,000 people in the EU. Most of these people suffer from diseases affecting less than one in 100,000 people.
- Between 5,000 and 8,000 distinct rare diseases exist, affecting between 6% and 8% of the population in total; in other words, between around 27 million and 36 million people in the EU.
- On an average, five new diseases are described every week in the medical literature.
- Symptoms of some rare diseases may appear at birth or in childhood, including spinal muscular atrophy, lysosomal storage disorders, and patent ductus arteriosus (PDA), familial adenomatous polyposis (FAP), and cystic fibrosis. More than half of rare diseases appear during adulthood, such as renal-cell carcinoma, glioma, and acute myeloid leukaemia.
- 80% of rare diseases have been identified as genetic origins, and affect between 3% and 4% of the humans at birth. Other rare diseases are due to degenerative and proliferative causes.
- Medical and scientific knowledge about rare diseases is lacking. The number of scientific publications about rare diseases continues to increase, particularly those identifying new syndromes. However, fewer than 1,000 diseases benefit from even minimal amounts of scientific knowledge. These tend to be the rare diseases that occur most frequently.

9.16 Application Procedure

9.16.1 *Pre-submission meeting*

The EMA strongly encourages sponsors/companies to request a pre-submission meeting prior to filing an application for orphan medicinal product designation. Pre-submission meetings for orphan designation are free of charge and are held mostly *via* teleconference, unless the sponsor/company has a strong preference to come to the agency in person. Follow-up teleconferences are also possible.

Sponsors have to take minutes of the meeting, which should be provided to the EMA within two weeks after the meeting. The agency will subsequently review the minutes within two weeks, and agree the final (amended) minutes with the applicant (sponsor).

Appointment of coordinators

Two coordinators [One for the Committee for Orphan Medicinal Product (COMP) member and one for the EMA scientific administrator] will be appointed for each application. The sponsor will be informed accordingly *via* e-mail.

9.16.2 *Submission*

Deadlines for submission of an orphan medicinal product designation application are published on the EMA website (www.ema.europe.eu).

9.16.3 *Validation*

The EMA secretariat will complete the validation of the application. In the event that the EMA requires additional data, information, or clarification to complete its validation, the sponsor will receive a validation issue letter and will be asked to respond within a three-month time limit. If no response from the sponsor is received within this time frame, the sponsor will be advised to withdraw the application and consider re-submission.

Once the validation process is successfully completed, a time-table to start the procedure for the evaluation will be forwarded to the sponsor for information.

9.16.4 *Evaluation*

During the evaluation phase, the EMA coordinator will work very closely with the COMP coordinators and appointed expert(s). The coordinators may gather information from Committee members on the disease state, availability of treatments, research status, etc.

A summary report will be provided based on the application. The summary report will include data reported in the sponsor's application, a critical review, and a conclusion.

Following agreement between the Agency coordinator and the COMP coordinator, the summary report will be circulated to the COMP members for comments. Members of COMP will forward comments to the Agency in accordance with the adopted time-table.

Following the COMP's first discussion, the sponsor may be invited to address the list of questions at the next meeting. The list of questions will be forwarded with the draft summary report to the sponsor after the first meeting. The sponsors may be invited to attend an oral explanation at the next COMP meeting.

Table 9.2:　Authorized applications for ATMPs.

Initial Evaluation of Marketing Authorisation Applications (MAA) for ATMP

	2009	2010	2011	2012	2013	Total
Submitted MAAs	3	1	2	3	1	10
Positive draft Opinion	1	0	1[i]	1[i]	2	5
						Corresponding to 4 ATMPs
Withdrawals	1	1	0	0	2	4
Ongoing MAAs						2

[i]Same product (Glybera).

The oral explanation lasts around one hour and includes the COMP discussion with the sponsor. The outcome of the discussion will be communicated to the sponsor immediately after the Committee has reached a conclusion.

9.16.5 *Opinion*

The COMP opinion, which may be favorable or unfavorable, is, wherever possible, reached by consensus.

If a negative outcome of the review of the application appears likely, the sponsor may withdraw the application before the COMP adopts the opinion. In such case, the sponsor will be informed immediately about the negative trend and advised on a possibility to withdraw the application by submitting a signed letter requesting a withdrawal by the end of the on–going COMP meeting.

9.16.6 *Decision*

The decision will be adopted by the Commission, within 30 days of its receipt of the COMP opinion and forwarded to the sponsor.

Following the EC decision on the designation, a public summary of opinion on orphan designation will be published on the EMA website.

9.17　The Hospital Exemption for Specific ATMPs

9.17.1 *Scope of the hospital exemption*

Most of the contributions from industry considered that the current scope is too broadly interpreted and discourages research in ATMP by pharma companies, thereby hindering the development of new products that could be used across the EU. In general, there appears to be a perception in the industry sector that the hospital exemption is being used to circumvent the requirements for MA. Thus, the most repeated suggestion from the industry sector was that the hospital exemption should not be permitted when there is an authorized product available. As per the type of conditions for which the hospital exemption should be permissible, the position of the industry sector was split: Some contributors considered that it should be limited to pathologies with few patients; others considered that it should be kept broad.

However, the predominant sentiment in contributions from academia is that the hospital exemption is a critical tool for the development of new innovative therapies. Reference was made to the fact that some of the institutions that are more actively involved in the research and development of advanced therapies are not driven by commercial interests and that, in any case, the majority of projects are focused on rare conditions with no significant market value. Many contributions from the non-industry sector considered that the current scope of the hospital exemption should be maintained or should be further expanded. However, some supported the restriction that the hospital exemption should not be applicable when there is an authorized medicinal product available.

The ATMP Regulation determines that medicinal products classified as ATMPs shall be regulated under the centralized European MA procedure. MA is granted by the European Commission following assessment by the EMA. Article 28 of the ATMP Regulation[9] defines an exemption from the central authorization requirement for ATMPs which are prepared on a non-routine basis and used within the same Member State in a hospital in accordance with a medical prescription for an individual patient, the so-called hospital exemption. Member States are required to implement this community requirement for a hospital exemption by putting in place the arrangements at the national level to meet the specific requirements set out in the ATMP Regulation.

The hospital exemption (Article 28) is applicable to all ATMPs that are

— Prepared on a non-routine basis;
— Prepared according to specific quality standards (equivalent to those for ATMPs with a centralized MA);
— Used within the same Member State;
— Used in a hospital;
— Used under the exclusive responsibility of a medical practitioner; and
— Comply with an individual medical prescription for a custom-made product for an individual patient.

The authorization on the basis of the hospital exemption is in the remit of the corresponding Member State. Therefore, the CAT is not formally involved in the hospital exemption authorization processes.

9.17.2 The hospital exemption for specific ATMPs in Germany

Hospital exemption as implemented in Germany is an option for ATMPs utilized for highly innovative treatments that are fulfilling the criteria set by Article 28 of the ATMP Regulation.[9]

One example may be the highly personalized patient–specific GTMPs that consist of autologous cells loaded with nucleic acids that are tumor-specific. For such a medicinal product, hospital exemption may be regarded as a suitable tool to support development and availability of these products, and thereby also providing specific treatment options for physicians and patients. Moreover, it also may be suitable to guide a particular ATMP into routine manufacturing toward a central MA. The hospital exemption procedure in Germany, which is performed by the Paul-Ehrlich-Institute (PEI), is set up to ensure compliance with community rules for safety and efficacy, put in place appropriate standards for QC of the manufacturing process including compliance with the good manufacturing practice (GMP) requirements, review of available data/information and a discussion on the benefit/risk balance.

9.18　From Preclinics to Clinics

9.18.1 Bridging the gaps from discovery to medicine

The regulatory requirements, model selection, and protocol development are paving the critical path for transition from preclinics into the application for clinical trials. A company or any contract organization involved which has a clear understanding of the nuances of the preclinical phase can extract more useful information that aids drug development and speeds overall progress to Phase I.

Selecting the appropriate model for a particular research protocol is perhaps the most important factor in a preclinical trial, especially for ATMPs like cell-based medicinal products (CBMPs). Yet, some Contract Research Organizations (CROs) do not have a lot of experience with animal-based studies, where even seemingly minor considerations, for example, having equal numbers of male and female mice, can have repercussions for getting through regulatory agencies.

In oncology, it is much more critical because malignant disease is enormously complex. You need to make sure you have the animal model that best represents a particular malignancy and will allow you to tease apart various drug effects.

Timing mostly depends on the model and tumor type. Obviously, the goal is to make the process as efficient as possible without compromising integrity and quality of the data. It is very important to know at the preclinical stage itself about how your clinical study will be designed.

Some issues that should be considered when selecting a model are whether it reproduces the major clinical symptoms of the human disease, whether the same cells and/or tissues are affected, whether the same genes and molecular pathways are involved, and whether the disease proceeds over a similar time compared to that in humans. In instances in which mice are not natural hosts of pathogens that infect humans, alternatives such as non-human primates may be better suited to study certain aspects of pathogenesis or to test novel therapeutics. Irrespecive of whether mice are 'good' or 'bad', they undoubtedly have a useful place in translational research. But it is important to realize where such animal models are inherently limited and to bridge the gaps between human patients and the animal model. The preclinical research determines the specifications (Do's/Don'ts) for Phase I clinical trial, which is in most cases designed for safety & tolerability.

9.19   Clinical Development of ATMPs

9.19.1   *Communication with authorities/agencies*

9.19.1.1   *National or International scientific advice*

According to Regulation (EC) No 726/2004, one of the tasks of the Agency is, where necessary, advising companies on the conduct of various tests and trials necessary to demonstrate the quality, safety, and efficacy of medicinal products. It covers the entire development process and can be used to provide advice on protocols for clinical trials. National Authorities throughout the European Community however retain the competence to review trials within their country and it should be remembered that there may be additional national requirements. The competent authorities (e.g., PEI) and agencies (e.g., FDA) highlight the importance of preparatory discussions with companies asking for scientific advice, especially when it is the first time for a company intended for scientific advice. These scientific advice pre-submission meetings (which should take place at least 1−2 months prior to the anticipated date of submission of the request) are a good opportunity for companies to obtain advice from the authority/agency on structure and content of the request as well as on procedural aspects, in order to get the best benefit from the scientific advice.

Once the initial pre-meeting has taken place, another pre-meeting is not required. It should be mentioned that any advice given is not legally binding with regard to any future CTA or MAA of the product concerned, but of course will be taken into account in the authorization process.

The question(s) posed by the company should be as precise and clear as possible. Such question(s) should address specific scientific issues concerning:

- Quality parameters and specifications of the IMP.
- Intended Pre-clinical studies.
- Clinical trials and indications.
- Biometry.
- PV and RM.

Also important to mention is that regulatory aspects should be addressed in a separate meeting, if necessary.

The decision on going national or international (e.g., EMA, EMA–FDA for parallel scientific advice) depends on the stage of development and the existing experience of the respective authority. Regulatory research within published assessment reports or former decisions and processes of approved medicinal products in the same indication or classification may help to find out the centers of excellence preferrably to achieve most reliable advice.

- The request for a scientific meeting should be forwarded as follows: A cover letter including the intention of the development.
- An authority-specific template filled with the requested basic information.
- A scientific briefing document providing the questions & company's position.
- Annexes (references and other supporting data).

For further information, please visit, e.g., Regulation (EC) No 726/2004 and Regulation (EC) No 470/2009 and the national or EMA/FDA homepages.

9.19.1.2 *Scientific advice meeting and follow up*

All meetings are successful, if prepared thoroughly! Therefore, the following steps should be introduced:

1. Include all research and marketing faculties in preparation of the questions and positions in the briefing document.
2. Rehearse the meeting before visiting the competent authority (CA).

3. Keep the minutes very seriously, as they will accompany the whole further development and approval process.

9.19.2 *CRO selection*

9.19.2.1 *Choose wisely the right CRO*

For many pharmaceutical and biotech companies, especially the smaller ones which are engaged in clinical trials outsourcing is not so much a choice, as it is a necessity. Clinical trials are often complex projects and it is not often feasible to conduct the whole process in-house, nor does it makes sense from a financial perspective. Therefore, it is very important to choose the right CRO. It is important to choose partners who are able to do the work and who can work well as a team. There are several issues to keep in mind when choosing a CRO.

9.19.2.2 *Selection/qualification criteria*

Before work at a CRO is initiated, a research team composed of members with a diversity of expertise should be involved in selecting which CRO will be performing the defined activities. This might also be called "qualifying" the CRO. It is generally recommended that a visit to the CRO's facility and meetings with management, scientists, and QA personnel be part of the process.

When selecting a CRO, due diligence requires establishing a predetermined set of criteria against which the CRO will be judged. These criteria range from regulatory compliance, areas of capability, location, and budget. There are several specific organizational and operational areas that should be evaluated during this process:

- **Policies and Procedures**: Comprehensive review of organizational structure, accreditation status, facility and equipment maintenance, QA procedures, and compliance with national and international guidelines.
- **Personnel Management**: Thorough review of staffing levels, job descriptions, training records, and observations of personnel performing work. Discussions should include scientific experience, capabilities, and expertise.
- **Facilities**: The physical structures should be inspected for quality and compliance. Required equipments, e.g., information technology (IT) should be well-maintained and meet the specifications for the outsourced work.
- **Security**: The confidentiality of the research performed by a CRO is critical. In addition to validated procedures for the security of electronic data and

correspondence, an inspection of facility security and intrusion deterrence system should be carried out.

- **Crisis Management**: CROs should have an effective crisis management plan that covers all potential circumstances and ensures effective communication with Sponsors.

9.19.2.3 *Review and ongoing evaluations*

CROs should be audited on a regular basis. Annual visits should be performed, but most CROs expect sponsor visits once every two to three years. Additionally, many sponsors opt to schedule visits that coincide with important study milestones.

During these visits, expectations can be reviewed and CRO records should be evaluated. Specific subjects to address during this assessment include significant changes in CRO staff, quality of data and communication, as well as regulatory or accreditation compliance issues.

Altogether, the selection of the right CRO for clinical trials is, among others, one of the most important steps for success.

9.19.3 *Selecting the right investigator*

A clinical trial must be supervised by a qualified person in accordance with applicable regulations and clinical guidelines. These qualifications may vary depending on the disease or therapeutic treatment under investigation, such as cancer research. One of the worst mistakes a sponsor can make is to hire someone who is not qualified to run the clinical trial. Such mistakes can be costly to the sponsor, participating patients, and the clinical investigator.

Therefore, one of the utmost important factors involving the success of a clinical research trial lies amongst the selection and evaluation of a clinical investigator. Clinical investigators perform the actual research used to support applications for new drugs, biologics, and medical devices. A clinical investigator may be a professional researcher operating out of a research institution such as a research hospital or university, or may be a practicing physician who also conducts clinical research.

The Clinical Trial Managers (CTMs) involved with the process of selecting and evaluating the clinical investigator must possess the skills and knowledge in the clinical research area in order to know what to look for in an individual.

What really counts in the selection and evaluation of the clinical investigator? Looking into different key areas and qualities which a successful investigator candidate should possess can make a clinical trial run more smoothly. A highly desirable clinical investigator should have knowledge in the research area, possess positive research practices and ethics, and will be unbiased to the clinical trial.

9.19.4 *Hosting an investigator meeting*

An Investigator meeting is a meeting that should be attended by all the participating Lead Investigators, Sub- and Co-Investigators and study site personnel, e.g., study coordinators and study nurses who have agreed to participate in a clinical trial. The purpose of the investigator meeting is to inform all the Investigators and the site staff about the IMP and the particularities of the clinical trial. There may also be some training in GCP and regulatory requirements. Investigator meetings are usually held just before the start of the trial, but when regulatory green light is given (from NCA and from the Lead Ethics Committee).

During this meeting, background information should be provided explaining why the clinical trial is conducted, the clinical endpoints of the clinical trial and the history of the study (if is not the first study), and the IMP itself. This information is very important for the investigators and helps them making their decisions during the conduct of the clinical trial.

The investigator meeting should be very interactive, meaning that all the participants should have the chance to ask questions, give feedback and offer other suggestions.

Note: The meeting itself should be held in a central and accessible location. Dedicated conference staff is essential. Someone from the sponsor or CRO should visit the venue prior to booking, to ensure facilities are as described in the brochure or on the internet. It should be checked that the meeting room is large enough and that the hotel bedrooms are up to the required standard.

For pan-European studies, it may be worth considering separate meetings in respective countries, or regional meetings as appropriate.

9.20 Request for Authorization for a Clinical Trial in the EU

For the CTA procedure, the guidance laid down in Article 9(8) of Directive 2001/20/ EC of the European Parliament and of the Council on April 4, 2001 relating to the implementation of GCP in the conduct of clinical trials on medicinal products (Directive 2001/20/EC) is valid.

The sponsor (applicant) may not start a clinical trial until the Ethics Committee has issued a positive opinion, as well as the CA of the Member State concerned has not informed the sponsor/applicant of any reasons for not approving the clinical trial.

For a given clinical trial, there may be several Member States concerned (multi-national clinical trials) which means that sponsor must apply in each single country, where the clinical trial will be conducted, for CTA.

As the different Member states in the European Union have a different view on the protocol, and the way it should be carried forward, it is possible that different feedback is given to the sponsor/applicant. According to International Conference on Harmonisation (ICH)–GCP, the study should be conducted under one protocol which means that all the different opinions of the different Members States have to be incorporated in one protocol versions.

9.20.1 *Request for CTA*

Before starting any clinical trial, one must submit a valid request for authorization to the CA of the Member State in which the clinical trial should be conducted. The authorization of a clinical trial by the NCA is valid for a clinical trial conducted in that Member State. This authorization is not to be considered as scientific advice on the development program of the tested IMP.

The submitted documents will be checked by the authority, e.g., at the PEI for formal compliance within 10 days after receipt of the CTA request. Non-compliances will be communicated to the sponsor within 10 days and must be answered within 14 days. If the request is without formal non-conformities, a confirmation of receipt will be sent to the sponsor, and the day after the receipt at the PEI, shall be the first day of the evaluation of the content by the PEI. The evaluation period is 30 days for allergens, vaccines, and biotechnology medicinal products, 60 days for biological products (of human/animal origin), and 90 days for GTMPs and GMOs. No fixed periods apply for xenogeneic cell therapeutics.

After the evaluations of the submitted documents, the applicant will either be notified about the reasons for rejection, or, if no reasons were communicated, the approval letter will be issued. If reasons for rejection were communicated, the sponsor will be granted a period of 90 days to answer the questions/comments by amending the request. After submission of the amendment, the PEI will have a period of 15 or 30 days, depending on the medicinal product, to evaluate the amendment (See Figure 9.2).

**Graphic display of the periods and process of clinical trial authorisations
for Allergens, Vaccines and Biotech Products**

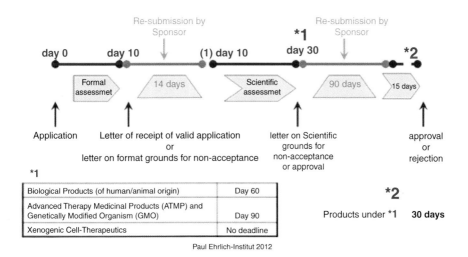

Figure 9.2:   Application procedure to PEI.

Source: www.pei.de.

   If the deficiency list is too exhaustive, the sponsor may also apply for
prolongation of the period. But this may vary from CA to CA. Important to mention is that some countries in the EU are following longer evaluation periods and
some other countries like Belgium and Austria have shorter timelines for approval
(Belgium has at present the shortest timelines within the EU with 28 days followed
by Austria with 30 days for approval).

9.20.2   *Application to the ethics committee (EC)*

The application to the Ethics Committee can be generally done in parallel to the
application to the competent authorities. In some European countries, the application can be done only after approval from the CA has been obtained. For country
specific requirements, the homepage of the local Ethics Committee should be vis-
ited. If an application is not valid, the Ethics Committee will inform the applicant
of the deficiencies.

Table 9.3: Average Processing Periods; Status as of 31.12.2011.

	30-Day Procedure		60-Day Procedure		90-Day Procedure	
	Target/ Days	Actual Days	Target/ Days	Actual Days	Target/ Days	Actual Days
Period up to the notification; additional documents needed/ confirmation of receipt	10	8	10	8	10	8
Answer period, sponsor	14	9	14	12	14	12
Valid application						
Period up to the notification of the grounds of non-acceptance of the contents/ authorization of the trial	30	25	60	47	90	76
Answer period, sponsor	90	42	90	42	90	67
Re-assessment response/period up to the authorization	15	12	30	20	30	26
Average of the total period (PEI & Sponsor); target and actual days	45 + 90	37 + 42	90 + 90	67 + 42	120 + 90	102 + 67

Source: www.pei.de.

All documents should carry the trial identification (EudraCT number, sponsor's protocol code number, date and/or version) as well as the version and/or date of the particular document submitted. The procedure for obtaining the EudraCT number: This number is described in the detailed guidance on the European clinical trials database.

The procedures for enrolment of clinical trial patients should be described in detail in the clinical trial protocol. When recruitment of subjects is planned to be

Table 9.4:   Distribution of scientific grounds of non-acceptance by products and part of the dossier; status as of 01.01.2013.

Product	Quality	Preclinical	Clinical	Viral Safety	Statistics
GTMPs	85.7	78.6	78.6	50.0	21.4
GMOs	71.1	73.7	78.9	50.0	31.6
SCTs	77.9	58.1	76.7	57.0	53.5

Source: www.pei.de.

by advertisement, copies of the material to be used should be attached, including any printed material. The procedures proposed for handling the responses to the advertisement(s) should be outlined.

9.20.3 *Substantial and non-substantial amendments*

Once a clinical trial has been approved by NCAs (e.g., PEI) and the Ethic Committees, changes to the clinical trial are frequently required to improve and maintain the integrity of the conduct of a clinical trial.

These changes are implemented *via* so called Amendments. Amendments are changes made to the clinical trial after NCA approval has been given. It must be distinguished between so called substantial and non-substantial amendments. Substantial amendments require approval and cannot be implemented until the relevant approvals are in place, except in the case of urgent safety measures.

A substantial amendment is defined as an amendment to the terms of the application, or to the protocol or any other supporting documentation, that is likely to affect to a significant degree:

- The safety or physical or mental integrity of the subjects of the study.
- The scientific value of the study.
- The conduct or management of the study; or
- The quality or safety of any IMP used in the trial.

For all studies, it is the responsibility of the sponsor to determine whether an amendment is substantial or not and this is sometimes very difficult as the definitions for substantial, as listed above, can be sometimes differently interpreted.

If the sponsor comes to the conclusion that the amendment is substantial, the change(s) must be included in the amendment, briefly explaining the reasons in each case, on the notice of amendment. The submitted documents that have been modified should show both the previous and new wording.

9.21 Author's Outlook on Clinical Trial Regulation

Upcoming Regulation in 2016/2017:

REGULATION (EU) No. 536/2014 OF THE EUROPEAN PARLIAMENT AND OF THE COUNCIL of 16 April 2014 on clinical trials on medicinal products for human use, and repealing Directive 2001/20/EC.

In 2016 or 2017 a new regulation for Clinical Trial Authorisation will come into effect. The new procedures for the authorisation of clinical trials should facilitate the inclusion of as many Member States as possible. Therefore, in order to simplify the procedures for the submission of an application dossier for the authorisation of a clinical trial, the multiple submission of largely identical information will be avoided and replaced by the submission of one application dossier to all the Member States concerned through a single submission portal. This new legal form of a Regulation should present advantages for sponsors and investigators, for example in the context of clinical trials taking place in more than one Member State.

The main characteristics of the new Regulation are:

- A streamlined application procedure via a single entry point, the EU portal.
- A single set of documents to be prepared and submitted for the application defined in Annex I of the Regulation;
- A harmonised procedure for the assessment of applications for clinical trials, which is divided in two parts. Part I is jointly assessed by all Member States concerned. Part II is assessed by each Member State concerned separately.
- Strictly defined deadlines for the assessment of clinical trial application;
- The involvement of the ethics committees in the assessment procedure in accordance with the national law of the Member state concerned but within the overall timelines defined by the Regulation.
- Simplified reporting procedures which will avoid submitting identical information separately to different Member States;
- Increased transparency for clinical trials and their outcomes;
- Clinical trials conducted outside the EU, but referred to in a clinical trial application within the EU, will have to comply with regulatory requirements that are at least equivalent to those applicable in the EU.

Source: Regulation (CTR) EU No 536/2014.

9.22   Development of Key Study Documents

Clinical trials should be designed, conducted, and analyzed according to sound scientific principles to achieve their objectives; and should be reported appropriately. The essence of rational drug development is to ask important questions and answer them with well-designed clinical trials. The primary objectives of any study should be clear and explicitly stated. Therefore, it is very important to work before hand in early development with consultants, scientific experts, and experienced investigators to develop the right study protocol. Selecting the right investigator for protocol assistance, development can be very challenging (please also see Section 9.19.3 "Selecting the Right Investigator").

It is also important to mention that the clinical trials are conducted serially. The logic behind serially conducted studies of a medicinal product is that the results of prior trials should/will influence the plan of later studies.

Data from an interim analyses or completed study will frequently prompt a modification of the development strategy. For example, results of a therapeutic confirmatory study may suggest a need for additional human pharmacology studies.

9.22.1   *Objectives of a clinical trial*

The objective(s) of a clinical trial should be clearly mentioned in the clinical trial protocol and should include exploratory or confirmatory characterization of safety and/or efficacy parameters.

9.22.1.1   *Design of a clinical trial*

The appropriate study design should be chosen to provide the desired information. Examples of study design include

— Parallel group,
— Cross-over,
— Dose escalation,
— Single blinded,
— Double blinded, etc. (See ICH E4, E6, E9, and E10).

Methods of monitoring adverse events by changes in clinical signs and symptoms and laboratory studies should be described (please also refer to ICH E3). The protocol should specify procedures for the follow-up of patients who stop treatment prematurely.

Safety Studies

For the first trials in humans (FIH), the dose that will be administered should be determined by careful examination of the prerequisite non-clinical PK, pharmacological, and toxicological evaluations (see ICH M3). Early non-clinical studies should provide sufficient information to support selection of the initial human dose and safe duration of exposure, and also provide information about physiological and toxicological effects of a new drug.

The objective(s) of the study should be clearly stated and may include exploratory or confirmatory characterization of safety and/or efficacy and/or assessment of PK parameters and pharmacological, physiological, and biochemical effects.

When nursing mothers are enrolled in clinical studies, their babies should be monitored for the effects of the drug.

Pharmacological and PK Studies

The basis and direction of the clinical exploration and development rests on the non-clinical PK and pharmacology profile, which includes information such as:

(a) Pharmacological basis of principal effects (Mode of action).
(b) Dose-response relationships and duration of action.
(c) Study of the potential clinical routes of administration.
(d) Systemic general pharmacology, including pharmacological effects on major organ systems and physiological responses.
(e) Studies of absorption, distribution, and metabolism, etc.

9.22.2 Preparation of the Investigator's Brochure (IB)

The purpose of writing an IB is to provide the participating investigators and other clinical trial study personnel involved in the clinical trial with information to facilitate their understanding of the rationale for, and their compliance with, key elements of the protocol. These key elements include the dose, dose frequency/dose interval, methods of administration (e.g., intravenous, oral, etc.) and safety monitoring procedures. An IB should be prepared from all available information/evidence that supports the rationale for the proposed clinical trial and the safe use of the IMP in the trial.

9.22.3 *Preparation of an Investigational Medicinal Product Dossier (IMPD)*

The IMPD is one of the core documents that compose the CTA. The IMPD provides quality and non-clinical data on the IMP, in addition to data from previous clinical trials and human experience to evaluate the benefits and risks associated with the administration of an IMP during the conduct of the clinical trial. The quality section of the IMPD, describing all aspects of the Chemistry, Manufacturing, and Control (CMC) of the product under investigation, plays an important role in ensuring safety and establishing the scientific relevance of the IMP along with already completed non-clinical and clinical studies. The nature of the information and the level of detail to be provided in an IMPD will vary depending on the product type [New Chemical Entity (NCE), Biologics, Cell, and GTPs] and the stage of clinical development. Several guidelines have been prepared by the EMA to provide further transparency on the content of the quality sections of IMPDs as detailed below.

The role of the CMC and the Regulatory Affairs department as well as other departments involved in compiling the information for an IMPD, is to keep safely the clinical trial subjects as the top priority for any study. Therefore, each CTA must provide the reviewers at the CA with the assurance that: (1) The study will not expose the subjects to unjustified risk and that; (2) The subjects may potentially benefit from the use of the IMP (with the exception of healthy volunteer studies, where the subjects are not necessarily expected to experience a clinical benefit from the IMP).

9.23 During the Conduct of a Clinical Trial

9.23.1 *Trial management & monitoring*

Appropriate planning before the trial and adequate oversight and monitoring during the trial will help ensure that safety of the trial subject is maintained throughout the trial and that there is accurate reporting of results at its conclusion.

Where trial management activities are contracted out to third parties, the sponsor must implement procedures to ensure appropriate oversight of all delegated functions. This can be achieved by:

(a) Assessing that individuals or organizations delegated with trial management functions are appropriately qualified and competent to perform those functions.

(b) Ensuring that all parties are aware of their roles and responsibilities (e.g., by clearly defining them in contracts and agreements).
(c) Maintaining lines of communication to ensure the obligations of all parties are being met (for example, by receiving progress reports).

The purpose of trial monitoring as defined in ICH–GCP is to ensure that:

- The rights and well being of trial participants are well protected.
- The reported trial data are accurate, complete, and verifiable from source documents.
- The conduct of the trial is in compliance with the currently approved protocol/amendments, with ICH–GCP, and with the applicable regulatory requirements.

The EMA has published a Reflection Paper on Risk-Based Quality Management in Clinical Trials stating: "Clinical research is about generating information to support decision making. The quality of information generated should therefore be sufficient to support good decision making. The adequacy of that quality can also be characterized by stating that it should be such that the decisions made would have been no different had the quality of data and information generated been perfect" (Reflection paper on risk-based quality management in clinical trials, August 4, 2011; EMA/INS/GCP/394194/2011).

9.23.2 *Data Monitoring Committee (DMC)*

A DMC should be considered for every trial, although one may not always be necessary.

The role of a DMC/Data and Safety Monitoring Board (DSMB) is to review the clinical trial data and to assess whether there are any severe safety issues which could lead to a stop of the clinical trial. If the clinical trial is a blinded clinical trial, the DMC/DSMB is the only group which can assess the clinical trial data unblinded. The sponsor and the participating investigators are kept blinded at any time.

The decision whether a DMC/DSMB should be implemented in a clinical trial, should be based on the potential risk of the drug and the patients who get the drug.

9.23.3 *Day to day monitoring*

9.23.3.1 *Day to day management should be carried out to check*

- That the data are consistent and in compliance with the clinical study protocol;

- That the case report form (CRF) are being completed by the responsible person and that no key data are missing in the CRF;
- That the data entered in the CRF are valid (range and consistency checks); and
- That the recruitment timelines are the expected ones and in line with the study timelines.

Above mentioned tasks are generally outsourced to a CRO, and therefore the CRO should be monitored regularly, e.g., by weekly/monthly telefon conferences with the CRO.

9.23.3.2 *On site monitoring/co-monitoring*

On site monitoring visits/co-monitoring visits should be also performed by the sponsor on a regular basis. For this, a co-monitoring plan should be set up; especially when many sites are involved as each single site cannot be monitored/co-monitored. For cause, audits are always possible, if an issue is persistent at a clinical trial site.

On site monitoring visits should be performed:

- To verify that the clinical trial site has the required documents in place to conduct the clinical trial.
- To ensure that the pharmacy and laboratory resources are still adequate.
- To check the compliance with the study protocol and review documents like the signed informed consent forms and patient's inclusion and exclusion criteria.
- To verify that all protocol relevant data have been transcribed in time to the case report form
- To identify study team training needs and other important items to ensure the proper trial conduct.

9.23.3.3 *Protection of personal data of the patient*

Protection of personal data of patients/subjects/healthy volunteers is laid down in EU legislation. It is a fundamental right of EU citizens. The policy ensures adequate personal data protection. It is fully compliant with applicable regulations in the EU, in particular Regulation (EC) No 45/2001 and Directive 95/46/EC. Here you can find ways and means to anonymize data and protect patients from identification.

In the context of the policy, clinical trial data refers to data and information listed in Annex I [according to ICH M4E (R1)] and Annex II (according to ICH E3).

9.24 Clinical Study Report and Publication

Pharmaceutical companies are legally required to disclose relevant data from clinical trials and other research to the appropriate national or regional regulatory authorities as part of the medicine development and approval process. After approval, companies have a continuing obligation to provide regulatory authorities with updated safety information on the medicine from clinical research/clinical trials and other sources. This ensures regulators/authorities (e.g., PEI) to assess the safety and effectiveness of medicines and monitor the safety.

The clinical study report (CSR) is a summary of the clinical trial results in which the clinical and statistical parts are integrated into one report incorporating tables, listings, and figures (TLFs). The CSR should provide an overview of the design and features of the study, and additional information on the plan, methods, and conduct of the study so that there is no doubt that the clinical trial was carried out in compliance with the ICH regulations. The report with its appendices should also provide enough individual patient data, including the demographic and baseline data, and details of analytical methods. Additionally, it is also of importance that all analyses made, tables, listings, and figures which are part of the text or of the appendix, bear a clear identification from which type/set of patients the analyses were generated.

Publication, but also non-publication of trial results can be motivated by several factors. Research reports may affect clinical practice, inform patients, influence future research, and prevent duplication of effort. Publication of clinical trial data also has important secondary effects. Authorship of papers in journals can establish reputations and enhance career prospects. Institutional or corporate reputations may also benefit. The productivity of academic departments is judged on their publication output, which also affects their chances of obtaining future funding. The peer-reviewed (and indexed "impact") journal has therefore become part of the process of academic appointments and promotions. And, of course, there are financial interests: Drug companies use publications to increase sales, while publishers make money both directly from journal sales and from spin-offs such as reprints and advertising. However, since most journals will not publish material that has already been published elsewhere, some companies have stated that results' summaries will not be posted if the trial is pending publication in a peer-reviewed journal. Journals have always accepted that publication of conference abstracts would not jeopardize subsequent full publications.

9.24.1 *The role of peer-review and traditional journals*

Publication in peer-reviewed journals is up to now the main mechanism for sharing findings among clinician physicians and researchers. Although they have not been through journal peer review, trial summaries prepared for regulatory reports are usually subjected to stringent QC mechanisms. The basic criterion of a peer-review is that there is a formalized process of peer-review prior to publication, so this presents a barrier to publication that acts as a QC filter. Typically, the journal editor will hand over a submitted paper to a certain number of qualified peers-recognized experts in the relevant field of the submitted paper. The reviewers will then submit detailed criticism of the paper along with a recommendation to reject or accept the paper with major/minor comments. It should be mentioned here that it is rare to get an acceptance during the first review round.

It is very common for authors/companies to submit a paper to a very prestigious journal first, and if they get finally rejected (after the first revision round), they take the road down until they find a journal that will accept it. This does not necessarily mean that the paper was of poor or poorer quality, as the most prestigious journals have a lot of submissions per month/year and can therefore select the most relevant or interesting clinical trials.

But there are also some limitations in terms of peer-reviews and this has to be taken into consideration. They may be prejudiced against studies that contradict their own research or their "own clinical trials". For this reason, editors often allow authors to request or recommend reviewers, or to request that certain people should not be asked to be reviewers. Each single journal has its own policy and this should be checked by the author of the paper/publication upfront.

References

1. Directive 2001/83/EC of the European Parliament and of the Council of November 6, 2001 on the Community code relating to medicinal products for human use (2001).
2. Lazarus, H.M., Haynesworth, S.E., Gerson, S.L., Rosenthal, N.S., and Caplan, A.I. Ex vivo expansion and subsequent infusion of human bone marrow-derived stromal progenitor cells (mesenchymal progenitor cells): Implications for therapeutic use. *Bone Marrow Transplant.* 16, 557–564 (1995).
3. Messina, C., *et al.* Prevention and treatment of acute GvHD. *Bone Marrow Transplant.* 41(Suppl 2), S65–S70 (2008).

 4. Otto, W.R., and Wright, N.A. Mesenchymal stem cells: From experiment to clinic. *Fibrogenesis & Tissue Repair* 4, 20 (2011).

 5. Le Blanc, K., *et al.* Mesenchymal stem cells for treatment of steroid-resistant, severe, acute graft-versus-host disease: A phase II study. *Lancet* 371, 1579–1586 (2008).

 6. Le Blanc, K., *et al.* Transplantation of mesenchymal stem cells to enhance engraftment of hematopoietic stem cells. *Leukemia* 21, 1733–1738 (2007).

 7. von Bonin, M., *et al.* Treatment of refractory acute GVHD with third-party MSC expanded in platelet lysate-containing medium. *Bone Marrow Transplant.* 43, 245–251 (2009).

 8. Nagaya, N., *et al.* Intravenous administration of mesenchymal stem cells improves cardiac function in rats with acute myocardial infarction through angiogenesis and myogenesis. *Am. J. Physiol. Heart Circ. Physiol.* 287, H2670–H2676 (2004).

 9. Union, O.J.o.t.E. Regulation (EC) No 1394/2007 of the European Parliament and of the Council of November 13, 2007 on advanced therapy medicinal products and amending Directive 2001/83/EC and Regulation (EC) No 726/2004. Official Journal of the European Union (2007).

10. Consumers, E.C.D.H. Medical Devices: Guidance document (2012).

11. Communities, O.J.o.t.E. Directive 2001/20/EC of the European Parliament and of the Council of April 4, 2001 on the approximation of the laws, regulations and administrative provisions of the Member States relating to the implementation of good clinical practice in the conduct of clinical trials on medicinal products for human use. (2001).

12. Directive 2004/23/EC of the European Parliament and of the Council of March 31, 2004 on setting standards of quality and safety for the donation, procurement, testing, processing, preservation, storage and distribution of human tissues and cells. (2004).

13. Halme, D.G., and Kessler, D.A. FDA regulation of stem-cell-based therapies. *N. Engl. J. Med.* 355, 1730–1735 (2006).

14. Liras, A. Future research and therapeutic applications of human stem cells: General, regulatory, and bioethical aspects. *J. Transl. Med.* 8, 131 (2010).

15. The Committee for Advanced Therapies (CAT) and the CAT Scientific Secretariat. Challenges with advanced therapy medicinal products and how to meet them. *Nat. Rev. Drug Discov.* 9, 195–201 (2010).

16. Regulation (EC) No 726/2004 of the European Parliament and of the Council of March 31, 2004 laying down Community procedures for the authorisation and supervision of medicinal products for human and veterinary use and establishing a European Medicines Agency. (2004).

17. Council, T.E.P.a.o.t. Directive 2001/18/EC of the European Parliament and of the Council on the deliberate release into the environment of genetically modified organisms and repealing Council Directive 90/220/EEC. (2001).

18. Food and Drug Administration: Title 21- Food and Drugs, Chapter I; Food and Drug Administration, Department of Health and Human Services, Sub-chapter D- Drugs for Human Use.

19. Food and Drug Administration; Code of Federal Regulation Title 21- Food and Drugs, Chapter I; Food and Drug Administration, Department of Health and Human Services, Sub-chapter F- Biologics, Part 600. Biological Products: General.

20. Astori, G., *et al.* Bone marrow derived stem cells in regenerative medicine as advanced therapy medicinal products. *Am. J. Transl. Res.* 2, 285–295 (2010).

21. Administration, F.a.D. Guidance for Industry: Regulation of Human Cells, Tissues, and Cellular and Tissue-Based Products (HCT/Ps). (2007).

22. Center for Biologics Evaluation and Research, Food and Drug Administration. Guidance for human somatic cell therapy and gene therapy, March 1998. *Hum. Gene Ther.* 9, 1513–1524 (1998).

23. Parson, A. The long journey from stem cells to medical product. *Cell* 125, 9–11 (2006).

24. Bieback, K., Kinzebach, S., and Karagianni, M. Translating research into clinical scale manufacturing of mesenchymal stromal cells. *Stem Cells Int.* 2010, 193519 (2011).

25. Gee, A. Mesenchymal stem-cell therapy in a regulated environment. *Cytotherapy* 3, 397–398 (2001).

26. Hyun, I. Allowing innovative stem cell-based therapies outside of clinical trials: Ethical and policy challenges. *J. Law Med. Ethics* 38, 277–285 (2010).

Pharmacovigilance and Look-Back Procedures

10

Stephanie Knoerzer, Josef M. Hofer, and Christine Guenther

10.1 Basic Principles of Pharmacovigilance for Advanced Therapy Medicinal Products (ATMPs)

The most prominent tasks in Pharmacovigilance of ATMPs, especially for autologous and allogeneic cell based medicinal products are

- Assurance of traceability;
- Active surveillance and adverse event/reaction reporting;
- Assessment and follow-up management.

Individual approaches and detailed product knowledge are the precondition for correct identification, detection and evaluation of product- and class-specific signals and events.

10.1.1 *Traceability*

The obligations on ATMPs to establish and maintain a system which ensures that the individual product and its starting and raw materials can be traced through the sourcing, manufacturing, packaging, storage, transport, and delivery are extremely high and always have to be discussed on a risk-based approach.[1]

10.1.2 *Active surveillance*

Active surveillance, in contrast to passive surveillance, seeks to ascertain completely the number of adverse events *via* a continuous pre-organized process. An example of active surveillance is the follow-up of patients who are treated with a particular drug, through a risk management program including specific educational material. Patients who get a prescription for this drug may be asked to complete a brief survey form and give permission for later contact. In general, it is more feasible to get comprehensive data on individual adverse event reports through an active surveillance system than through a passive reporting system.

10.1.3 *Pharmacovigilance and risk assessment in cell and gene therapy*

The special characteristics of cell-based medicinal product should be considered, taking into account the different levels of risk associated with each individual product and the proposed therapeutic use. The requirements of a Risk Management Plan (RMP) have to be considered in the light of relevant national and international legislation. For cell-based medicinal product, there are numerous adventitious agents (viral, bacterial, and other infectious diseases) that need to be evaluated, different associated medical devices and biomaterials have to be discussed and various malignancies and other potential long-term adverse effects have to be taken into account. The Guideline on Safety and Efficacy Follow-up and Risk Management of ATMPs should be consulted thoroughly.[2]

10.2 Qualified Person for Pharmacovigilance (QPPV)

The overall leadership in a company's Pharmacovigilance System is aggregated with the QPPV. The QPPV is a qualified and experienced person of a pharmaceutical company who ensures to conduct the regulatory compliance in regard to Pharmacovigilance as well as monitors the patient's safety. A QPPV responsible for a medicinal product approved in the EU must reside in Europe.

The role and the responsibilities of a QPPV are described in Table 10.1.

10.3 Pharmacovigilance during Development Phase

10.3.1 *Reporting procedure from clinical trials in Europe*

During clinical trials and all follow-up observational periods as well as within compassionate use programs, post-authorization safety or efficacy studies, all adverse reactions including severity, seriousness, and relatedness have to be reported.

Table 10.1:   Responsibilities of a QPPV.

Responsibilities of a QPPV:

Establishment and maintenance of a Pharmacovigilance system which ensures that information about all suspected adverse reactions is collected and evaluated in order to be accessible at least at one point within the community.

Oversight on all relevant aspects of the ongoing Pharmacovigilance system (e.g., compliance data, database operations, personnel training, contractual arrangements, quality control (QC) procedures, quality assurance (QA) procedures, internal audits).

Coordination of the collaboration with other departments in order to ensure the correct functioning of the Pharmacovigilance system.

Conduct of continuous overall risk — benefit evaluations of medicinal products under the Pharmacovigilance system.

Collection and collation of all suspected serious adverse reactions and, if applicable, reporting them to the relevant competent authorities in compliance with reporting timelines.

Collection and evaluation of serious quality defects of authorized medicinal products or Investigational Medicinal Products (IMPs).
[In collaboration with Qualified Person (QP)].

Coordination, documentation and reporting to authorities of recall procedures.
(In collaboration with QP).

Compilation of periodic safety update reports (PSURs) for competent authorities in compliance with reporting timelines.

QC of periodic reports and transmitted case reports regarding timelines and completeness.

Single contact point for competent authorities, also in terms of inspections, on a 24 hour basis.

Provision of information regarding risks or benefits of a medicinal product upon request by a competent authority.

Delegation of tasks to appropriately trained and qualified staff; documentation of this delegation.

Ensuring the provision and documentation of regular training and further education for members of staff involved in Pharmacovigilance procedures.

Obligation for continuing training in order to fulfill position requirements (including keeping abreast of current regulatory requirements).

The investigator should inform about all Serious Adverse Events (SAEs) immediately to the sponsor, having the overall responsibility. The sponsor needs to keep records of all Adverse Events (AEs) which are reported. These records should be submitted to the competent authorities in whose territory the clinical trial is being conducted. Figure 10.1 shows the process to be established to assure content- and time-adequate flow of information during development.

The Investigator has to report SAEs immediately, within 24 hours, to the sponsor, the sponsor has to notify the Ethics Committee and local authorities within

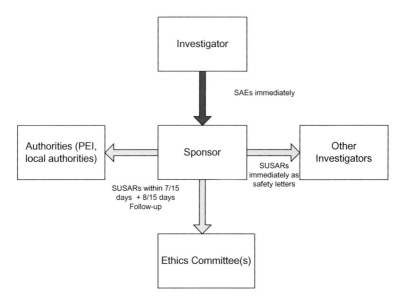

Figure 10.1: Flow chart which shows responsibilities and timelines of "detailed guidance on the collection, verification and presentation of adverse reaction reports arising from clinical trials on medicinal products for human use", e.g., in Germany.

seven or 15 days depending on its severity, with an eight or 15 days follow-up report. In addition, the Sponsor has to send a safety letter to all other Investigators of the study. Suspected Unexpected Serious Adverse Reactions (SUSARs) have to be reported *via* E2B–Form electronically into the EudraVigilance Database Management System (DBMS). DBMS is a web-based information system and it is designed to report in compliance with the International Conference on Harmonisation (ICH).

From July 2012, it became mandatory to provide all details of authorized product data according to the Extended EudraVigilance Medicinal Product Dictionary (XEVMPD).

10.3.2 *Development safety update report (DSUR)*

An annual DSUR is provided to give, e.g., a summary of collected risks and to evaluate newly occurred safety challenges of drugs and biologicals which are under investigation.

The following relevant information from post–authorization studies should also be included in the DSUR:

- Safety information from all ongoing clinical trials and other studies that the sponsor is conducting or has completed during the review period including:
  - Clinical trials using an investigational drug [i.e., human pharmacology, therapeutic exploratory and therapeutic confirmatory trials (Phase I–III)];
  - Clinical trials conducted using marketed drugs in approved indications [i.e., therapeutic use trials (Phase IV)];
  - Therapeutic use of an investigational drug [e.g., expanded access programs, compassionate use programs, particular patient use, single patient investigational new drugs (INDs), and treatment INDs]; and
  - Clinical trials conducted to support changes in the manufacturing process of medicinal products.[3]
- Information from long-term follow-up of subjects from clinical trials of IMPs should be included from ATMPs, even if the development program is completed.

During a clinical study, a Drug/Data Safety Monitoring Board (DSMB) is highly recommended, as specific medical review for Cell-Based Medicinal Products (CBMPs) is required.

10.3.3 *Responsibilities and tasks of a DSMB*

The DSMB members continuously review cumulative safety data and assess whether to recommend stopping the study due to unacceptable harm or to decide on the continuation, e.g., for the next dose level (See Table 10.2 for the summary of the responsibility).

The DSMB should be composed of

- Clinicians with expertise in the relevant indication/disease and broad medical knowledge.
- At least one biostatistician to be involved, who is knowledgeable about statistical methods for clinical trials, if the study is large enough. (Biostatistical tasks can also be outsourced to the CRO). In blinded studies, the DSMB biostatistician may be responsible for breaking the code for the DSMB members in interim analyses, as long as the study remains blinded for the investigators' and sponsors' study team.
- Toxicologists, epidemiologists, and clinical pharmacologists, for example, can be included in particular cases when such expertise appears important for informed interpretation of (interim) results. They can also be involved, without being

Table 10.2:   Summary of the responsibility of the DSMB.

Responsibilities of DSMB members:
Review of accumulated safety data.
Drawing of written summaries of safety.
To recommend stopping the study for unacceptable harm.

Responsibilities of a DSMB chairman:
Moderation of the DSMB meetings.
Providing and keeping DSMB meeting minutes.
Preparing the DSMB summaries of safety including a recommendation to stop the study
    due to unacceptable harm.

Responsibilities of a Statistical Expert:
Generate unblinded data to the members.
Providing unblinded data and safety evaluations for DSMB meetings.

---

regular members in the team, if specific issues have to be discussed. The decision on their involvement lies with the chairman of the DSMB.

10.4   Post Approval Pharmacovigilance

10.4.1   *Surveillance plan*

The pharmacovigilance plan should contain a specific surveillance plan. The plan should enable rapid identification of epidemiologically significant links, and should provide data for the assessment of long-term safety, e.g., of xenogeneic cell-based therapy.

The extent and duration of monitoring of the treated individuals should be justified. For cell-based medicinal products, it may be necessary to follow-up all recipients. It should be ensured that the medical records of the recipient contain all relevant information for both safety and maintenance of efficacy profiling. The information provided in the health records should be specified in the RMP. An adequate laboratory testing program with suitable validated methods should be in place to enable screening in case of adverse events. The active screening program requires the collection and archiving of appropriate body fluids (blood, plasma, and urine, etc.). These materials should be kept under adequate storage conditions for retrospective testing in the case of a diagnosed infection or a suspected infection, within an acceptable time period, after administration of the medicinal product.

The Marketing Authorization Holder (MAH) has to take provisions for the surveillance system, that all samples and records will be maintained or appropriately transferred to anyone agreed with the competent authority in the event that the establishment ceases operation. The plan may have to be modified according to new scientific information on the infectious agents and their epidemiology. The tests that should be performed on a regular basis has to be defined prior to marketing authorization (MA). It may be acceptable that certain tests will only be performed when clinically indicated (e.g., in the case of a suspected transmission of an infectious agent).

An efficient surveillance system allowing for the retrieval and linkage of the observation with the clinical records, the biological specimens and the source material, manufacturing, storage, and distribution should be in place and ready for use prior to MA.

It is important to provide adequate information about possible risks to close contacts and health care professionals involved in cell-based therapy. It is not always necessary or feasible to monitor on a routine basis. However, the events that would trigger the surveillance of the close contacts must be identified in advance. The system becomes operative, if the recipient is infected with agents and a risk of transmission cannot be excluded for close contacts and health care providers. All efforts should be made to adequately inform close contacts, if transmission of infectious agents cannot be excluded. It may be, in rare instances, necessary to collect blood samples of close contacts (e.g., family) prior to the procedure and store for retrospective testing. The MAH should be responsible for providing comprehensive information specific for the product to health care workers in order to ensure proper handling of the product, the treatment procedure and the follow-up.

10.4.2 RMP for ATMPs

At the moment, only few cell-based medicinal products requiring the complete system of pharmacovigilance have been marketed in the EU and the US. Nonetheless guidelines have been published by the European Medicines Agency (EMA) and the Food and Drug Administration (FDA), which govern the long-term follow-up of patients receiving cell-based products. The product characteristics of cell-based medicinal products need to be well established to receive appropriate data of toxicology and pharmacology.[7]

Guidance for the follow-up of patients receiving ATMPs is given in the guideline on safety and efficacy follow-up/risk management.[2] This overarching guideline for authorized ATMPs provides an overview on potential risks related to the unique characteristics of cell-based therapies and measures of intensified pharmacovigilance.

The risk assessment for Pharmacovigilance should consider the following topics and assess the potential influence on safety and efficacy:

- Risk to living donors (preconditioning/procurement of tissue or cells).
- Risks to patients related to quality characteristics (species and characteristics of cells, manufacturing aspects, and vectors used).
- Risks related to persistence of the product in the patient (potential risk of late complications as malignancies and autoimmunity).
- Risks to patients related to storage and distribution (cold-chain, stability, freezing/thawing procedures, and handling at the clinical site).
- Risks to health care provider and environmental risks (virus shedding, and risk of adventitious agents).
- Transmission of infectious/adventitious agents due to human origin of the starting material and ancillary materials (blood and transfusion components), and animal origin of ancillary materials (FCS of bovine origin, and Trypsin of porcine origin).
- Immunologic effects due to cellular components, transgenes, and other excipients.
- Human Leukocyte Antigen (HLA)-disparity (autologous *vs.* allogeneic) potentially causing graft-versus-host reaction and potential rejection of grafted cells.
- Reduction of efficacy may be relevant after repeated administration.
- Toxic effects of non-cellular components: Dimethylsulfoxide (DMSO) as a cryoprotectant may cause hypotension and shock if administered in higher dose (>1 ml/kg bw).
- The fate of the administered cells: Migration, homing, grafting, differentiation, and proliferation of the cells, persistence, vector persistence/integration/reactivation.
- Potential tumorigenicity of grafted cells which are able to divide and integrate into the patient's organism/transmission of tumor cells.
- Potential tumorigenicity of gene-modified cells in case of clonal evolution.[8] Genetic stability: Effect on functionality of cells and potential cancerogenic effect [no evidence so far in Mesenchymal Stem Cell (MSC)-treatment].

Special considerations in Gene-therapy: Risk related to integration of vector/gene,[9] including but not limited to:

- Potential and extent of chromosomal integration of a vector or gene.
- Capacity of a vector/gene for latency/reactivation and inadvertent replication.
- Persistence of the vector/gene product.
- Altered expression of host genes.

- Biodistribution to target/non-target organs/tissues/cells.
- Known interactions with treatment (present and past).

Specific pharmacovigilance measures for ATMP should be complemented by additional patient information with regard to:

- Mortality.
- Development of any new or recurrent cancer.
- Development of infections.
- Immunogenicity related reactions (caused by antibodies, cell-mediated immunity): Autoimmunity.

Additional measures, to be taken into consideration, for gene therapy products should be laid down in a pharmacovigilance plan. In essence, the tracking of the gene/vector sequence should be performed. Patient samples should be taken every three months up to five years and tested for vector sequences or expressed product. In case of cell-based gene therapy, immunologic parameters should be included additionally.

The Pharmacovigilance, the risk management and the traceability must be implemented for 30 years after the expiry date of the product.

10.4.3 *Periodic Benefit-Risk Evaluation Report (PBRER)*

A PBRER is a comprehensive, concise, and critical analysis of new or emerging information on the risks of the medicinal product, and on its benefit in approved indications, to enable an appraisal of the product's overall benefit–risk profile.[10] The PBRER should contain an evaluation of new information relevant to the medicinal product that became available to the MAH during the reporting interval, in the context of cumulative information by:

- Summarizing relevant new safety information that could have an impact on the benefit–risk profile of the medicinal product;
- Summarizing any important new efficacy/effectiveness information that has become available during the reporting interval;
- Examining whether the information obtained by the MAH during the reporting complies with previous knowledge of the medicinal product's benefit and risk profile; and
- Where important new safety information has emerged, conducting an integrated benefit–risk evaluation for approved indications.[10]

10.5　Pharmacovigilance Inspections

Inspections by national and supra-national authorities of companies already at the time of applying for clinical trial or marketing licenses are as important as the post approval surveillance of the Pharmacovigilance system. All activities either by cause or by routine are used to investigate whether organization, facilities and personnel are in compliance with the obligations or may pose a risk to public health.

The inspectors are empowered to visit all locations, including third parties involved, in connection with the product or the system. Their judgment decides on necessary implementation of corrective or preventive actions, on further pharmacovigilance or risk-minimization activities, on requirement for post-authorization safety studies (PASS) or on designation for additional monitoring.

Today routine inspection programs are running, e.g., in the EU generally at least once every four years for centrally approved products like ATMPs, prioritized by a risk-based approach. In order to re-establish the benefit–risk balance, pharmacovigilance-inspections may introduce non-statutory or statutory instruments, e.g., from educational measurement up to warning letters, infringement notices, penalties or in the worst case suspension or revocation of the MAs. All these measurements are part of an international and worldwide communication.

10.6　Reported Side-Effects of Cell-Therapy Products

In general, cell-based therapies are well tolerated and safe. Significant differences exist depending on the source and further manipulation of cells.

Immunologically inert cells as MSCs are associated with very few side-effects, whereas immunological active cells (T-cells, NK-cells, and others) may exert severe side-effects and even lethal effects have been reported in severe disease conditions [treatment of cancer with chimeric antigen receptor (CAR) T-cells].

1. Acute side effects after systemic administration of ATMPs comprise transient fever, chills, back pain or local reactions at the site of administration. Cardiac arrhythmia and pulmonary symptoms related to the lung passage after i.v. administration have been reported. After intramuscular administration of MSCs local pain requiring systemic analgesic treatment is common and antibiotic prophylaxis may be indicated. Safety concerns arise with innovative immune-therapies exerting intrinsic activity. T-cells and other immune-cells may cause severe side-effects relating to the activation of the patient's immune system. This may include acute reactions but also delayed side effects leading to cytokine release syndromes

and immunogenicity of the product. These reactions may pose the patient to a significant risk (even deaths have been reported). Repeated administration may have a negative effect on the efficacy by *in vivo* inactivation through induction of antibodies. Fatal outcomes resulting from lethal cytokine storms have been reported with genetically modified T-cells in patients with very severe cancer disease. Currently, the CAR technology is making significant progress and patient conditions are defined to cope with cytokine release syndromes.[5] An example of an apparently safe cell therapy are products based on MSCs. After administration to thousands of patients, a very favorable safety profile is reported.[6]

2. Severe chronic side effects attributable to cell-based therapies have not been reported for unmodified cells. The potential risk of transmission of infectious agents by cell-based therapies or an increase of infections due to potential immunomodulatory activity has not been confirmed. Special consideration is paid to potential tumorigenicity, but currently, after thousands of patients were treated, no increased risk for tumor formation has been reported. Donor-related safety issues have not been addressed so far.

Gene therapy products, depending on transient or permanent integration, carry additional risks and the vigilance program should monitor potential side effects[8] (please refer to chapter "Cell-Based Gene therapy") related to the genetic modification. Continuous optimization of vector technology, pharmaceutical development, and safety testing of gene-modified products is paving the way to a broader application for a large variety of diseases. This includes not only gene-replacement therapies (for example for inborn errors of metabolism), but also disease-modifying conditions and cancer treatment.

References

1. Art. 15 of the Regulation (EC) No 1394/2007 of the European Parliament and of the Council of November 13, 2007.
2. EMEA/149995/2008 Guideline on Safety and Efficacy Follow-up and Risk Management of Advanced Therapy Medicinal Products.
3. ICH Topic E2F, EMA/CHPM/ICH/3093/48/2008.
4. Wieczorck, A., and Uharek, L. Genetically modified T cells for the treatment of malignant disease. *Transfus. Med. Hemother.* 40, 388 (2013).
5. Lalu, M.M., McIntyre, L., Pugliese, C., Fergusson, D., Winston, B.W., Marshall, J.C., Granton, J., and Stewart, D.J. Safety of cell therapy with mesenchymal stromal cells (SafeCell): A systematic review and meta-analysis of clinical trials. October 25, 2012. DOI: 10.1371. www.plosone.org.
6. EMEA/149995/2008.

7. Braun, C.J, von Kalle, C., and Klein, C. Gene therapy for WAS: Long-term efficacy and genotoxicity. *Sci. Transl. Med.*, Mar 12, 2014.
8. Guideline EMEA/CHMP/GTWP/60436/2007.
9. ICH guideline E2C (R2).
10. EU-GMP guidelines Chapter 8 (under revision).

Personalized Cell Therapy — Biomarker & Companion Diagnostics

11

Ralf Huss

11.1 Introduction

Cell therapy and Regenerative Medicine are emerging therapeutic modalities in translational sciences comprising different technologies such as nanotechnology, innovative biomaterials, genetic engineering, and cellular therapeutics. While potential clinical indications as well as the market size for new drug developments are significantly increasing (considering the continuing high medical need), any new application would need to prove that its clinical efficacy and deployment is sustainable, more than being merely incremental and cost effective. In the context of cell therapy, biomarkers not only characterize the function, quality and safety/toxicity of a cell-based product (potency), but can also help identify those patients or cohorts who are most likely to benefit from such an innovative treatment modality (prediction or stratification) and allow monitoring efficacy in those patients who have been identified as potential responders. This is of pivotal importance for the development of drugs or drug candidates, which have not yet been approved, to foster early decisions on how to go forward and when to stop the development of less promising compounds or technologies. Presently, diverse and numerous technologies are available to identify and measure biomarkers. Tools such as "omics" platforms, modern imaging technologies and other technologies permit to measure many biomarkers *in vivo* and *ex vivo*. Intelligent clinical trial design is another valuable tool to validate and deploy biomarkers and to accelerate cost-saving drug development particularly in cellular therapies.

401

11.2 Biomarker

Generally in medicine, a biomarker is a metric characteristic that may reflect the severity or presence of some disease state. More generally, a biomarker is anything that can be used as an indicator of a particular disease state or some other physiological state of an organism. In 2001, a working group of the National Institute of Health (NIH) defined the biomarker as "a characteristic that is objectively measured and evaluated as an indicator of normal biological processes, pathogenic processes, or pharmacological responses to a therapeutic intervention". Biomarkers include genes, proteins, genetic variations, and differences in metabolic expression from different sources like body fluids, cells or tissues.

A biomarker can be a substance that is introduced into an organism as a means to examine organ function or other aspects of health. It can be a substance whose detection indicates a particular disease state, for example, the presence of an antibody may indicate an infection. More specifically, a biomarker indicates a change in expression or the state of a protein that correlates with the risk or progression of a disease or with the susceptibility of the disease to a given treatment. Biomarkers are characteristic biological properties that can be detected and measured in parts of the body like the blood or a tissue. They may indicate either normal or diseased processes in the body.[1] Biomarkers can be specific cells, molecules, genes, gene products, enzymes, or hormones. Complex organ functions or general characteristic changes in biological structures can also serve as biomarkers. Although the term biomarker is relatively new, biomarkers have been used in pre-clinical research and clinical diagnosis for a considerable time.[2]

Disease related biomarkers are as old as clinical laboratory medicine. Early examples include testing the blood glucose for (a) diagnosis and management of diabetes and (b) analyzing cardiovascular risk from cholesterol levels. The recent acceleration in biomarker activities has been caused by the availability of new genetic information and genomic technologies. Another driver is the need for better differential diagnosis systems as the number of targeted therapies, especially in the field of oncology, has increased. The same will apply for innovative approaches such as regenerative medicine.

Biomarker discovery has grown dramatically during the past decade, driven by an increasing demand in new therapeutic modalities such as regenerative medicine and the availability of powerful new "omics"-technologies, the increased utilization of new and untested targets in Pharma, and the opportunity to implement improved and validated biomarker assays.

In attempting to foster early attrition of unpromising compounds and also accelerate the time-to-market of innovative drugs and technologies, the pharmaceutical industry has focused more on mode-of-action (potency) and safety-related biomarkers than on disease-related biomarkers. Surrogate markers are needed to replace vague clinical endpoints particularly in emerging modalities such as regenerative medicine. Biomarkers are especially needed to identify the best fit for the individual need to the therapies in question.

11.3   Disease- and Drug-Related Biomarkers

As mentioned before, it is necessary to distinguish between *disease-related* and *drug-related biomarkers*. Disease-related biomarkers indicate the probable effect of treatment on the patient (risk indicator or predictive biomarkers), if a disease already exists (diagnostic biomarker), or how such a disease may develop in an individual case regardless of the type of treatment (prognostic biomarker). Predictive biomarkers help to assess the most likely response to a particular treatment type as in regenerative medicine, while prognostic markers show the progression of disease with or without treatment.[3] In contrast, drug-related biomarkers indicate whether a drug will be effective and/or safe in a specific patient and how the patient's body will process it.

In addition to long-known parameters, such as those included and objectively measured in a blood count, there are numerous novel biomarkers used in various medical specialties. Currently, intensive work is taking place toward the discovery and development of innovative and more effective biomarkers. These "new" biomarkers have become the basis for preventive medicine, that is, medicine that recognizes diseases or the risk of diseases early and provides specific counter-measures to prevent the progression of diseases. Biomarkers are key to personalized medicine, i.e., highly efficient treatment intervention in disease processes which could be personalized to suit specific patient requirements. The "classic" biomarker in medicine is a laboratory parameter that the doctor can use to make decisions in diagnosing and selecting an appropriate course of treatment.

According to Häupl T. *et al.*, prediction of response to treatment will become the most important aim of biomarker research in medicine. With the growing number of new biological agents, there is increasing pressure to identify molecular parameters that will not only guide the therapeutic decision but also help to define the most important targets for which new biological agents should be tested in clinical studies.[4]

In 1998, a study group of the NIH committed to the following definition for the biomarker: "A characteristic that is objectively measured and evaluated as an indicator of normal biologic processes, pathogenic processes, or pharmacologic responses to a therapeutic intervention". In the past, biomarkers were primarily physiological indicators such as blood pressure or heart rate. More recently, the biomarker is becoming a synonym for molecular biomarker, such as an elevated prostate specific antigen as the molecular biomarker for prostate cancer, or using enzyme assays in liver function tests. There has recently been heightened interest in the relevance of biomarkers in oncology, including the role of Kirsten rat sarcoma viral oncogene homolog (KRAS) in colorectal cancer (CRC) and other epidermal growth factor receptor (EGFR)-associated cancers. Currently, effective treatment is available for only a small percentage of cancer patients. In addition, many cancer patients are diagnosed at an advanced stage where the cancer has progressed too far to be treated successfully. Biomarkers have the ability in greatly enhancing cancer detection and drug development process. In addition, biomarkers will enable physicians to develop individualized treatment plans for their cancer patients, thus allowing doctors to tailor drugs specific to their patient's tumor type. By doing so, drug response rate will improve, drug toxicity will be limited and costs associated with testing various therapies and the ensuing treatment for side effects will decrease.[5]

11.4   Companion Diagnostics

Once a proposed biomarker has been validated, it can be used to diagnose the risk of a disease, presence of a disease in an individual, or to tailor treatments for the disease in an individual as companion diagnostics (choices of drug treatment or administration regimes). In evaluating potential cellular therapies, a validated biomarker may be used as a surrogate for a natural endpoint such as survival or irreversible morbidity. If a treatment alters the biomarker, which has a direct connection to improved health, the biomarker serves as a surrogate endpoint for evaluating clinical benefit. Some of the main areas in which molecular biomarkers are used in the drug development process are early drug development studies, safety studies, proof of concept studies, and molecular profiling.

Molecular biomarkers are increasingly important in early drug development studies. Particularly, it remains to be seen whether they will act as decisive tools in emerging modalities and be accepted by the market. For instance, they are used in phase I study for establishing doses and dosing regimen for future phase II studies. Pharmacodynamic (PD) biomarkers are commonly observed to respond (either decrease or increase) proportionally with dose. This data, in conjunction with safety data, help determine doses for phase II studies. In addition, safety molecular biomarkers have been used for decades both in pre-clinical and clinical research. Since these have become mainstream tests, they have been fully automated for both animal and human testing. Among the most common safety tests are those of liver function (e.g., transaminases, bilirubin, and alkaline phosphatase) and kidney function (e.g., serum creatinine, clearance of creatinine, and cystatin C). Others include markers of skeletal muscle (e.g., myoglobin) or cardiac muscle injury (e.g., CK–MB, troponin I or T), as well as bone biomarkers (e.g., bone-specific alkaline phosphatase).

11.5   Biomarker Requirements

For chronic diseases, whose treatment may require patients to take medications for years, accurate diagnosis is particularly important, especially when strong side effects are expected from the treatment. In such cases, biomarkers are increasingly becoming important, because they can not only make the diagnosis possible in the first place but also confirm a difficult diagnosis.[6] A number of diseases, in particular, chronic degenerative disorders often begin with an early, symptom-free phase. In such symptom-free patients, there may be more or less probability of actually developing the symptoms. In such cases, biomarkers help to identify high-risk individuals reliably and in a timely manner so they can either be treated before the onset of the disease or as soon as possible thereafter.[7,8] Here robust biomarker assays can be valuable tools to provide an early entry-point into the disease management, even of chronic diseases. This will certainly lower the threshold to meet the requirements for a marketing authorization (MA) if a sustainable efficacy can be shown early during the course of a disease.

In order to use a biomarker for diagnostics, the sample material must be easy to obtain. This may be a blood sample taken by a doctor, a urine or saliva sample, or extraction of a drop of blood similar to manner in which the diabetes patients extract from their own fingertips for regular blood-sugar monitoring.

For rapid initiation of treatment, the speed with which a result is obtained from the biomarker test is critical. A rapid test, which delivers a result after only a few minutes, is optimal. This makes it possible for the physician to discuss with the patient how to proceed and if necessary to start treatment immediately after the test. However, a predictive biomarker assay for patient stratification should be an *In vitro* diagnostic (IVD) test, which requires intensive clinical and regulatory validation steps.

Naturally, the detection method for a biomarker must be accurate and as easy to carry out as possible. The results from different laboratories may not differ significantly from each other, and the biomarker must naturally have proven its effectiveness for the diagnosis, prognosis, and risk assessment of the diseases in independent studies.

11.6　Biomarker Classification and Application

Biomarkers can be classified based on different parameters, either based on their characteristics such as imaging biomarkers (CT, PET, and MRI) or molecular biomarkers. Molecular biomarkers refer to non-imaging biomarkers that have biophysical properties, which allow their measurements in biological samples and include nucleic acid-based biomarkers such as gene mutations or polymorphisms and quantitative gene expression analysis, peptides, proteins, lipids metabolites, and other small molecules. Biomarkers can also be classified based on their applications such as diagnostic biomarkers, staging of disease biomarkers, disease prognosis biomarkers (cancer biomarkers), and biomarkers for monitoring the clinical response to an intervention (companion diagnostic). Another category of biomarkers includes those used in decision making in early drug development. For instance, PD biomarkers are markers of a certain pharmacological response, which are of special interest in dose optimization studies.[9]

11.7　Discovery of Biomarkers

Molecular biomarkers can be discovered using basic and acceptable platforms such as genomics and proteomics. Many genomic and proteomics techniques are available for biomarker discovery. Some of the recently used techniques are given in the following sections. Apart from genomics and proteomics platform biomarker assay techniques, metabolomics, lipidomics, glycomics, and secretomics are the most commonly used techniques in the identification of biomarkers.

11.7.1　*Genomics*

Genomics has been extensively used for biomarker discovery and identification. With approximately 30,000 genes in the human genome, realizing the clinical potential of genome scale information requires better methods of viewing, analyzing, and utilizing the complex, large-scale biomarker data. The availability of new platform technologies such as deep and high throughput sequencing has enabled researchers and scientists to make the next quantum leap. The genetic make-up of an individual influences the action of drugs in the same way as the design and manufacturing of a biological drug such as the therapeutic (stem) cells. The field of pharmacogenomics or pharmacogenomic biomarker deals with the influence of genetic variation, providing new methods to treat patients on an individual basis. The outcome of this research is known as personalized medicine.

11.7.2 Proteomics

On some occasions, proteomics is preferred as a more important tool than the gene expression analysis in understanding the complexities of human physiology and state of disease. Proteomics has immense potential in biomarker discovery, especially in the discovery of novel diagnostic and predictive biomarkers. Techniques include western blot, immunohistochemical staining, enzyme linked immunosorbent assay (ELISA) or mass spectrometry. Secretomics, a subfield of proteomics that studies secreted proteins and secretion pathways using proteomic approaches, has recently emerged as an important tool for the discovery of biomarkers. In what is now commonly referred to as proteogenomics, proteomic technologies are further used for improving gene annotations. Parallel analysis of the genome and the proteome facilitates the discovery of post-translational modifications and proteolytic events (comparative proteogenomics).

11.7.3 Metabolomics

The term metabolomics has been recently introduced to refer to the analysis of all metabolites in a biological sample. A related term, metabonomics, was introduced to refer specifically to the analysis of metabolic responses to drugs or diseases. Metabonomics has become a major area of research and is a study of complex system biology, used to identify the biomarkers for various diseases. It remains to be seen whether this sub-specialty will also prevail in the biomarker discovery in regenerative medicine.

11.7.4 Lipidomics

Lipidomics refers to the analysis of lipids. Since lipids have unique physical properties particular to cells and cell-based products, they have been traditionally difficult to study. However, improvements in new analytical platforms have made it possible to identify and quantify most of lipid metabolites from a single sample. Three key platforms used for lipid profiling include mass spectrometry, chromatography, and nuclear magnetic resonance (NMR).

11.7.5   *Tissue-based biomarkers*

One of the best established biomarker research areas is the discovery of biomarkers from tumor tissues. There is almost no cancer treatment being initiated without a diagnosis, either by conventional histopathological methods such as Hematoxylin and Eosin (H&E) staining or more complex immunohistochemistry and molecular tests. A cancer biomarker usually refers to a substance or process that is indicative of the presence of cancer in the body. A biomarker may be a molecule secreted by a tumor or a specific response of the body to the presence of cancer. Genetic, epigenetic, proteomic, glycomic, and imaging biomarkers can be used for diagnosis, prognosis, and epidemiology of cancer. Ideally, such biomarkers can be assayed in non-invasively collected body fluids like blood or serum.

Cancer biomarkers can also be used to determine the most effective treatment regime for a particular person's cancer,[10] an approach that would also be the principle for biomarker discovery and development in regenerative medicine. Because of differences in each person's genetic makeup, some people metabolize or change the chemical structure of drugs differently, which might be also true with the application of cell-based therapeutics or engineered biomaterials. In some cases, decreased or accelerated metabolism can create dangerous conditions in which high levels of the drug or drug metabolites accumulate in the body. As such, drug dosing decisions and appropriate formulations can benefit from screening for such biomarkers.

Cancer biomarkers have also shown utility in monitoring how well a treatment is working over time. Much research is going into this particular area, since successful biomarkers have the potential of providing significant cost reduction in patient care, as the presently available image-based tests such as CT and MRI for monitoring tumor status are very expensive.[11]

11.7.6   *Imaging biomarkers*

Many new biomarkers are being developed that involve imaging technology. Imaging biomarkers have many advantages. They are usually non-invasive and produce intuitive, multidimensional results. Yielding both qualitative and quantitative data, they are usually relatively comfortable for patients. When combined with other sources of information, they are not only very useful to clinicians seeking to make a diagnosis, but also in pharmacokinetic (PK) assay to monitor or trace substances *in vivo* to identify their metabolites or residuals in the body.

Another promising biomarker application is in the area of surrogate endpoints. In this application, biomarkers act as stand-ins for the effects of a drug on cancer progression and survival (typically for companion diagnostics). Ideally, the use of validated biomarkers would prevent patients from having to undergo biopsies and lengthy clinical trials to determine if a new drug or modality worked. In the current standards of care, the metric for determining a drug's effectiveness in the treatment of malignancies is to check if it has decreased cancer progression in humans, and ultimately whether it prolongs survival. However, successful biomarker surrogates could save substantial time, effort, and money, if failed drugs could be eliminated from the development pipeline before being brought to clinical trials. Not all biomarkers should be used as surrogate endpoints to assess clinical outcomes. Biomarkers can be difficult to validate and require different levels of validation depending on their intended use. If a biomarker is to be used to measure the success of a therapeutic intervention, the biomarker should reflect a direct effect of that intervention.[12–15]

11.8   Biomarker in Cell Therapy

Using biomedical approaches, a variety of new and innovative cell-based treatment modalities is used to regenerate and replace damaged tissues and organs utilizing stem cells.[16] Examples include the injection of stem cells or progenitor cells (cell therapies); inducing regeneration with biologically active molecules administered alone or as a secretion by infused cells (immunomodulation therapy); and transplantation of *in vitro* grown organs and tissues.[17,18]

Cell-based therapies and, in particular, stem cell-derived therapeutics are expected to revolutionize clinical medicine in the same way as monoclonal antibodies did. The clinical development of cellular therapeutics represents a new challenge for clinical scientists and pharmaceutical companies with regard to the current regulatory requirements for manufacturing, quality management (QM) and clinical trial execution. MA also requires the demonstration of more than incremental improvement compared to the current standards of care.

The development of a new therapeutic modality such as the (stem) cell therapeutics, as a pharmaceutical product, requires (i) The comprehensive characterization of the cell product *in vitro* (specification and potency assays); (ii) The identification of a patient population which is expected to benefit from the cell therapy; and (iii) The discovery of biomarker candidates to monitor the cell function *in vivo*. After the successful clinical validation of any biomarker candidate, a (stem) cell product can be matched to a patient cohort for a (semi) individualized treatment strategy as a step forward toward securing MA.

Stem cells represent a promising novel therapeutic modality for the treatment of devastating diseases with high unmet medical needs. Among the various types of stem cells, adult mesenchymal stromal cells (MSCs) emerged as cells with unique biological properties making them candidates for the treatment of autoimmune or inflammatory diseases or e.g., progressive organ failure.

MSCs have been isolated from virtually any tissue of the body including bone marrow, adipose tissue, muscle, liver, or pancreas. Since 1960s, bone marrow represents the most extensively studied source of MSCs. Bone marrow is a unique stem cell niche which hosts hematopoietic stem cells (HSCs), MSCs and endothelial precursor cells (EPCs). The interaction between HSCs and stromal cells as feeder cells is part of the microenvironment which maintains the stemness of HSCs, the so-called HSC niche. Bone marrow stromal cells regulate survival, self-renewal, migration, and differentiation of HSCs and precursor cells.[19] Thereby, direct cell–cell interactions, release of soluble factors such as growth factors, cytokines, or chemokines play an important role in the production of extracellular matrix molecules. At least three hematopoietic compartments in the bone marrow have been considered for involvement of cells potentially derived from MSCs as precursor cells: (i) Endosteal surface lining cells, primarily osteoblasts, (ii) Stromal niche containing, e.g., fibroblasts and reticular cells, and (iii) Adipocytes.

In the 1990s, Bianco *et al.* demonstrated that reticular cells[20] are similar, suggesting that marrow stromal cells, at least a portion of them in the bone marrow, are perivascular cells. Recently, the discovery of MSCs in a wide variety of tissues strengthened the hypothesis of stromal cells having perivascular characteristics.[21]

In conclusion, MSCs function as a key player in bone and bone marrow homeostasis. First, they are key regulators of hematopoiesis as crucial components of the hematopoietic niche and second, they maintain the cellular composition of the bone and bone marrow by their plasticity controlling the balance of adipogenesis and osteogenesis and replacement of adipocytes and osteoblasts. This differentiation capability is also used as a potency biomarker to predict their function *in vivo.*

Although many experts agree that cell-based therapy is still at its infancy and may be immature in certain areas, there is an increasing number of cellular therapy approaches in academia as well as industry with growing potential for tissue repair and organ protection. However, most knowledge on the biological function of cells in tissue repair and regenerative medicine has been collected from mouse models and those data seem difficult to transfer into clinical application in humans. Most preclinical and early clinical trials (phase I/II) have been based on the *in vitro* potential to differentiate bones, cartilages, and fat tissues and are therefore somehow related to tissue engineering approaches, but fail to have a sustainable effect *in vivo*. The same applies to pre-fabricated bone or cartilage tissue consisting of MSCs together with biomaterials.

11.9   Quality Management

Most of the regulatory authorities like the Food and Drug Administration (FDA) and the European Medicines Agency (EMA) acknowledge and take into account the increasing demand for new emerging modalities such as stem cell-based therapies in regenerative medicine. Therefore, it is not only pivotal to consider the implementation of biomarkers for patient stratification and the prediction of individual responses, but also in the use of validated assays to assess the quality of any product, either autologous or allogeneic. There are strict guidelines on the pharmaceutical development and clinical implementation of advanced therapeutics (e.g., Guidance for Industry on Human Somatic Cell Therapy, CBER, FDA).

11.10   Personalized Medicine

Biomarkers along with innovative treatment modalities (e.g., cellular therapies) have the potential to change the way medicine is practiced. Most of such changes have already improved patient treatment. Pharmacogenetics and pharmacogenomics are practical applications of biomarkers to examine how the genetic composition affects both disease predisposition and response to therapy, and take the promise of personalized medicine to a new era. Delivering the right drug to the right patient at the right dose.

Besides responder identification, advances in the knowledge of how individuals metabolize drugs or react to certain substances are also key to personalized medicine. But personalized medicine is not just about identifying optimal treatment modalities or dosages for individual patients. Some diagnostic tests can also determine the aggressiveness of a cancer or the state of a chronic degenerative disorder that might require early intervention with cell-based therapeutics. The number of diseases that can and will be precisely diagnosed and then treated with a highly personalized therapy will certainly increase dramatically in the near future. In order to effectively apply the personalized drug treatment paradigm on a broader basis, the already intensive biomarker activities have to be implemented during each step of research and drug discovery.

References

1. Mishra, A., and Verma, M. Cancer biomarkers: Are we ready for the prime time? *Cancers* 2(1), 190–208 (2010).
2. Jeanne R., and Molinaro, R.J. Cancer biomarkers: Surviving the journey from bench to bedside. Medical Laboratory Observer, March 2011.
3. Dienstmann, R., and Tabernero, J. BRAF as a target for cancer therapy. *Anticancer Agents Med. Chem.* 11(3), 285–295 (2011).
4. Häupl, T., Stuhlmüller, B., Grützkau, A., Radbruch, A., and Burmester, G.R. Does gene expression analysis inform us in rheumatoid arthritis? *Ann. Rheum. Dis.* 69(Suppl. 1), i37–i42 (2010).
5. *Biomarkers in Cancer: An Introductory Guide for Advocates.* Research Advocacy Network (2010).
6. Verma, M., and Manne, U. Genetic and epigenetic biomarkers in cancer diagnosis and identifying high risk populations. *Crit. Rev. Oncol. Hematol.* 60(1), 9–18 (2006).
7. Leong, P.P., Rezai, B., Koch, W.M., Reed, A., Eisele, D., Lee, D.J., Sidransky, D., Jen, J., and Westra, W.H. Distinguishing second primary tumors from lung metastases in patients with head and neck squamous cell carcinoma. *J. Natl. Cancer Inst.* 90(13), 972–977 (1998).
8. Terpos, E., Dimopoulos, M.A., Shrivastava, V. *et al.* High levels of serum TIMP-1 correlate with advanced disease and predict for poor survival in patients with multiple myeloma treated with novel agents. *Leuk. Res.* 34(3), 399–402 (2010).
9. Kroll, W. Biomarkers — predictive surrogate parameters — a concept definition. In Biomarker. (eds. Schmitz, G., Endres, S., and Götte, D). Schattauer, Germany (2008).
10. Sawyers, C.L. The cancer biomarker problem. *Nature* 452(7187), 548–552 (2008).
11. Schneider, J., Sidhu, M.K., Doucet, C., Kiss, N., Ohsfeldt, R.L., and Chalfin, D. Economics of cancer biomarkers. *Pers. Med.* 9(8), 829–837 (2012).
12. Price, C., and McDonnell, D. Effects of niobium filtration and constant potential on the sensitometric responses of dental radiographic films. *Dentomaxillofac. Radiol.* 20(1), 11–16 (1991).
13. Cohen, V., and Khuri, F. Progress in lung cancer chemoprevention. *Cancer Control* 10(4), 315–324 (2003). (Retrieved April 26, 2013).
14. The Biomarkers Consortium. Foundation for the National Institutes of Health.
15. Tevak, Z., Kondratovich, M., and Mansfield, E. US FDA and personalized medicine: *In vitro* diagnostic regulatory perspective. *Pers. Med.* 7(5), 517–530 (2010).
16. Riazi, A.M., Kwon, S.Y., and Stanford, W.L. (2009). Stem cell sources for regenerative medicine. *Methods Mol. Biol.* 482, 55–90 (2009).
17. Stoick-Cooper, C.L., Moon, R.T., and Weidinger, G. Advances in signaling in vertebrate regeneration as a prelude to regenerative medicine. *Genes Dev.* 21(11), 1292–1315 (2007).
18. Muneoka, K., Allan, C.H., Yang, X., Lee, J., and Han, M. Mammalian regeneration and regenerative medicine. *Birth Defects Res. Part C, Embryo Today: Rev.* 84(4), 265–280 (2008).
19. Dazzi, F., Ramasamy, R., Glennie, S., Jones, S.P., and Roberts, I. The role of mesenchymal stem cells in haemopoiesis. *Blood Rev.* 20, 161–171 (2006).

20. Bianco, P., Riminucci, M., Kuznetsov, S., and Robey, P.G. Multipotential cells in the bone marrow stroma: Regulation in the context of organ physiology. *Crit. Rev. Eukaryot. Gene Expr.* 9, 159–173 (2010).

21. Crisan, M., Yap, S., Casteilla, L., Chen, C.W., Corselli, M., Park, T.S., Andriolo, G., Sun, B., Zheng, B., Zhang, L., Norotte, C., Teng, P.N., Traas, J., Schugar, R., Deasy, B.M., Badylak, S., Buhring, H.J., Giacobino, J.P., Lazzari, L., Huard, J., and Peault, B. A perivascular origin for mesenchymal stem cells in multiple human organs. *Cell Stem Cell* 3, 301–313 (2008).

Mesenchymal Stem Cells 　　12

Ralf Huss

12.1　Stem Cells/Mesenchymal Stem or Stromal Cells (MSCs) for Therapy

Stem cells represent a promising therapeutic modality for the treatment of devastating diseases with high medical need. This has been proven already, for decades, during the clinical development and implementation of hematopoietic stem cells (HSCs) for the treatment of mostly hematological diseases, but also more recently to correct inborn metabolic diseases or as carrier ("shuttle") for various drugs or genes.

Amongst the various types of stem cells which became available as a therapeutic modality, adult MSCs emerged as particular cells with unique biological properties, also making them candidates for the treatment of autoimmune or inflammatory diseases or e.g., progressive organ failure.

In this chapter, the development of MSCs in the context of hematopoiesis and bone marrow transplantation, the *in vivo* origin in mesenchymal compartments, and the *in vitro* properties are highlighted. Proposed mode of action (MoA) of MSCs and deduced potential targets of MSC therapy are also discussed. Last but not least, an overview of the current status of cellular therapy approaches and future prospects regarding clinical testing of cells and technological opportunities are given.

MSCs only serve here as an example for a particular source of cells to develop cellular therapeutics, i.e., a type of second generation cell product after the clinical success of HSCs. However, the principle outlined in this chapter and this entire book is also applicable to other sources of cells (e.g., cells of the immune system), their modification (e.g., genetic engineering) and their manufacturing (e.g., quality by design and up-scaling).

12.2 The Development of MSCs

The history of stromal cells is in its essence the history of HSC research and stem cell transplantation. In the aftermath of World War II with its devastating nuclear experiences of Hiroshima and Nagasaki, it was recognized by the medical research community that spleen-derived cells could rescue and reconstitute hematopoiesis, after otherwise lethal irradiation or chemical myeloablation with destruction of the blood forming compartments.[1] Therefore, investigators and clinicians started to search for those reconstituting cells that have the capacity for life-long self-renewal and differentiation capacities into all blood lineages. The initial focus was undoubtedly on HSCs that could be easily isolated from bone marrow aspirates and "transplanted", like a blood transfusion, *via* peripheral venous access. But HSCs were only a small fraction of bone marrow-derived cells and Friedenstein *et al.* explored the biological potential of the transplantated "transitional epithelium".[2] That term described columnar cells lining the trabecular bone, particularly in areas of bone growth and remodeling. Soon after, it was further proposed that those "bone lining cells" were already common precursor cells for osteogenic and hematopoietic tissue, capable to form heterotopic bone marrow after transplantation.[2] Also Singer *et al.* observed immortalized cell clones that gave rise to both HSCs and cells of the marrow microenvironment.[3] These common progenitor cells could be cultured *in vitro* as adherent growing, spindle-shaped fibroblast-like cells that supported the viability, proliferation, and differentiation of HSCs in the culture dish. HSCs generally depend upon an intact "microenvironment" *in vivo* in the bone marrow and other sites of hematopoiesis, which is provided by those bone marrow "stromal cells". Stromal cells also secrete a variety of growth factors and cytokines, including TGF-β, which belongs to a family of factors that play a pivotal role in tissue remodeling, cell migration, and wound healing. Various experimental approaches have shown that high doses of human stromal cell-derived growth factors maintain human hematopoiesis in mice.

Based on all those observations and the heterogeneity of cell morphology and function, Maureen Owen and Arnold Caplan proposed the terms "marrow stromal cell" and "MSC", respectively, as a subtype of marrow cells also involved in mesengenesis (a term that describes the differentiation potential of MSCs into mature tissues like bone, cartilage or fat).[4,5]

However, some studies demonstrated the almost exclusive host origin of marrow stromal cells after complete allogeneic bone marrow transplantation,[6] while the hematopoiesis revealed a complete donor-derived chimerism, challenging the notion whether stromal cells are at all transplantable.

12.3 The Biology of MSCs

The hierarchical origin of MSCs is unknown but it is suggested that MSCs are mesodermal descendant of a pluripotent stem cell. The best characterized pluripotent stem cells are embryonic stem cells which are capable of giving rise to virtually all of the body's more than 200 cell types including mesodermal, endodermal, and ectodermal lineage. The only totipotent cell is the fertilized egg which can give rise to all cell types of an embryo and in addition supports its development *in utero* by building up the placenta and umbilical cord. Hypothetically, a pluripotent mesodermal stem cell has the capability to form precursor cells named hemangioblast and mesangioblast, again representing precursor cells for vascular or hematopoietic (intra-vascular) derivatives and vascular or extra-vascular mesodermal derivatives.[7] HSCs are considered to be multipotent stem cells with the potential to build up the entire blood and immune system. Endothelial precursor cells (EPCs) represent angiogenic cells forming blood vessels, whereby MSCs are precursors of mesenchymal lineages such as adipocytes, osteoblasts, chondrocytes, or myoblasts. MSCs reside in different mesenchymal compartments with bone marrow and perivascular zone of small blood vessels being the best characterized niches.

MSCs have been isolated from virtually any tissue of the body including bone marrow, adipose tissue, muscle, liver, or pancreas. Bone marrow represents the most extensively studied source of MSCs starting in the 1960s. Bone marrow is a unique stem cell niche hosting at least HSCs and MSCs, besides EPCs. The interaction between HSCs and stromal cells as feeder cells are part of the microenvironment maintaining "stemness" of HSCs, the so called HSC niche. Bone marrow stromal cells are candidates to regulate survival, self-renewal, migration, and differentiation of HSCs and precursor cells.[8] Thereby, direct cell–cell interactions, release of soluble factors such as growth factors, cytokines, or chemokines play an important role, as well as production of extracellular matrix molecules. At least three hematopoietic compartments in bone marrow have been discussed with involvement of cells potentially derived from MSCs as precursor cells: (i) Endosteal surface lining cells, primarily osteoblasts, (ii) Stromal niche containing, e.g., fibroblasts and reticular cells, and (iii) Adipocytes.[9]

The perivascular space has recently emerged as the most likely niche for MSCs.[10] The fact that vasculature may be the only common structure in tissues containing MSCs and the demonstration of perivascular origin of MSCs in bone marrow[11] supported the hypothesis that MSCs and perivascular cells, principally pericytes, are identical. The landmark study of Crisan *et al.* showed that pericytes can be identified by CD146, NG2, and platelet-derived growth factor receptor β (PDGF-Rβ) expression and absence of hematopoietic, endothelial, and myogenic markers *in vivo*.[11] In addition, after cell sorting for CD146+, CD34−, CD45−, CD56−, and CD144− pericytes, sorted cells were shown to have the capacity for *in vitro* expansion, multipotent *in vitro* or *in vivo* differentiation potential into the osteogenic, chondrogenic, adipogenic, and myogenic lineages at a clonal level and expressed markers typical for MSCs, such as CD10, CD13, CD44, CD73, CD90, CD105, and HLA class I and lacked expression of CD56, CD106, CD133, and HLA-DR.[10] Pericytes were isolated from various tissues including skeletal muscle, pancreas, adipose tissue, and placenta from multiple fetal and adult donors.

These findings suggest that walls of small blood vessels all over the body represent a reservoir for mesenchymal progenitor cells which are assumed to be the *in vivo* ancestors of the elusive MSC, which is established in *in vitro* long-term cultures. Thus, a viable model is that the perivascular region may be *in vivo*, if it is not the MSC niche. However, the physiological role of pericytes or MSCs as stem cells *in vivo* remains elusive. The perivascular model proposes MSCs as cells that stabilize blood vessels, sustain tissue and immunological homeostasis under physiological conditions and may function as local contributors to the repair process upon tissue damage.[10]

12.4 Properties of MSCs

According to the widely accepted scientific convention, plastic adherent cells isolated from bone marrow, adipose tissue and other sources are known as MSCs.[12] This term was popularized in the early 1990s by Arnold Caplan,[5] whereas in the 1980s these cells were termed osteogenic stem cells based on the work by Friedenstein,[2] but also the name marrow stromal stem cells has been proposed.[4] Furthermore, names such as mesenchymal progenitor cells and skeletal stem cells were also suggested.

12.4.1 *Nomenclature & definition*

In 2005, the International Society for Cellular Therapy (ISCT) published a statement proposing to call these cells multipotent mesenchymal stromal cells, while the term mesenchymal stem cell should be reserved for a subset of these (or other) cells that demonstrate stem cell activity.[12] This was based on the fact that *in vivo* demonstrations of long-term survival with self-renewal capacity and tissue repopulation with multi-lineage differentiation were still missing at that time. Nevertheless, the ISCT proposed to use the acronym MSC for both mentioned cell populations.

Additionally the terms "mesenchymal stromal cells" and "adult mesenchymal stromal cells" are widely used.

MSCs are plastic adherent fibroblast-like cells that can be isolated from a variety of mesenchymal tissues including bone marrow, adipose tissue, umbilical cord, umbilical cord blood, placenta, dental pulp, and others by density gradient centrifugation and/or enzymatic digestion.

In 2006, the ISCT published another position paper proposing three minimal criteria for defining MSCs[13]:

i. MSCs must be plastic-adherent when maintained in standard culture conditions using tissue culture flasks.

ii. A minimum of 95% of the MSC population must express CD105, CD73, and CD90, as measured by flow cytometry. Additionally, these cells must lack expression (maximum 2% positive) of CD45, CD34, CD14 or CD11b, CD79a or CD19 and HLA class II.

iii. The cells must be able to differentiate into osteoblasts, adipocytes, and chondroblasts under standard *in vitro* differentiation conditions.

Differentiation into osteoblasts is suggested to be demonstrated by staining with Alizarin Red or von Kossa staining, adipocyte differentiation by Oil Red O or Nile Red staining, and chondroblast differentiation by Alcian blue or collagen type II staining.

Since 2002, a number of MSC subtypes have been reported which show a wider differentiation potential than the classical MSC. These include, among others, human unrestricted somatic stem cell (USSC) from umbilical cord blood,[14] human very small embryonic-like stem cell (VSEL) from cord blood or bone marrow,[15] human bone marrow isolated adult multilineage inducible (MIAMI) cells,[16] and rodent and human multipotent adult progenitor cells (MAPCs) from bone marrow.[17]

The colony-forming unit-fibroblastic (CFU-F) assay was developed by Friedenstein in the 1960s/70s. Bone marrow cells were seeded at very low density in cultures containing serum and one to two weeks later discrete colonies of plastic adherent fibroblast like cells were observed. The clonogenic cell at the origin of each colony is called CFU-F. To date, this is the gold standard to estimate the number of clonogenic cells in a certain cell preparation and has been used for MSCs and MSC sub-populations isolated from various tissues.

Although proof of self-renewal has been missing for a long time,[12,13] it has been recently shown at least for bone marrow-derived MSCs sorted by antigen expression of CD146.[11]

12.4.2 *Cultivation of MSCs*

MSCs are usually isolated from bone marrow and umbilical cord blood by density gradient centrifugation and from various tissues by enzymatic digestion using a variety of protocols. Cells are plated on tissue culture plastic usually in standard medium (DMEM or alpha-MEM) containing 10% fetal calf serum (FCS). As not every batch FCS supports MSC growth, and also some batches do not support the *in vitro* trilineage differentiation potential, a number of FCS batches should be screened. Additionally, in some protocols growth factors like FGF-2, EGF, or PDGF are added to the medium. Usually, MSCs are cultured under normoxic conditions (20% O_2), but hypoxic conditions (3–5% O_2) have been shown to support proliferation and some other properties.[18] It is widely accepted that freshly isolated MSC cultures are very heterogenic and initially contain different sub-populations. During *in vitro* expansion, the variation of culture conditions can be selected for one or the other sub-population and as many different culture protocols are used even MSCs from the same tissue may differ from lab to lab. Additionally, properties of MSCs and their indication-specific suitability may be modulated over the course of cell expansion. Therefore, elaborated characterization of cell populations after expansion and a thorough quality control (QC) with the appropriate analysis before release is a prerequisite for a therapeutic use.

MSCs can be expanded up to about 35–50 population doublings, a number reflecting the Hayflick limit. Beyond this limit, cells grow larger, are less tightly packed and become senescent and also lose their differentiation potential. Therefore, cells for therapeutic use should be expanded only for a limited number of population doublings.

12.5 MoA of MSCs

MSCs represent a cell type that exhibits several advantages, making them promising candidates for application in the field of cell therapy or tissue engineering. MSCs are readily available due to their residence in virtually all tissues of the body and the ease of isolation of cells from tissues. In case of some tissues, like adipose tissue or placenta, they can be isolated from tissues which are subject to discard, i.e., there are neither ethical concerns nor concerns of harming the donor. In addition to the availability, MSCs are cultivated in standard cell culture systems as regards media, dishes, and other materials such as enzymes to release the cells from dishes. Cultivation of MSCs in serum-free and xeno-free media may be the exception in this respect, since there is no well–established medium available, but in development pipelines of media suppliers. MSCs are extensively expandable in *in vitro* culture which allows for yielding of tens or hundreds of thousands doses of MSCs from source material of a single donor in an allogeneic setting. Some tissues contain a high number of MSCs or MSC-like cells that facilitate usage of unexpanded cells in an autologous setting, i.e., for e.g., MSCs or MSC–like cells are isolated from adipose tissue and administered to patients immediately after the harvest and purification procedures. The autologous administration of MSCs may be performed intra-surgically.[19]

The administration route of MSCs has to be chosen specifically for the particular indication. MSCs were administered *via* both systemic and local routes ranging from most common intravenous injection/infusions to local intramuscular or intrathecal injections.[20] The traditional model of MSC pharmacokinetics (PK) after systemic administration, especially after intravenous injections/infusions, is that the cells get physically diluted in the lung capillary network and that the cells subsequently co–localize to the site of injury or inflammation following chemotactic gradients.[20] The process of MSC co–localization has also been termed "homing of MSCs". On a molecular level, chemokines, growth factors as well as adhesion molecules and their receptors have been discussed to play an important role in MSC co–localization. The model of MSC co–localization has been deduced from leukocyte trafficking, including the steps of rolling, adhesion, and para–cellular or trans–cellular transmigration from the luminal side of blood vessels into injured or inflamed tissues upon specific injury cues produced and secreted by the damaged tissue. The main difference between MSCs and leukocytes in their molecular endowment is lack of expression of selectin ligands on MSCs, which are known to mediate rolling of leukocytes on endothelial cells that express selectins.[21] Amongst the numerous discussed chemokines and chemokine receptors, the relevance of the CXC chemokine receptor type 4 (CXCR-4)-stromal cell–derived factor 1 (SDF-1) axis has extensively been evaluated in multiple disease models. As an example, overexpression of CXCR-4 on the surface of MSCs was shown to lead to migration of cells to ischemic myocardium and enhanced recovery of left ventricular function after systemic administration of cells. Interaction of integrin $\alpha 4/\beta 1$ (CD49d/CD29) on MSCs with vascular cell adhesion molecule 1 (VCAM-1), CD106 expressed on endothelial cell is an example for adhesion receptor interactions. Recently, reports suggesting systemic effects of MSCs, most probably independent of MSC co-localization at the site of injury, challenged the traditional homing model. In a model of myocardial infarction, MSCs retained in the pool of lung capillaries after intravenous administration were shown to reduce inflammatory response and scar size mainly by secreting a paracrine factor named TNF-α-induced protein 6 (TSG-6), suggesting a systemic effect of MSCs.[22] The therapeutic effect could be significantly reduced by silencing TSG-6 using siRNA and a similar, although not as pronounced, effect could be achieved by administration of recombinant TSG-6.[22]

In the early days of MSC research and in early preclinical experiments, MSCs were supposed to co-localize to the site of injury after administration and replace injured or dead cells by engraftment into the tissue and subsequent differentiation into mesenchymal lineages or even transdifferentiation into endodermal or ectodermal lineages. As early as in the 1980s and 1990s, following pioneering work by Alexander J. Friedenstein in the 1960s and 1970s, multilineage mesenchymal differentiation potential of MSCs has been demonstrated *in vitro* and *in vivo*.[4,5] Irrespective of the targeted organ or disease model, MSCs were found to co-localize, engraft and (trans-) differentiate into cardiomyocytes in the heart[23] or into renal tubule epithelial cells in a model of acute kidney injury.[24]

Meanwhile, the field of MSC research has undergone a paradigm shift and is close to reach a consensus on the primary MoA of MSCs which may be valid for many but not all disease settings. It has been suggested that MSCs primarily act *via* the release of paracrine or endocrine factors which create an environment facilitating and stimulating endogenous repair. Hallmark processes regulated by MSCs contributing to an environment for endogenous repair or regeneration include immunomodulation, stimulation of proliferation of resident tissue cells or local progenitor cells, inhibition of apoptosis, stimulation of angiogenic process, and induction of differentiation or re-differentiation processes (please see also Chapter 15 "Exosomes and their Therapeutic Applications").

12.5.1 *MicroRNAs (miRNAs) and exosomes*

miRNAs and exosomes have been identified as potential regulators of MSC fate and/or mediators of MSC effects, respectively. miRNAs, a class of single-stranded non-coding RNAs, modulate regulatory mechanisms of cellular functions in eukaryotic cells.[25] There is only little data on regulation of MSC fate by miRNAs with some studies focusing on the influence of miRNAs on MSC differentiation processes. For instance, miR-103 and miR-107 were found to be involved in acetyl-CoA and lipid metabolism which is important in adipogenic differentiation which can be induced by miR-143 regulating ERK5 as part of the leukemia inhibitory factor signaling cascade.[26] Cartilage development was found to be modulated by miR-140 which is supposed to inhibit HDAC4 potentially co-repressing Runx2. More research is required to get a basic understanding of miRNAs in the MoA of MSCs as well as the potential of miRNAs for MSC characterization.

Exosomes or microvesicles are 50–1,000 nm particles shown to be phospholipid vesicles consisting of e.g., cholesterol, sphingomyelin, and phosphatidylcholine which are secreted by a wide variety of cells including MSCs.[27] Exosome preparations can be obtained by collection of conditioned medium of MSCs and ultracentrifugation. Exosomes exhibit several surface adhesion molecules such as CD44, CD29, CD49d, CD49e, and CD73, but mostly lack expression of HLA Class I or HLA Class II, and have been found to contain proteins, mRNA, and miRNAs. In an Ischemia-reperfusion induced (IRI) model of acute kidney injury (AKI), it was shown that single administration of exosomes protected rats from AKI by inhibiting apoptosis and stimulating tubular epithelial cell proliferation.[27] RNase pretreatment of exosomes in this AKI study abrogated protective effects indicating a role of RNA as active pharmacological compound.

12.5.2 *In inflammation and immunity*

MSCs have been shown to exert strong immune modulatory and immunosuppressive effects *in vitro* and *in vivo*.[28] These effects of MSCs have been exemplarily demonstrated in multiple phase I or phase II clinical trials treating patients with severe or moderate graft-*versus*-host disease (GvHD) following allogeneic bone marrow transplantation.[29] *In vitro*, MSCs have been shown to interact with virtually all players of the human immune system resulting in a shift from pro–inflammatory to an anti-inflammatory profile. MSCs have been reported to inhibit T-cell proliferation and cytokine secretion, induce generation of regulatory T-cells, inhibit proliferation of natural killer (NK) cells and cytotoxicity, reprogram macrophages from pro-inflammatory toward an anti-inflammatory type, or for instance, inhibit differentiation and maturation of dendritic cells (DCs).[30] Most of the interactions between MSCs and immune cells are modulated by MSC-derived soluble factors but the field is far away from a thorough understanding of the mechanisms underlying such cellular interactions. Soluble factors derived from MSCs include indoleamine 2, 3-dioxygenase (IDO), an enzyme which degrades tryptophan as an important mitogen for T-cells and cytokines and growth factors such as interleukin (IL)-6, IL-10, or IL-1RA or transforming growth factor (TGF)-β, hepatocyte growth factor (HGF), insulin-like growth factor (IGF) but also low molecular weight factors such as prostaglandins E_2 (PGE$_2$) or nitric oxide (NO).

The outmost part of the immune modulatory effect of MSCs is based on soluble factors. However, there is evidence from Transwell experiments, separating immune cells and MSCs using a semi-permeable membrane, that cell−cell-interactions play an additional role in this respect. Cell surface molecules involved in MSC-mediated immunomodulation include Jagged-1 binding to Notch on immune cells, PD-1 pathway, VCAM-1 and inter-cellular adhesion molecule-1 (ICAM-1) binding to CD49d and CD11a on immune cells, respectively.[31] Expression of some of these factors on the surface of MSCs is only detectable after *in vitro* stimulation of MSCs by cytokines such as interferon (IFN)-γ and/or tumor necrosis factor (TNF)-α mimicking a pro-inflammatory environment. Some of the cell surface molecules have been described to be part of the immunological synapse at the interface of an antigen-presenting cell (APC) and T-cells and have been suggested to be involved in the interaction between MSCs and immune cells. In summary, the immune modulatory effects of MSCs are suggested to contribute to shift the microenvironment at the site of injury/inflammation from a pro-inflammatory to an anti-inflammatory milieu mainly by releasing soluble factors but also by direct MSC—immune cell interactions.

12.5.3 *In kidney disease*

In a milieu with damaged cells and high levels of inflammation, prompt attenuation or inhibition of cell death is obviously important besides creation of an anti-inflammatory milieu in order to facilitate tissue repair by surviving tissue cells and local resident progenitor cells. In this paragraph, MoA of MSCs in an acute disease model exemplified by toxic or IRI models of AKI is highlighted reflecting the multiple facets of MSC effects.[32] In a rat model of IRI-induced AKI, MSCs administered intra-arterially led to reduced inflammation in kidneys as determined by reduced expression levels of pro-inflammatory mediators and increased expression levels of anti-inflammatory mediators in kidneys as compared to control animals.[33] In addition to MSC-mediated immunomodulation, apoptotic index was significantly reduced in MSC-treated animals and at the same time, proliferation of kidney-resident cells was elevated indicating induction of repair processes. Kidneys of MSC-treated animals were histologically and functionally comparable to healthy animals in strong contrast to animals which were not treated or treated with fibroblasts as control cells. The authors discuss that MSCs in acute injury protect the kidney by release of paracrine factors mediating immunomodulation, protection from apoptosis, and induction of cell proliferation. In this study, immune cell infiltration into damaged kidneys was reduced and the cytokine expression profile in whole kidney switched from pro- to anti-inflammatory as indicated by up-regulation of expression of anti-inflammatory IL-10 and down-regulation of pro-inflammatory IL-1β, TNF-α, and IFN-γ. Candidate MSC-derived growth factors supposed to mediate tissue repair, induction of proliferation of kidney-resident cells, and other effects are amongst others HGF, IGF, and vascular endothelial-derived growth factor (VEGF).[34] The relevance of MSC-derived VEGF in therapeutic efficacy of MSCs in AKI was demonstrated by silencing VEGF expression of MSCs using siRNA which led to a decreased efficacy of MSCs.[31] Using a similar approach in a cisplatin model of AKI, the relevance of IGF-1 in MSC therapy has been demonstrated both *in vitro* and *in vivo*.[32] In addition to immune modulatory and repair-inducing effects of MSCs in AKI, reduction of fibrosis score and significant reduction of expression of fibrosis-associated factors such as TGF-β and plasminogen activator inhibitor (PAI)-1 has been demonstrated after long-term follow-up in rats. MSCs are known to exert pro-angiogenic effects; however, the role of these effects in AKI therapy is currently poorly understood but may also play a role. Interestingly, no or only a negligible number of MSCs are engrafted in acutely injured kidneys. In contrast, MSCs were detected for approximately up to three days in damaged kidneys and disappeared completely, i.e., MSCs were not found in the circulation or in any tissues or organs in a significant number. It has been suggested that MSCs undergo anoikis or apoptosis in the circulation.

The kidney has the potential to self-repair after injury to a certain extent. Recently, Humphreys and Bonventre showed by using different techniques that regeneration of tubules, which are most severely damaged after, e.g., IRI, by surviving tubular epithelial cells, is the primary repair mechanism in adult kidneys.[35] In the first study using genetic fate-mapping techniques to specifically label tubular epithelial cells, it was shown that 50% of labeled epithelial cells express proliferation marker Ki67 after IRI and two-third of epithelial cells had incorporated BromodeoxyUridine (BrdU) after complete repair, in contrast to only 3.5% of cells in not injured kidneys. Data indicates that surviving epithelial cells underwent proliferation to replace lost cells. A second study using DNA analog based technique confirmed the first study and gave further indications that epithelial proliferation after IRI occurred by proliferation of epithelial cells which were injured and dedifferentiated, and not by progenitor cells. In contrast to these findings, existence of renal progenitor cells which may contribute to renal repair has been proposed. In consideration of the natural self-repair mechanisms of the kidney and the therapeutic effects of MSCs in AKI, a conclusive hypothesis may be that MSCs create an environment which attenuates renal injury and facilitates endogenous repair mechanisms. MSCs may reduce local inflammation, protect surviving dedifferentiated tubular epithelial cells from apoptosis and stimulate their proliferation for replacement of dead cells. The influence of MSCs on the re-differentiation of propagated dedifferentiated epithelial cells [a process named mesenchymal-to-epithelial transition (MET) a reverse of epithelial-to-mesenchymal transition (EMT)] that injured epithelial cells can undergo upon injury is currently unknown, also the potential pro-angiogenic effects exerted by the MSCs.

12.5.4 *In organ fibrosis*

MSCs have been preclinically and clinically administered in various indications ranging from musculo–skeletal repair, neurological disorders, hematological malignancies, wound healing, autoimmune diseases, inflammatory diseases, tissue or organ transplantation, progressive organ failure, or fibrotic diseases. The underlying pathological mechanisms of those diseases are highly heterogeneous. However, there are some basic and common mechanisms which represent potential targets for MSCs as therapeutics. In an acute disease setting such as an AKI associated with inflammation and injury and loss of tubular epithelial cells, MSCs are suggested to exert immunomodulation, protection from apoptosis, and induction of cell proliferation indicating induction of repair processes by endogenous cells[26,36] as described in the paragraph potential MoA of MSCs above.

Potential targets in a chronic disease setting are illustrated in the following as exemplified by pulmonary fibrosis. Fibrosis is characterized by overgrowth and scarring of tissues accompanied by inflammation and excessive deposition of extracellular matrix (ECM) molecules such as collagens.[37] Fibrosis is a complex interplay of molecular cues and cells including bone marrow–derived cells, fibroblasts, dedifferentiated tissue cells such as epithelial cells, or immune cells, especially macrophages. Important molecular regulators of fibrosis include growth factors like PDGF, VEGF, TGF-β, or connective tissue growth factor (CTGF), interleukins like IL-13, IL-4, or IL-10, angiotensin II, endothelin-1, chemokines (MCP-1, MIP-1β), caspases, metallomatrix proteinases and their inhibitors as reviewed elsewhere.

The main cellular mediator of fibrosis is the myofibroblast, an active and contractile cell type found in inflammatory conditions with the capacity of proliferation and production of ECM compounds.[38] Myofibroblasts or activated fibroblasts have been found to originate from at least three different cell types: (1) Resident intrapulmonary fibroblasts are activated and differentiate into myofibroblasts, (2) Injured lung epithelial cells which underwent EMT or, as more recently proposed, injured endothelial cells which underwent endothelial-mesenchymal transition (EndMT), or (3) Bone marrow–derived circulating fibrocytes exhibiting morphological and molecular characteristics of HSCs, monocytes, and fibroblasts.

In an inflammatory environment, resident fibroblasts can be activated, migrate to sites of injury and turn into myofibroblasts characterized by increased contractility and expression of α-smooth muscle actin (α-SMA) and stress fibers. Important factors in this process are amongst others alternatively spliced fibronectin, PDGF, and TGF-β.

In case of EMT, epithelial cells are suggested to transform into fibroblast-like mesenchymal cells upon stress or wounding. Basement membrane beneath epithelial cells becomes leaky which is caused by proteolytic degradation (e.g., by metalloproteinases). Epithelial cells thereby lose their polarization and cell–cell-junctions accompanied by initiation of dedifferentiation processes, cell proliferation, and migration toward the interstitium. Transition of epithelial cells into mesenchymal cells involves factors such as TGF-β, epidermal growth factor (EGF), IGF-II, or fibroblast growth factor-2 (FGF-2) with TGF-β being the most prominent candidate factor. Fibroblast-type cells derived from EMT processes have been shown to produce ECM including collagens and contribute to fibrosis in different organs such as kidney or lung.

Fibrocytes have been described as bone marrow-derived circulating cells involved in reactive and reparative fibrosis which co-express markers of HSCs, monocytes, and fibroblasts. The surface antigen profile is unique since cells express, e.g., CD34, CD45, CD14, MHC class I and II, co-stimulatory molecules, diverse integrins and chemokine receptors, and mesenchymal markers including vimentin, fibronectin, or collagen I. Data from various animal models indicates that there is a causal link between fibrocyte accumulation and progressive tissue fibrogenesis after tissue damage or hypoxia.

Like many other organs such as kidney or liver, the lung has a potential for endogenous repair and recovery depending on the nature, duration, and severity of the injury stimulus.[39] Initially following injury, there is acute inflammation with recruitment of immune cells and activation of macrophages. Lung-resident or distal stem or progenitor cells such as MSCs are recruited to the sites of injury and inflammation. Epithelial cells, partially damaged and in the process of dedifferentiation *via* EMT begin to spread and migrate on ECM produced by themselves with involvement of diverse growth factors, cytokines, chemokines, and other molecules as described above derived from all different types of cells involved in the inflammation and repair processes. Signaling pathways such as sonic hedgehog, MAP kinase pathways, STAT3, and Wnt have been identified to function as important regulators of these processes. Cell proliferation to replace damaged or dead cells and subsequent differentiation of expanded cells into functional tissue cells such as epithelial cells is considered to be a crucial step in repair and wound healing processes.

Persistent injury stimuli may contribute to the pathology of fibrotic diseases. For instance, misdirected repair processes involving TGF-β and EMT may lead to fibrosis.

MSCs have been described to have beneficial therapeutic effects in multiple pre-clinical studies of lung fibrosis.[40] The MoA of MSCs in lung fibrosis has been elucidated to a minor extent so far. It has been described that administration of MSCs reduced inflammation, infiltration of immune cells, and expression of IFN-γ, and the proinflammatory cytokines, macrophage migratory inhibitory factor, and TNF-α. Collagen concentration in lungs was significantly reduced by MSC treatment, potentially mediated by inhibition of TGF-β activity and by increased matrix metalloproteinase levels and reduced levels of their endogenous inhibitors [tissue inhibitors of metalloproteinases (TIMPs)]. Interleukin-1 receptor antagonist (IL-1RA) has been suggested to be a key cytokine derived from MSCs in lung fibrosis studies mediating therapeutic effects by blocking IL-1 and TNF-α pathways of inflammation.

A crucial part of the MoA of MSCs is their capacity to release soluble factors involved in immunomodulation and induction of endogenous repair processes. Soluble factors in lung repair processes secreted by tissue cells and immune cells have been suggested to affect spreading and migration of epithelial cells and fibroblasts, wound closure, or re-establishing intact barrier function. Furthermore, TGF-β as soluble factor is involved in transition of epithelial cells to myofibroblasts, initiation of inflammatory responses, and excessive ECM deposition. The effect of MSCs on these processes is currently unknown; however, as known from various therapeutic approaches there is sufficient reason that MSCs may have therapeutically beneficial effects in the context of fibrosis. Furthermore, since MSCs are known to be immune modulatory and interact with virtually all cells of the immune system, MSCs may contribute to anti-fibrosis in down-regulation of immune cells at the site of injury, deactivation of macrophages or shifting macrophages from a pro- to an anti-inflammatory profile. The regulation of proliferation of tissue-resident cells involved in repair processes as well as the regulation of re-differentiation of cells toward functional epithelial cells is currently not known and requires more mechanistic pre-clinical studies. In conclusion, there is some body of indication that MSCs may represent a promising therapeutic approach to treat chronic diseases such as fibrotic diseases, although mechanisms and MoA are currently poorly understood and require further research.

Although many experts agree that MSC-based cell therapy is still at its infancy and maybe even too immature in certain areas, there is an increasing number of cellular therapy approaches in academia as well as industry with growing potential for tissue repair and organ protection. However, most knowledge on the biological function of MSC in tissue repair has been collected from mouse models and those data seem difficult to transfer into a clinical application in humans. Most pre-clinical and early clinical trials (phase I/II) have been based on the *in vitro* potential of MSC to differentiate into bone, cartilage, and fat tissue and are therefore somehow related to tissue engineering approaches, but failed to have a sustainable effect *in vivo*. The same applies to pre-fabricated bone or cartilage tissue consisting of MSCs together with biomaterials, e.g., for the treatment of severe osteoarthritis.

12.5.5 *In cardio-vascular diseases*

Nevertheless, the first "success" was reported in patients with acute myocardial infarction. After first attempts with CD34+ hematopoietic progenitor cells, bone marrow-derived MSCs were either injected *via* the intracoronary route[41] or systemically or directly into the myocardium. Most of those studies improved the left ventricular function and ejection fraction (EF) and patients could be discharged from the clinic earlier than their control groups. However, it could never be demonstrated that a single MSC ever differentiated *in vivo* into a contractile cardiomyocyte. Nevertheless, patients' benefit resulted from a faster and better scar formation in the infracted area and a smaller "area at risk" to maintain or even improve organ function. Whether this is due to a matrix or paracrine effect on residual cells in the myocardium is still unknown. However, several clinical trials have been performed to test the safety and efficacy of MSC transplantation.

MSCs albeit contribute to an improved microcirculation and the formation of new blood vessels (angiogenesis) that improve the hostile environment of the infracted area which counteracts inflammation, cell death, and loss of the ischemic tissue. This biological mechanism is currently used for the treatment of patients suffering from peripheral arterial disease (PAD) and critical limb ischemia (CLI). MSCs are either injected directly into the musculature of the affected limb or are given systemically. The long term clinical benefit of this approach still remains to be determined but it has already been proven that MSC therapy is safe for the surveillance time. This implies also the use of MSCs in wound healing to accelerate wound repair or even reconstitute the wound bed, e.g., after extended burns or in diabetic skin ulcers.

12.5.6 *In cancer therapy*

Recent developments also point toward the application of MSCs in cancer therapy.[42] Such an application can reach with the support of the hematopoietic recovery after myeloablative therapy *via* the direct interaction of MSCs with the tumor and the tumor environment[43] toward the delivery of therapeutic drugs or genes to cancer.[44,45] The homing, also of genetically modified MSCs,[46] to the tumor site and its special environment is most likely based on the composition of the inflammatory infiltrate and the tumor stroma itself.[47] This approach is currently been tested in a clinical trial for advanced cancer.[48] In the TREAT-ME 1 trial, the modified and pharmaceutically manufactured MSCs not only deliver a suicide gene to advanced gastrointestinal cancer including metastases after intravenous infusion, the activation of the therapeutic gene and its release in the tumor is tightly linked to specific promoter activation.[49] This certainly increases the local efficacy of otherwise toxic drugs and reduces unwanted off-target toxicity.

12.6 Clinical Applications

Since the incidence of differentiation of transplanted MSCs in the target tissue seems to be too low to explain some of the (pre) clinical improvements, other effects may significantly contribute to the biological function. MSCs secrete a vast number of different growth factors and cytokines that promote tissue regeneration, but also modulation of the immune system.

The ability of MSCs to modulate the immune system has been demonstrated manifold in different models and indications. MSCs may exert their immune modulatory functions by direct cell–cell contact or *via* soluble factors. Factors that are produced by MSCs also include members of the TGF-β family and respond to other cytokines like IFN-γ and TNF-α,[50] which allows a dynamic cross talk between MSCs and immune cells. MSCs have been shown to be anti-proliferative to stimulated T-cells in those diseases and shift the immune response rather to a state of tolerance [e.g., from MΦ1 to MΦ2 and proliferation of the regulatory T-cells (T$_{regs}$)]. Although inflammation is part of the body's natural defense system, its misdirection can lead to inevitable organ damage like in some autoimmune diseases. MSCs are currently under evaluation for the treatment for such disease conditions like inflammatory bowel disease, systemic lupus erythematosus, rheumatoid arthritis, type 1 diabetes or GvHD after allogeneic mismatched bone marrow transplantation.[29] Therefore, MSCs might even offer a therapeutic opportunity in solid organ transplantation and mediate a state of tolerance to reduce the need for immunosuppressive agents or protect β-islet allografts from rejection.[51]

The trophic and immune regulatory properties of MSCs also make them a potential therapeutic modality for neural repair like in multiple sclerosis, amyotrophic lateral sclerosis, Parkinson's disease or metachromatic leukodystrophy. MSCs have additionally been suggested for the treatment of spinal cord injury.[52]

Chronic liver diseases, either toxic, infectious or immune-mediated lead to an increase of fibrotic fibers and eventually cirrhosis, which is usually associated with irreversible liver failure. The anti-fibrotic effects of MSCs have already been demonstrated in animal models and first clinical trials are on its way, although advanced stages of liver fibrosis may not be suitable for cellular intervention, except for entire liver transplantation.

Like in the liver, there are also some studies revealing compelling benefits from the administration of MSCs in acute lung injury, obstructive airway disease and pulmonary fibrosis,[37] while there are also some concerns that MSCs might even worsen the pulmonary conditions, particularly after systemic intravenous administration of MSCs.

MSCs have also shown a therapeutic potential in AKI and chronic renal failure to reduce or alleviate the glomerular or tubular interstitial damage. MSC infusion has also been shown to significantly improve kidney function after IRI,[28] which is the major cause of acute renal failure in some unavoidable clinical situations like kidney transplantation or open heart surgery.

Currently, there are at least 170 clinical trials based on unmodified MSCs ongoing or completed (www.clinicaltrials.gov). Nevertheless, the research for the second generation of MSC therapies already started some years ago. Transgenic, biochemical, and priming/preconditioning methods are used to optimize MSC-based therapeutics. Therefore, two strategies are addressed: (1) Increasing the homing (co-localization) of MSCs to the target tissue, and (2) Enhancing the potency of MSCs.[53]

After transplantation, MSCs have been shown by many studies to follow chemo-attractants and to subsequently co-localize to sites of (tumor-associated) inflammation or to injured tissues. Other studies have shown that shortly after intravenous infusion, the majority of infused cells can be detected in the lung for a limited time. These differences might be explained by either different expansion protocols (as it has been proposed that during culture expansion, MSCs lose or change the expression of certain ligands and receptors which are critical for homing to target tissues) or by sensitivity and resolution of imaging methods.

To increase co-localization, transgenic, biochemical, and priming/preconditioning approaches have been performed. For example, the CXCR-4/SDF-1 axis has been improved by either overexpression of SDF-1 or CXCR-4 in rodent models of myocardial infarction,[20] whereas another study used hypoxic preconditioning of MSC (3% oxygen) to induce high expression of both SDF-1 chemokine receptors, CXCR-4 and CXCR-7 by activating HIF-1α.[54] A similar approach is to target the MSCs to a specific niche or tissue by modification or addition of adhesion receptors. Komarova et al. retrovirally induced expression of an artificial receptor that targets MSCs to ovarian tumors which highly express ErbB2.[55] This has also been done enzymatically and biochemically. Sackstein et al. enzymatically glycosylated the CD44 surface receptor on MSCs to induce E-selectin binding, as

E-selectin is highly expressed in bone marrow,[21] whereas Sakar *et al.* covalently coupled SialylLewisx (SLeX) moiety, a selectin ligand, onto the surface of MSCs through biotin–streptavidin chemical modifications.[56] Alternatively, antibodies[57] or precoating with antibodies *via* a palmitylated protein G have been used to enhance or induce co-localization to inflamed or specific tissues.[58]

The other line of investigation in optimizing MSC-based cell therapies is increasing their potency. This can be done either by enhancing the effective dose of MSCs by limiting cell death after application by overexpression of anti-apoptotic or otherwise protective proteins, or by overexpression or induction of expression of proteins which may act in a specific disease context. As an example, overexpression of the anti-apoptotic protein bcl-2 in rat MSCs resulted in reduced MSC apoptosis, increased cellular survival, and improved cardiac function in a rat left anterior descending ligation model *via* intracardiac injection.[59] This is in line with another study where MSCs overexpressing the heat shock protein Hsp70 have been shown to display higher viability and anti-apoptotic properties *via* increase of bcl-2 expression and to rescue heart functions from myocardial injury in a rat model.[60] Similar effects have been observed after overexpression of Akt-1, a protein involved in cellular survival pathways, by inhibiting apoptotic processes.[61] Notch-induced overexpression of glial cell–derived neurotrophic factor (GDNF), the most potent neurotrophic factor for dopaminergic neurons in MSCs is an example of a disease context-specific protein that has been used to enhance the potency of MSCs. The resulting genetically modified MSCs promoted recovery in a rat model of Parkinson's disease.[62] Other examples are VEGF which plays an important role in the renoprotective function of MSCs in AKI and IGF-1.[34]

All these and many other studies demonstrated some improvement of homing or efficacy of MSCs *in vitro* or in preclinical models. Nevertheless all used techniques manipulate the MSCs additionally to the manipulations anyways associated with extensive expansion *in vitro*. Transgenic overexpression results in mutations due to undirected insertions of the transgene into the genome. This could lead to either proliferation arrest and senescence or induction of tumorigenicity. Additionally influencing survival and apoptotic pathways and enzymatically or biochemically engineering MSCs is not without risk and the impact of therapy safety may be difficult to study. Therefore, at least characterization of genetic stability of the manipulated cells and potency assays might be necessary to minimize risks and batch to batch variability.

One step further goes the approaches which do not even use the MSC itself anymore. Based on the fact that the effects of administered MSCs are mainly mediated by paracrine and endocrine factors, some groups used MSC-derived exosomes or MSC-conditioned medium for their studies. In one of these studies, purified exosomes reduced infarct size in a mouse model of myocardial IRI.[63] Therefore, the authors concluded that MSCs mediate their cardioprotective paracrine effects by secreting exosomes. MSC-conditioned medium has been used in an *in vitro/ex vivo* rat myocardial reperfusion model and an *in vivo* pig myocardical infarction model.[64] Both studies could show some improvement. On the other hand, the use of conditioned media of human MSCs instead of cells as therapeutics is controversially discussed due to conflicting results.

MSCs offer therapeutic opportunities in many disease conditions with yet unmet medical need. Preliminary clinical trials have demonstrated that MSC therapy is safe and usually is well tolerated also in combination with biomaterials. Nevertheless, many fundamental questions remain open to develop MSC-based cell therapy including tissue engineering according to the present guidelines and regulations.

References

1. Till, J.E., and McCulloch, E.A. A direct measurement of the radiation sensitivity of normal mouse bone marrow cells. *Radiat. Res.* 14, 213–222 (1961).
2. Friedenstein, A.J., Petrakova, K.V., Kurolesova, A.I., and Frolova, G.P. Heterotopic of bone marrow. Analysis of precursor cells for osteogenic and hematopoietic tissues. *Transplantation* 6, 230–247 (1968).
3. Singer, J.W., Keating, A., Cuttner, J., Gown, A.M., Jacobson, R., Killen, P.D., Moohr, J.W., Najfeld, V., Powell, J., and Sanders, J. Evidence for a stem cell common to hematopoiesis and its *in vitro* microenvironment: Studies of patients with clonal hematopoietic neoplasia *Leuk. Res.* 8, 535–545 (1984).
4. Owen, M. Marrow stromal stem cells. *J. Cell Sci. Suppl.* 10, 63–76 (1988).
5. Caplan, A.I. Mesenchymal stem cells. *J. Orthop. Res.* 9, 641–650 (1991).
6. Simmons, P.J., Przepiorka, D., Thomas, E.D., and Torok-Storb, B. Host origin of marrow stromal cells following allogeneic bone marrow transplantation. *Nature* 328, 429–432 (1987).
7. Cossu, G., and Bianco, P. 2003. Mesoangioblasts — vascular progenitors for extravascular mesodermal tissues. *Curr. Opin. Genet. Dev.* 13, 537–542 (2003).
8. Dazzi, F., Ramasamy, R., Glennie, S., Jones, S.P., and Roberts, I. The role of mesenchymal stem cells in haemopoiesis. *Blood Rev.* 20, 161–171 (2006).
9. Bianco, P., Riminucci, M., Kuznetsov, S., and Robey, P.G. Multipotential cells in the bone marrow stroma: Regulation in the context of organ physiology. *Crit. Rev. Eukaryot. Gene Expr.* 9, 159–173 (2010).
10. Crisan, M., Yap, S., Casteilla, L., Chen, C.W., Corselli, M., Park, T.S., Andriolo, G., Sun, B., Zheng, B., Zhang, L., Norotte, C., Teng, P.N., Traas, J., Schugar, R., Deasy, B.M., Badylak, S., Buhring, H.J., Giacobino, J.P., Lazzari, L., Huard, J., and Peault, B.

A perivascular origin for mesenchymal stem cells in multiple human organs. *Cell Stem Cell* 3, 301–313 (2008).

11. Sacchetti, B., Funari, A., Michienzi, S., Di Cesare, S., Piersanti, S., Saggio, I., Tagliafico, E., Ferrari, S., Robey, P.G., Riminucci, M., and Bianco, P. Self-renewing osteoprogenitors in bone marrow sinusoids can organize a hematopoietic microenvironment. *Cell* 131, 324–336 (2007).

12. Horwitz, E.M., Le, B.K., Dominici, M., Mueller, I., Slaper-Cortenbach, I., Marini, F.C., Deans, R.J., Krause, D.S., and Keating, A. Clarification of the nomenclature for MSC: The International Society for Cellular Therapy position statement. *Cytotherapy* 7, 393–395 (2005).

13. Dominici, M., Le, B.K., Mueller, I., Slaper-Cortenbach, I., Marini, F., Krause, D., Deans, R., Keating, A., Prockop, D., and Horwitz, E. Minimal criteria for defining multipotent mesenchymal stromal cells. The International Society for Cellular Therapy position statement. *Cytotherapy* 8, 315–317 (2006).

14. Kogler, G., Sensken, S., Airey, J.A., Trapp, T., Muschen, M., Feldhahn, N., Liedtke, S., Sorg, R.V., Fischer, J., Rosenbaum, C., Greschat, S., Knipper, A., Bender, J., Degistirici, O., Gao, J., Caplan, A.I., Colletti, E.J., Almeida-Porada, G., Muller, H.W., Zanjani, E., and Wernet, P. A new human somatic stem cell from placental cord blood with intrinsic pluripotent differentiation potential. *J. Exp. Med.* 200, 123–135 (2004).

15. Kucia, M., Reca, R., Campbell, F.R., Zuba-Surma, E., Majka, M., Ratajczak, J., and Ratajczak, M.Z. A population of very small embryonic-like (VSEL) CXCR4(+)SSEA-1(+)Oct-4+ stem cells identified in adult bone marrow. *Leukemia* 20, 857–869 (2006).

16. D'Ippolito, G., Diabira, S., Howard, G.A., Menei, P., Roos, B.A., and Schiller, P.C. Marrow-isolated adult multilineage inducible (MIAMI) cells, a unique population of postnatal young and old human cells with extensive expansion and differentiation potential. *J. Cell Sci.* 117, 2971–2981 (2004).

17. Jiang, Y., Jahagirdar, B.N., Reinhardt, R.L., Schwartz, R.E., Keene, C.D., Ortiz-Gonzalez, X.R., Reyes, M., Lenvik, T., Lund, T., Blackstad, M., Du, J., Aldrich, S., Lisberg, A., Low, W.C., Largaespada, D.A., and Verfaillie, C.M. Pluripotency of mesenchymal stem cells derived from adult marrow. *Nature* 418, 41–49 (2002).

18. Dos Santos, F., Andrade, P.Z., Boura, J.S., Abecasis, M.M., da Silva, C.L., and Cabral, J.M. *Ex vivo* expansion of human mesenchymal stem cells: A more effective cell proliferation kinetics and metabolism under hypoxia. *J. Cell Physiol.* 223, 27–35 (2010).

19. Hicok, K.C., and Hedrick, M.H. Automated isolation and processing of adipose-derived stem and regenerative cells. *Methods Mol. Biol.* 702, 87–105 (2011).

20. Karp, J.M., and Leng Teo, G.S. Mesenchymal stem cell homing: The devil is in the details. *Cell Stem Cell* 4, 206–216 (2009).

21. Sackstein, R., Merzaban, J.S., Cain, D.W., Dagia, N.M., Spencer, J.A., Lin, C.P., and Wohlgemuth, R. *Ex vivo* glycan engineering of CD44 programs human multipotent mesenchymal stromal cell trafficking to bone. *Nat. Med.* 14, 181–187 (2008).

22. Lee, R.H., Pulin, A.A., Seo, M.J., Kota, D.J., Ylostalo, J., Larson, B.L., Semprun-Prieto, L., Delafontaine, P., and Prockop, D.J. Intravenous hMSCs improve myocardial infarction in mice because cells embolized in lung are activated to secrete the anti-inflammatory protein TSG-6. *Cell Stem Cell* 5, 54–63 (2009).

23. Toma, C., Pittenger, M.F., Cahill, K.S., Byrne, B.J., and Kessler, P.D. Human mesenchymal stem cells differentiate to a cardiomyocyte phenotype in the adult murine heart. *Circulation* 105, 93–98 (2002).

24. Morigi, M., Imberti, B., Zoja, C., Corna, D., Tomasoni, S., Abbate, M., Rottoli, D., Angioletti, S., Benigni, A., Perico, N., Alison, M., and Remuzzi, G. Mesenchymal stem cells are renotropic, helping to repair the kidney and improve function in acute renal failure. *J. Am. Soc. Nephrol.* 15, 1794–1804 (2004).

25. Lakshmipathy, U. and Hart, R.P. Concise review: MicroRNA expression in multipotent mesenchymal stromal cells. *Stem Cells* 26, 356–363 (2008).

26. Togel, F.E. and Westenfelder, C. Mesenchymal stem cells: A new therapeutic tool for AKI. *Nat. Rev. Nephrol.* 6, 179–183 (2010).

27. Gatti, S., Bruno, S., Deregibus, M.C., Sordi, A., Cantaluppi, V., Tetta, C., and Camussi, G. Microvesicles derived from human adult mesenchymal stem cells protect against ischaemia reperfusion-induced acute and chronic kidney injury. *Nephrol. Dial. Transplant.* 26, 1474–1483 (2011).

28. Togel, F., Hu, Z., Weiss, K., Isaac, J., Lange, C., and Westenfelder, C. Administered mesenchymal stem cells protect against ischemic acute renal failure through differentiation-independent mechanisms. *Am. J. Physiol. Renal Physiol.* 289, F31–F42 (2005).

29. Le Blanc, K., Frassoni, F., Ball, L., Locatelli, F., Roelofs, H., Lewis, I., Lanino, E., Sundberg, B., Bernardo, M.E., Remberger, M., Dini, G., Egeler, R.M., Bacigalupo, A., Fibbe, W., and Ringden, O. Mesenchymal stem cells for treatment of steroid-resistant, severe, acute graft-versus-host disease: A phase II study. *Lancet* 371, 1579–1586 (2008).

30. Nemeth, K., Leelahavanichkul, A., Yuen, P.S.T., Mayer, B., Parmelee, A., Doi, K., Robey, P.G., Leelahavanichkul, K., Koller, B.H., Brown, J.M., Hu, X., Jelinek, I., Star, R.A., and Mezey, E. Bone marrow stromal cells attenuate sepsis *via* prostaglandin E 2-dependent reprogramming of host macrophages to increase their interleukin-10 production. *Nat. Med.* 15, 42–49 (2009).

31. Newman, R.E., Yoo, D., LeRoux, M.A., and Nilkovitch-Miagkova, A. Treatment of inflammatory diseases with mesenchymal stem cells. *Inflamm. Allergy Drug Targets* 8, 110–123 (2009).

32. Imberti, B., Morigi, M., Tomasoni, S., Rota, C., Corna, D., Longaretti, L., Rottoli, D., Valsecchi, F., Benigni, A., Wang, J., Abbate, M., Zoja, C., and Remuzzi, G. Insulin-like growth factor-1 sustains stem cell-mediated renal repair. *J. Am. Soc. Nephrol.* 18, 2921–2928 (2007).

33. Humphreys, B.D., Valerius, M.T., Kobayashi, A., Mugford, J.W., Soeung, S., Duffield, J.S., McMahon, A.P., and Bonventre, J.V. Intrinsic epithelial cells repair the kidney after injury. *Cell Stem Cell* 2, 284–291 (2008).

34. Togel, F., Zhang, P., Hu, Z., and Westenfelder, C. VEGF is a mediator of the renoprotective effects of multipotent marrow stromal cells in acute kidney injury. *J. Cell Mol. Med.* 13, 2109–2114 (2009).

35. Humphreys, B.D. and Bonventre, J.V. Mesenchymal stem cells in acute kidney injury. *Annu. Rev. Med.* 59, 311–325 (2008).

36. Wynn, T.A. Cellular and molecular mechanisms of fibrosis. *J. Pathol.* 214, 199–210 (2008).

37. Westergren-Thorsson, G., Larsen, K., Nihlberg, K., Andersson-Sjoland, A., Hallgren, O., Marko-Varga, G., and Bjermer, L. Pathological airway remodelling in inflammation. *Clin. Respir.* J4 (Suppl 1), 1–8 (2010).

38. Crosby, L.M. and Waters, C.M. Epithelial repair mechanisms in the lung. *Am. J. Physiol. Lung Cell. Mol. Physiol.* 298, L715–L731 (2010).

39. Moodley, Y., Atienza, D., Manuelpillai, U., Samuel, C.S., Tchongue, J., Ilancheran, S., Boyd, R., and Trounson, A. Human umbilical cord mesenchymal stem cells reduce fibrosis of bleomycin-induced lung injury. *Am. J. Pathol.* 175, 303–313 (2009).

40. Ortiz, L.A., DuTreil, M., Fattman, C., Pandey, A.C., Torres, G., Go, K., and Phinney, D.G. Interleukin 1 receptor antagonist mediates the anti-inflammatory and anti-fibrotic effect of mesenchymal stem cells during lung injury. *Proc. Natl. Acad. Sci. U.S.A.* 104, 11002–11007 (2007).

41. Chen, S., Liu, Z., Tian, N., Zhang, J., Yei, F., Duan, B., Zhu, Z., Lin, S., and Kwan, T.W. Intracoronary transplantation of autologous bone marrow mesenchymal stem cells for ischemic cardiomyopathy due to isolated chronic occluded left anterior descending artery. *J. Invasive. Cardiol.* 18, 552–556 (2006).

42. Hayes-Jordan, A., Wang, Y.X., Walker, P., and Cox, C.S. Mesenchymal stromal cell dependent regression of pulmonary metastasis from Ewing's. *Front. Pediatr.* 2, 44 (2014).

43. Serakinci, N., Fahrioglu, U., and Christensen, R. Mesenchymal stem cells, cancer challenges and new directions. *Eur. J. Cancer* 50(8), 1522–1530 (2014).

44. Ďuriniková, E., Kučerová, L., and Matúšková M. Mesenchymal stromal cells retrovirally transduced with prodrug-converting genes are suitable vehicles for cancer gene therapy. *Acta Virol.* 58(1), 1–13 (2014).

45. Uchibori, R., Tsukahara, T., Ohmine, K., and Ozawa, K. Cancer gene therapy using mesenchymal stem cells. *Int. J. Hematol.* 99(4), 377–382 (2014).

46. Bao, Q., Zhao, Y., Niess, H., Conrad, C., Schwarz, B., Jauch, K.W., Huss, R., Nelson, P.J., and Bruns, C.J. Mesenchymal stem cell-based tumor-targeted gene therapy in gastrointestinal cancer. *Stem Cells Dev.* 21(13), 2355–2363 (2012).

47. Kidd, S., Spaeth, E., Klopp, A., Andreeff, M., Hall, B., and Marini, F.C. The (in)auspicious role of mesenchymal stromal cells in cancer: Be it friend or foe. *Cytotherapy* 10(7), 657–667 (2008).

48. Niess, H., Bao, Q., Conrad, C., Zischek, C., Notohamiprodjo, M., Schwab, F., Schwarz, B., Huss, R., Jauch, K.W., Nelson, P.J., and Bruns, C.J. Selective targeting of genetically engineered mesenchymal stem cells to tumor stroma microenvironments using tissue-specific suicide gene expression which suppresses growth of hepatocellular carcinoma. *Ann. Surg.* 254(5), 767–774 (2011).

49. Zischek, C., Niess, H., Ischenko, I., Conrad, C., Huss, R., Jauch, K.W., Nelson, P.J., Bruns, C. Targeting tumor stroma using engineered mesenchymal stem cells reduces the growth of pancreatic carcinoma. *Ann. Surg.* 250(5), 747–753 (2009).

50. Uccelli, A., Moretta, L., and Pistoia, V. Mesenchymal stem cells in health and disease. *Nat. Rev. Immunol.* 8, 726–736 (2008).

51. Ding, Y., Xu, D., Feng, G., Bushell, A., Muschel, R.J., and Wood, K.J. Mesenchymal stem cells prevent the rejection of fully allogenic islet grafts by the immunosuppressive activity of matrix metalloproteinase-2 and -9. *Diabetes* 58, 1797–1806 (2009).

52. Pal, R., Venkataramana, N.K., Bansal, A., Balaraju, S., Jan, M., Chandra, R., Dixit, A., Rauthan, A., Murgod, U., and Totey, S. *Ex vivo*-expanded autologous bone marrow-derived mesenchymal stromal cells in human spinal cord injury/paraplegia: A pilot clinical study. *Cytotherapy* 11, 897–911 (2009).

53. Wagner, J., Kean, T., Young, R., Dennis, J.E., and Caplan, A.I. Optimizing mesenchymal stem cell-based therapeutics. *Curr. Opin. Biotechnol.* 20, 531–536 (2009).

54. Liu, H., Xue, W., Ge, G., Luo, X., Li, Y., Xiang, H., Ding, X., Tian, P., and Tian, X. Hypoxic preconditioning advances CXCR4 and CXCR7 expression by activating HIF-1alpha in MSCs. *Biochem. Biophys. Res. Commun.* 401, 509–515 (2010).

55. Komarova, S., Roth, J., Alvarez, R., Curiel, D.T., and Pereboeva, L. Targeting of mesenchymal stem cells to ovarian tumors *via* an artificial receptor. *J. Ovarian. Res.* 3, 12 (2010).

56. Sarkar, D., Zhao, W., Gupta, A., Loh, W.L., Karnik, R., and Karp, J.M. Cell surface engineering of mesenchymal stem cells. *Methods Mol. Biol.* 698, 505–523 (2011).

57. Deng, W., Chen, Q.W., Li, X.S., Liu, H., Niu, S.Q., Zhou, Y., Li, G.Q., Ke, D.Z., and Mo, X.G. Bone marrow mesenchymal stromal cells with support of bispecific antibody and ultrasound-mediated microbubbles prevent myocardial fibrosis *via* the signal transducer and activators of transcription signaling pathway. *Cytotherapy* 13, 431–440 (2011).

58. Dennis, J.E., Cohen, N., Goldberg, V.M., and Caplan, A.I. Targeted delivery of progenitor cells for cartilage repair. *J. Orthop. Res.* 22, 735–741 (2004).

59. Li, W., Ma, N., Ong, L.L., Nesselmann, C., Klopsch, C., Ladilov, Y., Furlani, D., Piechaczek, C., Moebius, J.M., Lutzow, K., Lendlein, A., Stamm, C., R.K., and Steinhoff, G. Bcl-2 engineered MSCs inhibited apoptosis and improved heart function. *Stem Cells* 25, 2118–2127 (2007).

60. Chang, W., Song, B.W., Lim, S., Song, H., Shim, C.Y., Cha, M.J., Ahn, D.H., Jung, Y.G., Lee, D.H., Chung, J.H., Choi, K.D., Lee, S.K., Chung, N., Jang, Y., and Hwang, K.C. Mesenchymal stem cells pretreated with delivered Hph-1-Hsp70 protein are protected from hypoxia-mediated cell death and rescue heart functions from myocardial injury. *Stem Cells* 27(9), 2283–2292 (2009).

61. Gnecchi, M., He, H., Melo, L.G., Noiseux, N., Morello, F., de Boer, R.A., Zhang, L., Pratt, R.E., Dzau, V.J., and Ingwall, J.S. Early beneficial effects of bone marrow-derived mesenchymal stem cells overexpressing Akt on cardiac metabolism after myocardial infarction. *Stem Cells* 27(4), 971–979 (2009).

62. Glavaski-Joksimovic, A., Virag, T., Mangatu, T.A., McGrogan, M., Wang, X.S. and Bohn, M.C. Glial cell line-derived neurotrophic factor-secreting genetically modified human bone marrow-derived mesenchymal stem cells promote recovery in a rat model of Parkinson's disease. *J. Neurosci. Res.* 88, 2669–2681 (2010).

63. Lai, R.C., Arslan, F., Lee, M.M., Sze, N.S., Choo, A., Chen, T.S., Salto-Tellez, M., Timmers, L., Lee, C.N., El Oakley, R.M., Pasterkamp, G., de Kleijn, D.P., and Lim, S.K. Exosome secreted by MSC reduces myocardial ischemia/reperfusion injury. *Stem Cell Res.* 4, 214–222 (2010).

64. Timmers, L., Lim, S.K., Hoefer, I.E., Arslan, F., Lai, R.C., van Oorschot, A.A.M., Goumans, M.J., Strijder, C., Sze, S.K., Choo, A., Piek, J.J., Doevendans, P.A., Pasterkamp, G. and de Kleijn, D.P. Human mesenchymal stem cell-conditioned medium improves cardiac function following myocardial infarction. *Stem Cell Res.* 6, 206–214 (2011).

Next Generation Cell Therapies $\quad$ 13

Stefanos Theoharis

13.1 Introduction

Like other therapeutic technologies, cell therapies are in a constant state of evolution. As an example, monoclonal antibody therapeutics have been the subject of a continual progress from murine, to chimeric, humanized, fully human antibodies and currently continuing toward improved glycosylation, bi- and multi-specific antibodies, alternative antibody scaffolds and "armed" antibodies that carry anti-cancer agents. This progress yields better efficacy, specificity, and an improved safety profile. MSCs were first described by Arnold Caplan in the early 90s[1] and have proven a very popular therapeutic modality, having been the subject of at least 346 clinical trials in the past decade (registered with www.clinicaltrials.gov). There have so far been two conditional marketing authorizations (MA) for Prochymal[©] (see below). This chapter looks at the various technical improvements of the past, present and future that continue to drive the cell therapy field forward.

13.2 Early Products

The development of an entirely novel therapeutic technology is complex, due to the necessary optimization of all the inherent parameters necessary to achieve sufficient efficacy for clinical benefit and, ultimately, MA. This optimization process is inevitably the result of systematic experimentation and represents a lengthy process of change and evolution.

This book reviews the multiple aspects of pharmaceutical cell therapy development and it is by now obvious that multiple challenges are there to be overcome. Prochymal[©] (Remestemcel-L) is the original first generation of mesenchymal stem cell (MSC)-based therapeutics and is discussed extensively in subsequent chapters. It is based on MSCs from the bone marrow of donors, which is purified and expanded to yield thousands of doses. It was developed by Osiris Therapeutics, Inc. and is now owned by the Australian company Mesoblast Ltd. It has so far received conditional market approval in Canada and New Zealand for graft-*versus*-host disease (GvHD), and is being tested concurrently for several other indications. A vast amount of scientific literature has been built upon the groundwork laid by Prochymal©, aiming to exploit and enhance the therapeutic potential of MSCs through various improvements and modifications of the basic cell product.

13.3 First Improvements

The purification and expansion methodologies are now known to be critical and have the potential to fundamentally change the nature of the cells and, therefore, the resultant therapeutic product.

Multiple purification processes and methods have been tested and there are many notable examples where the selection of specific MSC sub-populations have yielded different cell types, sometimes with radically different characteristics. For example, by purifying MSCs expressing the marker Stro1, Paul Simmons was able to purify cells which may be progenitors of bone marrow MSCs that exist in an earlier stage of differentiation,[2] and were named Mesenchymal Precursor Cells (MPCs). This cell type is now in late-stage clinical development for multiple indications, including cardiac, vascular, and skeletal diseases.

The culturing conditions also have a profound effect on the biology of the cells. For example, Catherine Verfaillie, in 2001, developed a process to expand MSCs that results in a cell population with altered characteristics, called Multipotent Adult Progenitor Cells (MAPC).[3] These cells appear to have the ability to continuously self-renew and generate many thousands of doses from the same starting material. They are currently being developed under the brand name Multistem©.

13.4 Changes to the Characteristics of the Cells by Culture Conditions

Many additional methods that exploit alterations of culturing conditions to introduce changes in the nature and functionality have been published. These processes result in a "preconditioning" of the cells, rendering them more robust and potentially more responsive.

Production of MSCs under hypoxic (low oxygen) cell culture conditions has shown to enhance their capacity to treat ischemic disease, as they become adapted to hypoxia and resistant to hypoxic shock at the ischemic site.[4] Some evidence suggests that hypoxic culture conditions may mimic the bone marrow microenvironment more closely, and this may render bone marrow–derived MSCs better at targeting inflamed or ischemic sites, and resulting in higher levels of expression of anti-inflammatory cytokines.[5]

Likewise, introduction of pro-inflammatory cytokines in the cell culture medium has also shown potential in enhancing the immunomodulatory capacity of MSCs.[6–9] MSCs are known to respond to pro-inflammatory signals by secreting an array of immunomodulatory cytokines,[10] and are thus able to regulate the various immune cells. The expression of adhesion molecules on their surface enables them to attach and penetrate inflamed vasculature and reach the underlying site of inflammation.[11] Several pro-inflammatory cytokines, however, can also drive the cells toward certain differentiation pathways,[12] so it is crucial to maintain a tight control between preconditioning and differentiation.

Many of these methods can alter the functional and phenotypic characteristics of the cells, often to great extent, but their effects are often short-lived and, in many cases, not focused enough to generate sufficient therapeutic benefit.

13.5 Genetic Modification

13.5.1 Introduction

Of all the methodologies used to enhance the therapeutic potential of cells, genetic modification is unquestionably the most specific and controllable, and can yield products precisely engineered for each indication. Therapeutic genes can be delivered into the cells using a gene vector, resulting in permanent or transient expression of the gene, as per the requirements of the disease. Genetically modified MSCs (gmMSCs) have been therefore gaining popularity rapidly[13–15] and now represent a credible and promising new wave of MSC therapeutics. gmMSCs are already in clinical trials by apceth GmbH & Co. KG, and can now be considered a major step change and a true next generation in the field.

13.5.2 *Hematopoietic stem cell (HSC) engineering*

The genetic modification of various patient cell types is an established practice that offers great promise in multiple areas. Multiple cell types such as HSCs, or immune cells have been subjected to genetic modification for multiple purposes. In the case of HSC gene therapy, HSCs are isolated from patients suffering from genetic disorders (usually children) and transduced with an integrating virus, such as a retrovirus or lentivirus that carries the gene that the patient is missing or has a mutation. The correct gene is inserted in the genome of the HSCs and their progeny will from there carry the correct gene. This treatment therefore, potentially offers a lifelong cure for otherwise lethal childhood diseases. Bluebird bio, a company based in Cambridge, Massachusetts, has focused on HSC gene for such inherited diseases. Their first project on Cerebral Adrenoleukodystrophy[16] is currently in Phase II clinical trials and they have recently initiated early trials for β-thalassaemia.[17] In Italy, the Fondazione Telethon and Fondazione San Raffaele are now collaborating with GlaxoSmithKline (GSK) on a similar project for is Severe Combined Immunodeficiency that results from Adenosine Deaminase Deficiency (ADA-SCID).[18] Many more examples of this approach exist and are a certain cause for optimism for many patients.

13.5.3 *T-Cell engineering*

In addition to HSC gene therapy, T-cells have also received attention for the treatment of multiple diseases, including cancer, where T-cells are used to target, attack, and destroy tumor cells. Chimeric Antigen Receptor (CAR) modified T-cells currently used for immunotherapies are genetically modified to express a T-cell receptor against a specific antigen.[19–20] CD19, a marker on mature B-cells also found on malignant B-cells, is the first target where this approach has found success. The CAR expressed on these cells is generated against CD19 and is fused to co-stimulatory molecules and other protein fragments that increase its stability. So, in practice, CAR-T cell therapy is a form of gene therapy. The early clinical data from these efforts have been very promising. For example, data presented at the American Society of Hematology annual meeting in December 2013 showed that a total of 19 out of 22 Acute Lymphoblastic Leukemia (ALL) patients treated with Novartis/Penn University CAR-Ts targeting CD19 (known as CTL019) experienced complete remissions. Likewise, in a trial linked to Juno Therapeutics at the Memorial Sloan Kettering Cancer Center, 14 out of 16 patients suffering with advanced B-cell lymphoblastic leukemia experienced complete remissions. It must be noted that two patients from that clinical trial died, one due to cardiac and the second due to neurological complications that resulted from the cytokine release syndrome associated with the activation of T-cells against the tumor. The clinical trial was subsequently put on hold, until the recruitment criteria were amended to exclude patients with heart disease and other co-morbidities.

As the field moves beyond CD19 as a target, where specificity will be far more important, CAR structures will have to evolve considerably, in order to avoid toxicities associated with on target, off tumor immunity (e.g., for a target that is also expressed in some normal tissues, albeit at lower levels).

13.5.4 *Engineered MSCs*

The use of genetic modification on MSCs brings together the fields of cell and gene therapy and generates synergies in terms of efficacy and Mode of Action (MoA). By exploiting the well-defined tropism of MSCs to sites of inflammation, injury, or tumors, the transgene expression is targeted in the disease site, where it is needed.

There is virtually no limit to the new functions and uses that can be added to MSCs *via* genetic modification. For example, expression of Vascular Endothelium Growth Factor (VEGF)[22–23]; Hepatocyte Growth Factor (HGF)[24]; or the endothelial Nitric Oxide Synthase (eNOS) genes[25] have all been used to enhance therapeutic efficacy in ischemic disease in animal models. Likewise, genetic modification can be used to enhance tissue targeting, by expressing specific cell surface receptors, such as the CXCR4 chemokine receptor.[26]

The enormous potential of gmMSCs is also being exploited in oncology. An early report on gmMSCs for cancer therapy, described by Studeny *et al.*, used MSCs, transduced to express interferon IFN-β, to treat melanoma xenografts in mice *via* intravenous injection, leading to reduced tumor growth and prolonged survival of tumor-bearing mice.[27] To date, gmMSCs from various human, mouse, or rat tissues have been evaluated for tumor therapy in animal models, expressing a diverse array of therapeutic genes, including IFN-β, TRAIL, PEDF, IL-12, CX3CL1, VEGFR-1, iNOS, and HSV-TK.[28–29]

apceth GmbH & Co. KG, a company based in Munich that develops next generation MSC-based therapeutics, is the first company to initiate clinical trials with gmMSCs, based on the company's platform technology. The first product, called Agenmestencel, is based on MSCs that carry a suicide gene [Herpes Simplex Virus-Thymidine Kinase (HSV-TK)], driven by the RANTES promoter which is selectively activated in sites of inflammation, including tumors. The cells are therefore attracted into the tumors, where the suicide gene becomes expressed. HSV-TK activates the pro-drug ganciclovir to its active toxic form, so, when Agenmestencel-treated patients are given ganciclovir, it will become activated within the tumor and kill all the cells in the vicinity.[30]

13.6 Genetic Modification Technologies and Methodologies

There are multiple techniques being used to transfer genes to cells for therapeutic purposes. Viral vectors, such as the retrovirus and lentivirus, are popular, because they can yield stable genetic modification (transduction) of target cells. This is a very useful characteristic, as it means that cells can be transduced prior to expansion and all their progeny will also carry the therapeutic transgene.

Some viral vectors, such as the adenovirus and adeno–associated virus (AAV), non–viral chemical vectors such as liposomes and technologies such as electroporation, do not cause stable transduction. They result in transient gene expression, if this is what is desired, but their use in large-scale manufacturing is challenging, due to the requirement to transduce large amounts of cells at the end of the production process, rather than the beginning, rendering the process very expensive and labor intensive. Transposon-based systems, such as Sleeping Beauty and PiggyBac©, and gene editing technologies, such as zinc-finger nucleases (ZFNs), Transcription Activator-Like Effector Nucleases (TALENs) and the Clustered Regulatory Interspaced Short Palindromic Repeat (CRISPR) GeneArt© system also offer the possibility of stable integration into the host cell's genome. Such systems are potentially very useful for next generation cell therapies, but are still at early stages and, with the exception of ZFNs, have not yet entered the clinic.

Techniques that only lead to a transient gene expression have also been developed. For example, a transduction system whereby only the mRNA for the desired protein is added to cells will result in expression of a protein and when all the delivered mRNA is used, expression will cease. This method was used to express interleukin-10 (IL-10) in MSCs, as a therapeutic protein for inflammatory disease, alongside P-selectin glycoprotein ligand-1 (PSGL-1) and Sialyl-Lewisx (SLeX) to increase targeting inflamed vasculature.[21] This is a promising approach, although its scale-up is limited by the same cost restrictions as the non-stable gene transduction methods mentioned previously.

The most advanced therapeutic application of genetic modification relies on the use of conditional promoters to ensure that the expression of the therapeutic gene is limited to a particular site (e.g., an inflammatory environment) and not the entire body. This additional control is a second element of therapeutic specificity which, in combination with the natural homing characteristics of the cells, yields a very specific therapeutic effect. apceth's Agenmestencel takes advantage of this advancement, as mentioned above, to restrict expression of the therapeutic gene to tumors using the RANTES promoter and therefore restrict the anti-tumoral

Table 13.1:

MSC Evolution	Technology
First generation	1. Unmodified, purified by adhesion to cell culture flasks. 2. Cytokine pre-treatment. 3. Hypoxic culture conditions. 4. Cell selection.
Second generation	1. mRNA engineering. 2. Genetic modification (viral vectors). 3. Genetic modification (nuclease-based). 4. Genetic modification using conditional promoters.

therapeutic effect locally. The use of conditional promoters is clearly a promising development that further expands the use of engineered cells.

13.7 Summary

The development of gmMSC technology represents a significant advance and an important milestone in the progress of MSCs toward clinical efficacy and commercial success. The potential of this next generation of MSC therapeutics is obvious. Likewise, the genetic modification of cells such as HSCs and the development of many T-cell-based immunotherapies, which are driving the field of cell therapy forward, are already generating very promising results in the clinic. It is therefore an indispensable technology and a very useful addition to the field of cell therapy with the potential to yield many new products with better efficacy. Ultimately, the cell therapy field will be judged on the benefit it delivers to patients and this should therefore remain the prime aim of all stakeholders.

References

1. Caplan, A. Mesenchymal stem cells. *J. Orthop. Res.* 9, 641–650 (1991).
2. Gronthos, S., Zannettino, A.C., Hay, S.J., Shi, S., Graves, S.E., Kortesidis, A., and Simmons, P.J. Molecular and cellular characterisation of highly purified stromal stem cells derived from human bone marrow. *J. Cell Sci.* 116(Pt 9), 1827–1835 (May 1, 2003).
3. Reyes, M., and Verfaillie, C.M. Characterization of multipotent adult progenitor cells, a subpopulation of mesenchymal stem cells. *Ann. N. Y. Acad. Sci.* 938, 231–233 (Jun 2001).

4. Rosová, I., Dao, M., Capoccia, B., Link, D., and Nolta, J.A. Hypoxic preconditioning results in increased motility and improved therapeutic potential of human mesenchymal stem cells. *Stem Cells* 26(8), 2173–2182 (Aug 2008).

5. Tsai, C.C., Yew, T.L., Yang, D.C., Huang, W.H., and Hung, S.C. Benefits of hypoxic culture on bone marrow multipotent stromal cells. *Am. J. Blood Res.* 2(3), 148–159 (2012).

6. Bukulmez, H., Bilgin, A., Bebek, G., Caplan, A.I., and Jones, O. A125: Immunomodulatory factors produced by mesenchymal stem cells after *in vitro* priming with danger signals. *Arthritis Rheumatol.* 66(Suppl. 11), S163 (Mar 2014).

7. Carrero, R., Cerrada, I., Lledó, E., Dopazo, J., García-García, F., Rubio, M.P., Trigueros, C., Dorronsoro, A., Ruiz-Sauri, A., Montero, J.A., and Sepúlveda, P. IL1β induces mesenchymal stem cells migration and leucocyte chemotaxis through NF-κB. *Stem Cell Rev.* 8(3), 905–916 (Sep 2012).

8. Herrmann, J.L., Wang, Y., Abarbanell, A.M., Weil, B.R., Tan, J., and Meldrum, D.R. Preconditioning mesenchymal stem cells with transforming growth factor-alpha improves mesenchymal stem cell-mediated cardio protection. *Shock* 33(1), 24–30 (Jan 2010).

9. Kalwitz, G., Endres, M., Neumann, K., Skriner, K., Ringe, J., Sezer, O., Sittinger, M., Häupl, T., and Kaps, C. Gene expression profile of adult human bone marrow-derived mesenchymal stem cells stimulated by the chemokine CXCL7. *Int. J. Biochem. Cell Biol.* 41(3), 649–658 (Mar 2009).

10. Murphy, M.B., Moncivais, K., and Caplan, A.I. Mesenchymal stem cells: Environmentally responsive therapeutics for regenerative medicine. *Exp. Mol. Med.* 45, e54 (Nov 15, 2013).

11. Ren, G., Zhao, X., Zhang, L., Zhang, J., L'Huillier, A., Ling, W., Roberts, A.I., Le, A.D., Shi, S., Shao, C., and Shi, Y. Inflammatory cytokine-induced intercellular adhesion molecule-1 and vascular cell adhesion molecule-1 in mesenchymal stem cells are critical for immunosuppression. *J. Immunol.* 184(5), 2321–2328 (Mar 1, 2010).

12. Kotake, S., and Nanke, Y. Effect of TNFα on osteoblastogenesis from mesenchymal stem cells. *Biochim. Biophys. Acta.* 1840(3), 1209–1213 (Mar, 2014).

13. Myers, T.J., Granero-Molto, F., Longobardi, L., Li, T., Yan, Y., and Spagnoli, A. Mesenchymal stem cells at the intersection of cell and gene therapy. *Expert Opin. Biol. Ther.* 10(12), 1663–1679 (Dec 2010).

14. Meyerrose, T., Olson, S., Pontow, S., Kalomoiris, S., Jung, Y., Annett, G., Bauer, G., and Nolta, J.A. Mesenchymal stem cells for the sustained *in vivo* delivery of bioactive factors. *Adv. Drug Deliv. Rev.* 62(12), 1167–1174 (Sep 30, 2010).

15. Sanz, L., Compte, M., Guijarro-Muñoz, I., and Álvarez-Vallina, L. Non-hematopoietic stem cells as factories for *in vivo* therapeutic protein production. *Gene Ther.* 19(1), 1–7 (Jan 2012).

16. Cartier, N., Hacein-Bey-Abina, S., Bartholomae, C.C., Veres, G., Schmidt, M., Kutschera, I., Vidaud, M., Abel, U., Dal-Cortivo, L., Caccavelli, L., Mahlaoui, N., Kiermer, V., Mittelstaedt, D., Bellesme, C., Lahlou, N., Lefrère, F., Blanche, S., Audit, M., Payen, E., Leboulch, P., l'Homme, B., Bougnères, P., Von Kalle, C., Fischer, A., Cavazzana-Calvo, M., and Aubourg, P. Hematopoietic stem cell gene therapy with a lentiviral vector in X-linked adrenoleukodystrophy. *Science* 326(5954), 818–823 (Nov 6, 2009).

17. Cavazzana-Calvo, M., Payen, E., Negre, O., Wang, G., Hehir, K., Fusil, F., Down, J., Denaro, M., Brady, T., Westerman, K., Cavallesco, R., Gillet-Legrand, B., Caccavelli, L., Sgarra, R., Maouche-Chrétien, L., Bernaudin, F., Girot, R., Dorazio, R., Mulder, G.J., Polack, A., Bank, A., Soulier, J., Larghero, J., Kabbara, N., Dalle, B., Gourmel, B., Socie, G., Chrétien, S., Cartier, N., Aubourg, P., Fischer, A., Cornetta, K., Galacteros, F., Beuzard, Y., Gluckman, E., Bushman, F., Hacein-Bey-Abina, S., and Leboulch, P. Transfusion independence and HMGA2 activation after gene therapy of human β-thalassaemia. *Nature* 467(7313), 318–322 (Sep 16, 2010).

18. Aiuti, A., Cattaneo, F., Galimberti, S., Benninghoff, U., Cassani, B., Callegaro, L., Scaramuzza, S., Andolfi, G., Mirolo, M., Brigida, I., Tabucchi, A., Carlucci, F., Eibl, M., Aker, M., Slavin, S., Al-Mousa, H., Al Ghonaium, A., Ferster, A., Duppenthaler, A., Notarangelo, L., Wintergerst, U., Buckley, R.H., Bregni, M., Marktel, S., Valsecchi, M.G., Rossi, P., Ciceri, F., Miniero, R., Bordignon, C., and Roncarolo, M.G. Gene therapy for immunodeficiency due to adenosine deaminase deficiency, *N. Engl. J. Med.* 360(5), 447–458 (Jan 29, 2009).

19. Anurathapan, U., Leen, A.M., Brenner, M.K., and Vera, J.F. Engineered T-cells for cancer treatment. *Cytotherapy* 16(6), 713–733 (Jun 2014).

20. Wieczorek, A., and Uharek, L. Genetically modified T-cells for the treatment of malignant disease. *Transfus. Med. Hemother.* 40(6), 388–402 (Dec 2013).

21. Levy, O., Zhao, W., Mortensen, L.J., Leblanc, S., Tsang, K., Fu, M., Phillips, J.A., Sagar, V., Anandakumaran, P., Ngai, J., Cui, C.H., Eimon, P., Angel, M., Lin, C.P., Yanik, M.F., and Karp, J.M. mRNA-engineered mesenchymal stem cells for targeted delivery of interleukin-10 to sites of inflammation. Blood 122(14), e23–e32 (Oct 3, 2013).

22. Fierro, F.A., Kalomoiris, S., Sondergaard, C.S., and Nolta, J.A. Effects on proliferation and differentiation of multipotent bone marrow stromal cells engineered to express growth factors for combined cell and gene therapy. *Stem Cells* 29(11), 1727–1737 (Nov 2011).

23. Yang, J., Zhou, W., Zheng, W., Ma, Y., Lin, L., Tang, T., Liu, J., Yu, J., Zhou, X., and Hu, J. Effects of myocardial transplantation of marrow mesenchymal stem cells transfected with vascular endothelial growth factor for the improvement of heart function and angiogenesis after myocardial infarction. *Cardiology* 107(1), 17–29 (2007).

24. Su, G.H., Sun, Y.F., Lu, Y.X., Shuai, X.X., Liao, Y.H., Liu, Q.Y., Han, J., and Luo, P. Hepatocyte growth factor gene-modified bone marrow-derived mesenchymal stem cells transplantation promotes angiogenesis in a rat model of hind limb ischemia. *J. Huazhong Univ. Sci. Technolog. Med. Sci.* 33(4), 511–519 (Aug 2013).

25. Zhao, Y.D., Courtman, D.W., Deng, Y., Kugathasan, L., Zhang, Q., and Stewart, D.J. Rescue of monocrotaline-induced pulmonary arterial hypertension using bone marrow-derived endothelial-like progenitor cells: Efficacy of combined cell and eNOS gene therapy in established disease. *Circ. Res.* 96(4), 442–450 (Mar 4, 2005).

26. Cheng, Z., Ou, L., Zhou, X., Li, F., Jia, X., Zhang, Y., Liu, X., Li, Y., Ward, C.A., Melo, L.G., and Kong, D. Targeted migration of mesenchymal stem cells modified with CXCR4 gene to infarcted myocardium improves cardiac performance. *Mol. Ther.* 16(3), 571–579 (Mar 2008).

27. Studeny, M., Marini, F.C., Champlin, R.E., Zompetta, C., Fidler, I.J., and Andreeff, M. Bone marrow-derived mesenchymal stem cells as vehicles for interferon-beta delivery into tumors. *Cancer Res.* 62(13), 3603–3608 (Jul 1, 2002).

28. Bao, Q., Zhao, Y., Niess, H., Conrad, C., Schwarz, B., Jauch, K.W., Huss, R., Nelson, P.J., and Bruns, C.J. Mesenchymal stem cell-based tumor-targeted gene therapy in gastrointestinal cancer. *Stem Cells Dev.* 21(13), 2355–2363 (Sep 1, 2012).
29. Collet, G., Grillon, C., Nadim, M., and Kieda, C. Trojan horse at cellular level for tumor gene therapies. *Gene* 525(2), 208–216 (Aug 10, 2013).
30. Zischek, C., Niess, H., Ischenko, I., Conrad, C., Huss, R., Jauch, K.W., Nelson, P.J., and Bruns, C. Targeting tumor stroma using engineered mesenchymal stem cells reduces the growth of pancreatic carcinoma. *Ann. Surg.* 250(5), 747–753 (Nov 2009).

Cell-Based Gene Therapy   **14**

Sabine Geiger

14.1   Definition: What is Gene Therapy?

Gene therapy is the use of genetic material for therapeutic purposes. It is still mostly an investigational treatment that involves the introduction of recombinant nucleic acids into an individual's cells to prevent, cure or alleviate disease. From the beginning, gene therapy had a rocky course, but due to breakthrough successes during the last few years, gene therapy is now on its way to progressing from an exploratory therapy to an approved treatment.

Most commonly, DNA is introduced into cells or tissues by means of the so-called "vectors". From the very early beginnings of gene therapy until now, the choice of vector was and still remains one of the most crucial points to consider when planning a gene therapy treatment. To date, viruses that are genetically modified to be safe for the patient are the most frequently used type of vector in gene therapy clinical trials worldwide.

Once the genetic material has successfully been introduced into the target cell, the cellular machinery is used to express the transferred gene and to produce the encoded protein and consequently cure or alleviate the patient's disease.

Due to major scientific advances during the last decades and the progress of gene therapy from the bench to the bedside, three critical aspects have emerged for all gene transfer approaches which are also fundamental to further develop this novel and highly sophisticated therapy[1,2]:

1. Therapeutic gene: The affected gene causing the disease in question needs to be known, the condition well understood, and a functional copy of the dysfunctional gene must be available.

2. Gene therapy vector: Out of the possible choices, the optimal vector for the transfer of the reagents of interest needs to be chosen.
3. Target cell: The particular cells or tissues requiring therapy must be identified and be attainable.

14.1.1 *Somatic and germline gene therapy*

In gene therapy, two types of cells can be modified:

- Somatic cells, i.e., cells of the body, and
- Germ cells, i.e., sperm and eggs.

In the first case, genetic information introduced into somatic cells will be passed on only to the progeny of the modified cells. As somatic cells are non-reproductive, the effect of the transferred genetic material will end with that same individual who is receiving gene therapy. This approach is considered safer and more conservative compared to genetic modification of germ cells.

In the second case, genetic alteration of germ cells will lead to permanent changes in the treated individual's genome that will be passed on to future generations. This approach is a much more controversial one, raising serious ethical issues and to date still remains theoretical, as all other gene therapies that are performed today on humans are directed at somatic cells.

14.1.2 *In vivo versus Ex vivo gene therapy*

Somatic gene therapy can widely be categorized into

- *In vivo* gene therapy, and
- *Ex vivo* gene therapy (Figure 14.1).

In vivo gene therapy means genetic alteration of cells while they remain inside the living body. Usually, the viral vector carrying the genetic information for the desired therapeutic transgene is injected intravenously and can thus be transported to the target cells and tissues by the blood stream. One very successful current example of *in vivo* gene therapy is the CUPID (Calcium Up-Regulation by Percutaneous Administration of Gene Therapy in Cardiac Disease) Trial at Mount Sinai, New York, to treat heart failure.[3,4] Although the primary reasons leading to the disease are very diverse, heart failure is almost always associated with reduced activity of the sarcoplasmic reticulum Ca^{2+} ATPase (SERCA2a) mediating the transfer of Ca^{2+} into cellular Ca^{2+} stores from where it is released to induce contraction during systole. In the CUPID trial, patients are treated with an adeno-associated

In vivo gene therapy - direct delivery   **Ex vivo gene therapy - cell-based delivery**

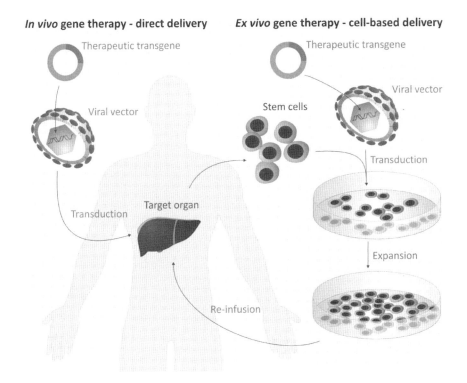

Figure 14.1: *In vivo versus ex vivo* gene therapy.

virus serotype 1 (AAV1) vector encoding the SERCA2a gene. The viral vector is injected into the coronary artery of the patients, delivering the gene directly to the dysfunctional cardiomyocytes to increase sarcoplasmic reticulum Ca^{2+} levels and cardiac contraction, thus rescuing the disease.

Ex vivo gene therapy, in contrast, describes the transfer of genetic material to the patient's cells outside of the body. The additional *in vitro* cultivation step allows for processes of selection, expansion or differentiation of the cells before or after genetic modification to enhance safety and efficacy of the therapy.[5] The principle of *ex vivo* gene therapy is straightforward: Initially, the cells of interest are harvested from the patient or a healthy donor. These could be stem, progenitor, or differentiated cells that come from various tissues including the bone marrow. These cells are then expanded *in vitro*, and (re-)injected into the patient after genetic modification and in some cases, selection of the transduced cells. Like this, depending on the cells used, a transient or stable graft of the transduced cells and their progeny expressing the therapeutic protein can be established in the patient, thereby curing or alleviating the underlying disease, without exposure of the patient to the gene therapy vector.

14.1.3 *Indications of gene therapy*

Originally conceptualized for the treatment of monogenic diseases like primary immune deficiencies (PID) or hematological diseases like beta-thalassemia or sickle cell disease, gene therapy nowadays is used for a broad range of indications,[93] such as cancer or infectious diseases in which the existing standard therapies have failed or are not working adequately.

14.2 Approaches

Most long-term follow-up data available to date stem from autologous cell-based gene therapy clinical trials, especially using hematopoietic cells. Due to the advanced clinical translation, this chapter will emphasize on the hematopoietic stem cell (HSC) therapy as a representative example of cell-based gene therapies. That said, most concepts and issues presented here are also applicable to other *ex vivo* cell and gene therapy approaches targeting a range of different kinds of somatic cells like multipotent stromal cells/mesenchymal stem cells (MSCs), neural stem/progenitor cells (NSPCs) or cardiac stem cells (CSCs).[5]

14.2.1 *Gene addition — Restoring cellular functions*

Gene therapy was initially established for the treatment of hereditary diseases caused by known single-gene defects like the PIDs or hemoglobinopathies. In these cases, a DNA encoding a functional copy of the gene that is mutated in the patient is added to the cells to compensate the missing or reduced function of the endogenous gene. This approach is called gene addition, as after gene therapy two copies of the gene, one defective and one functional, are present in the transduced cells. To date, gene addition to restore cellular functions and reconstitute dysfunctional lineages is the most commonly attempted gene therapy approach.[5,6]

The group of diseases that is the prototypic application example for gene addition therapies include PIDs and rare inherited blood disorders which result in an underdeveloped or inoperative immune system. Especially the forms of severe combined immune deficiency (SCID) are uniformly life-threatening for the patients. The standard treatment currently is allogeneic HSC transplant from a Human

Leukocyte Antigen (HLA)–matched donor with a success rate of about 70% for ADA-SCID [SCID due to a deficiency of the enzyme adenosine deaminase (ADA)].[7] However, these donors are available to only one-third of all patients, and transplantation with mismatched donors decreases the percentage of success markedly to approximately 43% due to immunological complications like graft rejection or graft-*versus*-host disease (GvHD).[8] Transplantation of autologous hematopoietic stem and progenitor cells (HSPCs) gene-modified to express a functional copy of the ADA gene offered a possibly life-saving alternative for patients lacking a suitable donor, and indeed ADA-SCID was the first PID to be treated with gene therapy in the early 1990s. With now close to 15 years of follow-up and more than 40 patients treated, the outcome of gene therapy for ADA-SCID is a brilliant success: The survival rate is 100% with no vector-related complications, and efficacy faring better than standard HSC transplantation.[9]

GlaxoSmithKline together with MolMed is currently working on the commercialization of ADA-SCID gene therapy.[10] Other examples of application of clinical gene addition therapy are X-linked SCID (SCID-X1), the most common form of human SCID[11] (compare Section 14.5 "Historical Milestones" for details about the clinical trial), chronic granulomatous disease (CGD),[12] and Wiskott-Aldrich syndrome (WAS).[13,50] In all of these clinical trials the results were mixed, with an unequivocal benefit of the treatment resulting in immune reconstitution in most of the subjects opposing the development of leukoproliferative disease in some of the patients a few years later.[8]

Another group of diseases that are predestinated for gene addition strategies are hemoglobinopathies like sickle cell disease (SCD) or beta-thalassemia. However, the globin gene locus is very complex and lineage-specific expression is needed, having hampered the development of a gene therapy vector for a long time.[8] Novel lentiviral vectors in contrast to their retroviral counterparts have the ability of transferring intact globin genes due to their rev-responsive element (RRE). Currently, clinical trials using lentiviral vectors to transduce HSPCs for the treatment of beta-thalassemia are being performed[14] or are advancing to the clinic in case of SCD.[15]

14.2.2 *Targeted integration — Gene editing*

The recent progress of designer endonucleases such as zinc finger nucleases (ZFNs), transcription activator-like effector nucleases (TALENs) and RNA-guided nucleases (CRISPR/Cas) has opened the door to the so far inaccessible field of targeted gene integration. As the quasi-random integration of retro- and lentiviral vectors into the host cell's genome bears the risk of potentially causing insertional mutagenesis, targeted integration of the transgene cassette into so–called "safe harbors" has been the Holy Grail since the early beginning of gene therapy.

The above-mentioned nucleases have the ability to introduce DNA double-strand breaks (DSB) at pre-selected genomic sites with high specificity and efficiency. Depending on the repair mechanism that the cell uses to mend the break in combination with a suitable DNA donor molecule, the result can be gene disruption, gene correction or gene editing.[5]

Whereas gene correction approaches aiming at targeting the transgene cassette into a putative "safe harbor" to date are still being optimized in development-stage studies,[16] gene disruption has been proven efficacious in a recent clinical trial.[17] 12 patients suffering from chronic aviremic HIV infection were treated with autologous CD4 T-cells in which the main co–receptor for HIV entry, the chemokine (C−C motif) receptor 5 (CCR5), had been disrupted by the use of ZFNs, thereby rendering the cells resistant to HIV infection. The results of the study were very impressive: The gene-modified cells readily engrafted in the patients and persisted with an estimated half-life of 48 weeks, suggesting that the cells are not rendered immunogenic by gene editing at the CCR5 locus; CD4 T-cell numbers increased in all patients, with gene-modified cells displaying a selective survival advantage to non–treated cells, indicating the feasibility of targeted genome editing to convey disease-resistance to cells.

14.2.3 Instructing novel cellular functions — Suicide gene therapy

One very sophisticated approach for the treatment of complex polygenic diseases like cancer in which the before-mentioned approaches would not be successful is suicide gene therapy. A transgene that is usually absent, from the cell's genome coding, for an enzyme that converts a pro–drug into a toxic metabolite is introduced into the cells.[18] Upon administration of the pro–drug, the enzyme that is now expressed by the transduced cells turns the pro–drug into its active, toxic form, subsequently killing not only the cells producing the enzyme, but also neighboring cells that are not expressing the transgene. This phenomenon is called bystander effect and has proven to be vital for the success of the therapy.[19] The most commonly used combination of pro–drug converting enzyme and corresponding pro–drug are the Herpes simplex virus thymidine kinase (HSV-tk) and ganciclovir (GCV).

One extremely successful example of a phase III clinical trial using this approach is the study published by Immonen *et al.* in 2004. In this trial, 36 patients suffering from malignant glioma received either standard therapy consisting of surgical resection of the tumor followed by radiotherapy or suicide gene therapy treatment.[20] In the latter approach, an adenoviral vector carrying the HSV–tk gene was injected into the wound bed after tumor excision, followed by intravenous GCV administration. All patients tolerated the treatment well, and suicide gene therapy proved to be clinically superior to standard treatment by yielding a statistically significant increase in mean survival rate from 39 to 70 weeks.

Another approach of suicide gene therapy is by using cells as vehicles transferring the pro–drug converting enzyme to tumor sites. Because of their intrinsic ability of homing to tumor sites, MSCs have shown to be the optimal candidates for this strategy, as they can seek and destroy tumor cells that are difficult to access by standard treatment methods. Several preclinical studies were paving the way for the first clinical evaluations of this innovative therapy.[21–23]

apceth GmbH was the first company to initiate a clinical trial in 2014, and is currently working on the commercialization of suicide gene therapy using MSCs.[24]

14.2.4 *Gene therapy vectors*

The selection of an appropriate vector and intelligent vector design are crucial steps in the development of a therapeutic strategy. For successful gene therapy to happen, a sufficient amount of a therapeutic transgene must be introduced into the target cells or tissue, without considerable toxicity[25] with maintained gene expression for a desired stretch of time.[18] To achieve this aim, the ideal gene therapy vector needs to be carefully chosen, well-designed and should meet the following criteria[26]:

- Easy production.
- Sufficient size capacity.
- Effective transduction of target cells.
- Controllable transgene expression.
- No immune response to viral vector or transgene after delivery.
- Minimized risk of insertional transformation.

Each vector system has different properties that determine its usability for particular gene therapy approaches. For monogenetic disorders, for example, long-term expression from even a relatively small number of transduced stem cells might be sufficient to achieve a benefit, whereas reconstitution of tumor suppressor genes for the treatment of cancer could require high-level, but maybe only transient expression.

Gene therapy vectors can be widely categorized into non-viral and viral vectors. As mentioned earlier, viral vectors are the most commonly used type of gene therapy vectors in clinical trials worldwide at present, with only the two groups i.e., adenoviral and retroviral vectors comprising more than 40% of vectors used in a total of 1996 gene therapy clinical trials.[27]

The second type of vectors is the so-called "non-viral" vectors, e.g., plasmid DNA, liposomes, organic polymers, and nanoparticles.[28,29] All of these non-viral types of vectors have the advantage of relatively easy large-scale production and minimal host immunogenicity compared to viral vectors; however, until recently low transfection efficiency and low levels of transgene expression are the major hurdles restricting the broader use of non-viral gene delivery. Latest advances in vector design and production have yielded transfection efficiencies comparable to those of viral vectors, raising hopes for the future of the field of non-viral gene transfer.

Because of the predominant position of viral vectors in current clinical trials, they will be discussed in greater detail.

14.3   Viral Vectors

Due to a deep understanding of virus biology gained during the last decades (compare Section 14.5 "Historical Milestones"), it has been possible to exploit the innate ability of viruses to introduce their genetic information into cells and utilize the cell machinery to produce viral proteins for gene therapy applications.[30] For improved safety, most viral genes necessary for replication were removed from the viral genome, thereby creating space for the therapeutic payload.

Within the field of viral vectors, one can distinguish between non-integrating viral vectors and integrating vectors (Table 14.1).

14.3.1   *Integrating viral vectors*

Generally, integrating vectors like gamma-retroviral or lentiviral vectors are used for gene therapy approaches when working with actively dividing cells like hematopoietic cells, because once integrated into the host cell's genome, the transferred information will be passed on to the progeny of the cell, thus promising life-long expression of the therapeutic protein.[26,34]

14.3.1.1   *Gamma-retrovirus*

Gamma-retroviruses belong to the family of Retroviridae, they are lipid-enveloped particles containing a homodimer of single-stranded, positive-sense mRNA genomes

Table 14.1: Main groups of viral vectors for gene therapy.[2,31−34]

	Adenoviruses	AAV	Gamma-Retrovirus	Lentivirus
Virion characteristics				
Genome	dsDNA	ssDNA	ssRNA (+)	ssRNA (+)
Capsid	Icosahedral	Icosahedral	Icosahedral	Icosahedral
Coat	Naked	Naked	Enveloped	Enveloped
Virion diameter	80–100 nm	20–25 nm	80–130 nm	80–130 nm
Genome size	35–38 kb	5 kb	7–10 kb	7–10 kb
Gene therapy characteristics				
Tropism	Dividing and non-dividing cells	Dividing and non-dividing cells	Dividing cells only	Dividing and non-dividing cells
Vector genome forms	Episomal	Episomal (>90%) Integrated (<10%)	Integrated	Integrated
Transgene expression	Transient	Potentially long lasting	Long lasting	Long lasting
Packaging capacity	7–8 kb	<5 kb	8 kb	8 kb
Main limitations	Capsid mediates strong inflammatory response	Small packaging capacity	Transduces dividing cells only; risk of insertional mutagenesis	Production scale-up complex
Main advantages	Extremely efficient transduction of most tissues	Non-inflammatory; non-pathogenic	Persistent gene expression in dividing cells	Persistent gene expression in most tissues

and measure 7–10 kb in size.[25] Their name originates from the way the viruses replicate: Once a host cell is infected, retroviruses reverse transcribe their RNA genome into DNA using their own reverse transcriptase, which depicts a "reverse" direction of genetic information.[35] This DNA is then integrated into the host chromatin by a viral integrase enzyme, and after integration, the cell machinery is exploited to produce the proteins needed to assemble new copies of the virus.

Each retroviral genome has two long terminal repeats (LTRs) flanking the three essential genes: gag, pol, and env which are coding for structural proteins, enzymes like reverse transcriptase and integrase, and the envelope protein that determines the host range, respectively.[25,26]

Gamma-retroviral vectors were among the first to be designed and established for gene therapy approaches, and thus were highly important tools for the development and improvement of viral vectors for gene therapy. Retroviral vectors based on Moloney Murine Leukemia Virus (M-MLV) were also amidst the first being tested in FDA-reviewed gene therapy trials.[6] One very well-known example of a clinical trial using such a retroviral vector is the French trial for SCID-X1 that resulted in the first definite cure of a disease by gene therapy being reported in 2000[36] (compare Section 14.5 "Historical Milestones" for details). However, the development of leukemia in five of the twenty patients treated in this trial overshadowed the spectacular success and led to increased research into the development of safer gamma-retroviral vectors. Self-inactivating (SIN) vectors that lack the strong enhancer elements in their LTRs mark one major milestone in that endeavor[37] (compare Section 14.4.2 "Strategies to Increase Safety" for details).

Another limitation that researchers have to face when working with retroviral vectors is that for the pre-integration complex (PIC) to be able to integrate into the chromatin, disruption of the nuclear membrane of the host cell is necessary. This implicates that transduction is strictly dependent on mitosis of the target cell just after the entry of the virus, and only actively dividing cells can successfully be transduced with retroviral vectors.[38,39]

14.3.1.2 *Lentivirus*

Lentiviruses such as the human immunodeficiency virus (HIV) got their name ("lentus" is Latin for "slow") due to the long incubation time of infection. They belong to the same family as gamma-retroviruses and mainly have the same structure and characteristics. The major advantage that distinguishes lentiviruses from their MLV-based counterparts though is that they are able to also infect non-dividing cells.[40] This is due to the fact that the PIC formed by lentiviruses is able to enter the nucleus through the nuclear pore complex without disturbing the nuclear membrane. Thus, cell division is not necessary for viral replication. Since HIV uses the T-cell surface marker CD4 as receptor for infection, HIV-derived vectors were originally developed for the transduction of lymphocytes.[41] The possibility of pseudotyping viral vectors with different envelopes such as the vesicular stomatitis virus glycoprotein (VSV-G) that enables viral entry into a very wide range of host cells thus expanding host tropism, significantly broadened the range of viable applications of gene therapy.[42] However, the drawback of such pseudotyped viral vectors is that the VSV-G is toxic to most mammalian cells, rendering the generation of stable producer cell lines and therewith large-scale production difficult.[43,44]

As the risk of insertional transformation is a big concern in all gene therapy approaches, especially in the development of novel viral vectors for clinical trials, thorough research into the safety profile of lentiviral vectors has been performed during the last few years, revealing a potentially safer integration profile compared to gamma-retroviral vectors.[45,46] Also, modifications in the lentivirus genome making it self-inactivating enhanced the safety profile and smoothed the way toward the conduct of clinical trials.[47,48]

Currently, lentiviral vectors are being tested in an increasing number of clinical trials, especially targeting hematopoietic stem cells (HSCs), with striking success so far. Examples include trials for X-linked adrenoleukodystrophy,[49] WAS,[50] metachromatic leukodystrophy,[51] and beta-thalassemia.[14]

14.3.2   *Non-integrating viral vectors*

Non-integrating viral vectors, such as adenoviral or AAV vectors, in contrast are mainly used for quiescent or slowly dividing cells, since after transduction, these vectors are not integrated into the genome, but reside in an extra–chromosomal state and are diluted with each cell division.

14.3.2.1   *Adenoviruses*

Members of the Adenoviridae family are 80–100 nm, non-enveloped double-stranded (ds) DNA viruses with an icosahedral capsid.[32,33] There are more than 50 different serotypes that usually cause mild respiratory infections in humans; only for immunocompromised patients the infection can be lethal. The adenovirus got its name in 1953, when it was first isolated from human adenoids.

As most cells in the human body express the corresponding receptors, adenoviruses undoubtedly are the most effective viruses in terms of *in vivo* delivery and expression of transgenes to date. Thus, adenoviral vectors are the most commonly used viral vectors in gene therapy trials worldwide, comprising close to 24% of all trials.[27] However, one major problem of adenoviruses that scientists have not been able to circumvent, even with the most highly sophisticated molecular strategies, up to now is the extremely high immunogenicity evoked against their capsid. This anti-adenovirus immunity limits the expression of transgenes in the human body to 1–2 weeks,[32] which is the reason why adenoviral vectors nowadays are used for applications where high-level short-term transgene expression is desired, e.g., oncolytic adenoviruses for the treatment of cancers,[52] or where immunity shall purposefully be induced like in the development of vaccines.[53]

In 2003, a recombinant adenovirus serotype 5 vector expressing wildtype-p53, Gendicine of Shenzhen SiBiono GeneTech (China), was the first gene therapy product approved for the use in humans.[54] Shenzhen obtained a drug license from the State Food and Drug Administration (SFDA) of China for the treatment of head and neck squamous cell carcinoma. However, the approval raised concerns about the efficacy of the treatment and the thoroughness of the regulatory process due to the fact that SFDA approved Gendicine without a standard Phase III clinical trial.[54,55]

14.3.2.2 AAV

The AAV belonging to the family of Parvoviridae is a small, non-pathogenic, non-enveloped virus with an average diameter of 20–25 nm and a single-stranded (ss) DNA genome of less than 5 kb.[2] It was first described in 1966 in a study about pathogens in the respiratory tract. It is replication defective and thus dependent on so-called helper viruses such as herpes simplex virus (HSV) or adenovirus for replication.

In recombinant AAV vectors, all viral coding sequences apart from the inverted terminal repeats (ITRs) that are necessary for packaging of the genome into the viral capsid have been removed to make space for the therapeutic gene, but still their maximum packaging capacity amounts to approximately 5 kb, which is half of what gamma-retro- and lentiviral vectors can carry, this is one major limitation for the use of AAV vectors in gene therapy approaches.

More than 10 different serotypes of AAV with different tissue tropisms have been discovered to date, with new serotypes being discovered every year. Out of those, AAV serotype 2 is the most extensively studied and most commonly used in clinical trials. However, pseudotyping the recombinant AAV2 vector genome into capsids of other serotypes to exploit their tissue tropism has become a common strategy.[34]

Another problem that scientists encounter when using AAV in gene transfer approaches is the induction of immune responses in the human body, either against the AAV vector component or the transgene product, or both. As most people are exposed to wild-type AAV during childhood and adolescence, the prevalence of neutralizing antibodies against AAV in the human population is more than 60%.[2]

To date, AAV vectors have been used in 109 clinical trials worldwide,[27] with the trial for the treatment of severe hemophilia B using an AAV vector expressing the human factor IX (FIX) cDNA, depicting a recent clinical success with therapeutic levels of FIX maintained for more than two years after a single injection.[2,56]

14.4 Safety Issues

As the expression of viral genes in the host cells is usually the reason for cellular toxicity and immunological complications associated with viral infections, transduction with recombinant viral vectors lacking these genes is typically well tolerated. However, problems that might be encountered using viral vectors in gene therapy approaches and that need to be considered are:

- Acute toxicity.
- Immune responses: Humoral immune reactions against the transgene or the viral vector, or both, and cellular immune responses against the transduced cells.
- Risk of insertional mutagenesis by integrating viral vectors.[25]

As adverse events due to insertional transformation by integrating vectors have posed a problem in several clinical trials so far, this important topic will be discussed in this chapter in more detail.

14.4.1 *Insertional transformation*

The risk of insertional mutagenesis to date is one of the major safety concerns for *ex vivo* gene therapy approaches using (stem) cells. Viral vectors like retroviral and lentiviral integrate their genetic information quasi-randomly into the host genome, with gamma-retroviruses tending to integrate near gene regulatory sites like transcriptional start sites, while lentiviruses have the presumably safer preference of integrating into actively transcribed genes.[57,58] Integration close to transcriptional control elements of genes can lead to their deregulation by the action of strong enhancer elements present in the viral LTRs, conveying a growth advantage to the affected clones, which in turn can lead to clonal expansion and malignancies.[5,8] Examples of such severe adverse events, in which the integration of a retroviral vector with strong enhancer elements in the LTRs close to a proto–oncogene lead to transactivation of that gene and in the end leukoproliferative disease are the clinical trials for SCID-X1,[11] CGD[12] and WAS.[13]

14.4.2 *Strategies to increase safety*

One constant frustration that gene therapy investigators had to deal with, from the beginning, was the incapacity of preclinical models to forecast the probability of adverse events caused by insertional mutagenesis in clinical trials.[59] With the development of novel large animal instead of mouse models that better represent the human system such as dogs, pigs, and non-human primates, of sophisticated *in vitro* assays[60] and integration site analysis,[61,62] it was possible to gain deeper insight into vector characteristics and a better understanding of the development of insertional transformation.[5]

Owing to these studies and the adverse events observed in clinical trials, it became clear that the major determinant of the risk of insertional transformation by a viral vector is the strength of the enhancer elements it contains. One very important strategy that has helped to considerably increase safety is improvements in the vector configuration. SIN vectors that have been gutted of the strong LTR enhancer elements, but use physiological internal promoters instead to drive transgene expression have been shown to be significantly safer compared to conventional retroviral vectors.[63,64] Also the inclusion of small boundary elements, so-called insulators, that minimize the interaction of the integrated DNA with the host chromatin, thus preventing trans-activation of neighboring genes as well as transgene silencing, has been demonstrated to increase safety.[65,66]

Another strategy to minimize the risk of insertional oncogenesis is targeted integration of the expression cassette into a pre-selected so-called "safe harbor". The recent development of designer nucleases like ZFNs or TALENs brought the possibility of site-specific, targeted integration into gene therapy's grasp.[5]

The introduction of suicide genes, such as the pro-drug converting enzyme HSV-tk, into gene therapy vectors represents one more strategy to increase safety and make gene therapy fail-safe. In case transduced cells cause adverse effects after being injected into the patient, treatment with the pro-drug (GCV) leads to the elimination of all transduced cells expressing the suicide gene that will convert the pro-drug into its active form.[5,18]

However, all of these safety improvements to date cannot abolish the need for conducting a clinical trial to ultimately assess the risk of a gene therapy procedure, always based on the ethical principle that the potential benefit to the patient easily outbalances the possible risks and limitations of the investigational therapy.

The overall safety outcome of close to 2,000 gene therapy clinical trials to date has been more than fulfilling expectations. Much more long-term safety data using viral vectors in gene therapy still need to be collected to make a conclusive assessment, but at least adenoviral vectors have been extensively shown to exhibit a satisfactory safety profile in humans.[18] An important fact that is often disregarded is that conventional alternative treatment strategies for cancer, immune deficiencies or blood diseases like HSC transplantation, radiation therapy or chemotherapy oftentimes have a more dangerous risk profile than gene therapy.[18]

14.5 Historical Milestones: The Rocky Road to Success

Over the past three decades the course of gene therapy has not been a stroll in the park, as a risk is inherent in any therapeutic approach so novel. It was marked by several highs and lows until 2012, when the first commercial gene therapy product was recommended by the European Union. This last section aims to picture some of the highlights, but also deep hits, on gene therapy's rocky road to success.

14.5.1 *The early ages*

Scientists caught a first glimpse of the amazing potential of genetic engineering in the late 1920s, after the discovery that genetic information encoding different properties can be transferred from one bacterium to another. Griffith described how a non-virulent bacterial strain is turned into a virulent type by a process which he called "transformation".[67] Avery *et al.* later found that genetic information is encoded by DNA and not protein, as the belief in the scientific community was at that time.[68] Just a few years later, it was unveiled that bacteriophages have the ability to transfer genetic material from one bacterium to another and thus modify the host bacteria's genetic features ("transduction").[69] In the 1960s, it was first described that genetic information can also be transferred *via* RNA[70] and that cells can stably acquire novel characteristics by chromosomal insertion of foreign genetic material and then pass them on to their progeny.[71]

It was also at that time that scientists started to exploit the unique potential of viruses as new tools for the delivery of genes into cells of interest, and for the first time thoughts about treating genetic diseases with that technique arose.[72,73]

Terheggen *et al.* were the first to perform a human gene therapy trial. In animal experiments, they had seen that infection of rabbit skin with Shope papilloma virus induced an arginase activity that was different from the rabbit arginase. Also, they had observed that laboratory personnel who had worked with Shope papilloma virus showed decreased levels of serum arginine that persisted over a long time, so the scientists deduced that the virus genome encoded an arginase.[74,75] Although the scientific community did not fully approve and asked for further experiments to be performed, the clinical study started in 1970, when two of three children in a German family with hyperargininemia and arginase deficiency suffering from a severe and progressive neurological disease were treated with wild-type Shope papilloma virus. The trial turned out negative: Neither were changes in arginine levels observed in any of the patients nor was the course of the disease altered in any way.[76–78] When the Shope papilloma virus genome was sequenced later on, it was discovered that the virus does not have a gene encoding arginase. Despite the failure of this clinical study, this was the beginning of the "golden age of molecular biology" since Terheggen and colleagues were the first attempting to exploit viruses for the transfer of genetic material into defective human cells.[78]

Due to the rapid scientific progress in the field of manipulating DNA paired with a deeper understanding of the molecular basis of genetic diseases, there was a lot of enthusiasm for gene therapy during the next decade, raising hopes that clinical success was up-coming.

14.5.2 *1980s*

In 1980, Martin Cline of the University of California, Los Angeles (UCLA) became the first to perform a clinical gene therapy trial for the treatment of beta-zero thalassemia, a terminal disease in which no functional hemoglobin beta chains can be produced in the patient's red blood cells, by delivering recombinant DNA, namely the functional human hemoglobin beta gene and the HSV-tk gene as a selection marker.[79–81] The scientific community again was split over the study — some called it premature as the exact same experiment had not yet been shown to work in mice. Cline again defended it as being the first of a series of experiments with the purpose of testing the delivery system and analyzing possible toxicities. "The patients were told that the likelihood of it working was very small" he said.[79] One patient was treated in Naples, Italy, and one in Israel after the UCLA team had gotten approval from both hospitals. However, the UCLA Institutional Review Board had not approved the experiments at the time of treatment, and in fact, months later decided that further animal data should be provided before they would approve. Also, in his application to the review committees, Cline did not mention that his therapy would involve the delivery of recombinant DNA. Five years after the trial, it was reported that no harm was done to the patients, but that there was also no discernible benefit.[81] Cline was sanctioned by the NIH later on for being in breach of federal regulations.[28,82,83] This episode clearly depicts that gene therapy on humans not only is a technically, but also ethically complex topic.

14.5.3 *1990s*

The first US Food and Drug Administration (FDA) — and Recombinant DNA Advisory Committee (RAC)-approved clinical study aiming at introducing foreign DNA into human cells happened in December 1988, when Rosenberg and colleagues used gene marking of tumor-infiltrating lymphocytes (TILs) to track these cells in cancer patients. They found that there were no adverse effects related to the injection of the cells, that the cells expressed the marker gene for two months in two patients, and that the cells could be recovered from the patients' tumors up to 64 days after injection.[84] These promising results led to the conduct of a subsequent clinical trial in which the scientists transduced TILs with tumor necrosis factor (TNF) and showed that there was no further tumor growth at the site of injection of the transduced cells.[85]

Around the same time, Michael Blaese and French Anderson got FDA approval for the treatment of two children with ADA-SCID, a life-threatening monogenetic disease in which a functional immune system is missing. The patients were treated with T lymphocytes that were retrovirally transduced to express the human ADA gene. Four years after treatment, T-cell levels had normalized, as had many cellular and humoral immune responses.[86] The effects were temporary and in one patient, Ashanti DeSilva, far more prominent than in the other.[28]

In the same issue of the journal "Science", Claudio Bordignon and colleagues reported about their clinical gene therapy trial that for the first time deployed genetically modified human HSCs to treat ADA-SCID. They were able to achieve successful gene delivery into long-lasting stem and progenitor cells and short-term and long-term reconstitution of the two patients' immune system, though they remained on enzyme replacement therapy.[87]

Those early years of gene therapy were marked by intriguing results on one side, by overoptimism and overenthusiasm followed by some clinical disappointments that were not surprising relating to the challenges and setbacks inherent in any approach that is novel on the other.

A major stroke of fate however was the death of 18-year-old Jesse Gelsinger in 1999 due to gene therapy associated toxicity. He suffered from a relatively mild form of ornithine transcarbamylase (OTC) deficiency and was a volunteer in a Phase I dose escalation study using adenovirus encoding the human OTC gene at the University of Pennsylvania. After receiving the highest dose of vector in the study (that other patients in this cohort had been able to tolerate), he developed a severe inflammatory response to the adenovirus and subsequently died of multi-organ failure, four days later.[88] Investigations revealed that several rules of conduct had been broken by the investigators about Dr. James Wilson: "They included Gelsinger in the study although his blood ammonia levels were too high, they did not inform the RAC about a change in their protocol, and failed to report a grade III severe adverse event (SAE) to the FDA".[28,88] Wilson and his colleagues apologized publicly for these mistakes, the University of Pennsylvania and Children's National Medical Center each paid more than $500,000 to the government, and Wilson was suspended from clinical research for five years, whereas two of his colleagues faced less severe constraints.[89,90]

14.5.4 *2000s*

After that dark episode of gene therapy, the scientific community was on a tear again when the group around Marina Cavazzana-Calvo and Alain Fischer at the Necker Hospital for Sick Children in Paris reported the first definitive cure of a disease by gene therapy. They treated two patients suffering from SCID-X1, a severe disease resulting in a premature block in T and NK cell development due to a mutation in the gene for the IL-2 receptor gamma chain (IL-2RG). Autologous CD34+ bone marrow cells had been transduced by a Moloney-derived retroviral vector to express the correct human IL2-RG gene[36] and injected back into the patients. Both patients had a complete restoration of their immune function and a full correction of their disease phenotype. In total, 20 children were treated in this study, but the spectacular success was overshadowed by the development of leukemia in five of the patients, among whom one died.[11] The integration of the retroviral vector that contained strong promoter/enhancer elements in the LTRs close to the LIM domain, only two (LMO2) proto-oncogene promoters had led to the transactivation of the gene, and uncontrolled proliferation of the transformed T-cells. However, as several children with ADA-SCID have been treated with a similar retroviral vector and none of the patients has developed leukemia to date, the current hypothesis postulates a synergistic effect of the integration close to LMO2 and the transgene itself in promoting clonal outgrowth.[6]

Despite this more than unsatisfactory outcome, gene therapy was still superior to the standard treatment of allogeneic bone marrow transplantation in terms of overall mortality (5% *vs.* 25%).[28] Also the trial was a success regarding efficacy: 18 of the 20 treated patients were still alive after a 10-year follow up, and in 17 patients, complete restoration of their immune function was achieved.[91]

In 2003, Carl June was the first to use a lentiviral vector in a clinical trial, assessing the safety profile of a conditionally replicating HIV-1-derived vector, expressing an antisense gene against the HIV-1 envelope.[92] Immune function improved in four of five patients, proving the lentiviral vectors as promising new tools for gene therapy.

Currently, almost 2,000 approved gene therapy clinical trials have been performed or are still ongoing,[93] among them the highly successful studies are the treatment of ADA-SCID,[94–96] Leber's congenital amaurosis,[97] chronic lymphoid leukemia,[98] hemophilia B,[56] Parkinson's disease,[99] advanced heart failure,[3] acute lymphoblastic leukemia,[100] metachromatic leukodystrophy,[51] WAS,[50] and HIV infection.[17]

These clinical success stories have led to a renascent fascination for and belief in gene therapy, and culminated in 2012, when the European Medicines Agency (EMA) for the first time recommended a gene therapy product, Glybera (alipogene tiparvovec), an AAV vector encoding the lipoprotein lipase (LPL) gene intended for the treatment of lipoprotein lipase deficiency, for approval in the European Union.[101,102] This depicted an important step in the field of gene therapy, paving the way for other gene and cell therapy products, so that this novel field of medicine can be made accessible for a greater number of patients with a broader spectrum of diseases in the future.

14.6 Synopsis and Outlook

Although the number of clinical gene therapy trials and their indications have increased rapidly over the last decade, the majority of current studies involve the use of the "prototypic" cell type for gene therapy applications, HSPCs; only very recently have other cell types such as NSPCs, CSCs and MSCs emerged and been explored in cell and gene therapy approaches.[5] Especially the latters have become an extremely attractive target for cell and gene therapy strategies. MultiStem® by Athersys, Inc. and Prochymal® initially developed by Osiris Therapeutics, Inc. are just two examples of MSC-based cell products being successfully used in Phase 2 and 3 clinical trials, respectively, for multiple indications.[103,104] However, these MSCs are non-modified and represent cell therapy products referred to as first generation. The more sophisticated next generation approaches involve the genetic modification of MSCs to increase specificity and efficacy of the therapy by improving the cells' characteristics customized for each specific indication.

In 2014, apceth GmbH was the first company to initiate a clinical trial worldwide using genetically modified MSCs for the treatment of advanced adenocarcinoma of the gastrointestinal tract.[24]

Since the development of a gene therapy approach, so entirely novel, is extremely complex and very expensive, extensive considerations of the crucial aspects such as the characteristics of the target cells or choice and delivery of the therapeutic gene is required.

In apceth's TREAT ME trial, the strategy of suicide gene therapy is being employed (compare Section 14.2 "Approaches"). MSCs are genetically modified to express the viral pro-drug converting enzyme HSV-tk that is harmless to humans. Upon systemic administration of the pro-drug GCV however, the enzyme expressed by the MSCs turns GCV into its toxic form, killing not only the cells expressing HSV-tk, but also neighboring cells. This phenomenon is a vital aspect of suicide gene therapy and is called bystander effect. However, it would be absolutely detrimental to achieve this effect throughout the whole patient's body. To minimize possible side effects and specifically target only the tumor cells, the scientists at apceth are combining cell-specific features and crafty vector technology in their approach. The well-defined intrinsic characteristic of MSCs of homing to inflammation and tumor sites, together with a vector construct that enables expression of HSV-tk, merely after induction of the promoter ensures stringently restricted killing of cells specifically at the tumor site.

To achieve this kind of inducible expression of the HSV-tk, apceth utilizes the RANTES (regulated upon activation, normal T-cell expressed and secreted) promoter that is activated by inflammatory cytokines such as TNF alpha (TNF-α) or interferon gamma (IFN-γ) present in virtually every neoplastic microenvironment.[105-107] This promoter is part of a gamma-retroviral vector that allows for highly efficient and also stable modification of the cells. Using an integrating viral vector for this application is of particular importance, as MSCs divide quite rapidly with doubling times between 24 and 40 hours,[108] and non-integrating vectors would be diluted with each cell division, and transgene expression reduced and eventually lost over time. Of the two possible choices of integrating viral vectors commonly used in gene therapy trials, apceth chose retroviral over lentiviral vectors for several practical reasons:

• MSCs divide relatively rapidly; therefore genetic modification by retroviral vectors that transduce dividing cells at high rates is sufficiently efficacious to achieve the desired transduction frequency.

• When performing clinical gene therapy trials, it is advisable to treat as many patients as possible with MSCs transduced with the same batch of viral supernatant to ensure optimal comparability of the outcomes. Using retroviral packaging cell lines such as PG13,[109] it is possible to generate up to 350 liters of viral supernatant per batch.[110] Such scale-up processes are much more difficult for lentiviral vectors, as to date, to the author's knowledge, there is no stable packaging cell line for lentiviral constructs, as the commonly used env protein VSV-G is toxic for most mammalian cells.[43,44]

• The lack of a stable producer cell line also brings along economic aspects: The production process of retroviral vectors is more cost-efficient compared to their lentiviral counterparts, mainly because the very expensive GMP-grade testing of the viral supernatant needs to be performed for each batch — bigger batch size equals lower total costs.

• Another important consideration is safety: For apceth's TREAT ME trial, it was decided to employ a SIN retroviral vector, and not a lentiviral vector. This decision might be surprising at a first glance because the integration profile of lentiviral vectors is presumably less prone to cause clonal dominance compared to that of retroviral vectors. The rationale behind it is straightforward though: First, SIN retroviral vectors using physiological internal promoters like RANTES have recently been shown to have a safe integration profile with no signs of insertional transformation in contrast to the outdated LTR-driven versions,[111] and second, the transduced cells live in the human body just for a few days before GCV is administered several times in a row and all transduced cells are killed off.

Apceth's current flagship products are genetically modified autologous MSCs used in the context of suicide gene therapy for the treatment of advanced cancer. However, the field of cell and gene therapy has been moving forward rapidly over the last years. For that reason, constant improvement of gene delivery technologies and of methods for cultivating large batches of cells, exploration of additional cell sources and diversification regarding the areas of application are vital to stay competitive. Especially regarding the field of gene transfer technologies, innovations go head over heels. Brand-new tools like, e.g., the CRISPR/Cas system that allows for targeted integration of the transgene of choice into safe harbors, thereby further reducing the risk of insertional transformation, are currently being improved and tested in preclinical models and will hopefully be available in optimized form for the use in clinical trials soon.

In light of the rapid progress and impressive success of the field of cell and gene therapy over the last few years, it will hopefully be possible to address many more indications with unmet medical need in the near future.

References

1. Kumar, A., Sharma, P., and Bhandari, A. Gene therapy: An updated review. *Eur. J. Biotechnol. Biosci.* 1(3), 42–53 (2014).
2. Mingozzi, F., and High, K.A. Immune responses to AAV vectors: Overcoming barriers to successful gene therapy. *Blood* 122(1), 23–36 (Jul 4, 2013).
3. Jessup, M., Greenberg, B., Mancini, D., *et al.* Calcium upregulation by percutaneous administration of gene therapy in cardiac disease (CUPID): A phase 2 trial of intracoronary gene therapy of sarcoplasmic reticulum Ca^{2+}-ATPase in patients with advanced heart failure. *Circulation* 124(3), 304–313 (Jul 19, 2011).
4. Greenberg, B., Yaroshinsky, A., Zsebo, K.M., *et al.* Design of a phase 2b trial of intracoronary administration of AAV1/SERCA2a in patients with advanced heart failure: The CUPID 2 trial (calcium up-regulation by percutaneous administration of gene therapy in cardiac disease phase 2b). *JACC Heart Fail.* 2(1), 84–92 (Feb 2014).
5. Naldini, L. *Ex vivo* gene transfer and correction for cell-based therapies. *Nat. Rev. Genet.* 12(5), 301–315 (May 2011).

6. Kay, M.A. State-of-the-art gene-based therapies: The road ahead. *Nat. Rev. Genet.* 12(5), 316–328 (May 2011).

7. Mukherjee, S., and Thrasher, A.J. Gene therapy for PIDs: Progress, pitfalls and prospects. *Gene* 525(2), 174–181 (Aug 10, 2013).

8. Kohn, D.B., Pai, S.Y., and Sadelain, M. Gene therapy through autologous transplantation of gene-modified hematopoietic stem cells. *Biol. Blood Marrow Transplant* 19(Suppl 1), S64–S69 (Jan 2013).

9. Cavazzana-Calvo, M., Fischer, A., Hacein-Bey-Abina, S., and Aiuti, A. Gene therapy for primary immunodeficiencies: Part 1. *Curr. Opin. Immunol.* 24(5), 580–584 (Oct 2012).

10. Molmed press release. MolMed enters an agreement with GSK for the manufacture of the Experimental gene therapy for compassionate use for ADA-SCID. (http://www. molmed.com/sites/default/files/uploads/press-releases/2347-molmed_enters_an_ agreement_with_gsk_for_the_manufacture_of_the_experimental_gene_therapy_for_ compassionate_use_for_ada-scid/2347_1385064344.pdf). (Retrieved Jun 10, 2014).

11. Hacein-Bey-Abina, S., Von Kalle, C., Schmidt, M., *et al.* LMO2-associated clonal T-cell proliferation in two patients after gene therapy for SCID-X1. *Science* 302(5644), 415–419 (Oct 17, 2003).

12. Stein, S., Ott, M.G., Schultze-Strasser, S., *et al.* Genomic instability and myelodysplasia with monosomy 7 consequent to EVI1 activation after gene therapy for chronic granulomatous disease. *Nat. Med.* 16(2), 198–204 (Feb 2010).

13. Braun, C.J., Boztug, K., Paruzynski, A., *et al.* Gene therapy for Wiskott-Aldrich syndrome — long-term efficacy and genotoxicity. *Sci. Transl. Med.* 6(227), 227ra33 (Mar 12, 2014).

14. Cavazzana-Calvo, M., Payen, E., Negre, O., *et al.* Transfusion independence and HMGA2 activation after gene therapy of human β-thalassaemia. *Nature* 467(7313), 318–322 (Sep 16, 2010).

15. Romero, Z., Urbinati, F., Geiger, S., *et al.* β-globin gene transfer to human bone marrow for sickle cell disease. *J. Clin. Invest.* pii, 67930 (Jul 1, 2013).

16. Lombardo, A., Cesana, D., Genovese, P., *et al.* Site-specific integration and tailoring of cassette design for sustainable gene transfer. *Nat. Methods* 8(10), 861–869 (Aug 21, 2011).

17. Tebas, P., Stein, D., Tang, W.W., *et al.* Gene editing of CCR5 in autologous CD4 T-cells of persons infected with HIV. *N. Engl. J. Med.* 370(10), 901–910 (Mar 6, 2014).

18. Wirth, T., and Ylä-Herttuala, S. Gene therapy used in cancer treatment. *Biomedicines* 2, 149–162 (2014).

19. Freeman, S.M., Abboud, C.N., Whartenby. K.A., *et al.* The "bystander effect": Tumor regression when a fraction of the tumor mass is genetically modified. *Cancer Res.* 53(21), 5274–5283 (Nov 1, 1993).

20. Immonen, A., Vapalahti, M., Tyynelä, K., *et al.* AdvHSV-tk gene therapy with intravenous ganciclovir improves survival in human malignant glioma: A randomised, controlled study. *Mol. Ther.* 10(5), 967–972 (Nov 2004).

21. Niess, H., Bao, Q., Conrad, C., *et al.* Selective targeting of genetically engineered mesenchymal stem cells to tumor stroma microenvironments using tissue-specific suicide gene expression suppresses growth of hepatocellular carcinoma. *Ann. Surg.* 254(5), 767–774 (Nov 2011).

22. Kim, S.W., Kim, S.J., Park, S.H., *et al.* Complete regression of metastatic renal cell carcinoma by multiple injections of engineered mesenchymal stem cells expressing dodecameric TRAIL and HSV-TK. *Clin. Cancer Res.* 19(2), 415–427 (Jan 15, 2013).

23. Martinez-Quintanilla, J., Bhere, D., Heidari, P., *et al.* Therapeutic efficacy and fate of bimodal engineered stem cells in malignant brain tumors. *Stem Cells* 31(8), 1706–1714 (Aug 2013).

24. apceth press release. apceth's ground-breaking first-in-man, first-in-class clinical trial in oncology with genetically modified mesenchymal stromal cells is now enrolling. (http://www.apceth.com/fileadmin/media/newsroom/press_releases/2014/PM_140131_en.pdf). (Retrieved June 10, 2014).

25. Kay, M.A., Glorioso, J.C., and Naldini, L. Viral vectors for gene therapy: The art of turning infectious agents into vehicles of therapeutics. *Nat. Med.* 7(1), 33–40 (Jan 2001).

26. Somia, N., and Verma, I.M. Gene therapy: Trials and tribulations. *Nat. Rev. Genet.* 1(2), 91–99 (Nov 2000).

27. Gene Therapy Clinical Trials Worldwide. Vectors Used in Gene Therapy Clinical Trials. *J. Gene Med.* (http://www.abedia.com/wiley/vectors.php). (Retrieved June 10, 2014).

28. Sheridan, C. Gene therapy finds its niche. *Nat. Biotechnol.* 29(2), 121–128 (Feb 2011).

29. Koirala, A., Conley, S.M., and Naash, M.I. A review of therapeutic prospects of non-viral gene therapy in the retinal pigment epithelium. *Biomaterials* 34(29), 7158–7167 (Sep 2013).

30. Macpherson, J.L, and Rasko J.E. Clinical potential of gene therapy: towards meeting the demand. *Intern. Med. J.* 44(3), 224–233 (Mar 2014).

31. Gene Therapy Net.com. Viral Vectors. (http://www.genetherapynet.com/viral-vectors.html). (Retrieved June 10, 2014).

32. Crystal, R.G. Adenovirus: The first effective *in vivo* gene delivery vector. *Hum. Gene Ther.* 25(1), 3–11 (Jan 2014).

33. Hay, R.T. Adenovirus DNA replication. In *DNA Replication in Eukaryotic Cells.* New York: Cold Spring Harbor Laboratory Press, 0-87969-459-9/96 (1996).

34. Thomas, C.E., Ehrhardt, A., and Kay, M.A. Progress and problems with the use of viral vectors for gene therapy. *Nat. Rev. Genet.* 4(5), 346–358 (May 2003).

35. Weiss, R.A. Retrovirus classification and cell interactions. *J. Antimicrob. Chemother.* 37(Suppl B), 1–11 (May 1996).

36. Cavazzana-Calvo, M., Hacein-Bey, S., de Saint Basile, G., *et al.* Gene therapy of human severe combined immunodeficiency (SCID)–X1 disease. *Science* 288(5466), 669–672 (Apr 28, 2000).

37. Yu, S.F., von Rüden, T., Kantoff, P.W., *et al.* Self-inactivating retroviral vectors designed for transfer of whole genes into mammalian cells. *Proc. Natl. Acad. Sci. USA* 83(10), 3194–3198 (May 1986).

38. Miller, D.G., Adam, M.A., and Miller, A.D. Gene transfer by retrovirus vectors occurs only in cells that are actively replicating at the time of infection. *Mol. Cell Biol.* 10(8), 4239–4242 (Aug 1990).

39. Roe, T., Reynolds, T.C., Yu, G., and Brown, P.O. Integration of murine leukemia virus DNA depends on mitosis. *EMBO J.* 12(5), 2099–2108 (May 1993).

40. Piller, S.C., Caly, L., and Jans, D.A. Nuclear import of the pre-integration complex (PIC): The Achilles heel of HIV? *Curr. Drug Targets* 4(5): 409–429 (Jul 2003).

41. Naldini, L., Blömer, U., Gallay, P., *et al*. *In vivo* gene delivery and stable transduction of non-dividing cells by a lentiviral vector. *Science* 272(5259), 263–267 (Apr 12, 1996).

42. Cronin, J., Zhang, X.Y., and Reiser, J. Altering the tropism of lentiviral vectors through pseudotyping. *Curr. Gene Ther.* 5(4), 387–398 (Aug 2005).

43. Stornaiuolo, A., Piovani, B.M., Bossi, S., *et al*. RD2-MolPack-Chim3, a packaging cell line for stable production of lentiviral vectors for anti-HIV gene therapy. *Hum. Gene Ther. Methods* 24(4), 228–240 (Aug 2013).

44. Chen, S.T., Lida, A., Guo, L., *et al*. Generation of packaging cell lines for pseudotyped retroviral vectors of the G protein of vesicular stomatitis virus by using a modified tetracycline inducible system. *Proc. Natl. Acad. Sci. USA* 93(19), 10057–10062 (Sep 17, 1996).

45. Schröder, A.R., Shinn, P., Chen, H., *et al*. HIV-1 integration in the human genome favors active genes and local hotspots. *Cell* 110(4), 521–529 (Aug 23, 2002).

46. Mitchell, R.S., Beitzel, B.F., Schroder, A.R., *et al*. Retroviral DNA integration: ASLV, HIV, and MLV show distinct target site preferences. *PLoS Biol.* 2(8), E234 (Aug 2004).

47. Zufferey, R., Dull, T., Mandel, R.J., *et al*. Self-inactivating lentivirus vector for safe and efficient *in vivo* gene delivery. *J. Virol.* 72(12), 9873–9880 (Dec 1998).

48. Dull, T., Zufferey, R., Kelly, M., *et al*. A third-generation lentivirus vector with a conditional packaging system. *J. Virol.* 72(11), 8463–8471 (Nov 1998).

49. Cartier, N., Hacein-Bey-Abina, S., Bartholomae, C.C., *et al*. Hematopoietic stem cell gene therapy with a lentiviral vector in X-linked adrenoleukodystrophy. *Science* 326(5954), 818–823 (Nov 6, 2009).

50. Aiuti, A., Biasco, L., Scaramuzza, S., *et al*. Lentiviral hematopoietic stem cell gene therapy in patients with Wiskott-Aldrich syndrome. *Science* 341(6148), 1233151 (Aug 23, 2013).

51. Biffi, A., Montini, E., Lorioli, L., *et al*. Lentiviral hematopoietic stem cell gene therapy benefits metachromatic leukodystrophy. *Science* 341(6148), 1233158 (Aug 23, 2013).

52. Di, Y., Seymour, L., and Fisher, K. Activity of a group B oncolytic adenovirus (ColoAd1) in whole human blood. *Gene Ther.* 21(4), 440–443 (Apr 2014).

53. Boyer, J.L., Sofer-Podesta, C., Ang, J., *et al*. Protective immunity against a lethal respiratory *Yersinia pestis* challenge induced by V antigen or the F1 capsular antigen incorporated into adenovirus capsid. *Hum. Gene Ther.* 21(7), 891–901 (Jul 2010).

54. Wirth, T., Parker, N., and Ylä-Herttuala, S. History of gene therapy. *Gene* 525(2), 162–169 (Aug 10, 2013).

55. Wilson, J.M. Gendicine: The first commercial gene therapy product. *Hum. Gene Ther.* 16(9), 1014–1015 (Sep 2005).

56. Nathwani, A.C., Tuddenham, E.G., Rangarajan, S., *et al*. Adenovirus-associated virus vector-mediated gene transfer in hemophilia B. *N. Engl. J. Med.* 365(25), 2357–2365 (Dec 22, 2011).

57. Wang, G.P., Levine, B.L., Binder, G.K., *et al*. Analysis of lentiviral vector integration in HIV+ study subjects receiving autologous infusions of gene modified CD4+ T cells. *Mol. Ther.* 17(5), 844–50 (May 2009).

58. Wu, X., Li, Y., Crise, B., and Burgess, S.M. Transcription start regions in the human genome are favored targets for MLV integration. *Science* 300(5626), 1749–1751 (Jun 13, 2003).

59. Nienhuis, A.W. Assays to evaluate the genotoxicity of retroviral vectors. *Mol. Ther.* 14(4), 459–460 (Oct 2006).

60. Modlich, U., Bohne, J., Schmidt, M., *et al.* Cell-culture assays reveal the importance of retroviral vector design for insertional genotoxicity. *Blood* 108(8), 2545–2553 (Oct 15, 2006).

61. Schmidt, M., Schwarzwaelder, K., Bartholomae, C., *et al.* High-resolution insertion-site analysis by linear amplification-mediated PCR (LAM-PCR). *Nat. Methods* 4(12), 1051–1057 (Dec 2007).

62. Paruzynski, A., Arens, A., Gabriel, R., *et al.* Genome-wide high-throughput integrome analyses by nrLAM-PCR and next-generation sequencing. *Nat Protoc.* 5(8), 1379–1395 (Aug 2010).

63. Montini, E., Cesana, D., Schmidt, M., *et al.* The genotoxic potential of retroviral vectors is strongly modulated by vector design and integration site selection in a mouse model of HSC gene therapy. *J. Clin. Invest.* 119(4), 964–975 (Apr 2009).

64. Zychlinski, D., Schambach, A., Modlich, U., *et al.* Physiological promoters reduce the genotoxic risk of integrating gene vectors. *Mol. Ther.* 16(4), 718–725 (Apr 2008).

65. Emery, D.W., Yannaki, E., Tubb, J., *et al.* Development of virus vectors for gene therapy of beta chain hemoglobinopathies: Flanking with a chromatin insulator reduces gamma-globin gene silencing *in vivo*. *Blood* 100(6), 2012–2019 (Sep 15, 2002).

66. Evans-Galea, M.V., Wielgosz, M.M., Hanawa, H., *et al.* Suppression of clonal dominance in cultured human lymphoid cells by addition of the cHS4 insulator to a lentiviral vector. *Mol. Ther.* 15(4), 801–809 (Apr 2007).

67. Griffith, F. The Significance of Pneumococcal Types. *J. Hyg. (Lond.)* 27(2), 113–159 (Jan 1928).

68. Avery, O.T., MacLeod, C.M., and McCarty, M. Studies on the chemical nature of the substance inducing transformation of pneumococcal types. Induction of transformation by a desoxyribonucleic acid fraction isolated from Pneumococcus type III. *J. Exp. Med.* 79(2), 137–158 (Feb 1944).

69. Zinder, N.D., and Lederberg, J. Genetic exchange in Salmonella. *J. Bacteriol.* 64(5), 679–699 (Nov 1952).

70. Temin, H.M. Mixed infection with two types of Rous sarcoma virus. *Virology* 13, 158–163 (Feb 1961).

71. Sambrook, J., Westphal, H., Srinivasan, P.R., and Dulbecco, R. The integrated state of viral DNA in SV40-transformed cells. *Proc. Natl. Acad. Sci. USA* 60(4), 1288–1295 (Aug 1968).

72. Tatum, E.L. Molecular biology, nucleic acids, and the future of medicine. *Perspect. Biol. Med.* 10(1), 19–32 (1966).

73. Rogers, S., and Pfuderer, P. Use of viruses as carriers of added genetic information. *Nature* 219(5155), 749–751 (Aug 17, 1968).

74. Rogers, S., and Moore, M. Studies of the mechanism of action of the Shope rabbit papilloma virus I. Concerning the nature of the induction of arginase in the infected cells. *J. Exp. Med.* 117, 521–542 (Mar 1, 1963).

75. Rogers, S. Shope papilloma virus: A passenger in man and its significance to the potential control of the host genome. *Nature* 212(5067), 1220–1222 (Dec 10, 1966).

76. Terheggen, H.G., Lowenthal, A., Lavinha, F., *et al.* Unsuccessful trial of gene replacement in arginase deficiency. *Z. Kinderheilkd.* 119(1), 1–3 (1975).

77. Rogers, S., Lowenthal, A., Terheggen, H.G., Columbo, J.P. Induction of arginase activity with the Shope papilloma virus in tissue culture cells from an argininemic patient. *J. Exp. Med.* 137(4), 1091–1096 (Apr 1, 1973).

78. Friedmann, T., and Rogers, S. Insights into virus vectors and failure of an early gene therapy model. *Mol. Ther.* 4(4), 285–288 (Oct 2001).

79. Wade, N. UCLA gene therapy racked by friendly fire. *Science* 210(4469), 509–511 (Oct 31, 1980).

80. Cline, M.J. Perspectives for gene therapy: inserting new genetic information into mammalian cells by physical techniques and viral vectors. *Pharmacol. Ther.* 29(1), 69–92 (1985).

81. Beutler, E. The Cline affair. *Mol. Ther.* 4(5), 396–397 (Nov 2001).

82. Dickson, D. Cline stripped of research grants. *Nature* 294(5840), 391–392 (Dec 3, 1981).

83. Dickson, D. NIH censure for Dr Martin Cline: Tighter rules for future research plans. *Nature* 291(5814), 369 (Jun 4, 1981).

84. Rosenberg, S.A., Aebersold, P., Cornetta, K., *et al.* Gene transfer into humans — immunotherapy of patients with advanced melanoma, using tumor-infiltrating lymphocytes modified by retroviral gene transduction. *N. Engl. J. Med.* 323(9), 570–578 (Aug 30, 1990).

85. Rosenberg, S.A., Anderson, W.F., Blaese, M., *et al.* The development of gene therapy for the treatment of cancer. *Ann. Surg.* 218(4), 455–463 (Oct 1993).

86. Blaese, R.M., Culver, K.W., Miller, A.D., *et al.* T lymphocyte-directed gene therapy for ADA-SCID: Initial trial results after 4 years. *Science* 270(5235), 475–480 (Oct 20, 1995).

87. Bordignon, C., Notarangelo, L.D., Nobili, N., *et al.* Gene therapy in peripheral blood lymphocytes and bone marrow for ADA-immunodeficient patients. *Science* 270(5235), 470–475 (Oct 20, 1995).

88. Hollon, T. Researchers and regulators reflect on first gene therapy death. *Nat. Med.* 6(1), 6 (Jan 2000).

89. Branca, M.A. Gene therapy: Cursed or inching towards credibility? *Nat. Biotechnol.* 23(5), 519–521 (May 2005).

90. Couzin, J., and Kaiser, J. Gene therapy. As Gelsinger case ends, gene therapy suffers another blow. *Science* 307(5712), 1028 (Feb 18, 2005).

91. Fischer, A., Hacein-Bey-Abina, S., and Cavazzana-Calvo, M. 20 years of gene therapy for SCID. *Nat. Immunol.* 11(6), 457–460 (Jun 2010).

92. Levine, B.L., Humeau, L.M., Boyer, J., *et al.* Gene transfer in humans using a conditionally replicating lentiviral vector. *Proc. Natl. Acad. Sci. USA* 103(46), 17372–17377 (Nov 14, 2006).

93. Gene Therapy Clinical Trials Worldwide. Indications Addressed by Gene Therapy Clinical Trials. *J. Gene Med.* (http://www.abedia.com/wiley/indications.php). (Retrieved June 10, 2014).

94. Aiuti, A., Cattaneo, F., Galimberti, S., *et al.* Gene therapy for immunodeficiency due to adenosine deaminase deficiency. *N. Engl. J. Med.* 360(5), 447–458 (Jan 29, 2009).

95. Ferrua, F., Brigida, I., and Aiuti, A. Update on gene therapy for adenosine deaminase-deficient severe combined immunodeficiency. *Curr. Opin. Allergy Clin. Immunol.* 10(6), 551–556 (Dec 2010).

96. Candotti, F., Shaw, K.L., Muul, L., *et al.* Gene therapy for adenosine deaminase-deficient severe combined immune deficiency: Clinical comparison of retroviral vectors and treatment plans. *Blood* 120(18), 3635–3646 (Nov 1, 2012).

97. Simonelli, F., Maguire, A.M., Testa, F., *et al.* Gene therapy for Leber's congenital amaurosis is safe and effective through 1.5 years after vector administration. *Mol. Ther.* 18(3), 643–650 (Mar 2010).

98. Porter, D.L., Levine, B.L., Kalos, M., *et al.* Chimeric antigen receptor-modified T-cells in chronic lymphoid leukemia. *N. Engl. J. Med.* 365(8), 725–733 (Aug 25, 2011).

99. LeWitt, P.A., Rezai, A.R., Leehey, M.A., *et al.* AAV2-GAD gene therapy for advanced Parkinson's disease: a double-blind, sham-surgery controlled, randomised trial. *Lancet Neurol.* 10(4), 309–319 (Apr 2011).

100. Brentjens, R.J., Davila, M.L., Riviere, I., *et al.* CD19-targeted T cells rapidly induce molecular remissions in adults with chemotherapy-refractory acute lymphoblastic leukemia. *Sci. Transl. Med.* 5(177), 177ra38 (Mar 20, 2013).

101. Miller, N. Glybera and the future of gene therapy in the European Union. *Nat. Rev. Drug Discov.* 11(5), 419 (May 2012).

102. Ylä-Herttuala, S. Endgame: Glybera finally recommended for approval as the first gene therapy drug in the European Union. *Mol. Ther.* 20(10), 1831–1832 (Oct 2012).

103. Lehmann, W. Athersys Inc. Press Release. Athersys Announces Results From Phase 2 Study of MultiStem® Cell Therapy for Ulcerative Colitis. (http://www.athersys.com/releasedetail.cfm?ReleaseID=842936). (Retrieved June 24, 2014).

104. Meldrum, J. Mesoblast press release. Mesoblast Provides Update On Clinical Programs Of Prochymal® For Crohn's Disease and Acute Graft Versus Host Disease. (http://ir.mesoblast.com/DownloadFile.axd?file=/Report/ComNews/20140429/01512252.pdf). (Retrieved June 24, 2014).

105. Lee, A.H., Hong, J.H., and Seo, Y.S. Tumour necrosis factor-alpha and interferon-gamma synergistically activate the RANTES promoter through nuclear factor kappaB and interferon regulatory factor 1 (IRF-1) transcription factors. *Biochem. J.* 350(Pt 1), 131 138 (Aug 15, 2000).

106. Hanahan, D., and Weinberg, R.A. Hallmarks of cancer. The next generation. *Cell* 144(5), 646–674 (Mar 4, 2011).

107. Grivennikov, S.I., and Karin, M. Inflammation and oncogenesis: A vicious connection. *Curr. Opin. Genet. Dev.* 20(1), 65–71 (Feb 2010).

108. Lu, L.L., Liu, Y.J., Yang, S.G., *et al.* Isolation and characterization of human umbilical cord mesenchymal stem cells with hematopoiesis-supportive function and other potentials. *Haematologica* 91(8), 1017–1026 (Aug 2006).

109. Miller, A.D., Garcia, J.V., von Suhr, N., *et al.* Construction and properties of retrovirus packaging cells based on gibbon ape leukemia virus. *J. Virol.* 65(5), 2220–2224 (May 1991).

110. EUFETS. Retroviral vectors. (http://www.eufets.com/Retroviral+vectors.php). (Retrieved June 25, 2014).

111. Stein, S., Scholz, S., Schwäble, J., *et al.* From bench to bedside: Preclinical evaluation of a self-inactivating gamma retroviral vector for the gene therapy of X-linked chronic granulomatous disease. *Hum. Gene Ther. Clin. Dev.* 24(2), 86–98 (Jun 2013).

Exosomes and their Therapeutic Applications

15

Ronne Wee Yeh Yeo and Sai Kiang Lim

15.1 Introduction

Exosome is essentially a class of extracellular vesicle (EV). Other classes of EVs are microvesicles, ectosomes, membrane particles, exosome–like vesicles, and apoptotic bodies. These different classes of EVs are defined by their biogenesis pathway, size, flotation density on a sucrose gradient, lipid composition, sedimentation force, and protein cargo (reviewed[1,2]). However, identifying the biogenesis pathway of an EV is technically challenging and may not always be practical. On the other hand, the other parameters while highly amenable to standard assay methodologies are not definitive and exclusive. Therefore, the different EVs as presently defined may not be distinct biological entities and this ambiguity has encumbered our understanding of the biology and functions of EVs.[3]

Of the classes of EVs, exosomes are presently the best characterized and are the only EVs known to have an endosomal origin, i.e., their biogenesis starts with the invagination of the endosomal membrane to form numerous intraluminal vesicles (ILVs) within a membrane vesicle. This larger vesicle known as multivesicular body (MVB) either fuses with lysosomes or plasma membrane. When MVB fuses with a lysosome, the ILVs are degraded and if MVB fuses with the plasma membrane, the ILVs are released as exosomes.[4] As a result of this endosomal origin, exosomes have lipid raft-enriched bilipid membrane.[5] In practice, exosomes are usually defined by technically amenable parameters, a diameter of 40–100 nm, a flotation density of 1.10–1.18 g/ml in a sucrose gradient, and exosome-associated markers such as Alix, Tsg101, the tetraspanins, CD9, CD63 or CD81.[6,7] The presence of exposed phosphatidylserine on exosome membranes remains controversial.[8–11]

477

Exosomes are secreted by many cell types including B cells,[12] dendritic cells (DCs),[13] mast cells,[14] T-cells,[15] platelets,[11] Schwann cells,[16] tumor cells,[17] skeletal muscles,[18] mesenchymal stem cells (MSCs),[19] human embryonic kidney cells,[20] various cancer cell lines,[21] and sperms.[22] Consequently, exosomes are found in extracellular fluid of these cells such as bronchial lavage fluid,[23] urine,[24, 25] saliva,[26] breast milk,[27] and blood.[25] The diversity of exosome-secreting cells indicates that exosome secretion is a conserved cellular function. This in turn implies that exosome has important biological functions, and four decades after its discovery,[28] exosomes were found to be important in mediating intercellular communication in many biological systems. For example, DCs when pulsed with tumor peptides secrete exosomes to mediate tumor suppression,[29] neurons secrete exosome during neurotransmission,[30, 31] oligodendrocytes secrete exosomes to inhibit myelin membrane biogenesis,[32] and exosomes from cardiomyocyte progenitor cells induce migration of endothelial cells.[33]

Exosomes carry a large diverse cargo that is reported to contain both proteins and RNA. The protein cargo includes a set of proteins that is conserved across exosomes from different cell sources, and these proteins include the tetraspanins (CD81, CD63, CD9), Alix and Tsg101. Exosomes also carry proteins and RNAs that reflect their cell sources and their physiological or pathophysiological states.[34] For example, exosomes from reticulocytes, unlike those from lymphocytes and DCs, are rich in transferrin receptors. They serve as "garbage bags" for the disposal of these transferrin receptors as the reticulocytes mature.[12, 35, 36] Exosomes from tumor cells also carry tumor antigens[17, 37–39] or tumor-specific microRNAs.[40] Similarly, exosomes from the epididymis are rich in proteins that are essential for the maturation of male gametes[22] and urinary exosomes secreted by kidney tubules carry aquaporin, a kidney-specific protein.[24] The cargo composition of exosomes is also modulated by its microenvironment. Exosomes secreted by tumor cells during hypoxia carry proteins that facilitate angiogenesis and metastasis.[41] The list of proteins and RNAs identified in exosomes are freely accessible at ExoCarta (http://www.exocarta.org) or Vesiclepedia (http://www.microvesicles.org). Because of the close association between the composition of exosomes and the physiological or pathological states of the secreting cells, exosomes are good sentinels of cellular health and pathology, and have become an attractive source of disease biomarkers (reviewed[42]).

15.2 Exosomes are Well-Positioned as Therapeutic Agents

Exosomes represent a non-canonical mode of intercellular communication that is distinct from conventional modes such as autocrine, juxtacrine, paracrine, endocrine, and exocrine. The main distinction lies in the complex structure and composition of exosomes that allow exosomes to target multiple molecules in multiple processes and multiple cell types simultaneously. For example, exosomes carry RNA, and both cytosolic and membrane proteins that could modulate extra- and intra-cellular activities. This modulation is facilitated by the bilipid membrane of exosomes which support the configuration of membrane proteins and enable the transport of luminal proteins or RNA through membrane fusion or endocytosis. This capacity to deliver a complex load to target cells and modify their activity underpins their promising therapeutic role. In addition, exosomes also have many desirable attributes of a drug delivery vehicle.[43,44] They are physiologically well-tolerated, as evidenced by their presence in many biological fluids. The encapsulation of proteins and nucleic acids within the "natural" cell-derived bilipid membranes of exosomes enhances the bioavailability of the cargo and facilitates the cellular internalization of the cargo by membrane fusion or endocytosis. Exosomes have been shown to deliver their cargo into the right cellular compartment to exert a functional response. For example, exosomes derived from DCs (also known as Dex) could modulate immune response by transferring peptide loaded MHC class I and II complexes to DCs.[45,46] Exosomes have also been shown to mediate intercellular transfer of mRNAs and miRNAs that resulted in the translation of the transferred mRNA in the recipient cells.[47] We have also demonstrated that MSC exosomes are internalized by H9C2 cardiomyocytes.[48]

Exosomes also possess the ability to home specific cell types. For example, melanoma exosomes have been reported to home preferentially sentinel lymph nodes to promote tumor metastasis.[49] Their membranes could also be modified to enhance cell type-specific targeting. For example, overexpression of a fusion gene consisting of a neuron-specific RVG encoding sequence and LAMP2B encoding an exosomal membrane protein in DCs resulted in the secretion of exosomes with RVG peptide on their membranes. These exosomes, after loading with siRNA, could cross the blood−brain barrier to knock down more than 60% of the siRNA-targeted gene in neurons, microglia, oligodendrocytes, and their precursors.[50] Together, these attributes of exosomes have positioned them as a promising "first-in-class" therapeutics that could potentially manipulate the activities of any cell type in the body through the introduction of exogenous cargo.

15.3   Exosomes with Intrinsic Therapeutic Activity

MSCs are presently the stem cell of choice for regenerative medicine as they can be easily isolated from adult tissues, expanded *ex vivo* and have a wide spectrum of therapeutic activities. As such, MSCs are currently the most clinically evaluated stem cells and it is not surprising that the first evidence of therapeutic stem cell-derived exosomes emerged from the studies of MSC secretions.

The ClinicalTrials.gov database lists more than 300 trials on the use of MSCs to treat a wide range of pathological conditions (http://www.clinicaltrials.gov/, accessed March 2013). These include cardiovascular diseases (e.g., acute myocardial infarction, endstage ischemic heart disease, or prevention of vascular restenosis), osteogenesisimperfecta (OI) or brittle bone disease, amyotrophic lateral sclerosis (ALS), lysosomal storage diseases (e.g., Hurler syndrome), steroid-refractory Graft-versus-Host Disease (GvHD), periodontitis, and bone fractures.[51] The therapeutic efficacy of transplanted MSCs was initially attributed to their homing and engraftment in injured tissues, and subsequent differentiation to repair and replace damaged tissues. However, studies in animal models and patients indicated that <1% of transplanted MSCs localize to the target tissue with most becoming trapped in the liver, spleen, and lungs.[52] Furthermore, evidence for differentiation of transplanted MSCs at the site of injury could not rule out the possibility of fusion with endogenous cells.[53–55] In fact, the efficacy of MSC transplantation in treating diseases in animal models and patients has been increasingly observed to be independent of engraftment or differentiation.[56–60] Consequently, MSC secretion is now implicated as the primary mediator of MSC-based therapies. Much of the initial attention on MSC secretion has been centered on small molecules such as growth factors, chemokines, and cytokines.[61] Although many candidates for mediating the therapeutic properties of MSCs have been proposed, none could sufficiently account for the efficacy of MSCs against such a diverse range of pathological conditions (reviewed[62]). Efforts to identify the therapeutic agent in MSC secretion were recently shifted from small molecules to EVs.

The intrinsic therapeutic potential of exosomes was revealed when MSC exosomes demonstrated cardioprotective effects. Timmers et al. first reported, in 2008, that MSC secretion mediated the cardioprotection of MSCs. They observed that after sterile filtration through a 0.2 μm filter, culture medium conditioned by human embryonic stem cell (hESC)-derived MSCs could reduce infarct size in pig and mouse models of acute myocardial ischemia/reperfusion (MI/R) injury.[63] This conditioned medium (CM) could also improve cardiac function in a pig model of myocardial ischemia by stimulating angiogenesis and preventing adverse myocardium remodeling.[64] Size fractionation of the CM subsequently revealed that the therapeutic activity resided in the 100–220 nm fraction. This fraction when purified by size-exclusion HPLC was found to be enriched in EVs that fulfilled the defining criteria of exosomes. It was able to reduce the infarct size in a mouse model of MI/R injury with an efficacy comparable to unfractionated CM19. Although our lab was the first to describe the secretion and therapeutic potential of MSC exosomes, Bruno *et al.* preceded us in describing the secretion of a population of EVs by MSCs which they termed "microvesicles" and its amelioration of glycerol-induced acute kidney injury (AKI).[65] As these microvesicles were not evaluated for exosome-associated properties and had an estimated diameter of 180 nm *versus* the 55–65 nm hydrodynamic radius[19] for the exosomes that we isolated, we postulated that these two populations of EVs are different.

In the last two years, MSC exosomes have been found to be efficacious in an increasing number of animal models for human diseases such as AKI,[65] cutaneous wound healing,[66] cerebral ischemia,[67] liver fibrosis and injury,[68, 69] and hypoxic pulmonary hypertension.[70] Recently, MSC exosomes were administered to a treatment-refractory grade IV acute GvHD patient. Her symptoms were dramatically alleviated and she remained stable for five months.[71] Apart from MSCs, exosomes from other stem cell sources, such as cardiosphere-derived cells (CDCs)[72] and neural stem cells (NSCs),[73] have also been reported to exhibit therapeutic potential. Studies that investigated the intrinsic therapeutic effects of exosomes are summarized in Table 15.1.

15.3.1 *Characteristics of MSC exosomes*

MSC exosomes fulfilled the defining characteristics of exosomes, i.e., bilipid membrane vesicles with a hydrodynamic radius of 55–65 nm and can be visualized by electron microscopy.[63, 74] They have a detergent-sensitive flotation density range of 1.10 g ml^{-1} to 1.18 g ml^{-1} in sucrose, and are enriched in exosome-associated protein markers such as CD9, CD81 and Alix, and membrane lipids such as cholesterol, sphingomyelin, and phosphatidylcholine.[19] They also contained small RNAs of <300 nucleotides (nts) that are enriched in pre-miRNAs.[48] Consistent with their encapsulation in a cholesterol-rich phospholipid vesicles, both exosomal proteins and RNAs are susceptible to enzymatic RNase or protease digestion only in the presence of a SDS-based lysis buffer, cyclodextrin, a cholesterol chelator, and phospholipase A2. These MSC exosomes were derived from endosomes formed through endosome derived from lipid raft, a membrane microdomain with high endocytic activity. Using transferrin (Tf) as a tracer for endocytosis, we have demonstrated that a small fraction of the internalized extracellular Tf recycled into MSC exosomes. Pulsing MSCs with labeled Tfs in the presence of chlorpromazine, an inhibitor of clathrin-mediated endocytosis, reduced the incorporation of Tfs in CD81-immunoprecipitate during the chase. Also consistent with their derivation from lipid rafts, MSC exosomes could be extracted with Cholera-toxin B chain (CTB) which targets GM1 ganglioside-enriched lipid rafts. Both Tf- or

Table 15.1: Summary of Studies that Investigated the Intrinsic Therapeutic Effects of Exosomes.

Date	EV Source	Purification Method	Disease Studied	Therapeutic Effect	Ref.
			MSC sources		
May 2009	MSC, human bone marrow	Ultracentrifugation	Mouse model of glycerol-induced AKI	Reduced tubular lesions, blood urea nitrogen and creatinine enhanced tubular cell proliferation	65
May 2010	MSC, hESC-derived	Size-exclusion HPLC	Mouse model of MI/R injury	Reduced infarct size	19
Nov 2012	MSC, human umbilical cord	PEG precipitation, size exclusion chromatography	Mouse model of hypoxia-induced pulmonary hypertension	Suppressed inflammation, prevented increase in ventricular systolic pressure, ventricular hypertrophy and pulmonary vascular remodeling	70
Mar 2013	MSC, human umbilical cord	Sucrose gradient ultracentrifugation	Mouse model of CCl₄-induced liver fibrosis	Inhibited hepatocyte apoptosis, alleviated fibrosis	68
Dec 2013	MSC, rat bone marrow	Sucrose gradient ultracentrifugation	Rat model of middle cerebral artery occlusion	Promoted neurite outgrowth of neurons and astrocytes	67
Apr 2014	MSC, human bone marrow	PEG precipitation, ultracentrifugation	Human GvHD	Reduced diarrhea volume, reduced cutaneous and mucosal GvHD severity	71

Date	Source	Isolation	Model	Outcome	Ref
Jun 2014	MSC, hESC-derived	Size-exclusion HPLC	Mouse model of CCl$_4$-induced liver injury	Reduced serum aspartate aminotransferase and alanine aminotransferase, reduced hepatic necrosis	69
Jun 2014	MSC, human umbilical cord	Sucrose gradient ultracentrifugation	Rat model of skin deep second degree burn wound	Promoted skin cell proliferation and re-epithelialization	66
Other stem cell sources					
Oct 2013	NSC line, human	Ultracentrifugation	N/A, *in vitro* assays	Improved wound closure in scratch assay, stimulated angiogenesis and neurite outgrowth	73
May 2014	CDCs, human	ExoQuick™	Mouse models of acute and chronic myocardial infarction	Improved left ventricle ejection fraction, reduced scar mass and proinflammatory cytokines	72

CTB-binding activity were found to co-localize with exosome-associated proteins such as CD81, CD91, Alix, and Tsg101.

15.3.2 *Biological activity of MSC exosomes correlates with their therapeutic activity*

An important corollary for the therapeutic potential of MSC exosomes is that the reported therapeutic efficacy of MSCs or MSC exosomes is underpinned by the biological activity of exosomes. As a first principle approach to elucidate the biological activity of MSC exosomes, we interrogated the proteome of MSC exosome by mass spectrometry and antibody array to identify 857 unique gene products (www.exocarta.org).[75] These proteins are distributed over a wide array of biochemical and cellular processes such as communication, structure and mechanics, inflammation, exosome biogenesis, tissue repair and regeneration, and metabolism. Many of the proteins are biochemically active enzymes or enzyme complexes. This wide distribution of protein function provides a molecular rationale for the widely ranging therapeutic efficacy of MSCs. However, the molecular mechanism of action of MSC exosomes in reducing specific tissue injury and enhancing tissue repair remains to be resolved. We propose that MSC exosomes have the potential to elicit injury-specific response. This potential is derived not only from the large complex exosome proteome but also from the enzyme-rich proteome. As enzymes are active only when their substrates are present, exosomal enzymes will be activated only in those injuries of tissue where substrates for the enzymes are present.

15.3.2.1 *Enhancing bioenergetics and redox homeostasis*

The first reported therapeutic efficacy of MSC exosomes is the reduction of infarct size in mouse model of acute MI/R injury.[74] MI/R injury is caused paradoxically by the restoration of blood and oxygen to ischemic heart tissue and is proportional to the duration of the ischemia. During ischemia, oxygen deprivation inhibits oxidative phosphorylation and consequently, aerobic ATP production. The heart which has the highest basal ATP consumption rate in a resting body derives most of its ATP from oxidative phosphorylation[76] and is particularly susceptible during ischemia. The lack of oxygen during ischemia disrupts ATP supply and curtails important ATP-dependent cellular activities such as muscle contraction, protein synthesis and turnover, gene transcription, ion pumps or transporters[77] leading to increasing deranged cellular activities that include loss of cellular homeostasis, accumulation of metabolic waste, and eventually cell death.[76, 78–81] While reperfusion to restore blood flow and oxygen supply could rescue most ischemic cells, reperfusion paradoxically exacerbates injury in severely ischemic cells. These cells are depleted from many rate-limiting metabolic enzymes such as those in fatty acid oxidation, glycolysis, and tricarboxylic acid cycle.[82] This depletion prevents the cells from utilizing the restored oxygen supply to produce ATP after reperfusion. We have proposed that MSC exosomes alleviate this depletion by delivering their cargo of active glycolytic enzymes and other enzymes like adenylate kinase and nucleoside-diphosphate kinase to increase ATP production.[43,75,83] Although we have not demonstrated directly that functional enzymes are physically transferred from MSC exosomes into reperfused myocardium to increase ATP production, we had demonstrated that MSC exosomes are endocytosed by H9C2 muscle cells and exposure to MSC exosomes increased ATP level in oligomycin-treated cells where oxidative phosphorylation was inhibited. More importantly, ATP level was also elevated in exosome-treated reperfused myocardium in a mouse model.[84]

15.3.2.2 *Immune regulation*

The immunomodulatory activity of MSCs through suppressive and regulatory effects on both adaptive and innate immune cells in an autologous and allogeneic manner has been widely documented.[85] For example, MSCs were reported to inhibit proliferation of mitogen-activated T-cells,[86–90] induce an anti-inflammatory tolerant phenotype in DCs, naive and effector T-cells and natural killer (NK) cells[91] and inhibit B cell proliferation.[92] Consequently, MSCs are being tested for therapeutic efficacy against immune diseases such as Crohn's disease[93] and type 1 diabetes.[94] In fact, MSC has been approved as the first "off-the-shelf" stem cell based pharmaceutical drug for the treatment of pediatric GvHD in Canada and New Zealand.

Despite the clinical success of MSC transplantation in ameliorating severe immune diseases, the mechanism for this therapeutic efficacy remains tenuous. Although MSCs have shown to exert effects on various immune cells, e.g., T-cells, antigen–presenting cells (APCs), NK cells, and B cells,[95–97] the physiological relevance of these effects to the amelioration of immune diseases remains unknown. It was previously thought that MSCs alleviate GvHD through the inhibition of T-cell proliferation.[87,89,90,98–101] However, in a subsequent long term follow up study of GvHD patients treated with MSCs, no correlation between *in vitro* suppression by MSCs in mixed lymphocyte cultures and outcome was observed.[102] Subsequently, it was postulated that MSC modulates both innate and adaptive immune cells (reviewed[103]) possibly through paracrine secretion of trophic mediators (reviewed[104,105]). A proteomic profiling of the MSC secretome revealed >200 proteins which include many potential immune modulators.[106]

Over the years, many secreted immune modulators have been proposed as the mediator of MSC immunomodulatory activity.[107] Two such modulators were interferon-γ (IFN-γ)[108–110] and indoleamine 2,3-dioxygenase (IDO).[111] However, it was subsequently reported that the immunomodulatory activity of MSCs was not compromised by a lack of IDO production caused by either defective IFN-γ receptor 1 or IDO inhibitors.[112] Also, murine MSCs generally lack the IDO activity found in human MSCs.[113, 114] Additionally, the implication of inducible nitric–oxide synthase (iNOS) and nitric oxide in the inhibition of T-cell proliferation by murine MSCs[115] could not be extended to human MSCs which have minimal expression level of iNOS mRNA.[116] MSCs are also known to secrete many generic immuno–modulating factors such as transforming growth factor (TGF)-β1, hepatocyte growth factor (HGF), hemeoxygenase 1, IL-6, prostaglandin E2 (PGE2), and HLA-G596.[117–127] It is unlikely that any of these molecules alone could be responsible for MSC-mediated immunoregulation. A more likely scenario is that several of these molecules worked synergistically to elicit the MSC-induced immune response. In this regard, exosomes with its complex cargo containing many of these immunomodulatory molecules represent a likely candidate as the immunomodulatory paracrine factor.

Consistent with this hypothesis, we observed in our animal studies that MSC exosomes attenuate injury induced inflammatory response. For example, they reduced white blood cell count and cardiac infiltration of neutrophils and macrophages within one to three days after MI/R injury.[128] In addition, MSC exosomes induced the expression of high levels of anti-inflammatory cytokines and attenuated the expression of pro-inflammatory cytokines in THP-1 monocytes, reminiscent of an M2 macrophage phenotype that promotes tissue repair and limit injury. Furthermore, they delayed the rejection of allogeneic skin grafts in mice with a concomitant increase in Tregs.[129] Finally, complement-mediated lysis of sheep red blood cells was inhibited by MSC exosomes in a CD59-dependent manner, suggesting that CD59 present on the exosome membrane could inhibit complement activation and the formation of the membrane attack complex.[43] These observations highlight the immunomodulatory role of MSC exosomes and support their potential use in the treatment of pathological conditions associated with immune dysregulation, such as autoimmune diseases and chronic inflammation.

15.3.2.3 *Activating pro-survival signaling pathways*

The kinases Akt and Erk1/2 belong to two of the most important survival signaling pathways, namely Ras/Raf/MEK/ERK (MAPK) and PTEN/PI3K/AKT/mTOR.[130] Activation of these pathways has been shown to be important in tissue repair and amelioration of tissue injury including MI/R injury,[131] sepsis,[132] and epithelial wound.[133] Specifically for the heart, these kinases are termed the Reperfusion Injury Salvage Kinases (RISKs) and their pharmacological activation through insulin, insulin-like growth factor-1 (IGF-1), TGF-β1, cardiotrophin-1 (CT-1), urocortin, atorvastatin, and bradykinin during post-ischemic reperfusion protects the heart from MI/R injury by exerting an anti-apoptotic effect.[131,134] Incidentally, ischemic postconditioning which consists of repeated interruptions of coronary blood flow following ischemia is effective in limiting reperfusion injury in animals[135] and humans,[136–139] and is also associated with activation of PI3K-Akt and ERK1/2 pathways. Inhibition of either pathway by small molecules abrogated the protective effect of ischemic postconditioning.[140]

CD73, an ecto 5'nucleotidase identified in the proteome of MSC exosomes,[43] is the only enzyme known to hydrolyze extracellular AMP to adenosine.[141] Adenosine is an activator of ERK and AKT that has been shown to reduce MI/R injury in animals[140,142] and clinical trials.[143,144] During tissue trauma such as shear stress-induced hemolysis of red blood cells, working skeletal muscle, perfused heart or isolated heart muscle cells under hypoxic conditions, ATPs and ADPs are released into the extracellular space (reviewed[145]). The half-life of extracellular ATP and ADP in the blood is estimated to be less than one second[146] and 3.2 minutes,[147] respectively. They are rapidly degraded by ecto-enzymes into AMP, which is the substrate for CD73. Consistent with the presence of enzymatically active CD73, exposure of H9C2 cardiomyocytes to MSC exosomes and AMP resulted in phosphorylation of ERK1/2 and AKT. This phosphorylation was abolished in the presence of theophylline, a non-selective antagonist of A1, A2A, A2B, and A3 adenosine receptors.[148] We also observed that MSC exosome treatment elevated pAKT levels in the reperfused myocardium of mice.[128]

15.3.3   *Advantages of exosome-based over cell-based therapies*

The discovery of exosomes as a mediator of MSC therapeutic activity represents a paradigm shift that could potentially transform MSC therapy from a cell- to a biologic-based therapeutics. Biologics are more amenable to the development of "off-the-shelf" formulations using rigorously regulated and monitored manufacturing processes. This will translate into safer and better products for timely delivery to patients. For a cell-based therapy, the need to preserve cell viability adds inordinate layers of regulatory oversight on the manufacture, storage, transport, and delivery/transplantation of the therapeutic agent. In addition, the use of viable cells as therapeutics carries unique risks and challenges. These include the high risk of occlusion in the distal microvasculature as demonstrated by the intra-arterial administration of MSCs in mice which resulted in pulmonary embolism and death in 25–40% of the animals.[149] Another is the viability of transplanted cells which is advantageous in providing long term therapeutic potency. However, in event of adverse activity or disease resolution, treatment may not be readily terminated and reversed, leading to increased risks of tumor formation and immune reactions. For stem cells such as MSCs, their differentiation potential could generate inappropriate and potentially deleterious cell types. For example, transplanted MSCs were thought to differentiate into cardiac sympathetic nerve sprouting and contribute to deleterious proarrhythmic side effects.[150–152] Other complications of MSC transplantation were a high frequency (51.2%) of ossifications and/or calcifications.[153] Therefore, transforming a cell-based therapy into one that is based on the secreted product of the cells carries distinct advantages.

15.4 Exosome Modification for Drug Delivery

The engineering of exosomes as drug vehicles to carry specific cargoes and homing signals is an emerging field of exosome-based therapeutics (reviewed[44, 154–156]). While synthetic bilipid vesicles or liposomes have already been used successfully to deliver both hydrophilic and lipophilic pharmaceutical drugs and protect drugs against premature transformation and elimination, it is increasingly recognized that there may be superior naturally-occurring delivery vehicles such as exosomes. Unlike synthetic liposomes, exosomes are generally well tolerated by the immune system, have a natural tissue tropism to enter specific cell types, and a long circulating half-life (reviewed[157]). Exosomes have been successfully loaded with a variety of exogenous therapeutic agents, such as siRNA, miRNA, protein or peptide and small molecule drugs using various means including incubation, electroporation, chemical-based transfection, and overexpression in exosome-secreting cells. Targeted exosome delivery to specific recipient cells could also be further enhanced through the engineered expression of homing proteins or peptides on exosome surface, or by harnessing the endogenous homing capacity exosomes secreted by specific cell types. However, exosome-based drug delivery technology is still in its infancy and its utility remains to be determined.

15.4.1 *Cell source*

A key consideration in the therapeutic applications of exosomes is the cell source. The ideal source would possess the following attributes: (1) A reproducibly high exosome yield, (2) Highly proliferative with an infinite expansion capacity, and (3) Produces immunologically inert exosomes. Based on these parameters, MSCs qualify as ideal candidate producers of both therapeutic exosomes and exosomes for drug delivery. As an exosome producer, we had reported that MSC produces at least 10 times more CD81+ vesicles than any of several other cell lines.[154] This production of exosome by MSC was inversely correlated with the age of the donor tissue with the most prolific producer being MSCs derived from hESCs followed by fetal tissues, umbilical cord, and adult bone marrow.[158] Furthermore, this capacity to produce therapeutic exosomes was not compromised when the MSCs were immortalized by over-expressing MYC and its differentiation potential was reduced. As MSCs, unlike many cell types, are reportedly immune privileged and could be transplanted in allogeneic recipients without immune suppression[159–162] and are highly suited for the production of immunologically inert exosomes. Indeed, MSC exosomes do not express MHC class I or II molecules, or co-stimulatory molecules.[129]

15.4.2 *Safety profile of exosomes*

The study of exosomes is relatively new and their physiological function has not been fully appreciated. Although exosomes have been shown to be therapeutic, they have also been implicated in a wide spectrum of diseases from cancers and degenerative diseases to infectious diseases. MSC exosomes have been implicated in multiple myeloma progression.[163] Exosomes secreted by tumor cells have been shown to be capable of enhancing tumor or metastatic phenotype.[164–166] They are also implicated in the formation of disease-associated protein aggregates such as alpha-synuclein aggregates in Parkinson's disease[53, 167] and amyloid beta protein aggregates ($A\beta$) in Alzheimer disease.[168] It was also reported that during infection, with diverse infectious agents such as scrapie, viruses, and bacteria, cells secrete exosomes containing the infectious agent or its products and thus provide potential route for disseminating the infection.[16, 29, 169–173] Therefore, even though exosomes represent a less complex subunit of a cell, they should still be subjected to rigorous tests for ominous biological agents that originate from their cell sources.

15.4.3 *Exosome purification*

Another manufacturing consideration is exosome purification. Exosomes are conventionally purified by ultracentrifugation, ultra-filtration, and gel filtration.[174–177] While these techniques result in exosome enrichment, the preparation is usually contaminated with other large particulate matter such as protein aggregates and cell debris. Additionally, this method is time-consuming, requires expensive equipment, and has poor scalability. We have previously reported that the purity of the exosome preparation could be greatly enhanced by size exclusion high performance liquid chromatography (HPLC).[19, 178] However, this method similarly requires expensive equipment, and has poor scalability, and product yield. While immuno–affinity chromatography[179, 180] is highly scalable and could potentially enhance the purity of the exosome preparations, none of the known exosome-associated antigens are exclusive to exosomes and immuno–affinity-based isolation protocols could still purify protein complexes and other EVs. In addition, the non-physiological salt or pH concentration needed to extract exosomes from the immuno–affinity column could affect the biological activity of the exosomes. Recently, novel methods of exosome purification have surfaced. One of them involves "salting out" exosomes from conditioned medium (CM) by titrating it with 0.1 M acetate to pH 4.75. Precipitation is observed as the CM becomes turbid, and an exosome pellet is obtained after centrifugation at 5,000 g.[181] Another technique involves the use of a microfluidic device consisting of ciliated micropillars with porous silicon nanowires on their sidewalls. This technology claims to preferentially trap exosomes while filtering smaller proteins and cellular debris, and the exosomes can be effectively released by dissolving the nanowires in phosphate buffered saline (PBS).[182] Nevertheless, the purity and integrity of the exosomes purified by these new methods remain to be validated. In short, to date, there is no ideal, scalable, and cost-effective method for the purification of exosomes.

15.5 Conclusion

As a therapeutic agent, exosomes straddle the space of biologics and cell therapeutics. It is essentially a bag of biologics that is more akin to a cell, but does not have the essence of a cell, i.e., viability. In many respects, exosome resemble a cell in having the combinatorial potency of many biologics protected in a membrane–like structure that could potentially deliver the biologics to and into target cells. The important differentiating factor between an exosome and a cell is the viability. The viability of a cell may be advantageous in providing a continuous supply of therapeutics without the need for repeated dosing. However, this advantage is a serious risk parameter as transplanted cells cannot be easily retrieved, killed or stopped in event of an adverse outcome. Also, unlike biologics, the potency of cell therapeutics does not always correlate to the dose of potent agent, but is dependent on the viability and therapeutic vitality of cells after transplantation. In contrast, exosome is not viable and repeated dosing would be required for prolonged treatments, but exosome-based treatments can be easily stopped when the disease has resolved or there are adverse effects. In conclusion, exosome-based therapeutics could potentially synergize the best of biologic- and cell-based therapies.

References

1. Thery, C., Ostrowski, M., and Segura, E. Membrane vesicles as conveyors of immune responses. *Nat. Rev. Immunol.* 9(8), 581–593 (2009).
2. Duijvesz, D., Luider, T., Bangma, C.H. *et al.* Exosomes as biomarker treasure chests for prostate cancer. *Eur. Urol.* 59(5), 823–831 (2011).
3. Simpson, R.J., and Mathivanan, S. Extracellular microvesicles: The need for internationally recognised nomenclature and stringent purification criteria. *J. Proteomics Bioinform.* 5(2), ii–ii (2012). doi: 10.4172/jpb.10000e10.
4. Simons, M., and Raposo, G. Exosomes — vesicular carriers for intercellular communication. *Curr. Opin. Cell Biol.* 21(4), 575–581 (2009).
5. Tan, S.S., Yin, Y., Lee, T., *et al.* Therapeutic MSC exosomes are derived from lipid raft microdomains in the plasma membrane. *J. Extracell. Vesicles* 2 (2013). doi: 10.3402/jev.v2i0.22614.
6. Wubbolts, R., Leckie, R.S., Veenhuizen, P.T., *et al.* Proteomic and biochemical analyses of human B cell-derived exosomes. Potential implications for their function and multivesicular body formation. *J. Biol. Chem.* 278(13), 10963–10972 (2003).
7. de Gassart, A., Geminard, C., Fevrier, B., *et al.* Lipid raft-associated protein sorting in exosomes. *Blood* 102(13), 4336–4344 (2003).
8. Zakharova, L., Svetlova, M., and Fomina, A.F. T-cell exosomes induce cholesterol accumulation in human monocytes *via* phosphatidylserine receptor. *J. Cell. Physiol.* 212(1), 174–181 (2007).
9. Keller, S., Konig, A.K., Marme, F., *et al.* Systemic presence and tumor-growth promoting effect of ovarian carcinoma released exosomes. *Cancer Lett.* 278(1), 73–81 (2009).
10. Carmo, A., Pedro, M., Silva, E., *et al.* Platelet-derived exosomes: a new vascular redox signaling pathway. *Crit. Care* 7 (Suppl 3), P117 (2003).
11. Heijnen, H.F., Schiel, A.E., Fijnheer, R., *et al.* Activated platelets release two types of membrane vesicles: Microvesicles by surface shedding and exosomes derived from exocytosis of multivesicular bodies and alpha-granules. *Blood* 94(11), 3791–3799 (1999).
12. Raposo, G., Nijman, H.W., Stoorvogel, W., *et al.* B lymphocytes secrete antigen-presenting vesicles. *J. Exp. Med.* 183(3), 1161–1172 (1996).
13. Zitvogel, L., Regnault, A., Lozier, A., *et al.* Eradication of established murine tumors using a novel cell-free vaccine: dendritic cell-derived exosomes. *Nat. Med.* 4(5), 594–600 (1998).
14. Raposo, G., Tenza, D., Mecheri, S., *et al.* Accumulation of major histocompatibility complex class II molecules in mast cell secretory granules and their release upon degranulation. *Mol. Biol. Cell* 8(12), 2631–2645 (1997).
15. Peters, P.J., Geuze, H.J., Van Der Donk, H.A., *et al.* Molecules relevant for T cell-target cell interaction are present in cytolytic granules of human T lymphocytes. *Eur. J. Immunol.* 19(8), 1469-1475 (1989).
16. Fevrier, B., Vilette, D., Archer, F., *et al.* Cells release prions in association with exosomes. *Proc. Natl. Acad. Sci. USA* 101(26), 9683–9688 (2004).
17. Wolfers, J., Lozier, A., Raposo, G. *et al.* Tumor-derived exosomes are a source of shared tumor rejection antigens for CTL cross-priming. *Nat. Med.* 7(3), 297–303 (2001).

18. Le Bihan, M.C., Bigot, A., Jensen, S.S., *et al.* In-depth analysis of the secretome identifies three major independent secretory pathways in differentiating human myoblasts. *J. Proteomics* 77, 344–356 (2012).

19. Lai, R.C., Arslan, F., Lee, M.M., *et al.* Exosome secreted by MSC reduces myocardial ischemia/reperfusion injury. *Stem Cell Res.* 4(3), 214–222 (2010).

20. Sokolova, V., Ludwig, A-K., Hornung, S., *et al.* Characterisation of exosomes derived from human cells by nanoparticle tracking analysis and scanning electron microscopy. *Colloids Surf. B, Biointerfaces* 87(1), 146–150 (2011).

21. Clayton, A., Al-Taei, S., Webber, J., *et al.* Cancer Exosomes Express CD39 and CD73, Which Suppress T Cells through Adenosine Production. *J. Immunol.* 187(2), 676–683 (2011).

22. Sullivan, R., Saez, F., Girouard, J., *et al.* Role of exosomes in sperm maturation during the transit along the male reproductive tract. *Blood Cells Mol. Dis.* 35(1), 1–10 (2005).

23. Admyre, C., Grunewald, J., Thyberg, J., *et al.* Exosomes with major histocompatibility complex class II and co-stimulatory molecules are present in human BAL fluid. *Eur. Respir. J.* 22(4), 578–583 (2003).

24. Pisitkun, T., Shen, R.F., and Knepper, M.A. Identification and proteomic profiling of exosomes in human urine. *Proc. Natl. Acad. Sci. USA* 101(36), 13368–13373 (2004).

25. Caby, M.P., Lankar, D., Vincendeau-Scherrer, C., *et al.* Exosomal-like vesicles are present in human blood plasma. *Int. Immunol.* 17(7), 879–887 (2005).

26. Kapsogeorgou, E.K., Abu-Helu, R.F., Moutsopoulos, H.M., *et al.* Salivary gland epithelial cell exosomes: A source of autoantigenicribonucleoproteins. *Arthritis Rheum.* 52(5), 1517–1521 (2005).

27. Admyre, C., Johansson, S.M., Qazi, K.R., *et al.* Exosomes with immune modulatory features are present in human breast milk. *J. Immunol.* 179(3), 1969–1978 (2007).

28. Pan, B.T., and Johnstone, R.M. Fate of the transferrin receptor during maturation of sheep reticulocytes *in vitro*: Selective externalization of the receptor. *Cell* 33(3), 967–978 (1983).

29. Pegtel, D.M., Cosmopoulos, K., Thorley-Lawson, D.A., *et al.* Functional delivery of viral miRNAs *via* exosomes. *Proc. Natl. Acad. Sci. USA* 107(14), 6328–6333 (2010).

30. Faure, J., Lachenal, G., and Court, M., *et al.* Exosomes are released by cultured cortical neurones. *Mol. Cell. Neurosci.* 31(4), 642–648 (2006).

31. Lachenal, G., Pernet-Gallay, K., Chivet, M., *et al.* Release of exosomes from differentiated neurons and its regulation by synaptic glutamatergic activity. *Mol. Cell. Neurosci.* 46(2), 409–418 (2011).

32. Bakhti, M., Winter, C., and Simons, M. Inhibition of myelin membrane sheath formation by oligodendrocyte-derived exosome-like vesicles. *J. Biol. Chem.* 286(1), 787–796 (2011).

33. Vrijsen, K.R., Sluijter, J.P.G., Schuchardt, M.W.L., *et al.* Cardiomyocyte progenitor cell-derived exosomes stimulate migration of endothelial cells. *J. Cell. Mol. Med.* 14(5), 1064–1070 (2010).

34. Simpson, R.J., Jensen, S.S., and Lim, J.W. Proteomic profiling of exosomes: Current perspectives. *Proteomics* 8(19), 4083–4099 (2008).

35. Thery, C., Zitvogel, L., and Amigorena, S. Exosomes: Composition, biogenesis and function. *Nat. Rev. Immunol.* 2002; 2 (8): 569–579 (2002).

36. Stoorvogel, W., Kleijmeer, M.J., Geuze, H.J., *et al.* The biogenesis and functions of exosomes. *Traffic* 3(5), 321–330 (2002).

37. Andre, F., Schartz, N.E., Movassagh, M., *et al.* Malignant effusions and immunogenic tumour-derived exosomes. *Lancet* 360(9329), 295–305 (2002).

38. Dai, S., Wan, T., Wang, B., *et al.* More efficient induction of HLA-A*0201-restricted and carcinoembryonic antigen (CEA)-specific CTL response by immunization with exosomes prepared from heat-stressed CEA-positive tumor cells. *Clin. Cancer Res.* 11(20), 7554–7563 (2005).

39. Clayton, A., Mitchell, J.P., Court, J., *et al.* Human tumor-derived exosomes selectively impair lymphocyte responses to interleukin-2. *Cancer Res.* 67(15), 7458–7466 (2007).

40. Taylor, D.D., and Gercel-Taylor, C. MicroRNA signatures of tumor-derived exosomes as diagnostic biomarkers of ovarian cancer. *Gynecol. Oncol.* 110 (1), 13–21 (2008).

41. Park, J.E., Tan, H.S., Datta, A., *et al.* Hypoxic tumor cell modulates its microenvironment to enhance angiogenic and metastatic potential by secretion of proteins and exosomes. *Mol. Cell. Proteomics* 9(6), 1085–1099 (2010).

42. Diederick, D., Theo, L., Chris, H.B., *et al.* Exosomes as biomarker treasure chests for prostate cancer. *Eur. Urol.* 59(5), 823–831 (2010).

43. Lai, R.C., Yeo, R.W., Tan, S.S., *et al.* Mesenchymal stem cell exosomes: The future MSC-based therapy? In *Mesenchymal Stem Cell Therapy*. New York: Humana Press (2012).

44. Lai, R.C., Yeo, R.W., Tan, K.H., *et al.* Exosomes for drug delivery — a novel application for the mesenchymal stem cell. *Biotechnol. Adv.* 31(5), 543–551 (2013).

45. Thery, C., Duban, L., Segura, E., *et al.* Indirect activation of naive CD4+ T-cells by dendritic cell-derived exosomes. *Nat. Immunol.* 3(12), 1156–1162 (2002).

46. Andre, F., Chaput, N., Schartz, N.E., *et al.* Exosomes as potent cell-free peptide-based vaccine I. Dendritic cell-derived exosomes transfer functional MHC class I/peptide complexes to dendritic cells. *J. Immunol.* 172(4), 2126–2136 (2004).

47. Valadı, H., Ekstrom, K., Bossios, A. *et al.* Exosome-mediated transfer of mRNAs and microRNAs is a novel mechanism of genetic exchange between cells. *Nat. Cell Biol.* 9(6), 654–659 (2007).

48. Chen, T.S., Lai, R.C., Lee, M.M., *et al.* Mesenchymal stem cell secretes microparticles enriched in pre-microRNAs. *Nucleic Acids Res.* 38(1), 215–224 (2010).

49. Hood, J.L., San, R.S., and Wickline, S.A. Exosomes released by melanoma cells prepare sentinel lymph nodes for tumor metastasis. *Cancer Res.* 71(11), 3792–3801 (2011).

50. Alvarez-Erviti, L., Seow, Y., Yin, H., *et al.* Delivery of siRNA to the mouse brain by systemic injection of targeted exosomes. *Nat. Biotechnol.* 29(4), 341–345 (2011).

51. Giordano, A., Galderisi, U., and Marino, I.R. From the laboratory bench to the patient's bedside: An update on clinical trials with mesenchymal stem cells. *J. Cell. Physiol.* 211(1), 27–35 (2007).

52. Phinney, D.G., Prockop, D.J. Concise review: Mesenchymal stem/multipotent stromal cells: The state of transdifferentiation and modes of tissue repair — current views. *Stem Cells* 25(11), 2896–2902 (2007).

53. Ferrand, J., Noel, D., Lehours, P., *et al.* Human bone marrow-derived stem cells acquire epithelial characteristics through fusion with gastrointestinal epithelial cells. *PLoS One* 6(5), e19569 (2011).

54. Spees, J.L., Olson, S.D., Ylostalo, J., *et al.* Differentiation, cell fusion, and nuclear fusion during *ex vivo* repair of epithelium by human adult stem cells from bone marrow stroma. *Proc. Natl. Acad. Sci. USA* 100(5), 2397–2402 (2003).

55. Vassilopoulos, G., Wang, P.R., and Russell, D.W. Transplanted bone marrow regenerates liver by cell fusion. *Nature* 422(6934), 901–904 (2003).

56. Prockop, D.J. "Stemness" does not explain the repair of many tissues by mesenchymal stem/multipotent stromal cells (MSCs). *Clin. Pharmacol. Ther.* 82(3), 241–243 (2007).

57. da Silva Meirelles, L., Caplan, A.I., and Nardi, N.B. In search of the *in vivo* identity of mesenchymal stem cells. *Stem Cells* 26(9), 2287–2299 (2008).

58. Dai, W., Hale, S.L., Martin, B.J., *et al.* Allogeneic mesenchymal stem cell transplantation in postinfarcted rat myocardium: Short- and long-term effects. *Circulation* 112(2), 214–223 (2005).

59. Noiseux, N., Gnecchi, M., Lopez-Ilasaca, M., *et al.* Mesenchymal stem cells overexpressing Akt dramatically repair infarcted myocardium and improve cardiac function despite infrequent cellular fusion or differentiation. *Mol. Ther.* 14(6), 840–850 (2006).

60. Iso, Y., Spees, J.L., Serrano, C., *et al.* Multipotent human stromal cells improve cardiac function after myocardial infarction in mice without long-term engraftment. *Biochem. Biophys. Res. Commun.* 354(3), 700–706 (2007).

61. Caplan, A.I., and Dennis, J.E. Mesenchymal stem cells as trophic mediators. *J. Cell. Biochem.* 98(5), 1076–1084 (2006).

62. Yeo, R.W., Lai, R.C., Tan, K.H., *et al.* Exosome: A novel and safer therapeutic refinement of mesenchymal stem cell. *Exosomes Microvesicles* 1(7), 1–12 (2013).

63. Timmers, L., Lim, S-K., Arslan, F., *et al.* Reduction of myocardial infarct size by human mesenchymal stem cell conditioned medium. *Stem Cell Res.* 1, 129–137 (2008).

64. Timmers, L., Lim, S-K., Hoefer, I.E., *et al.* Human mesenchymal stem cell-conditioned medium improves cardiac function following myocardial infarction. *Stem Cell Res.* 6(3), 206–214 (2011).

65. Bruno, S., Grange, C., Deregibus, M.C., *et al.* Mesenchymal stem cell-derived microvesicles protect against acute tubular injury. *J. Am. Soc. Nephrol.* 20(5), 1053–1067 (2009).

66. Zhang, B., Wang, M., Gong, A., *et al.* HucMSC-exosome mediated-Wnt4 signaling is required for cutaneous wound healing. *Stem Cells* (2014).

67. Xin, H., Li, Y., Liu, Z., *et al.* MiR-133b promotes neural plasticity and functional recovery after treatment of stroke with multipotent mesenchymal stromal cells in rats via transfer of exosome-enriched extracellular particles. *Stem Cells* 31(12), 2737–2746 (2013).

68. Li, T., Yan, Y., Wang, B., *et al.* Exosomes derived from human umbilical cord mesenchymal stem cells alleviate liver fibrosis. *Stem Cells Dev.* 22(6), 845–854 (2013).

69. Tan, C.Y., Lai, R.C., Wong, W., *et al.* Mesenchymal stem cell-derived exosomes promote hepatic regeneration in drug-induced liver injury models. *Stem Cell Res. Ther.* 5(3), 76 (2014).

70. Lee, C., Mitsialis, S.A., Aslam, M., *et al.* Exosomes mediate the cytoprotective action of mesenchymal stromal cells on hypoxia-induced pulmonary hypertension. *Circulation* 126(22), 2601–2611 (2012).

71. Kordelas, L., Rebmann, V., Ludwig, A.K., *et al.* MSC-derived exosomes: A novel tool to treat therapy-refractory graft-versus-host disease. *Leukemia* 28(4), 970–973 (2014).

72. Ibrahim, A.G., Cheng, K., and Marban, E. Exosomes as critical agents of cardiac regeneration triggered by cell therapy. *Stem Cell Rep.* 2(5), 606–619 (2014).

73. Sinden, J., Stevanato, L., and Corteling, R. Stem cell microparticles. *Google Patents* PCT/GB2013/050879 (2013).

74. Lai, R.C., Arslan, F., Lee, M.M., *et al.* Exosome secreted by MSC reduces myocardial ischemia/reperfusion injury. *Stem Cell Res.* 4, 214–222 (2010).

75. Lai, R.C., Tan, S.S., the, B.J. *et al.* Proteolytic potential of the MSC exosome proteome: Implications for an exosome-mediated delivery of therapeutic proteasome. *Int. J. Proteomics* 2012, 971907 (2012).

76. Rosano, G.M., Fini, M., Caminiti, G., *et al.* Cardiac metabolism in myocardial ischemia. *Curr. Pharm. Des.* 14(25), 2551–2562 (2008).

77. Frank, A., Bonney, M., Bonney, S., *et al.* Myocardial ischemia reperfusion injury. *Semin. Cardiothorac. Vasc. Anesth.* 16(3), 123–132 (2012).

78. Inserte, J., Garcia-Dorado, D., Ruiz-Meana, M., *et al.* Effect of inhibition of Na+/Ca2+ exchanger at the time of myocardial reperfusion on hypercontracture and cell death. Cardiovasc. Res. 55(4), 739–748 (2002).

79. Garnier, A., Fortin, D., Delomeïnie, C., *et al.* Depressed mitochondrial transcription factors and oxidative capacity in rat failing cardiac and skeletal muscles. *J. Physiol.* 551(2), 491–501 (2003).

80. Jennings, R.B., and Reimer, K.A. The cell biology of acute myocardial ischemia. *Annu. Rev. Med.* 42, 225–246 (1991).

81. Gurusamy, N., Goswami, S., Malik, G., *et al.* Oxidative injury induces selective rather than global inhibition of proteasomal activity. *J. Mol. Cell. Cardiol.* 44(2), 419–428 (2008).

82. Li, X., Arslan, F., Ren, Y., *et al.* Metabolic adaptation to a disruption in oxygen supply during myocardial ischemia and reperfusion is underpinned by temporal and quantitative changes in the cardiac proteome. *J. Proteome Res.* 11(4), 2331–2346 (2012).

83. Lai, R.C., Yeo, R.W., Tan, K.H., *et al.* Mesenchymal stem cell exosome ameliorates reperfusion injury through proteomic complementation. *Regen. Med.* 8(2), 197–209 (2013).

84. Crisan, M., Corselli, M., Chen, C.W., *et al.* Multilineage stem cells in the adult: A perivascular legacy? *Organogenesis* 7(2), 101–104 (2011).

85. Marigo, I., and Dazzi, F. The immunomodulatory properties of mesenchymal stem cells. *Semin. Immunopathol.* 33(6), 593–602 (2011).

86. Potian, J.A., Aviv, H., Ponzio, N.M., *et al.* Veto-like activity of mesenchymal stem cells: Functional discrimination between cellular responses to alloantigens and recall antigens. *J. Immunol.* 171(7), 3426–3434 (2003).

87. Tse, W.T., Pendleton, J.D., Beyer, W.M., *et al.* Suppression of allogeneic T-cell proliferation by human marrow stromal cells: Implications in transplantation. *Transplantation* 75(3), 389–397 (2003).

88. Bartholomew, A., Sturgeon, C., Siatskas, M., *et al.* Mesenchymal stem cells suppress lymphocyte proliferation *in vitro* and prolong skin graft survival *in vivo. Exp. Hematol.* 30(1), 42–48 (2002).

89. Di Nicola, M., Carlo-Stella, C., Magni, M., *et al.* Human bone marrow stromal cells suppress T-lymphocyte proliferation induced by cellular or nonspecific mitogenic stimuli. *Blood* 99(10), 3838–3843 (2002).

90. Le Blanc, K., Tammik, L., Sundberg, B., *et al.* Mesenchymal stem cells inhibit and stimulate mixed lymphocyte cultures and mitogenic responses independently of the major histocompatibility complex. *Scand. J. Immunol.* 57(1), 11–20 (2003).

91. Aggarwal, S., and Pittenger, M.F. Human mesenchymal stem cells modulate allogeneic immune cell responses. *Blood* 105(4), 1815–1822 (2005).

92. Corcione, A., Benvenuto, F., Ferretti, E., *et al.* Human mesenchymal stem cells modulate B-cell functions. *Blood* 107(1), 367–372 (2006).

93. Newman, R.E., Yoo, D., LeRoux, M.A., *et al.* Treatment of inflammatory diseases with mesenchymal stem cells. *Inflamm. Allergy Drug Targets* 8(2), 110–123 (2009).

94. Wu, H., and Mahato, R.I. Mesenchymal stem cell-based therapy for type 1 diabetes. *Discov. Med.* 17(93), 139–143 (2014).

95. Le Blanc, K., and Ringden, O. Immunobiology of human mesenchymal stem cells and future use in hematopoietic stem cell transplantation. *Biol. Blood Marrow Transplant.* 11(5), 321–334 (2005).

96. Aggarwal, S., and Pittenger, M. Human mesenchymal stem cells modulate allogeneic immune cell responses. *Blood* 105, 1815–1822 (2005).

97. Meisel, R., Zibert, A., Laryea, M., *et al.* Human bone marrow stromal cells inhibit allogeneic T-cell responses by indoleamine 2, 3-dioxygenase-mediated tryptophan degradation. *Blood* 103, 4619–4621 (2004).

98. Groh, M.E., Maitra, B., Szekely, E., *et al.* Human mesenchymal stem cells require monocyte-mediated activation to suppress alloreactive T-cells. *Exp. Hematol.* 33(8), 928–934 (2005).

99. Krampera, M., Glennie, S., Dyson, J., *et al.* Bone marrow mesenchymal stem cells inhibit the response of naive and memory antigen-specific T-cells to their cognate peptide. *Blood* 101(9), 3722–3729 (2003).

100. Majumdar, M.K., Keane-Moore, M., Buyaner, D., *et al.* Characterization and functionality of cell surface molecules on human mesenchymal stem cells. *J. Biomed. Sci.* 10(2), 228–241 (2003).

101. Rasmusson, I., Ringden, O., Sundberg, B., *et al.* Mesenchymal stem cells inhibit the formation of cytotoxic T lymphocytes, but not activated cytotoxic T lymphocytes or natural killer cells. *Transplantation* 76(8), 1208–13 (2003).

102. von Bahr, L., Sundberg, B., Lonniesm, L., *et al.* Long-term complications, immunologic effects, and role of passage for outcome in mesenchymal stromal cell therapy. *Biol. Blood Marrow Transplant.* 18(4), 557–564 (2012).

103. Le Blanc, K., and Mougiakakos, D. Multipotent mesenchymal stromal cells and the innate immune system. *Nat. Rev. Immunol.* 12(5), 383–396 (2012).

104. Tolar, J., Le Blanc, K., Keating, A., *et al.* Concise review: hitting the right spot with mesenchymal stromal cells. *Stem Cells* 28(8), 1446–1455 (2010).

105. Lai, R.C., Yeo, R.W.Y., Tan, S.S., *et al.* Mesenchymal stem cell exosomes: The future MSC-based therapy? In *Mesenchymal Stem Cell Therapy.* New York: Springer (2013).

106. Sze, S.K., de Kleijn, D.P., Lai, R.C., *et al.* Elucidating the secretion proteome of human embryonic stem cell-derived mesenchymal stem cells. *Mol. Cell. Proteomics* 6(10), 1680–1689 (2007).

107. Ghannam, S., Bouffi, C., Djouad, F., *et al.* Immunosuppression by mesenchymal stem cells: Mechanisms and clinical applications. *Stem Cell Res. Ther.* 1(1), 2 (2010).

108. Rasmusson, I., Ringden, O., Sundberg, B., *et al.* Mesenchymal stem cells inhibit lymphocyte proliferation by mitogens and alloantigens by different mechanisms. *Exp. Cell Res.* 305(1), 33–41 (2005).

109. Kang, H.S., Habib, M., Chan, J., *et al.* A paradoxical role for IFN-γ in the immune properties of mesenchymal stem cells during viral challenge. *Exp. Hematol.* 33(7), 796–803 (2005).

110. Krampera, M. Role for interferon-γ in the immunomodulatory activity of human bone marrow mesenchymal stem cells. *Stem Cells* 24, 386–398 (2006).

111. Meisel, R., Zibert, A., Laryea, M., *et al.* Human bone marrow stromal cells inhibit allogeneic T-cell responses by indoleamine 2, 3-dioxygenase-mediated tryptophan degradation. *Blood* 103(12), 4619–4621 (2004).

112. Gieseke, F., Schütt, B., Viebahn, S., *et al.* Human multipotent mesenchymal stromal cells inhibit proliferation of PBMCs independently of IFNγR1 signaling and IDO expression. *Blood* 110(6), 2197–2200 (2007).

113. Djouad, F., Charbonnier, L-M., Bouffi, C., *et al.* Mesenchymal stem cells inhibit the differentiation of dendritic cells through an interleukin-6-dependent mechanism. *Stem Cells* 25(8), 2025–2032 (2007).

114. Ren, G., Su, J., Zhang, L., *et al.* Species variation in the mechanisms of mesenchymal stem cell-mediated immunosuppression. *Stem Cells* 27(8), 1954–1962 (2009).

115. Sato, K., Ozaki, K., Oh, I., *et al.* Nitric oxide plays a critical role in suppression of T-cell proliferation by mesenchymal stem cells. *Blood* 109(1), 228–234 (2007).

116. Ren, G., Su, J., Zhang, L., *et al.* Species variation in the mechanisms of mesenchymal stem cell-mediated immunosuppression. *Stem Cells* 27(8), 1954–1962 (2009).

117. Chabannes, D., Hill, M., Merieau, E., *et al.* A role for heme oxygenase-1 in the immunosuppressive effect of adult rat and human mesenchymal stem cells. *Blood* 110, 3691–3694 (2007).

118. Di Nicola, M., Carlo-Stella, C., Magni, M., *et al.* Human bone marrow stromal cells suppress T-lymphocyte proliferation induced by cellular or non-specific mitogenic stimuli. *Blood* 99, 3838–3843 (2002).

119. Djouad, F., Charbonnier, L., Bouffi, C., *et al.* Mesenchymal stem cells inhibit the differentiation of dendritic cells through an interleukin-6-dependent mechanism. *Stem Cells* 25, 2025–2032 (2007).

120. Jiang, X., Zhang, Y., Liu, B., *et al.* Human mesenchymal stem cells inhibit differentiation and function of monocyte derived dendritic cells. *Blood* 105, 4120–4126 (2005).

121. Nasef, A., Mazurier, C., Bouchet, S., *et al.* Leukemia inhibitory factor: Role in human mesenchymal stem cells mediated immunosuppression. *Cell. Immunol.* 253, 16–22 (2008).

122. Nasef, A., Zhang, Y., Mazurier, C., *et al.* Selected Stro-1-enriched bone marrow stromal cells display a major suppressive effect on lymphocyte proliferation. *Int. J. Lab. Hematol.* 31, 9–19 (2009).

123. Nemeth, K., Leelahavanichkul, A., Yuen, P., *et al.* Bone marrow stromal cells attenuate sepsis *via* prostaglandin E2-dependent reprogramming of host macrophages to increase their interleukin-10 production. *Nat. Med.* 15, 42–49 (2009).

124. Raffaghello, L., Bianchi, G., Bertolotto, M., *et al.* Human mesenchymal stem cells inhibit neutrophil apoptosis: A model for neutrophil preservation in the bone marrow niche. *Stem Cells* 26, 151–162 (2008).

125. Selmani, Z., Naji, A., Zidi, I., *et al.* Human leukocyte antigen-G5 secretion by human mesenchymal stem cells is required to suppress T lymphocyte and natural killer function and to induce CD4+ CD25 high Foxp3+ regulatory T cells. *Stem Cells* 26, 212–222 (2008).

126. Spaggiari, G., Abdelrazik, H., Becchetti, F., *et al.* MSCs inhibit monocyte derived DC maturation and function by selectively interfering with the generation of immature DCs: Central role of MSC-derived prostaglandin E2. *Blood* 113, 6576–6583 (2009).

127. Xu, G., Zhang, Y., Zhang, L., *et al.* The role of IL-6 in inhibition of lymphocyte apoptosis by mesenchymal stem cells. *Biochem. Biophys. Res. Commun.* 361, 745–750 (2007).

128. Arslan, F., Lai, R.C., Smeets, M.B., *et al.* Mesenchymal stem cell-derived exosomes increase ATP levels, decrease oxidative stress and activate PI3K/Akt pathway to enhance myocardial viability and prevent adverse remodeling after myocardial ischemia/reperfusion injury. *Stem Cell Res.* 10(3), 301–312 (2013).

129. Zhang, B., Yin, Y., Lai, R.C., *et al.* Mesenchymal stem cells secrete immunologically active exosomes. *Stem Cells Dev.* (2014).

130. Steelman, L.S., Chappell, W.H., Abrams, S.L., *et al.* Roles of the Raf/MEK/ERK and PI3K/PTEN/Akt/mTOR pathways in controlling growth and sensitivity to therapy-implications for cancer and aging. *Aging (Albany NY)* 3(3), 192–222 (2011).

131. Hausenloy, D.J., and Yellon, D.M. New directions for protecting the heart against ischaemia-reperfusion injury: Targeting the reperfusion injury salvage kinase (RISK)-pathway. *Cardiovasc. Res.* 61(3), 448–460 (2004).

132. McDunn, J.E., Muenzer, J.T., Rachdi, L., *et al.* Peptide-mediated activation of Akt and extracellular regulated kinase signaling prevents lymphocyte apoptosis. *FASEB J.* 22(2), 561–568 (2008).

133. Yin, J., Xu, K., Zhang, J., *et al.* Wound-induced ATP release and EGF receptor activation in epithelial cells. *J. Cell Sci.* 120(Pt 5), 815–825 (2007).

134. Hausenloy, D.J., and Yellon, D.M. Reperfusion injury salvage kinase signalling: Taking a RISK for cardioprotection. *Heart Fail. Rev.* 12(3–4), 217–234 (2007).

135. Zhao, Z-Q., Corvera, J.S., Halkos, M.E., *et al.* Inhibition of myocardial injury by ischemic postconditioning during reperfusion: Comparison with ischemic preconditioning. *Am. J. Physiol. Heart Circ. Physiol.* 285(2), H579–H588 (2003).

136. Staat, P., Rioufol, G., Piot, C., *et al.* Postconditioning the human heart. *Circulation* 112(14), 2143–2148 (2005).

137. Lønborg, J., Kelbæk, H., Vejlstrup, N., *et al.* Cardioprotective effects of ischemic postconditioning in patients treated with primary percutaneous coronary intervention, evaluated by magnetic resonance/clinical perspective. *Circ. Cardiovasc. Interven.* 3(1), 34–41 (2010).

138. Yang, X.C., Liu, Y., Wang, L.F., *et al.* Reduction in myocardial infarct size by postconditioning in patients after percutaneous coronary intervention. *J. Invasive Cardiol.* 19(10), 424–430 (2007).

139. Thibault, H., Piot, C., Staat, P., *et al.* Long-term benefit of postconditioning. *Circulation* 117(8), 1037–1044 (2008).

140. Zhao, Z.Q., and Vinten-Johansen, J. Postconditioning: Reduction of reperfusion-induced injury. *Cardiovasc. Res.* 70(2), 200–211 (2006).

141. Colgan, S.P., Eltzschig, H.K., Eckle, T., *et al.* Physiological roles for ecto-5'-nucleotidase (CD73). *Purinergic Signal* 2(2), 351–360 (2006).
142. Gross, E.R., and Gross, G.J. Ligand triggers of classical preconditioning and postconditioning. Cardiovasc. Res. 70(2), 212–221 (2006).
143. Forman, M.B., Stone, G.W., and Jackson, E.K. Role of adenosine as adjunctive therapy in acute myocardial infarction. *Cardiovasc. Drug Rev.* 24(2), 116–147 (2006).
144. Headrick, J.P., and Lasley, R.D. Adenosine receptors and reperfusion injury of the heart. *Handb. Exp. Pharmacol.* (193), 189–214 (2009). doi: 10.1007/978-3-540-89615-9_7.
145. Luthje, J. Origin, metabolism and function of extracellular adenine nucleotides in the blood. *Klin. Wochenschr.* 67(6), 317–327 (1989).
146. Chekeni, F.B., Elliott, M.R., Sandilos, J.K., *et al.* Pannexin 1 channels mediate/'find-me'/signal release and membrane permeability during apoptosis. *Nature* 467(7317), 863–867 (2010).
147. Luthje, J., and Ogilvie, A. Catabolism of Ap4A and Ap3A in whole blood. The dinucleotides are long-lived signal molecules in the blood ending up as intracellular ATP in the erythrocytes. *Eur. J. Biochem.* 173(1), 241–245 (1988).
148. Jacobson, K.A. Introduction to adenosine receptors as therapeutic targets. *Handb. Exp. Pharmacol.* (193), 1–24 (2009). doi: 10.1007/978-3-540-89615-9_1.
149. Furlani, D., Ugurlucan, M., Ong, L., *et al.* Is the intravascular administration of mesenchymal stem cells safe? Mesenchymal stem cells and intravital microscopy. *Microvasc. Res.* 77(3), 370–376 (2009).
150. Chang, M.G., Tung, L., Sekar, R.B., *et al.* Proarrhythmic potential of mesenchymal stem cell transplantation revealed in an *in vitro* coculture model. *Circulation* 113(15), 1832–1841 (2006).
151. Pak, H.N., Qayyum, M., Kim, D.T., *et al.* Mesenchymal stem cell injection induces cardiac nerve sprouting and increased tenascin expression in a swine model of myocardial infarction. *J. Cardiovasc. Electrophysiol.* 14(8), 841–848 (2003).
152. Price, M.J., Chou, C.C., Frantzen, M., *et al.* Intravenous mesenchymal stem cell therapy early after reperfused acute myocardial infarction improves left ventricular function and alters electrophysiologic properties. *Int. J. Cardiol.* 111(2), 231–239 (2006)
153. Breitbach, M., Bostani, T., Roell, W., *et al.* Potential risks of bone marrow cell trans plantation into infarcted hearts. *Blood* 110(4), 1362–1369 (2007).
154. Yeo, R.W., Lai, R.C., Zhang, B., *et al.* Mesenchymal stem cell: An efficient mass producer of exosomes for drug delivery. *Adv. Drug Deliv. Rev.* 65(3), 336–341 (2013).
155. Johnsen, K.B., Gudbergsson, J.M., Skov, M.N., *et al.* A comprehensive overview of exosomes as drug delivery vehicles- endogenous nanocarriers for targeted cancer therapy. *Biochim. Biophys. Acta* 2014.
156. Marcus, M.E., and Leonard, J.N. Fed exosomes: Engineering therapeutic biological nanoparticles that truly deliver. *Pharmaceuticals (Basel)* 6(5), 659–680 (2013).
157. Yoo, J-W., Irvine, D.J., Discher, D.E., *et al.* Bio-inspired, bioengineered and biomimetic drug delivery carriers. *Nat. Rev. Drug Discov.* 10(7), 521–535 (2011).
158. Chen, T.S., Yeo, R.W.Y., Arslan, F., *et al.* Efficiency of exosome production correlates inversely with the developmental maturity of MSC donor. *J. Stem Cell Res. Ther.* 3(3), 145 (2013).
159. Le Blanc, K., and Pittenger, M.F. Mesenchymal stem cells: Progress toward promise. *Cytotherapy* 7(1), 36–45 (2005).

160. Brooke, G., Cook, M., Blair, C., *et al.* Therapeutic applications of mesenchymal stromal cells. *Semin. Cell Dev. Biol.* 18(6), 846–858 (2007).

161. Bernardo, M.E., Pagliara, D., Locatelli, F. Mesenchymal stromal cell therapy: A revolution in regenerative medicine? *Bone Marrow Transplant.* 47(2), 164–171 (Feb 2012).

162. Salem, H.K., and Thiemermann, C. Mesenchymal stromal cells: Current understanding and clinical status. *Stem Cells* 28(3), 585–596 (2010).

163. Roccaro, A.M., Sacco, A., Maiso, P., *et al.* BM mesenchymal stromal cell-derived exosomes facilitate multiple myeloma progression. *J. Clin. Invest.* 123(4), 1542–1555 (2013).

164. Hao, S., Ye, Z., Li, F., *et al.* Epigenetic transfer of metastatic activity by uptake of highly metastatic B16 melanoma cell-released exosomes. *Exp. Oncol.* 28(2), 126–131 (2006).

165. Peinado, H., Aleckovic, M., Lavotshkin, S., *et al.* Melanoma exosomes educate bone marrow progenitor cells toward a pro-metastatic phenotype through MET. *Nat. Med.* 18(6), 883–891 (2012).

166. Meckes, D.G.Jr., Shair, K.H., Marquitz, A.R., *et al.* Human tumor virus utilizes exosomes for intercellular communication. *Proc. Natl. Acad. Sci. USA* 107(47), 20370–20375 (2010).

167. Bernardo, M.E., Pagliara, D., and Locatelli, F. Mesenchymal stromal cell therapy: A revolution in regenerative medicine? *Bone Marrow Transplant.* 47(2), 164–171 (2012).

168. Rajendran, L., Honsho, M., Zahn, T.R., *et al.* Alzheimer's disease beta-amyloid peptides are released in association with exosomes. *Proc. Natl. Acad. Sci. USA* 103(30), 11172–11177 (2006).

169. Fevrier, B., Vilette, D., Laude, H., *et al.* Exosomes: A bubble ride for prions? *Traffic* 6(1), 10–17 (2005).

170. Porto-Carreiro, I., Fevrier, B., Paquet, S., *et al.* Prions and exosomes: From PrPc trafficking to PrPsc propagation. *Blood Cells Mol. Dis.* 35(2), 143–148 (2005).

171. Bhatnagar, S., and Schorey, J.S. Exosomes released from infected macrophages contain Mycobacterium aviumglycopeptidolipids and are proinflammatory. *J. Biol. Chem.* 282(35), 25779–25789 (2007).

172. Lenassi, M., Cagney, G., Liao, M., *et al.* HIV Nef is secreted in exosomes and triggers apoptosis in bystander CD4+ T-cells. *Traffic* 11(1), 110–122 (2010).

173. Vallhov, H., Gutzeit, C., Johansson, S.M., *et al.* Exosomes containing glycoprotein 350 released by EBV-transformed B cells selectively target B cells through CD21 and block EBV infection *in vitro. J. Immunol.* 186(1), 73–82 (2011).

174. Denzer, K., Kleijmeer, M.J., Heijnen, H.F., *et al.* Exosome: From internal vesicle of the multivesicular body to intercellular signaling device. *J. Cell Sci.* 113(Pt 19), 3365–3374 (2000).

175. Zitvogel, L., Regnault, A., Lozier, A., *et al.* Eradication of established murine tumors using a novel cell-free vaccine: Dendritic cell derived exosomes. *Nat. Med.* 4(5), 594–600 (1998).

176. Lamparski, H.G., Metha-Damani, A., Yao, J-Y., *et al.* Production and characterization of clinical grade exosomes derived from dendritic cells. *J. Immunol. Methods* 270(2), 211–226 (2002).

177. Simpson, R.J., and Mathivanan, S. Extracellular microvesicles: The need for internationally recognised nomenclature and stringent purification criteria. *J. Proteomics Bioinform.* 5, 2 (2012).

178. Lai, R.C., Arslan, F., Tan, S.S., *et al.* Derivation and characterization of human fetal MSCs: An alternative cell source for large-scale production of cardioprotective microparticles. *J. Mol. Cell. Cardiol.* 48(6), 1215–1224 (2010).

179. Clayton, A., Court, J., Navabi, H., *et al.* Analysis of antigen presenting cell derived exosomes, based on immuno-magnetic isolation and flow cytometry. *J. Immunol. Methods* 247(1–2), 163–174 (2001).

180. Mathivanan, S., Lim, J.W.E., Tauro, B.J., *et al.* Proteomics analysis of A33 immunoaffinity-purified exosomes released from the human colon tumor cell line LIM1215 reveals a tissue-specific protein signature. *Mol. Cell. Proteomics* 9(2), 197–208 (2010).

181. Brownlee, Z., Lynn, K.D., Thorpe, P.E., *et al.* A novel "salting-out" procedure for the isolation of tumor-derived exosomes. *J. Immunol. Methods* (2014).

182. Wang, Z., Wu, H.J., Fine, D., *et al.* Ciliated micropillars for the microfluidic-based isolation of nanoscale lipid vesicles. *Lab Chip* 13(15), 2879–2882 (2013).

Commercial and Business Aspects of Cell Therapy — Start-Up to Market

16

Stefanos Theoharis

16.1 Introduction

The last decade has been transformational in the field of cell therapy and a large number of crucial milestones have been achieved.[1] Many new treatments based on cells have entered the clinic, of which some have by now garnered marketing authorization (MA), and many of these therapeutic technologies have been the subject of a significant effort by the scientific community to study, understand, and improve therapeutic outcomes. With continuous improvements and an ever evolving understanding of how to develop safe and efficient cell therapeutics, it is likely that the pharmaceutical industry is currently witnessing the first makings of a new revolution in healthcare.

For the cell therapy field to fulfill its potential, companies and research institutions must successfully bridge the gap between the lab, where their cell therapy innovations originate, and the market, where patients are in need, often a significant unmet medical need. Here, the old "bench to bedside" cliché applies well. For all pharmaceuticals, this is a long, complex, and expensive process, fraught with risk and uncertainty. This is more so the case for cell therapies that work differently and, being an emerging technology, have relatively limited clinical proof of concept (POC), so far, compared with established therapeutic modalities such as small molecules and biologics.

16.2　Financing and Funding Operations

To bring a cell therapy product to market, the investigators must develop a discovery to manufacture a drug, a product that can be manufactured consistently and reproducibly for a global market and they must conduct regulated clinical trials to prove that it is safe and effective. These topics are discussed in this book in great detail and it becomes evident that such activities are considerably expensive. Most cell therapy companies are still in development stages, many already in clinical development. Their only source of finance funding for their activities is through investors, partnerships, and research grants.

16.2.1　*Investment*

Companies attract investors by offering to sell them a percentage of the company for an agreed company valuation. The investors subsequently become shareholders of the company, alongside its founders and the company therefrom belongs to all the shareholders. The two main types of investors are public and private.

16.2.1.1　*Private investors*

This list includes venture capital (VC), private Equity (PE), or so called "Angel Investors", high net worth individuals acting alone or organized in groups, investing directly in a company. VC investors are a very common source of early capital, as well as subsequent funding rounds. Many large pharmaceutical companies are also active in VC investments, in their areas of interest, through their own Corporate Venture Capital (CVC) or Corporate Venture Funds (CVFs).

Crowd funding is a new trend that helps companies attract multiple (often hundreds, or thousands) of private investors. It is a relatively new and largely untested scheme which has so far not made a significant impact in life sciences.

16.2.1.2　*Public investors*

Public investors buy shares in the companies whose shares are listed in public stock markets. For a company to offer its shares in the public markets, it must first perform an Initial Public Offering (IPO). A public company can subsequently issue and sell new shares, either in "secondary" public offerings in the markets, or directly to private investors. Many cell therapy companies, especially those in the more expensive, later stages of clinical development, have opted to enlist their shares in public markets. Table 16.2 is a list of some notable companies in the cell therapy space and also contain information about their ownership. Conditions in 2013 and 2014 have been particularly fertile for companies wishing to go the IPO route, following years of difficult market conditions, due to many reasons, one of them being the JOBS ("Jumpstart Our Business Start-ups") Act, voted by congress in the US in 2013 to facilitate access to capital for small companies (https://www.sec.gov/spotlight/jobs-act.shtml).

16.2.1.3 *Investment approaches*

Most investors, public or private, will mitigate their risk by spreading their funds in a broad portfolio of companies, assuming that if many of those companies succeed, the Return on Investment (ROI), will be greater than the total capital invested, yielding a net profit. They invest in different types of companies with different risk profiles, to further mitigate their risk. More investment flows to low-risk investments, and a smaller percentage ends up elsewhere. Cell therapies are considered risky, as they are still relatively in early-stage. Due to the scarcity of early-stage funding, the preclinical and early clinical stages are often referred to as the "valley of death" in our industry. Cell therapy companies must traverse this valley burdened with a relative lack of POC. This is, of course, feasible as evidenced by the growing number of companies in the field.

There are advantages and disadvantages to both public and private investment. Table 16.1 lists some of them. Companies and investors need each other, but it is crucial that the expectations, needs, and time horizon of each party are clearly understood and aligned as best as possible, to ensure that this symbiotic relationship is mutually beneficial.

16.2.2 *Non-dilutive public grants*

New investment into a company dilutes its existing investors, as they now have to share a smaller slice of a larger pie with the new investors. This is a compromise worth making, of course, because companies need the funds. Another way to finance drug development without diluting the investors is through public research from government organizations, charities, and research organizations. Large organizations like the National Institutes of Health (NIH) in the US, the European Union in Europe and a wide variety of institutes and charities contribute in billion each year to research, and some of that funding is increasingly being directed toward cell and gene therapies. In addition, specialist funding bodies have emerged that focus on cell therapies, such as the California Institute for Regenerative Medicine (CIRM).

Cell therapy companies have so far successfully raised about 60% from private investors, 20–25% from public grants and 15–20% from the public markets. Less

Table 16.1:

Private Investment	Public Investment
• Most common source of early finance. • Relatively small number of investors. • Investors intimately knowledgeable of company, management, and strategy. • Alignment on company strategy. • Investors are very close to company and its management. • Industry network of investors.	• Available capital from downstream share offerings, or specialist private investors. • Possible to raise enough capital for late-stage clinical development and marketing of own products. • Possible to benefit from share price increases when things go well.
• Relatively limited funding capacity, often dictated by individual funding strategies. • Potentially different investment time horizons. • Some dependence on macroeconomic factors (investors must also raise funds).	• Investors may have unrealistic expectations that will influence share price. • IPOs are expensive, as are downstream reporting obligations. • Strong dependence on macroeconomic, cyclical, and sector-related factors. • Share price will decline when things are not going well.

than 20% of cell therapy companies are public, mostly the larger companies with late-stage pipelines (data from Alliance for Regenerative Medicine report, 2013).

16.2.3 *Partnering*

Major pharmaceutical companies represent several important links in the chain of pharmaceutical development, as they have the financial strength and drug development experience required to bring new drugs to the market. In addition, they have the manufacturing capabilities and marketing infrastructure necessary for a product to reach the market. As a result, many early stage biopharmaceutical companies rely on partnerships with big pharmaceutical companies to finance and perform large, expensive, late-stage clinical trials and subsequent marketing of their products. Equally, big pharmaceutical companies are in constant need for novel, effective, and innovative therapeutics and understand that it is not possible to generate everything in-house. Partnering deals are therefore common. As with investors, pharmaceutical companies must manage and mitigate their risk and, as a result, late-stage, low-risk products such as small molecule drugs and antibodies take precedence, while early-stage cell therapies only represent a small amount of deals and deal values. In fact, at the time of writing, most pharmaceutical companies are yet to partner in the cell therapy space. A few, however, have and the deals are listed in Table 16.2.

Table 16.2:

Big Pharma Company	Partner	Deal Summary	Date
Genzyme	Osiris Therapeutics	(Terminated) Bone marrow mesenchymal stem cells (MSCs) for multiple indications	Nov 4, 2008
Novartis	Univ. Minnesota	Hematopoietic stem cells (HSCs) for haematological cancers (HSC835)	N.A.
Pfizer	Athersys	Bone marrow MAPC cells (Multistem®) for inflammatory bowel disease	Dec 21, 2009
GSK	San Raffaele & Telethon Institute	Gene-modified HSCs for ADA-SCID and other genetic diseases	Oct 18, 2010
Teva (Cephalon)	Mesoblast	Bone marrow MSC progenitor cells (MPCs) for multiple indications	Dec 7, 2012
Novartis	Univ. Pennsylvania	Chimeric antigen receptor (CAR)-CD19 T-cells for blood cancers	Aug 6, 2012
Celgene	Bluebird Bio and MD Anderson Cancer Centre	CAR-CD19 T-cells for blood cancers	Mar 21, 2013
Merck Serono	Opexa	T-cell induced tolerance for multiple sclerosis (MS)	May 2, 2013
Novartis	Regenerex	HSC transplantation for induction of tolerance to solid organ transplantation	Sep 6, 2013
Janssen (J&J)	DC Prime	Allogeneic dendritic cell (DC) therapy for oncology	Oct 3, 2013
Janssen (J&J)	Capricor	Allogeneic cardiac progenitor cells (CPCs) for myocardial infarction	Jan 6, 2014
Servier	Cellectis	Allogeneic T-cells for leukemia and solid tumors	Feb 17, 2014
GSK	Adaptimmune	T-Cell Receptor (TCR)-modified T-cells for cancer	June 2, 2014
Pfizer	Cellectis	Allogeneic T-cells for multiple targets	Jun 18, 2014
Janssen (J&J)	Transposagen	Allogeneic T-cells for multiple targets	Nov 24, 2014

Partnering a product does provide some assurance that it will be developed rapidly with high standards and will thus have the best chance of reaching the market. It is important to note, however, that while partnering is non–dilutive, in most instances, the licensee will own the majority of the inherent value and downstream market potential of the asset. So, it is in fact, a considerable dilution, albeit, of a different kind.

16.3 Cell Therapy Commercial Landscape

16.3.1 *Overview*

Cell Therapy is a diverse field that encompasses many different types of therapeutic platforms. The distinctions between them are often unclear. Furthermore, different names are being used to describe the various activities and uses of cells, including regenerative medicine, tissue engineering, cell therapy, gene therapy, or even (adoptive or cellular) immunotherapy.

It is therefore becoming increasingly challenging to define and categorize the various efforts in specific categories. It is more helpful to refer to the cell type being used and the desired use. The following graphic (Figure 16.1) provides a summary of the main cell types currently in clinical trials and the applicable indications.

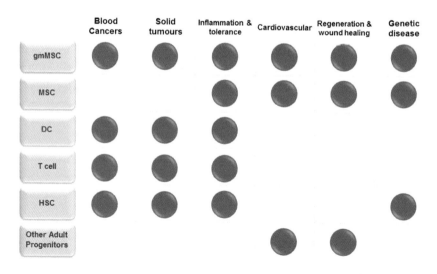

Figure 16.1

The figure excludes pluripotent stem cells (PSCs), such as embryonic stem cells (ESCs) or induced PSCs (iPSCs). Furthermore, other specialized cell types can be used for specific indications, according to their individual characteristics. Some of the uses described in the figure necessitate the use of genetic modification to achieve the desired function. For example, T-cells can either be selected based on their specificity, or genetically modified to express TCRs or CARs against specific tumor antigens.

Of all these therapies, most are still in clinical trials. Some pioneering products are, however, approved for the market and are being discussed later.

16.3.2 *Company landscape*

The list of companies active in the cell therapy space has been steadily and rapidly increasing, as new technologies and intellectual property are being generated and developed. Table 16.3 lists some of the main players in the field, currently conducting clinical trials and their ownership status.

Table 16.3:

Company	Description	Public/Private
Aastrom	Autologous MSC treatments for cardiovascular disease.	Public
Activartis	DC immunotherapy for cancer based on LPS adjuvant.	Private
Adaptimmune	T-cells carrying increased affinity engineered TCRs for cancer and infectious disease.	Private
Advanced Cell Technology (ACT)	Human ESCs (hESCs) derived without destruction of the embryo. Focus on dry Age-Related Macular Degeneration (AMD) and Stargardt's Muscular Dystrophy.	Public
Allocure	Allogeneic MSC therapy for acute kidney injury (AKI).	Private
apceth	Next-generation gene modified MSC-based treatments for multiple indications and GMP contract manufacturing activities for cell therapy products (CTPs).	Private
Argos	Personalized DC therapy for cancer using tumor-derived antigen from patients.	Public
Athersys	Allogeneic MSC-based treatment (MAPC) for multiple indications.	Public
Avita Medical	Autologous skin technology, including the Spray-On-Skin®.	Public

(Continued)

Table 16.3: (*Continued*)

Company	Description	Public/Private
BioHeart	Myoblast progenitor and adipose–derived stem cells for cardiovascular disease.	Public
BioTime	Therapeutic cell products based on pluripotent cells and research reagents.	Public
Bluebird Bio	*Ex-vivo* gene therapy of genetic diseases and T-cell therapy.	Public
BrainStorm	Autologous bone marrow cells for neurodegenerative disease.	Private
Capricor	Allogeneic CPCs.	Public
Cardio3	Bone marrow MSCs which are reprogrammed as myocardial precursor cells and other therapeutics for cardiac disease.	Public
Cell Medica	Anti-viral T-cell therapy for EBV and CMV infections in immunosuppressed patients and anti-cancer therapy.	Private
Cell Therapy Ltd	MSC technologies for cardiac and skeletal diseases and platelet therapies for wound healing.	Private
Cellectis	Allogeneic CAR T-cell technology using genome editing. Platform based on nuclease gene editing also available as research reagents.	Private
Cytori	Autologous adipose-derived minimally manipulated MSC therapies for cardiac disease and cosmetic applications.	Public
DaVinci Biosciences	Several cell-based technologies for spinal cord injury, cardiovascular disease, neurological disease, arthritis and sports injuries, and autoimmune disease.	Private
DC Prime	Allogeneic DC-based cancer vaccines for leukaemia and solid tumors.	Private
Dendreon	Provenge® approved for prostate cancer is the first DC-based cancer vaccine. Pipeline of products based on Provenge® or other DC vaccines.	Public
DiscGenics	Progenitor cell and tissue engineering technology for intervertebral disk disease.	Private
Fibrocell	Autologous fibroblast treatment for aesthetic and medical applications.	Public
Gamida Cell	Metal chelator chemistry for HSC expansion and other progenitor and MSC-based technologies for multiple indications.	Private
Immunocellular Therapeutics	DC-based vaccine for brain tumors and other diseases, using multiple cancer antigens.	Public

(*Continued*)

Table 16.3: *(Continued)*

Company	Description	Public/Private
Intrexon	Synthetic biology focus for health, food, energy, and consumer products. Endometrial Regenerative Cells (ERCs) for organ regeneration through acquisition of Medistem.	Public
JCyte	Cell therapies for Retinitis Pigmentosa (RP), AMD and other retinal diseases.	Private
Juno Therapeutics	T-cell-based cancer vaccine using CAR technology from the Fred Hutchinson Cancer Center, Memorial Sloan-Kettering Cancer Center, and Seattle Children's Research Institute.	Private
Kite Pharma	Autologous T-cell-based CAR therapeutics	Public
Medipost	Largest cord blood bank in Korea. Allogeneic cord blood MSCs for various indications. Cartilage regeneration product (Cartistem) approved in Korea.	Public
Mesoblast	MSC (Prochymal®) and MPC technology for multiple indications. Prochymal® conditional approval for graft-*versus*-host disease (GvHD) in New Zealand and Canada.	Public
Neostem	Group of companies with a portfolio of different cell therapy technologies and GMP contract manufacturing activities for CTPs.	Public
NW Biotherapeutics	Personalized DC-based cancer vaccine using patient-derived tumor antigens.	Public
Opexa	T-cell based therapeutics for autoimmune disease, such as MS.	Public
Organogenesis	Cell-based regenerative medicine products. Two approved products, Apligraf® (non-healing skin ulcers) and GINTUIT® (oral soft tissue regeneration)	Private
Organovo	3D tissues and organs for therapeutic and research applications.	Public
Osiris Therapeutics	Originator of Prochymal® (sold to Mesoblast) and Osteocel® (approved bone graft, sold to NuVasive). Owns Grafix® and Ovation® for wound and soft tissue repair and Cartiform® for articular cartilage injury.	Public
Pluristem	Placenta-derived MSCs (PLX®) for multiple indications.	Public
Promethera	Allogeneic liver-derived CTPs for liver diseases and drug screening.	Private

(Continued)

Table 16.3: (*Continued*)

Company	Description	Public/ Private
Q Therapeutics	Glial restricted progenitor cells for neurodegenerative disease.	Public
ReNeuron	Allogeneic neural stem cell (NSC) treatments for stroke and critical limb ischemia.	Public
Rhinocyte	Autologous progenitor cell therapies for neurodegenerative diseases and spinal cord injuries.	Private
SanBio	Allogeneic cell treatments for neurological, ocular, and inflammatory disease.	Private
StemCells, Inc.	Neural progenitor cells for CNS disorders, such as Pelizeaus−Merzbacher Disease, a childhood demyelination disorder and spinal cord injury.	Public
Stemedica	Mesenchymal, NSCs and retinal pigment epithelium (RPE) progenitor cells for various diseases.	Private
Stratatech	Artificial skin and next generation, genetically modified tissues for wound healing.	Private
t2cure	Autologous MSC-based therapy for cardiovascular indications.	Private
TheraBiologics	NSC-mediated brain cancer therapies by targeted delivery of anti-cancer agents to cancer sites.	Private
TiGenix	Commercial product for cartilage disorders (Chondrocelect®). MSC technology for inflammatory diseases from merger with Cellerix.	Public
Viacyte	Encapsulated pancreatic beta-cell precursors for diabetes.	

16.3.3 *Commercial CTPs*

A significant number of CTPs exist on the market. Table 16.4 is a list of major cell-based products currently on the market.

The majority of these products are various permutations of artificial skin, cartilage, or bone grafts. They are based on patient-derived cells, cultured, differentiated, and formed under specific conditions, often using proprietary biologically active matrices or membranes, to support and guide the tissue formation. Such products are most commonly used in severe cases, when few other treatment alternatives are available.

Only two products in the above list are what may be called "true" cell therapeutics, where the purified cells themselves are the only ingredient in the preparation which are the active therapeutic and are thus highlighted in the table. They both

Table 16.4:

Product	Company	Indication
Apligraf	Organogenesis	Skin/wound healing
BioDfactor	BioDlogics (Amedica)	Skin/wound healing
BioDfence	BioDlogics (Amedica)	Skin/wound healing
Carticel	Genzyme (Sanofi), sold to Aastrom (2014)	Cartilage
Cartistem	Medipost	Cartilage
ChondroCelect	TiGenix	Cartilage (EU)
Dermagraft	Advanced Biohealing (Shire), sold to Organogenesis (2014)	Skin/wound healing
Epicel	Genzyme (Sanofi), sold to Aastrom (2014)	Skin/wound healing
Grafix	Osiris	Skin/wound healing
laViv	Fibrocell	Skin/wound healing (cosmetic)
MACI	Genzyme (Sanofi), sold to Aastrom (2014)	Cartilage (EU)
Osteocel	Allosource/NuVasive, bought from Osiris Therapeutics (2008)	Bone
Prochymal®	**Osiris Therapeutics, sold to Mesoblast (2013)**	**GvHD (Canada, New Zealand conditional approval)**
Provenge®	**Dendreon Corp**	**Advanced prostate cancer**
PureGen	Alphatec Spine	Bone
ReCell	Avita Medical	Skin/wound healing (spray-on)

represent considerable milestones and case studies in the field and therefore warrant some additional analysis.

Prochymal®

Prochymal® (Remestemcel-L) is the first commercial version of MSC therapeutics. It is an allogeneic, off-the-shelf product developed by Osiris Therapeutics for a variety of inflammatory, respiratory, and cardiovascular indications. It has been a pioneering product in the cell therapy field, reaching phase III clinical trials for several indications; it has generated some early POC and even garnered conditional marketing approvals for GvHD in New Zealand and Canada (2012). Osiris has also developed Osteocel®, a bone graft for non-union bone fractures, based on allogeneic MSCs and bone, sold to NuVasive in 2008 and Grafix®, a three-dimensional cellular matrix, designed for application directly to acute and chronic wounds, including diabetic foot ulcers and burns, approved in 2013. In 2013, the company sold all rights to Prochymal® and associated intellectual property to Mesoblast.

Provenge®

The second cell therapy in the list is Provenge® (Sipuleucel-T), an autologous DC-based product developed and marketed by Dendreon Corp., for prostate cancer. It is generated by isolation of mononuclear cells from the blood of patients, activated against the prostatic acid phosphatase (PAP) antigen that is normally present on prostate cancer cells, under special culture conditions. This process results in the maturation and activation of the cells into DCs, the professional antigen presenting cells (APCs) of the immune system, against the particular antigen. When reinfused in the patient, they activate and direct the patient's own immune response against PAP-carrying tumor cells.

16.4 Commercial Considerations

16.4.1 *Target product profile (TPP)*

The business model of a cell therapy company will inevitably rely on the nature of the product, but there are a number of crucial decisions to be made. The TPP is a document often used to describe the final product and the decisions that have gone into it.

The source of the starting cell material is of crucial importance. Cells, like organs must be matched to the immune system of the recipient, to avoid either rejection or GvHD. This limitation can be overcome by using the patient's own cells (autologous). This is done by collecting the cells from the patient's blood or tissues, expanding them in culture and modifying them, if necessary, before using them to treat the patient. Based on this exact principle, for instance, DC immunotherapies, such as Provenge® are manufactured by isolating immature DCs (monocytes) from the blood of each patient and priming them against a particular target, such as a cancer protein. They are then cultured and infused back into the patient, where they will activate the appropriate effector cells to find and kill tumor cells that display the target protein. Most T-cell-based therapeutics and most adult progenitor cells must, for the same reasons, be patient-derived, or matched with the patient's immune system. Some new technologies may offer a way to avoid this, with various levels of success and ease of use, but for now this remains a limitation.

MSCs are more straightforward to use, as they do not need to be matched. They are isolated from various tissues from the patient (autologous) or a donor (allogeneic), such as bone marrow, adipose tissue, umbilical cord, placenta, and others, expanded and used to treat the patient. Allogeneic use has been one of the reasons why they gained popularity from early-on and remain a very popular cell type for therapeutic use, currently the subject of almost 350 clinical trials. Next generation MSCs, like the ones apceth is currently testing in clinical trials for the first time, are genetically modified. This involves an extra step which confers additional and improved functionality to the cells.[2]

16.4.2   Autologous vs. allogeneic cell therapy

In order to deliver patient-derived autologous cell therapies to patients, a company requires facilities where it can isolate cells from each patient, purify, expand them, package them, and then send them to a treatment center, or hospital, where the patient will receive the treatment. This entire process must be performed reasonably close to the patient. Each of those patient-derived cell preparations is a separate batch that must be produced, tested, and then released for infusion into patient by a Qualified Person (QP). It must then be transported to the place where the patient can be treated, sometimes across country borders and time zones. This must often happen fast, as many autologous treatments are not cryopreserved. This process therefore necessitates the establishment and maintenance of multiple manufacturing centers and a very efficient distribution network, capable of serving a global market. It also results in some added inconvenience to the patient.

On the other hand, cells, such as MSCs, can be readily obtained and used from donors (allogeneic). Hundreds or even thousands of doses can be prepared from each donor and frozen, to be used when needed. New processes have also opened the possibility to develop allogeneic treatments from some other cell types. Such technical developments have the potential to transform the field and the way by which many cell therapies are delivered to patients, but are still at early stages of development. In the future, therefore, the choice between autologous and allogeneic products may become a crucial consideration for many more companies and research organizations. Both processes have advantages and disadvantages, as shown in the Table 16.5.

16.4.2.1   Autologous cell products

Autologous production processes are an easy start for early-stage investigators who wish to move their new cell therapy to the clinic and generate some first POC. It may be impractical and expensive to set up and optimize a large-scale manufacturing process for a small Phase I or Phase II clinical trial, but, this may ultimately prove to be an expensive and cumbersome business model for a global market. The process must be extensively scaled out, for thousands or hundreds of thousands of patients around the world. Furthermore, cells derived from patients may be of lower quality

Table 16.5:

Autologous	Allogeneic
• Easy to manufacture in small scale. • No need for long-term storage. • Perceived safety. • Simple manufacturing (can be automated in small scale).	• Standardized and consistent product. • Commercially attractive. • Controllable quality and quantity of cells. • Product available "off the shelf" (easy for doctors to use). • Safety due to consistency. • Fewer tests necessary on patients. • Simple scale-up. • Automation possible. • Cheaper on a large scale.
• High variability across patients (quality and quantity of cells). • Less attractive to Big Pharma. • Challenging scale-up (scale-out). • Holding up manufacturing space. • Patients not always keen to undergo procedure. • Patient has to wait for product (progressive disease?) • More expensive in large scale. • Immunological matching is still necessary for many. • It may not be possible to expand all cell types enough in order to treat multiple patients.	• Storage required. • Unknown variability between donors (can be controlled and tested by using 2−3 donors in early stages).

and quantity compared to those from a young and healthy donor. Their critical characteristics may be subject to great variability. In addition, for the duration the cell product is being manufactured, the patient's disease is progressing, often rapidly, and this is time lost for the patient.

16.4.2.2 *Allogeneic cell products*

Allogeneic manufacturing processes refer to the use of cells from a donor to treat one, or multiple patients. The process can theoretically deliver hundreds or thousands of doses from a single donor, rendering this an "off-the-shelf" product that can be stored and available for immediate use. The amount of cell doublings is an important factor, as the cells must retain their integrity and function. Development of a large, scalable process, capable of serving a global market, may be an added but necessary step in the early investigative steps of a new product. Furthermore, the cryopreservation conditions and formulation of the product must be optimized and the resulting shelf-life must be carefully studied and considered as part of the manufacturing, storage, and distribution planning.

16.4.2.3 *Discussion*

Any cell product that can be manufactured using allogeneic methods and offered "off-the-shelf" will be commercially more attractive than the same or equivalent patient-derived autologous product. The cell therapy industry exists because of the prevalence of many major unmet medical needs for better and safer treatments for patients who have very few, or no options available to them. To achieve their full potential, cell therapies must be made available to a mass market and allogeneic products are the easiest path toward that reality.

16.4.3 *Cost of goods sold (COGS)*

As a general rule, cell therapies are more expensive to produce than most traditional pharmaceuticals. Manufacturing costs are often referred to as the COGS, in accounting terms, and Sales revenues minus COGS is known as Gross Profit. A good measurement of profitability is the ratio of gross profit to sales, also known as the Gross Margin. Naturally, all companies aim to maintain high gross margins by maximizing sales and reducing manufacturing costs. For the last few decades, the pharmaceutical industry has been very successful in optimizing the production process for biologic medicines, such as monoclonal antibodies and reducing COGS, which is now estimated somewhere between 1–5%, depending on the production capacity and output. In contrast, Provenge®, the only cell product where such information exists, is sold at a price of $94 per treatment and for the full year 2013, the COGS represented over 55% of sales. Crucially, however, 12 months ago the COGS were closer to 70%. Off-the-shelf products and a constant increase in global manufacturing capacity will continue to reduce COGS, as it has for biologics.

16.4.4 *Pricing and reimbursement*

Pricing and reimbursement are important considerations that inform the valuation of products as well as the selection of indications and patient populations to treat. The cost *vs.* efficacy of a given drug, also known as the Incremental Cost-Effectiveness Ratio (ICER), is a fairly exact science and is calculated in standardized and sophisticated methodologies by different reimbursement agencies around the world.[3] Each new drug is compared with the existing standard of care in each country.

The equation used to determine the ICER of each new drug is:

$$ICER = (C1 - C2)/(E1 - E2)$$

where C1 and E1 are the cost and effect in the intervention or treatment group and C2 and E2 are the cost and effect in the control care group. Costs are usually described in monetary units while benefits/effect in health status is measured in terms of quality-adjusted life years (QALYs) gained or lost.[4] QALY in turn is a quantification of disease burden, as opposed simply to life years added. It, therefore, takes into account quality of life, hospitalization, disability, and other parameters that determine the impact of a drug or treatment on the patient and the healthcare system. To achieve this, each life year gained is multiplied with a number known as a utility value that determines how far the patient is from "perfect" health. So, a year gained in perfect health would represent a QALY of 1. A year in poor health (e.g., bedridden) would be less than 1 (e.g., 0.5). There are generally accepted utility values for various conditions, adjusted for the costs of healthcare provision in each country.

A new drug could therefore only be as expensive compared to existing drugs, as the actual benefit to the patient. For example, many indications, such as paediatric and diseases of old age also place a financial burden on carers and families, especially in chronic diseases that require lengthy but frequent care. Even when the burden on the carer is not calculated, small improvements in the utility value can yield considerable ICER. Conversely, small survival benefits as achieved by many novel cancer treatments, often measured in months, may not. Moreover, when the patent of a drug expires, the drug can be copied by others. Such copy drugs are known as generics, or, in the case of biologic drugs, biosimilars and are priced at a discount to the original. Any improved next-generation versions of the original must therefore yield improvements of the same magnitude as the discount of the generic to simply justify the same price tag as the original. So, if the generic is priced at a 30% discount to the original, the next generation drug will require an ICER of 1.3 to maintain the price of the original. For additional information on the use of QALY measurements readers should read the review by Weinstein, Torrance and McGuire.[5]

16.5 Summary

The complexity, variation and high COGS of CTPs determine their potential profitability, as they must be priced within the limits that global healthcare systems can withstand. This is compounded by the rising cost of healthcare, a worrying trend for governments and patients who need access to better medicines but must control the rate of cost increases, so, in addition to high manufacturing costs, cell therapies must eventually also overcome pricing pressures to be commercially successful. To do this, the cell therapy field must target patients and indications of high unmet medical need that represent a considerable burden on public health systems, and generate cost/benefit ratios that are greatly superior to prevailing standards of care. The ever increasing popularity of the field suggests that an increasing number of investigators, investors, and patients are convinced that this is a feasible proposition.

References

1. Mason, C., *et al.* Cell therapy industry: Billion dollar global business with unlimited potential. *Regen. Med.* 6(3), 265–272 (2011).
2. Zischek, C., Niess, H., Ischenko, I., Conrad, C., Huss, R., Jauch, K.W., Nelson, P.J., and Bruns, C. Targeting tumor stroma using engineered mesenchymal stem cells reduces the growth of pancreatic carcinoma. *Ann. Surg.* 250(5), 747–753 (Nov 2009).
3. Weinstein, M.C., and Stason, W.B. Foundations of cost-effectiveness analysis for health and medical practices. *N. Engl. J. Med.* 296(13), 716–721 (Mar 31, 1977).
4. Fanshel, S., and Bush, J.W. A health status index and its application to health services outcomes. *Oper. Res.* 18, 1021–1066 (1970).
5. Weinstein, M.C., Torrance, G., McGuire, A. QALYs: The basics. *Value Health* 12(Suppl 1), S5–S9 (Mar 2009).

Index

AAV, 460
Acceptance criteria, 219
Active Pharmaceutical Ingredient (API), 176
adenoviruses, 457
administration route, 421
adsorption, distribution, metabolism, and excretion (ADME), 39
advanced therapies, 2, 26
advanced therapy medicinal products (ATMP), 3, 27
airlocks, 101
allogeneic products, 118
Ancillary Materials, 192
Angel Investors, 504
aphoresis, 123
Assay Development, 205
autologous, 118

Batch Record Review, 331
bio-distribution, 40
biomarker, 401, 402
bone marrow transplantation, 416
buffy-coat, 123
business model, 2

CAPA, 65
cancer therapy, 429
carrier-based systems, 131
cell and gene therapy, 1
cell banking, 317
cell therapy products (CTPs), 25
cell-based gene therapies, 452
cell-based therapeutics, 2

cellular and tissue-based products, 319
Center for Biologics Evaluation and Research (CBER), 28
Certificate of analysis, 259
certification scheme, 10
Change control management, 64
Chimeric Antigen Receptor (CAR) modified T-cells, 442
ChondroCelect®, 149
Classification, 10
clean room, 97
clean room design, 99
clean room grades, 100
cleaning and disinfection, 105
CliniMACS®, 126
Code of Federal Regulations (CFR), 51
coding system- Information Standard for Blood and Transplant (ISBT) 128, 160
companion diagnostics, 401, 404
Corporate Venture Capital (CVC), 504
Corporate Venture Funds (CVFs), 504
Cost of goods sold (COGS), 517
Crowd funding, 504
cryo-conservation/cryopreservation, 322

design qualification (DQ), 113
development safety update report (DSUR), 392
Deviation, 64, 304
diagnostic biomarker, 403
differentiation, 419
discovery stage, 31

disease management, 405
doublings, 420
drug delivery vehicle, 479
Drug/Data Safety Monitoring Board (DSMB), 393
Drug Master File (DMF), 200
Drug Product, 177
Drug Substance, 177

ELISA, 209
ELISpot, 210
endotoxin, 255
EN ISO 14644-1, 101
Environmental Risk Assessment (ERA), 20
epithelial-to-mesenchymal transition (EMT), 425
European Commission, 13
European Regulation (EC) 1394/2007 on ATMPs, 92
Excipient, 202
exosome, 423, 477
extracellular vesicle (EV), 477

FACS, 127
Failure Mode Effects Analysis (FMEA), 62
FDA, 11
fibrocytes, 427
financing, 504
first generation, 445
Flow cytometry, 208

gamma-retroviral vectors, 144
gene addition, 452
gene editing, 453
Gene Therapy (GT), 351, 449
gene therapy products (GTPs), 25
gene therapy vector, 450
genetic engineering, 415
genetic modification, 441, 443
genetic stability, 140
Genetically modified MSCs (gmMSCs), 441
genomics, 406
genotoxicity, 42
germ cells, 450
Glybera®, 151
Good documentation practice, 76

Good Manufacturing Practice (GMP), 51
good laboratory practice (GLP), 35
gowning, 104
graft-*versus*-host disease (GvHD), 423

hematopoiesis, 415
hematopoietic stem cell (HSC), 415, 441
Herpes simplex virus thymidine kinase (HSV-tk), 454
homing of MSCs, 421
hospital exemption, 10, 366
HVAC (Heating, Ventilation, and Air Conditioning) system, 102

Identity, 229
Impurities, product related, 231
Impurities, process related, 232
immunomodulation, 424
Incremental Cost-Effectiveness Ratio (ICER), 517
Infectious disease marker (IDM), 185
Initial Public Offering (IPO), 504
insertional mutagenesis, 461
installation qualification (IQ), 113
integrating vectors, 456
International Conference on Harmonization of Technical Requirements for Registration of Pharmaceuticals for Human Use (ICH), 28
In vitro diagnostic (IVD) test, 405
ISO 9001, 50
investigational ATMP, 9
isolator technique, 116

Karyotyping, 213, 261

lentiviral vectors, 144
lentivirus, 457, 458
lipidomics, 407
Lipopolysaccharide (LPS), 253

MACS, 125
Magnetic-activated cell sorting (MACS), 125
marketing authorization (MA), 503

master cell bank (MCB), 140, 319
material, 318
Matrix validation, 282
media fills, 163
mesenchymal stromal cells (MSCs), 2, 410, 415, 418
metabolomics, 407
microenvironment, 416
microvesicles, 423, 481
miRNAs, 422
Mixed lymphocyte reaction (MLR), 211
mode of action (MoA), 33, 415
Monocyte Activation Test (MAT), 254
MSC-based cell therapies, 432
MSC exosomes, 486
Multipotent Adult Progenitor Cells (MAPC), 440
Multistem©, 440
multivesicular body (MVB), 477
mycoplasma, 257

next generation cell therapies, 439
No Observed Adverse Effect Level (NOAEL), 42
non–clinical development, 26
non–integrating viral vectors, 459
non-rodent models (NRMs), 33
non-viral vectors, 456
Nucleic-acid Amplification Technique (NAT), 214

operational qualification (OQ), 113
Organization chart, 67
Out of specification (OOS), 304

particle monitoring, 102
partnering, 506
performance qualification (PQ), 113
pericytes, 417
Periodic Benefit-Risk Evaluation Report (PBRER), 397
personalized medicine, 411
personnel and material flow, 103
Pharmaceutical Quality System (PQS), 54
pharmacokinetics (PK), 39
pharmacovigilance, 21, 389
pluripotent stem cell, 417

PMDA, 12
Potency, 240
predictive biomarkers, 403
pricing, 517
private equity (PE), 504
Process validation, 162
Prochymal©, 439
producer cell, 139
Product release, 325
Product Specification File, 342
Product Quality Review (PQR), 66
product specifications, 29
prognostic biomarker, 403
proof-of-concept, 39
proteomics, 407
PROVENGE®, 150
Purity, 230
Pyrogens, 253

Qualification, 81
Qualified Person, 325, 328
Qualified Person for Pharmacovigilance (QPPV), 390
quality-adjusted life years (QALYs), 518
Quality Agreement, 203
Quality Assurance (QA), 50
quality by design, 11
Quality Control, 173
Quality Management (QM), 49
Quality Management System (QMS), 53
Quality Risk Management (QRM), 62

Raw materials, 192
RANTES, 468
Rapid microbiological methods (RMM), 249
rare diseases, 364
Recombinant DNA Advisory Committee (RAC), 464
recombinant nucleic acid, 27
Reference sample, 269
regulations, 9
regulatory affairs, 19
regulatory principles, 9
regulatory requirements, 11
reimbursement, 517

replication competent viruses, 141
Retention sample, 269
retrovirus, 456, 457
Return on Investment (ROI), 505
risk analysis, 113
Risk Management Plan (RMP), 19
risk quantification (RQ), 113
risk-based approach, 11, 13
RNA-guided nucleases (CRISPR/Cas), 453
Round robin test, 307

scale-up, 95
scientific advice, 10
second generation, 445
self-inactivating (SIN)-LTR, 142
severe combined immune deficiency (SCID), 452
Sipuleucel-T, 150
Site Master File (SMF), 61
small and medium-sized enterprises (SMEs), 356
Soft Agar Colony Formation Assay, 212
Somatic cell therapy (SCT), 351
somatic cells, 450
Stability, 272
starting material, 120
stem cell niche, 417
Sterility test, 242
storage rooms and warehouses, 111
Strol, 440
suicide gene therapy, 454
Summary of Product Characteristics, 19
surrogate endpoint, 404
surveillance plan, 394
Suspected Unexpected Serious Adverse Reactions (SUSARs), 392

T-cell engineering, 442
target cell, 450
Target product profile (TPP), 514
The Center for Biologics Evaluation and Research (CBER), 362
The Committee for Advanced Therapies (CAT), 356
therapeutic gene, 449
tissue engineered products (TEPs), 351
traceability, 389
Training effectiveness, 69
transcription activator-like effector nucleases (TALENs), 453
transduction, 463
transportation, 160
TREAT ME trial, 468
tumor-infiltrating lymphocytes (TILs), 464
tumorigenicity, 42, 140, 259

user requirement specification, 113

Validation, 83
vectors, 449
venture capital (VC), 504
viability, 239
viral vectors, 444

warehouses, 111
working cell bank (WCB), 140, 319

X-linked SCID (SCID-X1), 453

zinc finger nucleases (ZFNs), 453